AMERICAN

PHARMACY

ROBERT J. PHELAN
45 Hamilton Street
Holyoke, Massachusetts

Contributors

Roy A. Bowers, Ph.D.
Dean, College of Pharmacy,
Rutgers University

Edward Armond Brecht, Jr., Ph.D.
Dean and Professor of Pharmacy,
University of North Carolina

Elmon Lamont Cataline, Ph.D.
Dean, University of New Mexico
College of Pharmacy

Henry George DeKay, Ph.D.
Professor of Pharmacy,
Purdue University

Melvin F. W. Dunker, Ph.D.
Professor of Pharmaceutical Chemistry,
Wayne State University

Perry Albert Foote, Ph.D.
Dean, College of Pharmacy,
University of Florida

Noel E. Foss, Ph.D.
Dean, School of Pharmacy,
University of Maryland

Karl John Goldner, Ph.D.
Professor of Pharmacy,
University of Tennessee

James Wilson Jones, Ph.D.
Professor of Pharmacy, College of
Pharmacy, State University of Iowa

William Reese Lloyd, Jr., Ph.D.
Associate Professor of Pharmacy,
College of Pharmacy, University
of Texas

Alfred N. Martin, Ph.D.
Professor of Physical Pharmacy,
Purdue University

Elmer Michael Plein, Ph.D.
Professor of Pharmacy,
University of Washington

William Arthur Purdum, Ph.D.
Vice President in charge of Production
and Development, Burrough Brothers
Manufacturing Co.; Professor of Hospital Pharmacy, University of Maryland

Sidney Riegelman, Ph.D.
Associate Professor of Pharmacy and
Pharmaceutical Chemistry, University
of California

Thomas Dudley Rowe, Ph.D.
Dean and Professor of Pharmacy,
University of Michigan College
of Pharmacy

Donald M. Skauen, Ph.D.
Professor of Pharmacy, School of
Pharmacy, University of Connecticut

Joseph Barnett Sprowls, Jr., Ph.D.
Dean, Temple University School
of Pharmacy

Mitchell John Stoklosa, A.M.
Professor of Pharmacy,
Massachusetts College of Pharmacy

Allen I. White, Ph.D.
Dean, School of Pharmacy,
Washington State University

Louis C. Zopf, D.Sc.
Dean, College of Pharmacy,
State University of Iowa

AMERICAN PHARMACY

Textbook of Pharmaceutical Principles, Processes and Preparations

Edited by

JOSEPH B. SPROWLS, JR., PH.D.
Dean, School of Pharmacy,
Temple University, Philadelphia

FIFTH EDITION

1960

Philadelphia • Montreal

J. B. LIPPINCOTT COMPANY

FIFTH EDITION—*Second Printing*

Copyright © 1960, *by* J. B. LIPPINCOTT COMPANY

Copyright by J. B. LIPPINCOTT COMPANY, 1945, 1948, 1951, 1955

> This book is fully protected by copyright and, with the exception of brief extracts for review, no part of it may be reproduced in any form without the written permission of the publishers.

The use of portions of the text of the *United States Pharmacopeia,* Sixteenth Revision, official October 1, 1960, is by permission received from the Board of Trustees of the United States Pharmacopeial Convention. The said Board is not responsible for any inaccuracies of the text thus used.

Permission to use for comment parts of the text of *The National Formulary,* Eleventh Edition, in this volume has been granted by the Council of the American Pharmaceutical Association. The American Pharmaceutical Association is not responsible for any inaccuracy of quotation or for any errors in the statement of quantities or percentage strength.

The use in this volume of certain portions of the text of *New and Nonofficial Drugs* is by virtue of permission received from the Council on Pharmacy and Chemistry of the American Medical Association. The said Council is not responsible for the accuracy of transpositions or excerpts taken from texts under its authority, or for false implications that may arise by reason of the separation of excerpts from the original context.

Distributed in Great Britain by
Pitman Medical Publishing Co., Limited, London

Library of Congress Catalog Card No. 60-12042

Printed in the United States of America

DEDICATED TO THE MEMORY OF
RUFUS ASHLEY LYMAN, M.D., and
GEORGE URDANG, Ph.G., D.Sc. Nat., Sc.D. (h.c.)
*Editor and Technical Editor, respectively, of
the first four editions*

Preface to Fifth Edition

More than fifteen years have passed since a dedicated group of pharmaceutical educators gathered together to introduce a new concept in textbook writing for pharmacy. Since then, pharmacy has lost by death two men who have been active in planning and editing the previous editions—Dr. Rufus A. Lyman and Dr. George Urdang. But the challenge of American Pharmacy lives on—the challenge to prepare a textbook suitable for use by students beginning their professional training in pharmacy yet alive with the most recent scientific and technical advances in the field.

Once more the overwhelming task of revision has been completed. The text has been completely reset to agree with the Sixteenth Revision of the *United States Pharmacopoeia,* the Eleventh Edition of the *National Formulary,* and the latest edition of *New and Nonofficial Drugs.* The extensive material dealing with the preparation of parenteral products has been covered in a separate chapter with the addition of a new author to cover the material on solutions. Numerous illustrations have been added or replaced in order that the student may become familiar with machinery and apparatus which are in current use.

Helpful suggestions have been received from users of the book. These have been gratefully received and many have led to specific improvements. The Editor looks forward to a continuation of such unsolicited advice. It is hoped that the Fifth Edition will be a worthy successor to those which have felt the guiding hand of the beloved Dr. Lyman.

JOSEPH B. SPROWLS, JR.

GEORGE URDANG, Ph.G., D. Sc.Nat., Sc.D. (h.c.)
*Lately Professor Emeritus, School of Pharmacy, University of Wisconsin;
Director, American Institute of the History of Pharmacy*

Introduction to American Pharmacy

SEPARATION OF PHARMACY FROM MEDICINE
DEVELOPMENT OF INDEPENDENT PHARMACY
THE FIELD OF THE PHARMACIST
PHARMACEUTICAL LITERATURE
ASSOCIATIONS IN AMERICAN PHARMACY
THERE IS A FUTURE IN PHARMACY

Pharmacy has been defined as the art and the science of recognizing, identifying, collecting, selecting, preparing, safeguarding, testing, evaluating and dispensing all substances of whatever kind and combination used in preventive or curative medicine.

Pharmacy was an integral part of medicine as long as preparative pharmaceutical technics were simple and what we today call the basic sciences of medicine and pharmacy were still undeveloped. It became an independent branch of medicine when an increasing variety of drugs and the growing complexity of compounding demanded specialists thoroughly familiar with the technics concerned. This specialization proved to be especially fruitful when chemistry and physics entered their modern phase, that of systematic research.

SEPARATION OF PHARMACY FROM MEDICINE

Pharmacy, as an independent branch of medicine, was born on European soil when, in 1240, the Emperor of the Holy Roman Empire, Frederick II of Hohenstaufen, issued the last of a series of edicts regulating the hygienic conditions in the Two Sicilies and separating pharmacy from medicine. It was the recognition of the importance to society of an independent profession of drug specialists that found its expression in the special place granted and the special tasks assigned to pharmacy within the program of public welfare promulgated in Sicily in the early 13th century.

The need for protection of the people from fraud and ignorance had become evident. It could be met only by a group of skilled professionals who could be entrusted with, and made responsible for, the adequate administration, the preparation and the dispensing of drugs. It is this social role of pharmacy that has made the profession subject to innumerable laws and regulations in all countries of the western world and has determined both the duties and the privileges granted to pharmacists.

A new profession of technicians rather than of scientists was intended by the edict of 1240. What was called science remained with the physicians. At that time, medical knowledge was comprised of little more than some mutilated remnants of antique wisdom and the employment of these remnants within the definite boundaries of a rigid medical and therapeutic doctrine.

DEVELOPMENT OF INDEPENDENT PHARMACY

It is but natural that, under such circumstances as prevailed until the late 17th and to some extent even the late 18th century, the universities taught materia medica in the general frame of a "system" that was as speculative as it was time-honored. The pharmacists attending European universities from the 15th to the 18th centuries studied medicine primarily. A few French universities, especially Montpellier, offered academic courses for pharmacists as early as the late 16th century. Even then, however, it was pharmacy as a part of dogmatic medicine, not as an art and a science of its own, that was taught.

Thus, for centuries after the establishment of pharmacy as a profession in its own right, it was a literature conceived and compiled by physicians that formed the basis not only of the work of the pharmacists but also of the information and the instruction available to them. Even when, near the end of the 15th century, an Italian pharmacist, Manlius de Bosco, wrote his *Luminare Majus* (greater light), intended to secure uniformity in the preparation of compounded medicaments and to spread light on the origin and the nature of the simple drugs used, his book represented of necessity a compilation based on the writings of earlier medical authors—Greeks, Romans, Italians and Arabs.

It was in 1498, at Florence, that for the first time a formulary was compiled especially for a European political unit and made obligatory for the physicians and the pharmacists of this territory, thus establishing the concept as well as the reality of what we since have called "official pharmacopeias." The Florentine book owed its origin to the request of the Florentine apothecaries. It was compiled, however, by a commission of physicians. It was not until the late 18th century that pharmacists were given an active and an increasingly important part in the preparation of the official pharmacopeias.

This change, when it did come, came for good reasons. During the 17th and especially the 18th centuries, empirical data more and more were supplemented, if not superseded, by scientific findings and reasoning, and it was pharmacists who played an extraordinary part in the progress achieved. That was by no means a matter of chance. In pharmacy, the young science of chemistry found the laboratories, the equipment, the men and the readiness necessary for its cultivation. The elite in pharmacy developed into the leaders of the scientific world of their time. The average pharmacist developed from an empirical technician into a scientific one.

It was in the late 18th century that the various branches of pharmacy gradually assumed the places they now occupy. Retail pharmacy has remained the most obvious representative of the profession. However, its service to society is supported, expanded and to some extent even made possible by organized pharmaceutical education, pharmaceutical research, pharmaceutical industry, wholesale druggists and pharmaceutical journalism. Today, we can think of pharmaceutical education developing the mental capacity of the body pharmaceutic, manufacturing industry and wholesale business feeding the body, research taking care of the necessary oxygen to keep the body alive and alert, and the journals representing the nerve system connecting all individual parts and activities and conveying the necessary information and stimulation.

It has been this concept of one body pharmaceutic comprising pharmaceutical production, distribution and education as its interdependent branches that has resulted in an institution of highest factual as well as moral importance: the American Foundation for Pharmaceutical Education, established in 1942. This foundation has been sponsored by all national associations holding membership in the National Drug Trade Conference, or, in other words, by organized American pharmacy as a whole.

With annual contributions, especially on the part of the manufacturers and the wholesalers, continuously replenishing the original fund, large amounts have been spent every year "to uphold and improve pharmaceutical education ... by aiding colleges of pharmacy and students therein" (quoted from the Foundation's certificate of incorporation). The success of this support has been great as well as significant. It has helped the adequate development of a number of schools. It has made it possible for a number of students to reach their educational goals. It has promoted scientific research for the sake of society. Finally, it has proved that free enterprise in a democracy is able and willing to meet requirements of a social nature and to give talent a chance irrespective of the financial resources of the individual.

THE FIELD OF THE PHARMACIST

It is, naturally, pharmaceutical education that is the foundation for all the branches of pharmacy. In the obligatory 5-year course (6 years in a few instances), the accredited American schools of pharmacy have to give to their students the fundamentals of knowledge, professional responsibility, insight and outlook. What a student later builds upon these fundamentals depends on his personal inclinations and special opportunities.

Pharmacy being a special answer to special needs of society, it must be as definite in its character as these needs and as flexible as possible in adaptation to the constant changes in the means and the methods of protection and restoration of health brought about by scientific progress and by changes in the structure of society.

In the modern fight against disease and all the circumstances which are or may be detrimental to health, drugs of botanic and animal origin as well as chemicals and biologicals are employed, and the technics used in pharmacy are based on physical and mathematical laws and considerations. Hence, it is the sciences of botany, zoology, chemistry and biochemistry, bacteriology and finally mathematics and physics with which the pharmacist has to become familiar not only in their fundamentals but also in their application to pharmacy. He must be conversant, furthermore, with the elements of pharmacology, which is the science of the action of drugs on the living body as well as the ways of testing and measuring this action. He must familiarize himself with medical terminology, for, being expected to co-operate with the physician, the pharmacist must understand the physician's language and his patterns of thought. A rather recent development has led to the teaching of "pharmaceutical administration," i.e., the economics of pharmacy, in the colleges of pharmacy.

All over the world and in all kinds of human activity, teamwork, reliance upon and co-operation with each other are required from everyone who hopes to be considered a responsive and responsible member of human society. The education of the pharmacist in his undergraduate study, as well as in his specifically pharmaceutical graduate work, aims definitely at giving the student an unusual capacity for teamwork.

It is his teamwork with the physician on the one hand and the public authorities on the other that makes the activity of the retail pharmacist useful to society and a source of personal satisfaction to himself. It is his teamwork with the representatives of all the sciences mentioned above and, last but not least, of medicine, that offers the research pharmacist special opportunities to advance human knowledge and to benefit humanity besides satisfying his own personal, social and financial ambitions.

PHARMACEUTICAL LITERATURE

Among the books and the periodicals making up the abundant literature of pharmacy, the official books of standards which are endowed with legal authority are naturally the most important and, therefore, sometimes are called significantly the "bibles of pharmacy." The United States of America has two such "official" or legally enforced pharmaceutical standards. The first is the *United States Pharmacopeia* (hereinafter referred to as *U.S.P.*), the first edition of which appeared in 1820 "by the authority of the Medical Societies and Colleges." The second is the *National Formulary* (hereinafter referred to as *N.F.*), the first edition of which was published by the American Pharmaceutical Association in 1888. Both books were conceived and edited as private enterprises of American physicians and/or pharmacists. They were made the legal standards for the examination of drugs by the Pure Food and Drugs Act of 1906. It was the ninth edition of the *U.S.P.* (eighth decennial revision) and the third edition of the *N.F.* which in this way received full legal recognition.

The drugs listed in the *U.S.P.* are determined by organized American medicine and, therefore, restricted to those thought to have stood the test of modern research, pharmacologic experiment and clinical experience. The scope of the *N.F.* is determined by organized American pharmacy and includes drugs the efficiency of which is not always recognized by modern official medicine, but which have had long and customary use.

There is a kind of national formulary presented by organized American medicine which has appeared annually since 1907 under the title *New and Nonofficial Remedies* (changed to *New and Nonofficial Drugs* with the 1960 issue) and hereinafter referred to as the *N.N.D*. This book, edited by the Council on Pharmacy and Chemistry of the American Medical Association, lists and gives more or less concise descriptions of those articles and brands accepted by the Council.

These three books are presented to the American student of pharmacy as those bearing the seal of authoritative approval. They do not, by any means, cover the whole field. Pharmacy enjoys an abundant literature which goes back for centuries. In the course of his study, the student is expected not only to become acquainted with that part of this literature which he has to know for some immediate purpose, but also to get the feeling of the pulse vibrating in these old and new books and to learn how to employ and to enjoy them.

Since it is impossible to understand the present and to plan intelligently for the future without having a sound knowledge of the past, the student will have to become acquainted with the historical development of pharmacy—not only with events themselves, but also with their motives; not only with the great pharmacists and their work as such, but also with the meaning of their contributions to society; not only with the scientific and the professional sides of pharmacy, but also with the economic development and conditions. Fortunately, books on the history of pharmacy are now available which can be used as a solid basis on which to build.

ASSOCIATIONS IN AMERICAN PHARMACY

Like almost everything in this country, the development leading to the present state of pharmacy has been the product not of governmental coercion but of given circumstances. It has been the result of the free decision and the free action and reaction of free men. In the last few decades, steps were taken and legally enforced as to the prerequisites and the educational requirements for a pharmaceutical career. This process is still going on. It has made and will continue to make the younger pharmaceutical generation in the United States of America the equals of the graduates of the best schools of pharmacy in Europe.

It is due to the suddenness of this development that, at the present time, American pharmacy lacks the homogeneity forced upon the profession in Continental Europe by governmental rules through many centuries. There are still in the United States, side by side, stores and men representing very diverse stages of development and professional standing. The direction, however, is definite, and the time is not far away in which the American profession of pharmacy will be represented by a homogeneous group of practitioners earning the fruits of their higher learning on the ground prepared for them by the foresight of broadminded and forward-looking predecessors.

Group goals such as the progress of pharmacy for the sake of society can be achieved only by concerted action. Such action in turn requires the exchange of opinion and the consent of the majority of those concerned, or at least of their active members. In other words, in a democracy people must unite in order to consolidate their ideas and to achieve the realization of their goals, and finally to defend their achievements. The way to progress goes through the associations.

American pharmacy recognized this truth at a comparatively early period. In 1821, the first local American pharmaceutical association, the Philadelphia College of Pharmacy (called the College of Apothecaries in the first year of its existence), was founded, the school being only one of the association's activities. In 1852, the all-comprehensive national pharmaceutical corporation, the American Pharmaceutical Association, was founded, and it is not without symbolic meaning that it was organized in the building of the Philadelphia College of Pharmacy.

It is due to the initiative of the American Pharmaceutical Association that the idea of state pharmaceutical associations was conceived and realized. There are now state associations in all states of the Union, holding the members of the profession together and working hand in hand with the governmentally appointed pharmacists of the state boards of pharmacy who constitute the pharmaceutical licensing and supervising agencies. The secretaries of the state associations as well as the members of the state boards, on their part, are organized in special national associations, allowing concerted planning and exchange of opinion.

In 1870, the schools of pharmacy organized the Conference of Schools of Pharmacy, which, after a period of inactivity in the next decade, was followed in 1900 by a new organization. Originally named the Conference of Pharmaceutical Faculties, it has been known since 1925 as the American Association of Colleges of Pharmacy. Cooperation between the boards and the schools of pharmacy is secured by annual joint meetings, started in 1904, of their national associations and joint district meetings, the first of which were held in 1927. The American Council on Pharmaceutical Education, founded in 1932, is entrusted with the task of accrediting the schools of pharmacy on the basis of established requirements.

The aims of the following organizations are characterized sufficiently by the names of the groups concerned: the National Conference on Pharmaceutical Research, founded in 1922 (defunct since 1941); the Plant Science Seminar, founded in 1923 (title changed to American Society of Pharmacognosy in 1959); and the Pharmaceutical Syllabus Committee, founded in 1910, and since 1946, continued as a standing committee on curriculum of the American Association of Colleges of Pharmacy. Scientific pharmacy is represented further by a special subsection within the American Association for the Advancement of Science. The past of pharmacy and the place of the profession in society or, in other words, the history and the sociology of pharmacy, are made the subjects of research, teaching, information and propagation by the American Institute of the History of Pharmacy, which was founded in 1941.

In 1883, the National Retail Druggists' Association was founded as a representative of the commercial interests of the independent pharmaceutical retailers within the world of business and business legislation. It was discontinued in 1887 and revived in 1898 under the name National Association of Retail Druggists. The American chain-drugstore proprietors organized themselves in 1933 into the National Association of Chain Drug Stores. Other groups bound together by specific interests within the practice of pharmacy are the American College of Apothecaries, which was founded in 1940 and the membership of which is restricted to pharmacists who comply with special requirements as to the professional appearance and the conduct of their stores, and the American Society of Hospital Pharmacists, which was established in 1942.

The pharmaceutical wholesalers are organized in the National Wholesale Druggists' Association, founded as the Western Wholesale Drug Association in 1876 and taking its present name in 1882, and in the Federal Wholesale Druggists' Association, founded in 1912. The pharmaceutical manufacturers have grouped themselves in a number of organizations: the American Pharmaceutical Manufacturers' Association, founded in 1908 as the American Association of Pharmaceutical Chemists; the American Drug Manufacturers' Association, founded in 1912 as the National Association of Manufacturers of Medicinal Products; and the Proprietary Association of America, founded in 1881. In 1958 the first two named organizations merged their interests into a single organization called the Pharmaceutical Manufacturers Association (PMA).

As a kind of roof organization, the National Drug Trade Conference, founded in 1912, offers the representatives of retail, wholesale, manufacturing and educational pharmacy a forum in which to meet, to explain and to bridge differences of opinion and policy, and to decide upon common action for common or compromise goals.

There have been complaints about an overorganization of American pharmacy:

however, there is scarcely anything in the life of the profession which does not receive adequate care and attention within one or more of the existing associations. At any rate, there is no stagnation in American pharmacy—there is a place for everyone to follow his personal inclinations and his special interests, to expand and to defend them and to make them useful to society and to himself within the frame of his chosen profession.

THERE IS A FUTURE IN PHARMACY

Individual business is still the keynote of American life. There is no doubt, however, that the idea of collective responsibility is gaining ground. If some adjustment is to come, it will affect the health professions first. Health insurance in one or another form may make the medical support of a greater or lesser part of the people a matter of organized economy instead of a voluntary decision by the individual. Whatever system may be chosen, there is nobody to replace the educated pharmacist as the responsible agent for the distribution of the drugs to be supplied.

Life is movement and action, surprising and crushing those who are unprepared, and a wonderful adventure if, in the segment of life in which we have decided to work, we are prepared as individuals and as groups to meet the vicissitudes to be expected in general, but which are unforeseeable in particular. The American student of pharmacy is offered all means of such preparation and organization.

A vast field of work, success and genuine satisfaction is waiting in pharmacy for those who are willing to take advantage of its potentialities and opportunities.

Contents

Introduction to American Pharmacy . . . . *George Urdang*   ix

PART ONE
Fundamental Principles and Processes

1. Metrology . . . . *Edward Armond Brecht, Jr.*   1
   - The Metric System 1
     - Length in the Metric System 2
     - Area in the Metric System 2
     - Volume in the Metric System 2
     - Weight in the Metric System 2
   - The English Systems 3
     - Historical Background 3
   - Weight 6
     - Balances and Weights 6
     - Technic of Weighing 10
   - Volume 11
     - Technic of Measuring Liquids 12

2. Specific Gravity and Specific Volume . . . . *Elmon Lamont Cataline*   15
   - Specific Gravity 15
     - Determination of Specific Gravity 16
     - Specific Gravity of Liquids 17
     - Specific Gravity of Solids 19
     - Specific Gravity of Powders 20
   - Specific Volume 20
   - Density 21

3. Heat and Refrigeration . . . . *James Wilson Jones*   22
   - General Considerations 22
   - Practical Sources of Heat 24
     - Solid Fuels 24
     - Liquid Fuels 24
     - Gas Fuels 25
     - Electricity 26
   - Fuel Values 26
   - Measurement of Heat 26
     - Thermometer Scales 27
     - Special Thermometers 28
   - Regulation and Distribution of Heat 29
     - Necessity for Regulating and Distributing Heat 29
     - Methods of Regulating and Distributing Heat 29

3. HEAT AND REFRIGERATION—(*Continued*)
    Applications of Heat 32
    Processes Involving Chemical Changes 33
        Inorganic Materials 33
        Organic Materials 33
    Processes Involving Physical Changes 34
    Vaporization 35
        Vaporization Below the Boiling Point 35
        Vaporization at the Boiling Point 36
        Effect of Stirring on the Rate of Vaporization 36
    Evaporation 37
        Concentration of Solutions by Evaporation 37
        Hoods 37
    Vapor Pressure 38
    Boiling Point 39
        Pressure and Boiling Point 39
        Boiling-Point Determination 40
    Melting Point 41
    Humidity 41
    Distillation 42
        Registration of Stills 47
    Sublimation 47
    Lyophilization 47
    Desiccation 48
    Exsiccation 50
    Refrigeration, Congealing Point and Freezing Point 52
        Refrigeration 52
        Congealing Point 53
        Freezing Point 53

4. PURIFICATION AND CLARIFICATION .... *William Reese Lloyd*   54
    Preliminary Survey 54
    Standards and Tests 54
        General 54
        Specific 55
    States of Matter 55
        The Gaseous State 56
        The Liquid State 56
        The Solid State 57
    Separation of Gases 57
    Separation of a Gas from a Liquid 58
    Separation of Liquids 58
        Immiscible Mixtures 58
        Soluble Mixtures 59
    Separation of a Liquid and a Solid 68
        Separation of Insoluble Mixtures 68
        Separation of Soluble Mixtures 73
        Separation of Components of Solutions 74
        Separation of Colloids 75

4. PURIFICATION AND CLARIFICATION—(*Continued*)
    Separation of Solids 75
        Conversion to the Vapor Phase 76
        Conversion to the Liquid Phase 76
        Crystallization 77
        Miscellaneous Methods 78
    Clarification 78

5. PHYSICAL AND CHEMICAL SUBDIVISION OF DRUGS .... *James Wilson Jones* 79
    Comminution 79
        Methods of Comminution 80
        Mechanical Aids in Comminution 82
    Precipitation 85
        Types of Precipitates 87
        Collection of Precipitates 87
        Washing Precipitates 87
    Granulation 89
    Separation of Particle Sizes 89

6. SOLUTIONS .... *Karl John Goldner* 92
    General Considerations 92
    Factors Affecting Solubility 93
    Effect of Other Substances on Solubility 94
    Expression of Solubility 95
    Percentage Solutions 96
    Solutions of Liquids in Liquids 98
    Solutions of Gases in Liquids 98
    Solvents for Pharmaceutical Use 99
    Properties of Solutions 101
        Determination of pH 104
    Buffer Solutions 105

7. COLLOIDS, EMULSIONS AND SUSPENSIONS .... *Melvin F. W. Dunker* 107
    General Considerations 107
    Colloids 108
        History 108
        The Colloidal State 109
        Preparation of Colloidal Dispersions 112
            Condensation Methods 113
            Dispersion Methods 114
        Properties of Colloidal Dispersions 114
            Optical Differences 114
            Size Differences 116
            Deviations from Solution Laws 117
            Electric Properties 118
        Precipitation of Colloids 119
        Lyophilic Colloids 120
        Protection 120

7. Colloids, Emulsions and Suspensions—(Continued)

- Gels ... 121
- Aerosols ... 122
- Adsorption ... 124
- Surface Films—Surface-Active Agents ... 127
- Foams ... 130
- Emulsions ... 131
  - Introduction ... 131
  - Formation and Stability ... 132
    - Surface and Interfacial Tension ... 132
    - Viscosity ... 133
    - Hydration Theory ... 134
    - Adsorbed Films ... 134
    - Oriented Wedge Theory ... 135
    - Mixed Emulsifiers ... 135
    - Solid Emulsifiers ... 135
    - Volume Effect ... 136
    - Inversion ... 137
    - Electric Charge ... 137
    - Globule Size ... 138
  - Emulsifying Agents ... 138
  - Recognizing Types of Emulsions ... 140
  - Preparation of Emulsions ... 141
    - Agitation by Hand ... 141
    - Mechanical Agitation ... 141
    - Large-Scale Emulsifications ... 141
  - Creaming ... 142
  - Cracking or De-emulsification ... 142
  - Effect of Electrolytes on Emulsion Stability ... 143
  - Transparent and Chromatic Emulsions ... 144
- Suspensions ... 144
- Some Applications of Colloids, Emulsions and Suspensions in Pharmacy ... 146

8. Extraction .... *Noel E. Foss* 149

- General Considerations ... 149
- History ... 149
- Purposes of Extraction ... 151
- Theory of Extraction ... 151
  - Extraction of Dried Drugs ... 152
  - Extraction of Substances from Liquids ... 154
- Solvents Used in Extraction ... 155
- Extraction Apparatus ... 157
- Methods of Extraction ... 163
  - Maceration ... 163
  - Decoction, Infusion and Digestion ... 165
  - Percolation ... 166
- Recovery of Menstrua ... 171
- Extraction by Immiscible Solvents ... 171

PART TWO
PHARMACEUTICAL PREPARATIONS

9. **WATERS** .... *Roy A. Bowers*   175
    - Introduction 175
    - Standards for Water 175
    - Aromatic Waters 176
    - Official Aromatic Waters 180
    - Storage and Preservation of Aromatic Waters 181

10. **SYRUPS AND JUICES** .... *Edward Armond Brecht, Jr.*   182
    - Syrups 182
    - Syrups of *U.S.P. XVI* 184
    - Syrups of *N.F. XI* 188
    - Juices 193
    - Juices of *U.S.P. XVI* 193

11. **SOLUTIONS** .... *Mitchell John Stoklosa*   195
    - Solutions (Liquores) 195
      - History 195
      - General Considerations 195
      - Solutions Prepared by Simple Solution 198
      - Solutions Prepared by Chemical Reaction 209
      - Solutions Prepared by Simple Solution with Sterilization 216
      - Solutions Prepared by Extraction 221
      - Unofficial Solutions 222

12. **PARENTERAL PREPARATIONS** .... *Joseph Barnett Sprowls, Jr.*   224
    - Historical 224
    - Advantages and Uses of Parenterals 225
    - General Considerations 226
    - Preparation of Injections 227
      - Filling of Ampuls and Vials 230
      - Sealing Ampuls 233
      - Sterilization 234
      - Sterility Testing 240
      - Labeling 241
    - List of Official Parenterals 241
      - United States Pharmacopeia 241
      - National Formulary 243

13. **INFUSIONS AND DECOCTIONS** .... *William Arthur Purdum*   245
    - Infusions 245
    - Nonofficial Infusions 247
    - Decoctions 247

14. **MUCILAGES, CREAMS, GLYCEROGELATINS, GLYCERITES AND COLLODIONS** .... *Elmer Michael Plein*   249
    - Mucilages 249

14. Mucilages, Creams, Glycerogelatins, Glycerites and Collodions—(Continued)

- History 250
- General Considerations 250
- Properties and Uses of Mucilages 252
- Creams 252
  - History 253
  - General Considerations 253
  - Properties and Uses of Creams 253
- Glycerogelatins 254
  - History 254
  - General Considerations 254
  - Storage 255
- Glycerites 255
  - History 255
  - General Considerations 255
  - Storage 256
- Collodions 256
  - History 256
  - General Considerations 257
  - Storage 257

15. Mixtures, Suspensions, Magmas, Gels and Jellies .... *Alfred N. Martin* 259

- Mixtures 259
  - Official Mixtures 260
  - Solubilizing Agents in Mixtures 260
- Suspensions 262
  - Properties of Suspensions 263
  - Dispersion Stabilizers and Other Constituents 263
  - Formulation and Preparation of Suspensions 265
  - Official Suspensions 266
- Magmas, Gels and Jellies 269
  - Inorganic Gels: Official Magmas and Gels 270
  - Recent Investigations of Antacids 272
  - Organic Gels: Official Jellies and Recent Investigations 273
  - Recent Investigations 274

16. Emulsions .... *Alfred N. Martin* 276

- History of Emulsions 276
- Purpose of Emulsification 277
  - Emulsions for Internal Use 277
  - Emulsions for External Application 279
- Composition of an Emulsion 279
  - The Aqueous Phase 279
  - The Oil Phase 279
  - The Emulsifying Agent 280
- Preparation of Emulsions 285
  - Devices and Machines for Emulsification 285
  - Methods of Emulsification 287

16. EMULSIONS—(*Continued*)
    Emulsifying Agents for Internally Used Products 291
    Emulsifying Agents for Externally Used Products 293
    Finely Divided Solids as Emulsfiying Agents 297
  Deterioration and Preservation of Emulsions 298
  Official Products 300

17. SOAPS, LINIMENTS, LOTIONS, OLEATES AND SPRAYS .... *Allen I. White* 303
  Soaps 303
    Definition 303
    History 303
    Manufacture 304
    Properties 305
    Uses 306
    Official Soaps 306
  Liniments 308
    Classification 308
  Dentiliniments 310
  Petroxolins 310
  Lotions 310
  Oleates 312
  Sprays 313

18. OINTMENTS, CERATES, PLASTERS AND CATAPLASMS .... *Louis C. Zopf* 315
  Ointments 315
    General Considerations 315
    Application 317
    Classification 317
    Preparation 334
    Packaging, Storage and Labeling 336
    Comments on Some *U.S.P.* and *N.F.* Ointments 338
  Cerates 340
    History 340
    Use 340
    Preparation 340
    Storage and Packaging 341
  Pastes 341
    History 341
    Use 341
    Preparation 342
    Storage and Packaging 343
  Plasters 343
    Use 344
    Preparation 344
    Comments 345
  Cataplasms 345

19. SUPPOSITORIES .... *Sidney Riegelman* 347
  Definition and General Considerations 347
  History 348

Contents

19. SUPPOSITORIES—(Continued)
    - Factors Affecting Drug Action via Rectal Administration 348
    - Suppository Bases 351
    - Manufacture of Suppositories 363

20. SPIRITS AND ELIXIRS .... *Thomas Dudley Rowe* 367
    - Spirits in General 367
      - History 367
    - Official Spirits 368
    - Elixirs 369
      - History 370
      - Classification of Elixirs 370
      - Unofficial Elixirs 374

21. VINEGARS, TINCTURES, FLUIDEXTRACTS, FLUIDGLYCERATES AND
    EXTRACTS .... *William Arthur Purdum* 376
    - Vinegars (Aceta) 376
    - Tinctures 377
      - Tinctures of the *U.S.P.* 380
      - Tinctures of the *N.F.* 382
    - Fluidextracts 388
      - Fluidextracts of the *U.S.P.* 391
      - Fluidextracts of the *N.F.* 392
    - Nonofficial Fluidextracts 393
    - Fluid Glycerates 394
    - Extracts 395
      - Extracts of the *U.S.P.* 397
      - Extracts of the *N.F.* 398
      - Nonofficial Extracts 401

22. RESINS AND OLEORESINS .... *Noel E. Foss* 402
    - Resins 402
      - History 402
      - Comments on the Resins 402
      - Natural Resins 404
      - Synthetic Resins 404
    - Oleoresins 404
      - History 405
      - Comments on the Oleoresins 405

23. POWDERS, CAPSULES AND RELATED DOSAGE FORMS .... *Perry Albert Foote* 408
    - Powders 408
      - Dispensing Powders 410
      - Special Problems in Compounding Powders 412
      - *U.S.P.* Powders 414
      - *N.F.* Powders 414
    - Capsules 416
      - Hard Capsules 417
      - Dispensing Capsules 418

23. POWDERS, CAPSULES AND RELATED DOSAGE FORMS—(Continued)

      Special Problems with Capsules 420
      Elastic Capsules 422
      Pearls and Globules 424
      Official Capsules 425
  Wafers, Cachets, Konseals 425
  Oil-Sugars 426
  Candy Medication 426
  Triturations 426

24: MASSES, PILLS, TROCHES AND TABLETS .... *H. George DeKay* 428

  Masses 428
  Pills 429
      Preparation of Pills 430
      Industrial Production of Pills 432
      Pill Coating 433
  Pills of the *U.S.P.* 434
  Pills of the *N.F.* 434
  Nonofficial Pills 434
  Troches 435
      Extemporaneous Preparation of Troches 435
  Tablets 436
      Weighing the Ingredients 438
      Mixing the Ingredients 438
      Granulating the Mixture 438
      Compressing the Tablet 439
      Compressed Tablet Triturates 441
      Dispensing Tablets 442
      Sublingual or Buccal Tablets 443
  Molded Tablets 443
      Preparation of Molded Tablet Triturates 444
      Hypodermic Tablets 445
      Abbreviations Commonly Used for Tablets 446
  Pill and Tablet Coating 446
      Methods of Application of Coatings 446
      Enteric Coating of Pills and Tablets 447
  Official Tablets 449
  List of Official Tablets 449
      United States Pharmacopeia 449
      National Formulary 451

25. EFFERVESCENT SALTS .... *H. George DeKay* 454

  The Official Effervescent Salt 455
  Methods of Manufacture 455
      Preparing the Formula 456
      Preparing and Mixing the Ingredients 456
      Moistening and Granulating 457

xxiv Contents

25. EFFERVESCENT SALTS—(*Continued*)
    Drying the Moist Granules 459
    Packaging and Storing 460
    Coloring Effervescent Salts 460

26. RADIOACTIVE PHARMACEUTICALS ....*Donald M. Skauen* 462
    Fundamental Concepts 462
    Methods of Production of Radioactive Isotopes 464
        The Cyclotron 464
        The Nuclear Reactor 465
    Methods of Detection 465
    Units of Measurement 465
    Type of Radiation 465
    Radioactive Hazards and Protection Therefrom 466
    Radioisotopes in Pharmacy and Medicine 466
    Procurement of Radioactive Isotopes 471
    Distributors 472

INDEX 473

PART ONE

Fundamental Principles and Processes

EDWARD ARMOND BRECHT, Jr., Ph.D.
Dean and Professor of Pharmacy, University of North Carolina

1
Metrology

THE METRIC SYSTEM	THE ENGLISH SYSTEMS	WEIGHT
LENGTH	HISTORICAL BACKGROUND	BALANCES AND WEIGHTS
AREA	LENGTH	TECHNIC OF WEIGHING
VOLUME	VOLUME	VOLUME
WEIGHT	WEIGHT	TECHNIC OF MEASURING LIQUIDS

Metrology is the science of weights and measures. In pharmacy, a perfect intellectual command of this subject is indispensable since even an apparently minor error may account for the difference between life and death.

Two complete systems of weights and measures are used in American pharmacy: the metric and the English systems.

THE METRIC SYSTEM

The metric system was originated by a committee of French scientists soon after the French Revolution of 1789. It has several advantages. It is based on the decimal system, and to express any measurement in another unit it is necessary only to move the decimal point. The primary units of volumes and weight are derived from the primary unit of length, the meter, which is based on a natural standard, the earth's quadrant. It has a scientific nomenclature: the names of the divisions and the multiples of the primary units are self-defining, and the units have names which were selected to avoid words which have other meanings. It has gained world-wide scientific acceptance.

The use of the metric system in the United States was legalized by an act of Congress in 1866. Since 1893, the U.S. Bureau of Standards has defined all weights and measures in terms of metric units. The metric system is the official system used in the *U.S.P.* and the *N.F.*, and many non-official formularies use it. It is much used in prescriptions, and physicians of the Armed Forces are required to use the metric system exclusively. In 1943, the Council on Pharmacy and Chemistry of the American Medical Association adopted a resolution to use only the metric system to express dosages in its publications. The use of the metric system is legalized in all of the countries of Europe and South America, and in many of them its use is compulsory for all purposes. It is used universally in science.

The names of the divisions and the multiples of a primary unit are derived from the name of the primary unit by the use of prefixes.

Latin prefixes are used for decimal parts:

deci-	=	0.1
centi-	=	0.01
milli-	=	0.001
micro-	=	0.000,001

Greek prefixes are used for multiple parts:

deka- = 10
hecto- = 100
kilo- = 1,000
(myria- = 10,000, rare)
(mega- = 1,000,000, rare in pharmacy)

LENGTH IN THE METRIC SYSTEM

The primary unit of length is the *meter*. It was defined originally as 1/10,000,000 of the earth's quadrant—the distance from the North Pole, through Paris, to the equator. This distance on the earth's surface serves as the natural standard of the metric system. However, later measurements showed that an error was made by the committee of scientists, the quadrant of the meridian being 10,002,288.3 meters, so the meter is now defined as the distance between 2 marks on a platinum-iridium alloy bar, known as the International Prototype Meter, at 0° C. This standard was accepted by an international committee in 1889. The bar is kept in a vault on neutral territory given by the French government in the Park of St. Cloud at Sèvres, France. The U.S. Bureau of Standards has 2 accurately calibrated copies of the International Prototype Meter.

Metric Table of Lengths

10 millimeters (mm.) = 1 centimeter (cm.)
10 centimeters (cm.) = 1 decimeter (dm.)
10 decimeters (dm.) = 1 meter (M.)
10 meters (M.) = 1 dekameter (Dm.)
10 dekameters (Dm.) = 1 hectometer (Hm.)
10 hectometers (Hm.) = 1 kilometer (Km.)

The abbreviations of the units with Greek prefixes must be capitalized to distinguish them from the abbreviations of the units with Latin prefixes. For very small measurements, in microscopy, the *micron* is used. This word is derived from the Greek word for "small" and its length is one millionth of a meter or one thousandth of a millimeter. The abbreviation of a micron is the Greek letter μ (pronounced "mew").

AREA IN THE METRIC SYSTEM

Surface can be measured by the square of a unit of length, i.e., square foot, sq. cm., cm.^{2}, etc. The metric unit of surface is the *are*, which is the area of 10 meters squared (10 M.)^2. This measure is not used in pharmacy.

VOLUME IN THE METRIC SYSTEM

Volume can be measured by the cube of a unit of length, i.e., cubic foot, cu. cm., cm.^{3}, etc. The metric system has 2 primary units of volume, one for measuring dry volume for solids and the other for wet volume for liquids. This duplication is similar to the use of bushels for dry volume and gallons for wet volume in the English systems.

The metric unit of dry volume is the *stere,* which is the cube of 1 meter (1 M.)^3. This unit is not used in pharmacy.

The metric unit of wet volume is the *liter,* which originally was defined as the volume of one tenth meter cubed (0.1 M.)^3 or 1 cubic decimeter. The liter has been defined since 1889 as the volume occupied by 1 kilogram of pure water at its maximum density, 4° C., and at standard atmospheric pressure, 760 mm. of mercury. Due to an error in the construction of the original standards, the liter is equal to 1.000028 dm.^{3} This error is negligible in ordinary measurements.

Metric Table of Volumes

10 milliliters (ml.) = 1 centiliter (cl.)
10 centiliters (cl.) = 1 deciliter (dl.)
10 deciliters (dl.) = 1 liter (L.)
10 liters (L.) = 1 dekaliter (Dl.)
10 dekaliters (Dl.) = 1 hectoliter (Hl.)
10 hectoliters (Hl.) = 1 kiloliter (Kl.)

The *milliliter* frequently is called the *cc.*, the abbreviation for *cubic centimeter*. They were intended to be exactly equal, but, due to the error mentioned above, they denote volumes which are slightly different. In former editions of the official compendia in which the cc. was used as the standard unit of volume, confusion was avoided by specific statements that cubic centimeter was used as the exact equivalent of milliliter. In U.S.P. XV and N.F. X, and in subsequent volumes, the milliliter was adopted as the standard unit of volume.

WEIGHT IN THE METRIC SYSTEM

The metric unit of weight is the *gram,* which was defined originally as the weight of the cube of one hundredth meter (0.01 M.)^3, or 1 cubic centimeter, of pure water, at its maximum density, 4° C., in a vacuum. Since 1889, the gram has been defined as one thousandth of the International Prototype Kilogram, which is kept with the International Prototype Meter. The U.S. Bureau of Standards has 2 accurately calibrated copies of the International Prototype Kilogram.

Metric Table of Weights

10 milligrams (mg.) = 1 centigram (cg.)
10 centigrams (cg.) = 1 decigram (dg.)
10 decigrams (dg.) = 1 gram (Gm.)
10 grams (Gm.) = 1 dekagram (Dg.)
10 dekagrams (Dg.) = 1 hectogram (Hg.)
10 hectograms (Hg.) = 1 kilogram (Kg.)

In American pharmacy, *Gm.* has been adopted as the abbreviation for gram to distinguish it from the abbreviation of another common unit of weight, the grain (gr.). The abbreviations, g. and gm., sometimes seen, should not be used for gram.

A kilo means a kilogram. A metric pound is 500 Gm., a little more than the common English pound. The microgram is important as a very small unit of weight, especially in the definitions of units for vitamins and antibiotics. It is one millionth of a gram, and the *U.S.P.* and the *N.F.* have adopted mcg. for its abbreviation. In the field of chemistry, the abbreviation for microgram is the Greek letter gamma, γ, and *gamma* is another name for the unit. In physics, the abbreviation $\mu g.$ also has been used.

1,000 micrograms(mcg.) = 1,000 gammas(γ)
= 1 milligram(mg.)

It is customary, in using the metric system, to use decimals rather than fractions to express parts of a unit, and to use only one unit to express a specific amount, i.e., 6.4 dg. (*not* 6⅖ dg. *or* 6 dg. 4 cg.).

THE ENGLISH SYSTEMS

HISTORICAL BACKGROUND

The history of English weights and measures can be traced back to antiquity. The Hebrew historian Josephus credits the invention of weights and measures to Cain, the tiller of the land and the first builder of a city, supposedly about 3875 B.C. Among other references to weights and measures, the Bible states (Lev. 19:35, 36): "Ye shall do no unrighteousness in judgment, in measures of length, of weight, or of quantity. Just balances, just weights, a just ephah and a just hin, shall ye have . . ."

Although prehistoric weights, believed to be 7,000 years old, are still in existence, the Babylonian Assyrians usually are credited with the invention of a system of weights and measures. The Babylonian weights and measures were adopted, with varying changes, by succeeding civilizations. The Indian *pala,* averaging 581 grains; the Chinese *tael,* averaging 578 grains; the Etruscan unit of 579 grains—all closely approximate the Babylonian *talent* of 580 grains.

By a similarity of names, divisions and sizes of the units, although many of these characteristics gradually were changed through each transition, the evolution of modern weights and measures can be traced from Babylon through Egypt and Greece to the Roman Empire. Both France and England became colonies of the Roman Empire, and received systems of weights and measures.

The earliest known system of weights used in England was based on the tower pound, equal to 5,400 modern grains. (This system may have been introduced by the Saxons.) The charter of A.D. 1225 meant the tower pound when it stated that there should be one weight, one measure and one quarter of corn in all the realm. The tower pound of 12 ounces, used in the Mint until 1526, and a corresponding merchants' pound of 15 ounces were used until gradually they were replaced by troy and avoirdupois weights.

Both troy and avoirdupois weights were introduced into England from France, probably at the beginning of the 14th century, a time when trade between the two countries flourished. Both systems show derivation from Roman weights. The abbreviation for pound is lb. because the pound was called *libra* in Latin. Ounce comes from the Latin *uncia,* meaning one twelfth.

Troy weight, *pois de troie,* first was mentioned in an inventory of 1399 to 1400. Troy weight was mentioned in the English statutes of 1414 and 1423, indicating that it was known and used by the goldsmiths. It became well established in the trade of precious metals and drugs. Apothecaries' weight was derived from troy weight by dividing the ounce in a different fashion; compare apothecaries' weight, page 5, with troy weight:

Troy Weight

24 grains (gr.)   = 1 pennyweight (dwt.)
20 pennyweights = 1 ounce (oz. t.)
12 ounces   = 1 pound (lb. t.)

The troy pound of 5,760 grains was legalized in the United States in 1828 to be used as the standard unit in the Mint. Troy weight is used for the buying and the selling of precious metals.

The word "avoirdupois" was used first in a law of 1335, but it was used as a general term meaning "weighable things." A law of 1533 required that meats be sold by avoirdupois weight.

The English colonists brought avoirdupois and apothecaries' weights to the New World, and these constitute the English weights now used in the United States. In England, avoirdupois weight has been designated as "imperial weight" since 1824, and the use of apothecaries' weight based on the troy pound was discontinued in 1858 under authority of the medical act.

Vestiges of Roman measures are shown in English measure by the apothecaries' abbreviations, Cong. or C., for gallon, from the Latin *congius;* O. for pint, from *octarius,* etc. The size of the gallon was subject to several variations in England. The United States uses the wine gallon of 231 cubic inches which was established by confusion in 1496 and confirmed in 1707 under Queen Anne. The English abandoned this gallon in 1824 when they adopted imperial volume, which they now use.

Imperial Volume (British)

60 minims (min.) = 1 fluid drachm (fl. dr.)
 8 fluid drachms = 1 fluid ounce (fl. oz.)
20 fluid ounces   = 1 pint (O. or pt.)
 8 pints   = 1 gallon (C. or gal.)

The imperial gallon is defined as the volume occupied by 10 imperial pounds of pure water at 62° F. and a barometric pressure of 30 inches.

The ancients obtained their measures of length from the human body. The fathom (6 feet) was the distance from tip to tip of the fingers with the arms expanded. One half fathom constituted the ell or arm, the distance from the breastbone to the end of the middle finger with the arm expanded. One half ell was 1 cubit, one half cubit was 1 span, one third span was 1 palm, and one fourth palm was 1 finger. These units were used to measure length.

Distance was measured by the pace. The Roman pace, a double step, was equal to 5 feet. The Roman mile of 1,000 paces did not differ greatly from the modern mile. The inch was named from *uncia* (see p. 3). The yard was a comparatively recent introduction from the Saxons, the original word being *gyrd,* meaning the girth or circumference of a man. It was standardized at 3 feet. From this background were derived the English measures of length.

Because the English systems of weights and measures were developed gradually over a period of many centuries, they lack the uniformity and the integration found in the metric system.

In the United States, English units are used almost exclusively to measure lengths and distances. The following abbreviated table is sufficient in pharmacy.

English Table of Lengths

12 inches (in.) = 1 foot (ft.)
 3 feet (ft.)   = 1 yard (yd.)

Apothecaries' fluid measure is a second system used by the pharmacist for measuring volume. It is used frequently in prescriptions. It is derived from the layman's volume measure known as U.S. Wine Measure, differing in adding small units which are necessary for potent medicines and omitting some of the larger units. Units with the same name have the same volume.

Apothecaries' Fluid Measure

60 minims (♏︎)   = 1 fluidram (fℨ)
                                    (or fluid drachm)
 8 fluidrams (fℨ)   = 1 fluidounce (f℥)
                                    (or fluid ounce)
16 fluidounces (f℥) = 1 pint (O.)
 8 pints (O.)   = 1 gallon (Cong. or C.)

Apothecaries' weight is used only in the filling of prescriptions:

Apothecaries' Weight

20 grains (gr.) = 1 scruple (℈)
3 scruples (℈) = 1 dram (ʒ) (or drachm)
8 drams (ʒ) = 1 ounce (℥)
12 ounces (℥) = 1 pound (℔)

It is also useful to remember that 1 dram = 60 grains, 1 ounce = 480 grains, and 1 pound = 5,760 grains.

Avoirdupois weight is used in the United States for all common transactions involving weight. The pharmacist buys and sells by avoirdupois weight, except in selling drugs on prescription.

Avoirdupois Weight

4371½ grains (gr.) = 1 ounce (oz.)
16 ounces (oz.) = 1 pound (lb.)

Thus, 1 pound = 7,000 grains.

The grain of both systems has the same value, and this provides a basis for the interconversion of the other units.

In using the English systems, it is customary to use fractions to express parts of units and to express measurements in largest whole units, i.e., 2 ft. 6 in. instead of 2.5 ft. In prescriptions written in the English system, numbers are written in Roman numerals, and the numerals follow the abbreviations or the symbols for the units.

Approximate Equivalents. It frequently is necessary to convert a weight or a measurement from units of one system to units of another. Such a calculation requires an equivalent of the 2 units. Approximate equivalents are used because the exact equivalents would require too many digits to be used conveniently and assume deceptive accuracy. The following equivalents are accurate to within 0.1 per cent, excepting the one converting kilograms to pounds (which has an 0.18 per cent error and is included on the basis of common usage).

Approximate Equivalents

Length

1 inch (in.) = 2.54 centimeters (cm.)
1 meter (M.) = 39.37 inches (in.)

Volume

1 milliliter (ml.) = 16.23 minims (♏)
1 fluidounce (f℥) = 29.57 milliliters (ml.)
1 pint (O.) = 473 milliliters (ml.)

Weight

1 grain (gr.) = 64.8 milligrams (mg.)
1 gram (Gm.) = 15.43 grains (gr.)
1 ounce (oz.) = 28.35 grams (Gm.)
1 ounce (℥) = 31.1 grams (Gm.)
1 pound (lb.) = 454 grams (Gm.)
1 kilogram (Kg.) = 2.2 pounds (lb.)

*Accurate Equivalents**

1 inch, U.S. and British = 25.4 millimeters, exactly
1 gallon, U.S. = 3.7853 liters
1 gallon, British imperial = 4.5460 liters
1 pound, U.S. avoirdupois and British imperial = 453.59237 grams, exactly
1 grain = 64.79891 milligrams, exactly

Household Measures. Although medicines are prepared in the pharmacy with professional accuracy, they are administered in the home with available measures, called household measures. For household purposes, the American Standards Association has established the American Standard Teaspoon with a volume of 4.93 ± 0.24 ml. The National Bureau of Standards recognizes this same volume (1⅓ f℥) as corres-

---

* In 1959 agreement was reached in a uniform redefinition of the inch and the pound by the English-speaking nations: the United States, the United Kingdom, Australia, Canada, New Zealand and the Union of South Africa. The new inch (based on the international yard, 1 yard = 0.9144 meter) is about 2 parts per million shorter than the former U.S. inch (1 inch = 25.4000508 millimeters) and 2 parts per million longer than the former British inch (1 inch = 25.399956 millimeters). The new standard of length does not apply to geodetic surveys within the United States, which will continue to be based on the former definition until desirable and expedient to readjust the basic geodetic survey networks.

The new international pound differs by only about 1 part in ten million from the former standards (1 U.S. lb. = 453.5924277 grams, and 1 British imperial lb. = 453.5924338 grams).

ponding more closely with the actual capacities of "measuring" spoons and silver teaspoons. Studies have shown that "teaspoons" may have capacities varying from 3 to 8 ml., but 5 ml. is the most realistic average.*

Household Measures

1 teaspoonful	=	5 ml. or 1⅓ f℥
1 dessertspoonful	=	10 ml. or 2⅔ f℥
1 tablespoonful	=	15 ml. or 4 f℥
1 wineglassful	=	60 ml. or 2 f℥
1 teacupful	=	120 ml. or 4 f℥
1 glassful	=	240 ml. or 8 f℥

The drop sometimes is included in the household measures. Since its volume is extremely variable, it ought to be avoided as a measure of potent medicines, because the size of a drop depends not only on the nature of the liquid but also on the size and the shape of the dropping surface. For the specifications of the international standard dropper, see page 13.

WEIGHT

Weight is the quantity of matter as determined from the action of gravity on it.

In physics, the following distinction is made: mass is the *quantity* of matter, regardless of gravitational effect, and weight is the *force exerted* by a quantity of matter when it is acted upon by gravity. When this distinction is made, mass is the better term for specifying a quantity of matter because gravity is not a constant value on the earth's surface. Weight, as the term is used in physics, can be determined by a spring balance, like the kind used to weigh ice. With a spring scale, a body which weighs 1,000 Gm. at Panama will be found to weigh 1,000.7 Gm. at Key West, Fla., 1,002.2 Gm. at Cambridge, Mass. and 1,004 Gm. at St. Michael, Alaska, due to the changes in the value of gravity. Mass is determined by comparing the weight of a body with the weight of a standard body by using a balance. By this method, the quantitative value of gravity is canceled, and it will be found that the body has a mass of 1,000 Gm. at each of the 4 locations. In ordinary practice, both methods are used, and, in each case, the result is termed the weight of the body.

Another factor involved in weighing is the buoyant effect of air. The apparent weight of an object (in air) is always less than its absolute weight as determined in a vacuum. A brass body having a weight of 100 Gm. in air will have a weight of 100.014 Gm. in a vacuum. The relationship between apparent weight and absolute weight is governed by Archimedes' principle (p. 16). Weighings are corrected for the buoyant effect of air only when extreme accuracy is required.

Balances and Weights

Balances: Hand Balance. The apparatus used for weighing is the *balance* (Fig. 1).

---

* Some references list a (medicinal) teaspoon equivalent to 4 ml. or 1 f℥ and a dessertspoon equivalent to 8 ml. or 2 f℥. These volumes may be measured with special spoons or medicine glasses, but the availability of these measures is problematical. There are also plastic spoons made specifically for administering medicines which measure the standard teaspoonful of 5 ml. It is noteworthy that, in France (the source of the metric system), the *Codex Medicamentarius Gallicus* states the 5 ml. and the 10 ml. equivalents to be official.

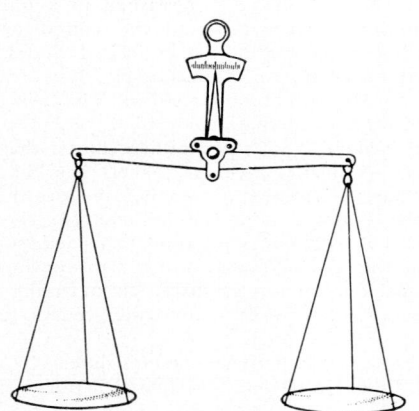

Fig. 1. Hand balance.

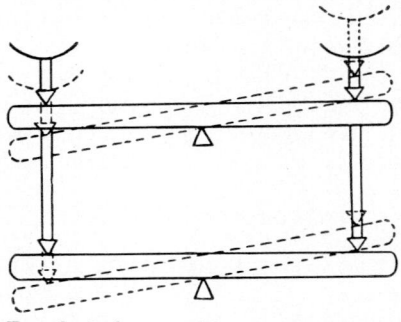

Fig. 2. Balance with parallel beams.

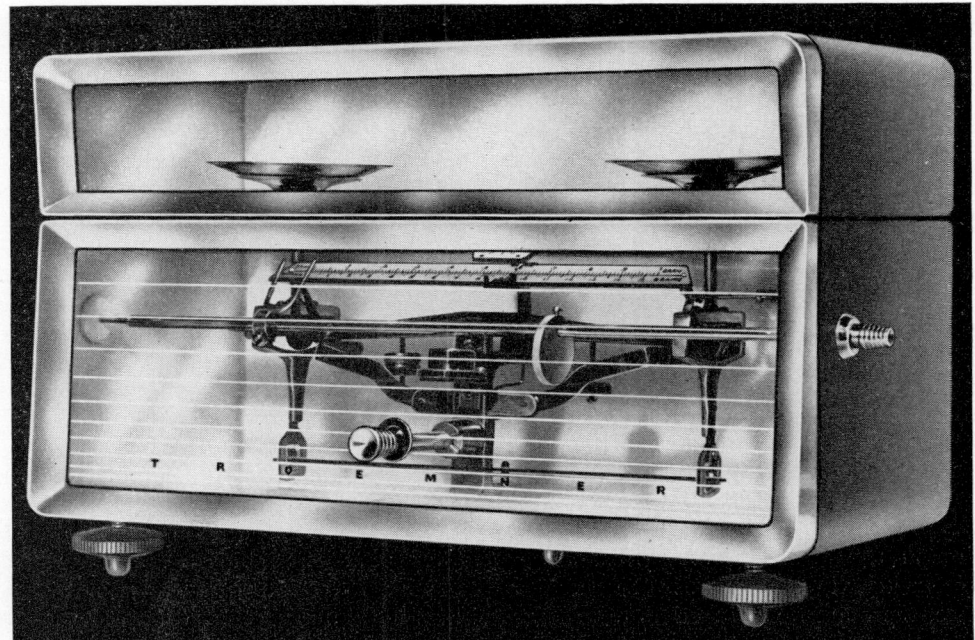

Fig. 3. Troemner prescription balance.

It frequently is called a scale. Since scale originally meant, and also still means, either pan of a balance, "scales" is a better term. In its simplest form, a balance consists of a horizontal beam with a pan suspended at each end, supported in the middle, and equipped with a pointer to indicate the equilibrium position. These parts are embodied in the hand balance, a type that has been used for more than 4,000 years.

At equilibrium, the physical law of moments states:

$$W_1 L_1 = W_2 L_2$$

In the equal arm balance, L_1 and L_2 are equal, therefore:

$$W_1 = W_2$$

This law also shows that a given weight exerts twice as much force if it is twice as far from the fulcrum. This direct proportion is the basis of the graduated beam found on many balances.

BALANCE WITH PARALLEL BEAMS. Since the hand balance is unwieldy in actual use, it has been refined in many ways, but the basic principle is retained in modern balances. Placing the pans above the beam gives readier access to them. However, the pans cannot be attached rigidly because they would tilt with the beam, and an object in one position on a pan would exert more force than if it were in another position closer to the fulcrum. Both trou-

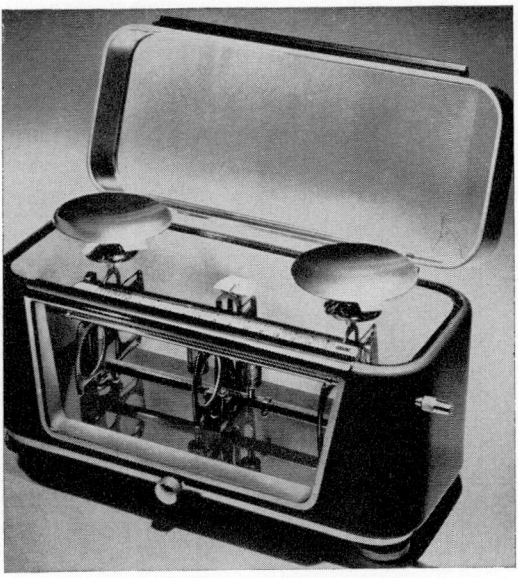

Fig. 4. Torsion prescription balance.

bles are remedied by adding a second beam parallel with the first (Fig. 2).

TROEMNER PRESCRIPTION BALANCE. Accuracy is increased by using sharp knife-edges for the fulcrum and the pan suspensions. The knife-edges are made of hardened steel or agate, and the plane surfaces in contact with the knife-edges are made of the same materials. The knife-edges are protected from wear by pan supports which prevent friction excepting at those times when the balance is in actual use. The delicate mechanism is protected from dust and chemicals by enclosure in a boxlike case, often of glass. These features are represented in the modern Troemner prescription balance (Fig. 3).

TORSION PRESCRIPTION BALANCE. The torsion prescription scale (Fig. 4) eliminates friction at the knife-edges by substituting tautly stretched steel bands. In such a balance, there are no knife-edges to become dull. An added advantage in this type of balance is the ability to balance the pans, preliminary to making a weighing, by raising or lowering either side of the balance, using the steel bands' tension to overcome the slight overweight of either pan.

A good prescription balance ought to satisfy the following requirements: the 2 arms of the beam should be exactly equal in length; this is true when it is possible to interchange the positions of 2 balanced weights without any change of balance resulting. The pans should be suspended properly: proper pan suspension is tested by changing the positions of balanced weights to various areas of each pan; no change of balance should occur. The sensitivity should be sufficient to indicate a change of balance when 2 mg. is added to either pan. The balance should have a capacity to weigh quantities as great as 120 Gm. Finally, a graduated beam is a

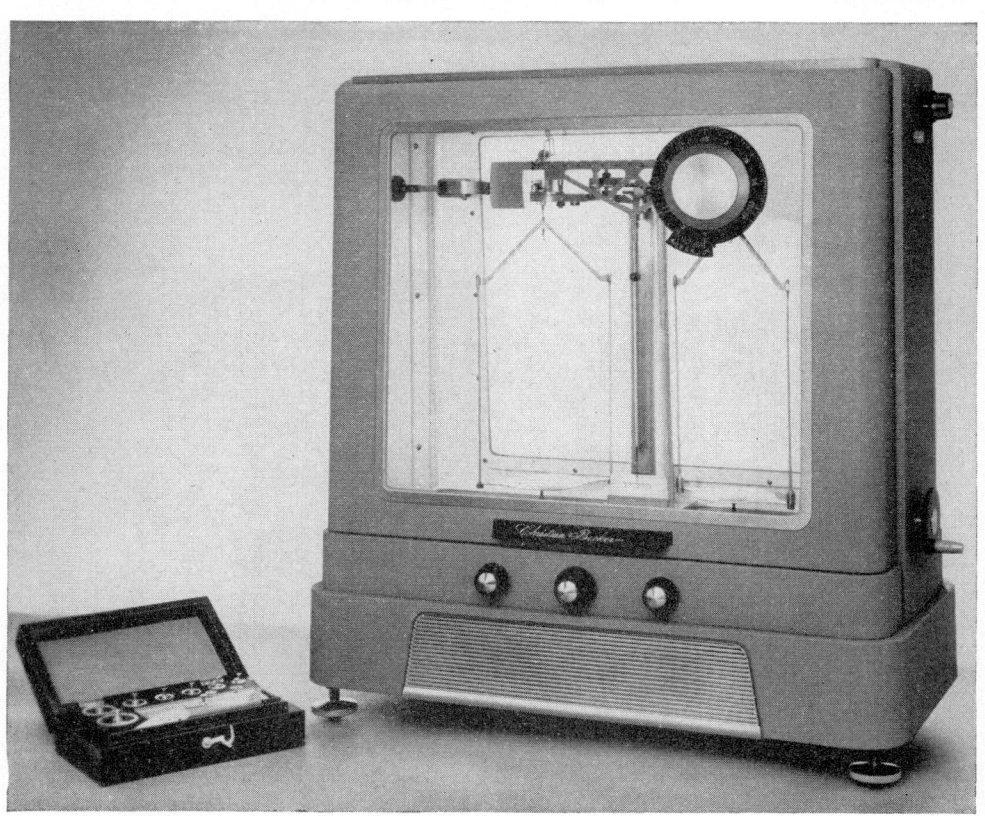

FIG. 5. Chainomatic analytical balance. Other types use a vertical pole or a horizontal bar instead of a drum to regulate the chain.

great convenience in eliminating the necessity for handling weights less than 1 Gm., but it may be the source of error if the rider inadvertently is left in an improper position.

The sensitivity is the smallest weight which will cause a perceptible deviation of the pointer. This terminology is so indefinite that it is better to evaluate the quality of a balance by its *sensitivity reciprocal* which is the smallest weight which will cause the pointer to deviate by one scale division. However, it must be recognized that a balance is capable of better accuracy than its sensitivity reciprocal when it is used carefully.

The National Formulary XI includes specifications for the testing of a prescription balance.

The National Bureau of Standards and nearly all state governments require that the maximum maintenance sensitivity reciprocal of a Class A prescription balance shall be 0.2 grain (13 mg.) and for a Class B balance shall be 0.5 grain (32 mg.). The latter must be labeled with the following or its equivalent: "Class B. Not to be used for weighing loads of less than 10 grains."

ANALYTICAL BALANCE. For more accurate work, an analytical balance is used (Fig. 5). In appearance, it closely resembles the hand balance. It is an instrument designed and constructed with great precision. Increased sensitivity is obtained by reducing the friction of moving parts to a minimum and by raising the center of gravity of the moving parts to a position just slightly below the fulcrum.

COUNTER BALANCE. For less accurate work, when quantities as great as 10 lb. are to be weighed, a counter balance is used (Fig. 6). It is constructed like a prescription balance, but it is larger and its construction is stronger. Such a balance has a capacity of 4.5 Kg. (10 lb.) and a sensitivity of 100 mg. (1½ gr.).

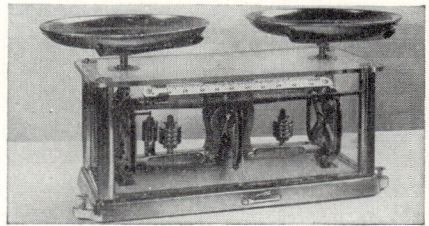

Fig. 6. Counter balance.

SOLUTION BALANCE. For manufacturing purposes, a solution scale is convenient (Fig. 7). It has a capacity of 20 Kg. (or 45 lb.) and a sensitivity of 1 Gm. It is a balance of the unequal arm, compound lever type. It can be obtained with the beams graduated in metric, avoirdupois, troy or both metric and avoirdupois units.

Weights. Equally as important as the balance in the weighing process are the mass standards, the weights (Fig. 8). Any inaccuracy in either nullifies the accuracy of the other. Good weights commonly are made of polished brass. Often they are made in 2 pieces, so that the knob can be unscrewed to permit adjustment of the weight. To increase resistance to corrosion, they may be lacquered or plated with nickel, chromium, gold or platinum. Weights of high accuracy are also made of stainless alloys. Metric weights of less than 1 Gm. are made of aluminum or platinum, and apothecary weights of less than one half scruple are

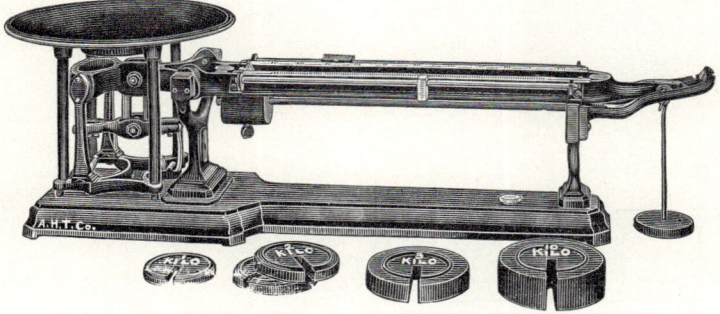

Fig. 7. Solution balance.

made of aluminum, a light metal being preferred to increase the size. Good weights are purchased in covered blocks with a hole of appropriate size and shape for each weight. A forceps is kept with the weights to eliminate handling them with the fingers. Coin weights of the apothecaries' system are illustrated on the basis of wide use in earlier times and historical interest. The use of coin weights is not recommended in the *National Formulary* because they can be handled conveniently only with the fingers which quickly causes a loss in accuracy. Counter weights of avoirdupois units are available in blocks of brass weights or piles of iron weights.

Technic of Weighing

In making a weighing, it is customary to place the weights on the right pan of the balance and the substance to be weighed on the left. All graduated beams are attached on this basis. Also, this position is more convenient for transferring powders from bottles to the pan. A left-handed operator will find it useful to learn to handle a spatula with the right hand.

When the weights on both pans are equal, a balance is said to be at equilibrium or *in balance*.

Balance may be determined by several methods. *Down balance* consists of adding the substance until the weights are overbalanced. Although this method is rapid, it is greatly inaccurate; if used at all, it must be used judiciously. *Fixed balance* is a more nearly accurate method, in which the pointer remains at the central position when the beam is made free to swing. *Swinging balance* is most accurate, and is indicated when the pointer swings an equal number of divisions to both sides of the central position.

Good technic in the weighing process is important to both accuracy and prolonged usefulness of the equipment. The following rules may serve as guides:

The balance should be located in a well-lighted place, as free as possible from vibration, dust, moisture and corrosive vapors.

The balance cover should be kept down except when the balance is in use.

The balance should be kept clean at all times. Any chemical spilled upon the bal-

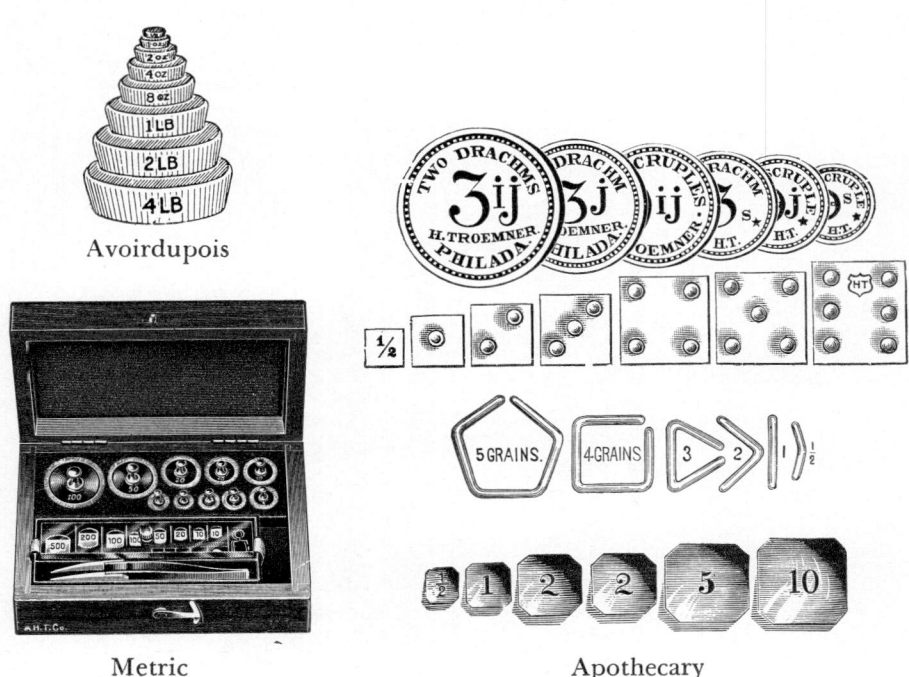

Fig. 8. Weights: avoirdupois, metric and apothecary.

ance should be removed immediately with a soft brush or a clean, dry towel.

The pans should be protected from wear and corrosion by using powder papers routinely and tared watch glasses or stoppered bottles for corrosive substances.

The knife-edges or steel bands should be protected from jarring and unnecessary wear by supporting the pans at all times except when equilibrium is being tested. Weights and materials should never be added to or removed from the pans unless the pans are supported. The pan support is controlled by the knob at the front of the balance.

Weights should be protected from dust and corrosion by keeping them in covered boxes.

Weights should be handled only with a forceps. Fingerprints not only increase their weight but also accelerate corrosion.

If the weights require cleaning, it should be done with a soft, clean towel. If this is not sufficient, a paste of precipitated calcium carbonate and glycerin may be used, to be followed by cleaning with a moistened towel and drying.

To avoid mistakes in totaling the weights, they are totaled 3 times: as they are placed on the balance, from the vacant positions in the weight box and as they rest on the pan.

VOLUME

Volume is space. It is possible to specify an amount of matter by the space which it occupies, just as it is possible to specify the amount by its weight. It is customary to specify amounts of liquids by volumes and solids by weights. However, there are many exceptions to this generalization. The pharmacist buys many liquids by weight (glycerin, acids, oils). He sells them by volume.

An important factor in the accuracy of an instrument for measuring volume is the surface area of the liquid in it (Fig. 9); the accuracy is increased as the surface area is decreased, because a perceptible difference in the height of the liquid represents a smaller volume. At the same time, as the surface is decreased, the convenience of transferring a liquid to and from the instru-

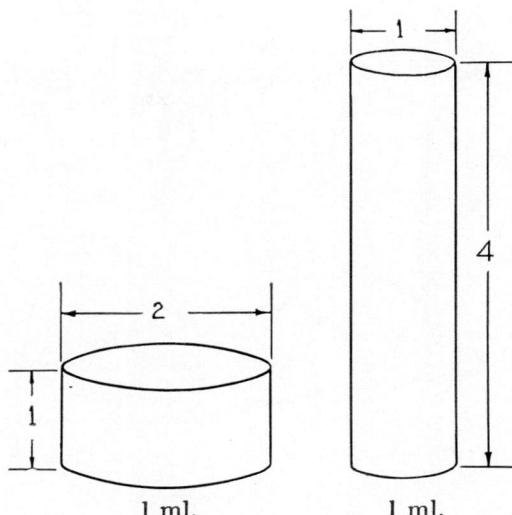

FIG. 9. Relation of surface area to volume.

ment is decreased. Therefore, there must be a compromise between accuracy and convenience.

Since it is seldom possible to pour all of a liquid from a vessel, a distinction must be made between *receiving capacity*, the true volume, and *delivery capacity*, the true volume plus an allowance for the liquid (water as a standard) which will adhere to the vessel. Unless specified otherwise, graduated vessels are calibrated to show delivery capacities. Volumetric flasks are an exception, usually being graduated to show receiving capacity. Some volumetric flasks and pipets have double calibrations, showing both receiving and delivery capacities.

Conical graduates (Fig. 10) are used most

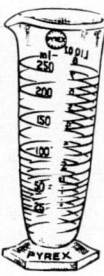

FIG. 10. Conical graduate.

12   Metrology

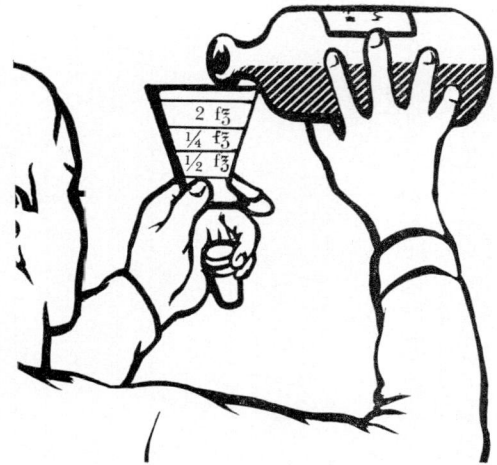

Fig. 11. Measuring technic.

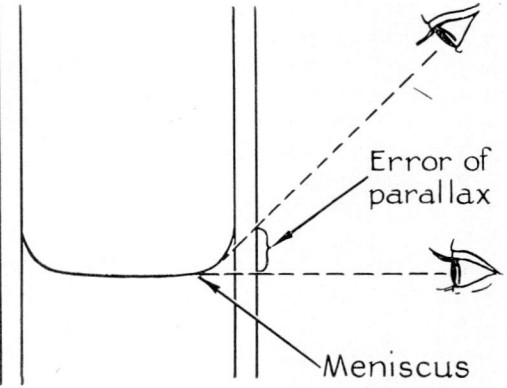

Fig. 12. Error of parallax.

frequently for measuring volumes in pharmacy. Many apparatus catalogs list them as *pharmaceutical graduates*. They possess several advantages. The wide mouth is convenient for filling and emptying and for cleaning and drying. A low center of gravity gives stability. Conical graduates usually are graduated in both metric and apothecary units.

Technic of Measuring Liquids

Good technic in measuring liquids involves the following points (Fig. 11): the graduate is held at the bottom with the thumb and the forefinger and supported on the curved middle finger of the left hand. The bottle is grasped with the right hand so that the label of the bottle will be up while pouring: this prevents drippings from soiling the label. The stopper of the bottle is removed with the little finger of the left hand. The graduate is then raised level with the eyes to minimize the error in reading (error of parallax, Fig. 12). The liquid is poured into the graduate until the bottom of the meniscus exactly reaches the required mark, which should be level with the eyes.

Cylindrical graduates (graduated cylinders) (Fig. 13) can be used somewhat more accurately than conical graduates. The uniform diameter makes it possible to judge volumes between graduation markings more accurately. They usually are graduated only in metric units, but they are available with both metric and apothecary graduations.

Important changes in the legal requirements for graduates and effective in nearly all states were announced in the National Bureau of Standards Handbook 44—Second Edition, effective July 1, 1956 for all new equipment. Previous graduates and graduated cylinders, which may be used for their normal life, were out of conformity with one or more of the following: (1) The smallest graduation may not be less than $1/5$ and not more than $1/4$ of the capacity of the graduate. (2) A graduate for a capacity of 4 fluid drams or less may not be conical (must be cylindrical). (3) A graduate for a capacity of 4 fluid drams or less may not have a dual scale (both apothecaries' and metric graduations). These requirements apply to pre-

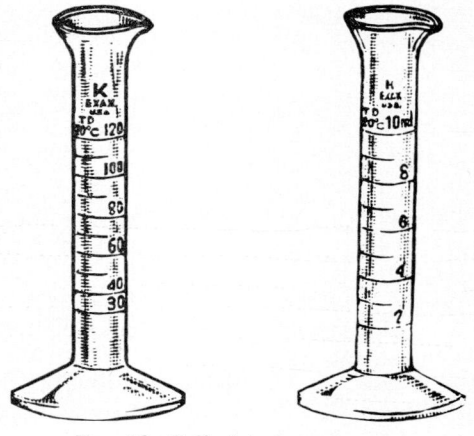

Fig. 13. Cylindrical graduates.

Volume   13

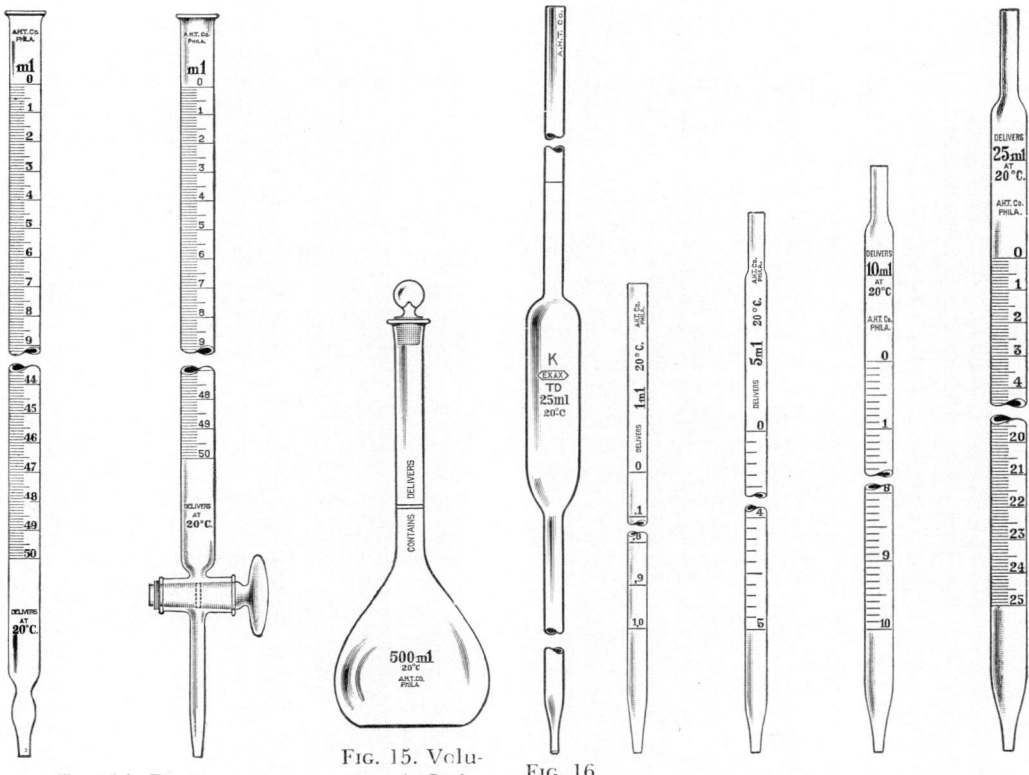

Fig. 14. Burets.   Fig. 15. Volumetric flask.   Fig. 16. Pipet.   Fig. 17. Graduated pipets.

scription work. These changes enforce good pharmaceutical practice against attempting to measure small volumes in large graduates.

Burets (Fig. 14) are used for the very accurate measurement of volumes, as in volumetric analysis.

Volumetric flasks (Fig. 15) are used to measure specific volumes accurately, especially for preparing solutions in quantitative analysis.

Pipets (Fig. 16) provide a means for greatest accuracy in measuring volume, by affording the smallest surface to the liquid. Ordinarily, a pipet is used to measure only one specific volume, e.g., a 25-ml. pipet. They are sometimes called transfer pipets. Graduated pipets are used to measure different volumes with the same pipet. A pharmacist would find especially useful for measuring small volumes a 10-ml. pipet graduated in tenth milliliters and a 1-ml. pipet graduated in hundredth milliliters (Fig. 17).

The official specifications for volumetric apparatus are stated in *U.S.P. XVI*.

U.S.P. XVI gives the international specifications for an official medicine dropper (Fig. 18). Such a dropper has a delivery tip with an outside diameter of 3 mm. From it, when held in a vertical position, 20 drops of water weigh 1.0 Gm. A 10 per cent tolerance is allowed. This represents an effort to standardize the drop as a unit of volume. However, even with the same dropper, the volume of a drop will vary for different liquids, depending on the surface tension, the viscosity and the density of the liquid. A drop should not be used as a measure for

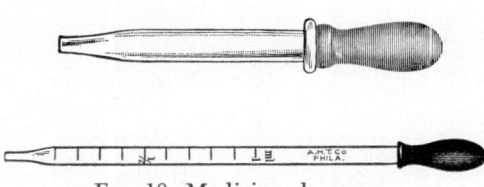

Fig. 18. Medicine droppers.

medicine until its volume has been determined in each specific case.

BIBLIOGRAPHY

Berriman, A. E.: Historical Metrology, London, Dent, 1953.

Ellis, B.: On weights and measures, from "Report of the Secretary of State upon Weights and Measures" by John Quincy Adams, J. Phila. Coll. Pharm. (Am. J. Pharm.) **2**:111–135, 188–205, 1831.

———: Weights and measures in history, Chemist & Druggist **110**:816–833, 1929.

Goldstein, S. W., and Mattocks, A. M.: Professional equilibrium and compounding precision, J. Am. Pharm. A. (Pract. Ed.) **12**:214–216, 293–295, 310, 362–364, 421–423, 485, 1951. (The 5 parts collected in a reprint are available at 20 cents from the American Pharmaceutical Association, Washington, D. C.)

Gray, S. F.: On Weights, J. Phila. Coll. Pharm. (Am. J. Pharm.) **1**:174–193, 1830.

Griffinhagen, G.: Pharmaceutical balances, J. Am. Pharm. A. (Pract. Ed.) **17**:152–153, 1956; Pharmaceutical weights, *ibid.*, **17**:240–241, 1956.

LaWall, C. H.: Balances, Am. Druggist **88**: No. 4, 68–69, 118–119, 1933.

National Council of Teachers of Mathematics: The Metric System of Weights and Measures, New York, Bureau of Publications, Teachers Coll., Columbia Univ., 1948.

Scattergood, G. M.: Standards for Rx glassware, J. Am. Pharm. A. (Pract. Ed.) **19**:36–37, 1958.

Smith, R. W.: The Federal Basis for Weights and Measures, National Bureau of Standards Circular 593, Washington, 1958.

ELMON LAMONT CATALINE, Ph.D.
Dean, University of New Mexico College of Pharmacy

2

Specific Gravity and Specific Volume

SPECIFIC GRAVITY
   DETERMINATION OF SPECIFIC GRAVITY
   SPECIFIC GRAVITY OF LIQUIDS
SPECIFIC GRAVITY OF SOLIDS
SPECIFIC GRAVITY OF POWDERS
SPECIFIC VOLUME

SPECIFIC GRAVITY

The fact that objects of identical size and shape frequently show considerable difference in weight is familiar to everyone. For example, brass candlesticks are considerably heavier than those made of glass, though they may be of about the same size and the same shape. If, from each material, a person cuts a cube 1 centimeter on a side and weighs it, he will find that the brass cube weighs about 8.5 Gm., whereas the glass cube weighs about 3 Gm. It can be seen, therefore, that brass is about 2.8 times as heavy as glass. Thus one might compare materials and construct tables indicating the relationships of weights of one centimeter cubes of various substances. However, for practical purposes such a table would be needed for every material with which one wished to compare other materials, and the number of tables would be indefinitely large. It is far simpler to select some one substance as a *primary standard* with which all materials can be compared, and thus arrive at a single table. Table 1 is illustrative of such listings. More extensive tables are to be found in the reference books of pharmacy, chemistry, and physics.

Because distilled water is common and easily purified, it has been selected as the primary standard. The ratio of the *apparent weight* of a given volume of a substance to that of an equal volume of distilled water is called the *apparent specific gravity* of the substance.

By apparent weight is meant the weight determined in air. Air tends to buoy up objects in it, the extent of the buoyant effect depending in part on the volume of the object being weighed. The larger the object, the more the buoyant effect. Thus, weighings made in air will be accurate only when the volume of the object being weighed is the same as that of the weights used. Such is seldom the case. Furthermore, the buoyant effect depends in part on the barometric pressure. As the barometric pressure increases, the density of the air increases, the buoyant effect becomes

TABLE 1. SPECIFIC GRAVITIES OF SOME FAMILIAR SUBSTANCES

SUBSTANCE	SPECIFIC GRAVITY
Ether	0.715
Alcohol	0.816
Water	1.000
Aluminum	2.70
Iron	7.86
Mercury	13.5
Gold	19.3

greater and the apparent weight becomes smaller. Thus, to determine the *true weight* of an object, the apparent weight must be corrected. Formulas for making this correction may be found in the reference books mentioned earlier. Their derivations and uses are beyond the scope of this discussion.

When the true weights have been determined for both the substance of unknown specific gravity and an equal volume of distilled water, then they may be used to determine the *true specific gravity* in the usual manner (described later in this chapter). Alternatively, one may first determine the apparent specific gravity (specific gravity in air) and then convert it to true specific gravity (specific gravity *in vacuo*) by the use of the following formula:

$$S_t = S_a - 0.0012 (S_{air} - 1)$$

where S_t = true specific gravity.
S_a = apparent specific gravity.

It should be noted that it is unnecessary to determine true specific gravity except in very exact work.

The specific gravity of a pure substance is always the same at any given temperature and barometric pressure and is a *constant* of the substance. In conjunction with other constants, specific gravity is of considerable use in medicine, pharmacy and chemistry, as well as many other fields. In diseases such as diabetes mellitus (sugar diabetes) and certain kidney disorders, the specific gravity of the urine is greater than normal and the diagnoses of such diseases nearly always include a determination of the specific gravity of the urine. In the commercial manufacture of salts used in medicine and pharmacy, it is seldom that the concentrations of some of the reagents employed are expressed in terms of per cent. Rather, they commonly are designated by specific gravity, as, for example, "sulfuric acid, sp. gr. 1.84." This method is used because specific-gravity determinations are carried out more readily than are most chemical analyses.

The specific gravities of solutions of the common acids and bases and other substances in water can be found in the handbooks of chemistry and physics. The *U.S.P.* *XVI* includes a table in which the percentage of alcohol in solution in water, both by weight and by volume, is related to specific gravity (pp. 1102–3). In addition, the monographs of the *U.S.P.* and the *N.F.* usually include a statement of specific gravity of the substances described when it may be useful in controlling the strength or the purity.

DETERMINATION OF SPECIFIC GRAVITY

The Greek scientist Archimedes (287–212 B.C.) was the first to recognize that substances can be differentiated on the basis of their differing specific gravities. In his treatise, *Of Floating Matter,* he recorded the principle which bears his name and which, in effect, states that "a body immersed in a fluid is buoyed up by a force equal to the weight of fluid displaced by the body." On this basis, Archimedes devised methods for distinguishing gold from other metals.

In the first centuries of the Christian era, the scholars of the Greek school at Alexandria devised a kind of hydrometer which they used for determining the specific gravities of liquids. Later, the Arabs, who were among the first experimentalists, devoted much attention to the determination of specific gravity. According to Gerland and Traumüller (*Geschichte der physikalischen Experimentierkunst,* Leipzig, 1899, p. 57 ff.), a 12th-century Arabic table of specific gravities contains amazingly accurate data for gold, mercury, copper, lead, sea water and blood. For their determinations, the Arabs made use of the balance and the pycnometer.

To the French pharmacist Antoine Baumé (1728–1804) is due the credit for the development of the modern hydrometer which he employed in the determination of the specific gravities of many liquids. The so-called Westphal balance (Fig. 20) is, in fact, one of the many inventions of the ingenious German apothecary Carl Friedrich Mohr (1806–1879). This instrument, which was described by Mohr in 1848, later was improved on and manufactured by the mechanician Westphal; to be correct, it should be called the Mohr-Westphal balance.

Archimedes' principle forms the basis for most methods for the determination of specific gravity. From this principle it is seen that a body whose volume is 1 ml. and, therefore, displaces 1 ml. of a fluid, is buoyed up by a force equal to the weight of 1 ml. of the fluid. If this weight is greater than that of the body, the body will float in the fluid; if it is less, the body will sink. When the buoyant force and the weight of the body are equal, the body will float indifferently in the fluid and the specific gravity of the fluid and the body are the same. Therefore, the specific gravity of a body may be determined by finding a fluid of known specific gravity in which it will float indifferently. Indeed, this method is used to a limited extent, but is rather cumbersome for most purposes.

Since the specific gravity of a substance indicates how many times heavier a given volume of that substance is than an equal volume of water, most methods for the determination of specific gravity are designed to determine the weights of equal volumes of the unknown and water. Having determined these, the specific gravity is calculated by the following formula:

$$\text{Sp. gr.} = \frac{Wx}{Ws}$$

where Wx is the weight of a given volume of the substance being investigated, and Ws is the weight of an equal volume of water.

It should be noted that temperature has a marked effect on specific gravity. Most substances expand when heated and contract on cooling. A rise in temperature usually is accompanied by a decrease in specific gravity, and the reverse is true when the substance is cooled. For instance, 1 Gm. of water measures 1 ml. at 4° C., the temperature at which water has the greatest weight per unit volume, although, at 80° C., 1 Gm. of water measures about 1.03 ml. Therefore, it is always necessary to indicate the temperature at which the determination is made and it has become customary to determine specific gravities at arbitrary *standard* temperatures. The *U.S.P.* and the *N.F.* have established 25° C. as the standard temperature unless otherwise stated. In the case of alcohol, the *U.S.P.* and the *N.F.* give 15.56° C. (60° F.) as the temperature at which the specific gravity is to be determined. The latter temperature is the standard established by the U.S. Revenue Department for all determinations of the specific gravity of alcohol.

Specific Gravity of Liquids

Hydrometer Method. The hydrometer (from the Greek, *hydor,* water, and *metron,* measure) consists of a double bulb to which is attached a long, thin stem (Fig. 19). Shot or mercury is placed in the lower bulb and the upper bulb is left empty. This assures that the instrument will assume an upright position in a liquid. In the stem is a scale constructed by placing the hydrom-

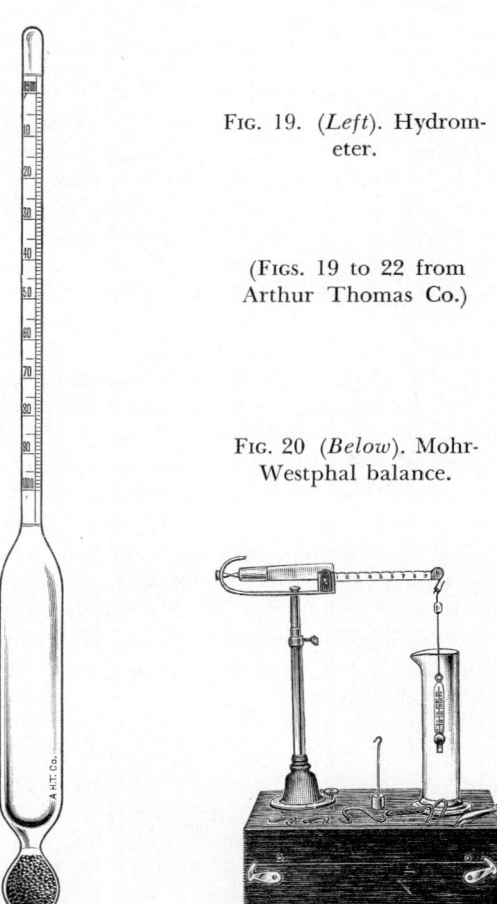

Fig. 19. (*Left*). Hydrometer.

(Figs. 19 to 22 from Arthur Thomas Co.)

Fig. 20 (*Below*). Mohr-Westphal balance.

eter in liquids of varying specific gravities and noting the points to which it sinks. Since the scale would need to be extremely long if the hydrometer were to cover the normal range of specific gravities of the commonly used liquids (0.700–2.000), it is customary to construct the instrument so that its scale covers only a portion of this range, usually 0.200 specific gravity unit. Hydrometers are furnished in sets of differing ranges, making it possible to determine the specific gravity of any liquid, provided that it falls within the range mentioned above.

To determine the specific gravity of a liquid, one selects a hydrometer which floats in the liquid with the scale partially submerged. The reading at the point of contact of the surface of the liquid with the scale is the specific gravity.

In addition to those hydrometers which read specific gravity directly, there are a number of other types used for special purposes. Among these are: (1) the *Baumé hydrometer* which is graduated in arbitrary "degrees," (2) the *Twaddle hydrometer*, likewise graduated in arbitrary "degrees" which, however, are different from those of the Baumé hydrometer, (3) the *lactometer*, used in testing milk and (4) the *alcoholometer*, for determining the amount of alcohol in a sample.

The Mohr-Westphal Balance. The construction and operation of this instrument is understood best by reference to Figure 20. The balance consists of an upright member supporting a beam on a knife-edge. The right-hand part of the beam has 9 notches and, suspended from a hook at the far end, a plummet. The plummet usually displaces 5 ml. at 15° C. Attached to the left end of the beam are a counterpoise and a sharp point, the latter being matched by a sharp point attached to the frame. A leveling device is located at the base. When the balance is level, the counterpoise balances the plummet in air and the 2 sharp points come to rest directly opposite each other. The balance is supplied with a set of 4 pairs of horseshoe-shaped weights. The individual weights are of 5 Gm., 0.5 Gm., 0.05 Gm. and 0.005 Gm.

To determine the specific gravity of a liquid, the plummet is immersed in it and one of the large weights is suspended from the hook. If the specific gravity is greater than 1, the plummet will displace a weight of liquid greater than 5 Gm., the 5-Gm. weight will be insufficient to counteract the buoyant force on the plummet and the right end of the beam will be higher than the left. It then is necessary to add more weights in order to bring the beam to equilibrium. First, the other large weight is placed in one after another of the numbered notches until the beam is brought as near equilibrium as possible. The process is repeated, using one weight from each pair. When all 5 weights have been placed properly, the sharp points will be exactly opposite each other, when the balance is at rest. The first large weight, suspended from the hook, represents a specific gravity of 1. The other large weight represents the first decimal place of the specific gravity, the next smaller weight the second decimal place, the next smaller the third and the smallest weight the fourth decimal place. Thus, the specific gravity is read directly to 4 decimal places.

When the specific gravity of the liquid is less than 1, the plummet will be buoyed up by a force of less than 5 Gm., and the large weight, if suspended from the hook, will be more than sufficient to counteract the buoyant force and therefore is not necessary. Only 4 weights will be needed, one of each size. The determination is carried out as described above. The large weight represents the first decimal place and the others the second, the third and the fourth in the order of their sizes.

The Mohr-Westphal balance is comparatively accurate; the determination is simple and rapid. Its major disadvantage is that a rather large sample is required. If only very small samples are available, other methods must be employed.

The Specific Gravity Bottle or Pycnometer. The most accurate method for determining the specific gravity of liquids is that which makes use of the pycnometer (from the Greek, *pycnos*, thick, dense, and *metron*, measure) (Fig. 21). This instrument is simply a bottle so constructed as to make it possible to weigh identical volumes of liquids.

To determine the specific gravity of a liquid, the clean, dry, empty pycnometer is first assembled, as shown in Figure 21,

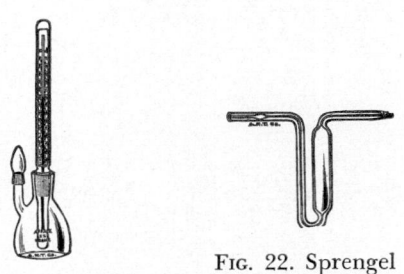

FIG. 21. Pycnometer.   FIG. 22. Sprengel tube.

and weighed accurately. It then is filled with water at a temperature slightly below that at which the determination is to be made, the thermometer is inserted and the temperature allowed to rise. As the temperature increases, the water expands, and some is forced out of the capillary tube. When the proper temperature has been reached, the excess water is removed from the capillary tube with a piece of filter paper or other bibulous material, the cap fitted to the tube and the whole weighed accurately. Although the temperature may still rise, the cap prevents evaporation of the water forced into it, and the weight remains constant. Thus, the weighing may be at a temperature different from that desired but the weight of water will remain the same. The difference between the weight of the empty bottle and the bottle filled with water is the weight of water which the bottle holds.

The pycnometer is then emptied, dried and filled with the liquid to be tested, following the directions given above, and the whole is weighed. The weight of the liquid is obtained by subtracting the weight of the empty pycnometer from the weight of the bottle and the liquid.

The specific gravity is calculated by dividing the weight of the liquid by the weight of water. Since the same bottle was used in both determinations and the temperature was the same, it is obvious that the volumes were identical.

Sprengel Tube. A device useful for determining the specific gravities of viscous materials such as oils and other materials which render the cleaning of a pycnometer difficult is the Sprengel tube (Fig. 22). Because of its size, it may be employed when only small amounts of liquids are available. Tubes similar to the one illustrated are made easily by drawing out and bending glass tubing. They are inexpensive and may be discarded after use.

SPECIFIC GRAVITY OF SOLIDS

Since most of the solid bodies for which one wishes to determine the specific gravity are of irregular shape, it usually is impossible to ascertain their volumes directly. Therefore, methods for determining the specific gravities of such bodies usually involve an indirect determination of the volume by finding either the volume of liquid which the body will displace or the apparent loss in weight when the body is immersed in a liquid.

The Displacement Method. The solid object is weighed in air. A graduated cylinder (metric) or buret is filled partially with water or other liquid in which the solid is insoluble and which has a specific gravity less than that of the solid (so that the latter does not float), and the volume is noted. The solid is immersed in the liquid, and again the volume is noted. The difference in the two volumes is equal to the volume of the solid in cubic centimeters and is numerically equal, in grams, to the weight of the water displaced. The specific gravity is found by dividing the weight of the solid in air by the weight of the water displaced.

Of course, the accuracy of this method is only as great as the operator's accuracy in reading the graduated tube. However, it is an excellent method for rapid estimation.

The Apparent Loss of Weight Method. To find the apparent loss of weight of a body in water, it is necessary only to weigh the body in air, immerse it in water and weigh again. However, when the solid is soluble in or lighter than water, the method must be modified as indicated below. These modifications are listed according to the type of solid being investigated.

1. SOLIDS INSOLUBLE IN, AND HEAVIER THAN, WATER. The solid object is weighed in air on an analytical balance. Then it is attached to the beam by means of a fine thread, immersed in a beaker of water which rests on a small bench or support so arranged that it does not interfere with the free movement of the balance pan, and weighed. The difference in the 2 weights is the apparent loss of weight in water and is equal to the weight of water displaced by the solid. The specific gravity is found by dividing the weight in air by the apparent loss of weight in water.

2. SOLIDS SOLUBLE IN, AND HEAVIER THAN, WATER. If the solid is soluble in water, it is necessary to select a liquid of known specific gravity in which it is insoluble. Since the weight of the amount of liquid displaced is proportional to its specific gravity, the apparent loss of weight of the solid when immersed in the liquid may be converted into the weight the solid would have lost, if it had been possible to weigh it in water, by the use of the following proportion:

Sp. gr. of liq. : Sp. gr. water =
   Loss wt. in liq. : Loss wt. in water

If, for example, a liquid of specific gravity 0.75 was used and the apparent loss of weight in it was 15 Gm., the apparent loss of weight in water would be calculated

$$0.75 : 1 = 15 : x$$

$x = 20$ Gm., the apparent loss of weight in water

The specific gravity then is found by dividing the weight in air by the calculated apparent loss of weight in water.

3. SOLIDS INSOLUBLE IN, AND LIGHTER THAN, WATER. Since such solids float on water, it is necessary to attach a sinker to them in order that they may be immersed completely. To determine the specific gravity of such a solid, one proceeds as follows: weigh the solid in air, weigh the sinker alone in water, attach the sinker to the solid, weigh both in water. By keeping the sinker always in water, its weight remains constant. To find the apparent loss of weight of the solid, subtract the weight of both solid and sinker in water from the combined weight of the solid in air and the sinker in water. The weight of the solid in air is then divided by its apparent loss of weight in water.

4. SOLIDS SOLUBLE IN, AND LIGHTER THAN, WATER. The specific gravity of such solids is determined by combining methods 2 and 3, using a liquid in which the solid is insoluble and calculating the apparent loss of weight in water from the apparent loss of weight in the liquid selected.

SPECIFIC GRAVITY OF POWDERS

The specific gravity of powdered materials may be determined by means of the pycnometer. Fill the pycnometer with water and weigh (I). Empty the pycnometer, place a weighed quantity of the powder in it, fill with water and weigh again (II). To the weight of the pycnometer filled with water, add the weight of the powder (III). From this *calculated weight* (III), subtract the weight of the pycnometer containing the powder and filled with water (II). The remainder is the weight of the water displaced by the powder. The specific gravity then is obtained by dividing the weight of the powder by the weight of water displaced.

SPECIFIC VOLUME

Specific volume is defined as the ratio of the volume of a given weight of a substance to the volume of an equal weight of water. Therefore, it is the volume per unit weight of substance and may be expressed as

$$\text{Sp. vol.} = \frac{V}{W}$$

Since specific gravity may be expressed as

$$\text{Sp. gr.} = \frac{W}{V}$$

it is seen that specific volume is the reciprocal of specific gravity.

There are 2 methods available for the determination of specific volume. First, one may measure the volumes of equal weights of the substance and water. The specific volume then is found by dividing the volume of the substance by the volume of the water. However, since it is impossible to measure volumes as accurately as weights may be determined, a more accurate determination of specific volume consists of determining the specific gravity and dividing this into 1. Tables of specific gravity, listing most of the common substances, are readily available, making it unnecessary to determine the specific gravity in most instances when one wishes to ascertain the specific volume.

Specific volume is of use in some pharmaceutical calculations, among which is the determination of the volume occupied by a given weight of a liquid of known specific gravity. For instance, if one wished to know what volume 100 Gm. of glycerin would occupy, he would calculate as follows:

Sp. gr. of glycerin $= 1.25$

Sp. vol. of glycerin $= \dfrac{1}{1.25} = 0.8$

that is, each gram of glycerin will occupy 0.8 ml. 100 Gm. $\times$ 0.8 $=$ 80 ml., the volume occupied by 100 Gm. of glycerin.

DENSITY

The density of a substance is defined as the ratio of the mass of the substances to its volume. (For a discussion of mass, see page 6.)

When mass and volume are expressed in metric units, the numerical value of the density of a substance is equal to its specific gravity. For example, a 1-cc. cube of cast iron weighs about 7.25 Gm. Its density is 7.25 Gm. per cc., and its specific gravity is 7.25. In the English system of weights and measures, this relation does not exist. Water has a specific gravity of 1, but its density is 62.4 pounds per cubic foot. The specific gravity of cast iron is about 7.25; its density is about 452 pounds per cubic foot.

Because it is far more convenient to use specific gravity, density is seldom used in pharmacy. It is sometimes employed in chemistry and physics and is commonly used in the practice of engineering.

BIBLIOGRAPHY

Jenkins, G. L., Christian, J. E., and Hager, G. P.: Quantitative Pharmaceutical Chemistry, ed. 5, pp. 385–404, New York, McGraw-Hill, 1957.

Lange, N. A.: Handbook of Chemistry, ed. 9, pp. 1113–1190, 1727, 1750, also var. tables, Sandusky, O., Handbook Publishers Inc. 1956.

Stocking, C. H., and Cataline, E. L.: Arithmetic of Pharmacy, ed. 8, pp. 19–34, New York, Van Nostrand, 1952.

JAMES WILSON JONES, Ph.D.

Professor of Pharmacy, College of Pharmacy, State University of Iowa

3

Heat and Refrigeration

GENERAL CONSIDERATIONS
PRACTICAL SOURCES OF HEAT
FUEL VALUES
MEASUREMENT OF HEAT
    THERMOMETER SCALES
    SPECIAL THERMOMETERS
REGULATION AND DISTRIBUTION OF HEAT
APPLICATIONS OF HEAT
PROCESSES INVOLVING CHEMICAL CHANGES
PROCESSES INVOLVING PHYSICAL CHANGES
VAPORIZATION
EVAPORATION

VAPOR PRESSURE
BOILING POINT
MELTING POINT
HUMIDITY
DISTILLATION
SUBLIMATION
LYOPHILIZATION
DESICCATION
EXSICCATION
REFRIGERATION, CONGEALING POINT
    AND FREEZING POINT

GENERAL CONSIDERATIONS

The applications of heat in the practice of pharmacy are manifold. Crude vegetable drugs must be deprived of their moisture for the purposes of preservation and grinding, and, in some instances, for developing certain medicinal properties to the exclusion of others. The separation of volatile constituents from vegetable drugs and chemical mixtures; the melting of fats preparatory to the compounding of ointments, suppositories and other solid pharmaceuticals; the sterilization of equipment and medicinal products; the analysis of drugs and chemicals—these are but a few of the processes in which heat is required.

According to an early theory, heat was a material called *caloric,* which, in some undescribed manner, was able to penetrate bodies. A hot body contained a large amount of caloric while a cold body contained a smaller amount in accordance with the degree of coldness. To accept this theory, it was necessary to assume that the caloric was different from other matter in that it possessed neither mass nor inertia.

Modern theory states that heat is a form of energy. According to this theory, the molecules, the atoms and the electrons in all bodies are in constant motion, and the particles in bodies at elevated temperatures have larger amounts of kinetic energy than those in bodies at lower temperatures. Based on this theory, the production of heat by friction can be explained as follows:

When one body slides over another, the particles of the contacting surfaces are caused to vibrate at an increased rate. Some of the mechanical energy necessary to move one surface over the other is transformed into kinetic energy of the surface particles. This form of energy is called heat. The *quantity* of heat is the amount of kinetic energy possessed by the minute subdivisions of matter.

Heat produced by friction once was used by people to produce fire by rubbing pieces of wood together until the kindling temperature was attained or by striking a piece of steel on flint rock. On the other hand, the production of heat by friction has widespread detrimental aspects. The life of any machine is dependent to a large degree upon how effectively friction and the heat produced therefrom can be minimized. This problem is the basis of the huge lubricant industry, which has developed concurrently with the increased adoption of machines in all industries.

The greatest source of heat for usable purposes is derived from chemical reactions. A chemical reaction involves the interchange of the ionic components of 2 molecules or the union of elements from their metallic or nonionized state. These reactions are accompanied ordinarily by a mild to vigorous increase in the movement of molecules and atoms, which is manifested as heat. When a dilute, ionized acid is added to a dilute, ionized base, the average amount of heat liberated is a constant (K) for each gram-molecular weight of water formed. For example, when 1 gram-molecular weight of sulfuric acid reacts with 2 gram-molecular weights of sodium hydroxide, both in dilute solutions, 2 gram-molecular weights of water are formed according to the reaction

$$H_2SO_4 + 2NaOH \rightarrow Na_2SO_4 + 2H_2O + 2K$$

The system on the left has a total latent heat energy greater than the latent heat energy of the system on the right, and the reaction proceeds because energy can be liberated.

Another example of the evolution of heat through the formation of a new chemical compound is found in the hydration or slaking of lime. When water is added to a lump of quicklime, hydration results in the formation of calcium hydroxide.

$$CaO + H_2O \rightarrow Ca(OH)_2$$

If the water is added carefully, calcium hydroxide will be obtained as a very fine, dry powder. Sufficient heat is evolved in this hydration process to cause severe burns. Since heat is liberated, this is known as an exothermic reaction.

Some substances absorb heat when they dissolve in water. This property is common to many ammonium and potassium salts. When potassium iodide is dissolved in water, the solution may become cold enough to cause condensation of atmospheric moisture on the outside of the container. Any process in which heat is absorbed is said to be endothermic. However, most solids and liquids and all gases evolve heat when they dissolve in water.

The above examples illustrate very briefly that chemical and physical processes are accompanied by the liberation of heat energy. However, these sources of heat are impractical, insufficient and too costly for fulfilling the requirements of pharmaceutical, industrial and home uses.

Combustion. This process affords the largest share of heat for practical use the world over. Combustion means burning or rapid oxidation with the emission of heat. When combustion takes place in the presence of air or pure oxygen, a flame is produced. However, combustion takes place in instances where atmospheric oxygen is not available and no flame is produced (as illustrated by the underground burning of peat and coal beds which, in some instances, has taken place over a long period of time). The flame produced is visible evidence of combustion in which gases are at the ignition point and are undergoing union with oxygen to form water and carbon dioxide. The illumination produced by a flame is due to carbon particles within the flame which have been heated to incandescence but have not reached a position in the flame where oxygen is available to them. If a fuel composed of carbon, hydrogen and oxygen (such as alcohol) is ignited, a complete combustion process can be represented as follows:

$$C_2H_5OH + 3O_2 \rightarrow 2CO_2 + 3H_2O$$

This equation shows that carbon dioxide and water are the products of complete combustion, which takes place only if sufficient oxygen is present to combine with all the hydrogen and the carbon of the fuel. The flame of alcohol is almost colorless because no carbon is liberated to be heated to incandescence. On the other hand, the flame of kerosene, when burning from a wick as in an ordinary lamp, is highly luminous because the high temperature produced decomposes some of the gases to produce carbon. The liberated carbon is then heated to incandescence and glows until it reaches the outer fringe of the flame, where it too will combine with oxygen and pass into the atmosphere as carbon dioxide. If insufficient oxygen is present, the carbon is oxidized only partially, and carbon monoxide is formed. Some carbon may escape oxidation completely and pass into the atmosphere as soot. The latter condition prevails to a large extent when coal or wood is first ignited. Gases liberated from the fuel are decomposed so rapidly that insufficient oxygen for complete combustion can reach them. Consequently, large amounts of carbon and carbon monoxide escape, the free carbon being visible as smoke. Therefore, the appearance of smoke indicates incomplete combustion and a waste of potential heat energy.

PRACTICAL SOURCES OF HEAT

The various solid, liquid and gaseous fuels and electricity afford the practical sources of heat.

Solid Fuels

The most important of the solid fuels are wood, coal, charcoal and coke.

Wood was once the most universally used of all fuels due to its wide distribution and a lack of knowledge of other fuels. However, the current demand for this fuel is small since more convenient and more economical fuels are available.

Coal is one of the most economical of all fuels if properly used and is available in 2 forms.

Anthracite or hard coal contains as high as 95 per cent of carbon and, due to the absence of vaporizable organic compounds, burns with a clean, intensely hot flame.

Bituminous or soft coal contains as much as 25 per cent of hydrocarbons, which makes it easier to ignite. However, it burns with a considerable loss of unoxidized carbon when first ignited in the ordinary combustion chamber. Proof of this is the dense smoke which appears when the combustion chamber is recharged. When the hydrocarbons in the surface layer of the coal have been eliminated, the remaining carbon burns with a nonluminous, hot flame. As combustion progresses downward through the coal bed, the hydrocarbons in the lower layers are volatilized more slowly and are burned almost completely as they pass through the flame.

Charcoal is produced by the destructive distillation of wood. It might be considered the by-product in the production of wood tar, creosote and other volatile wood products. Charcoal is available in various forms, a common form being compressed, brick-shaped lumps. After being kindled with a hot flame, it burns with a nonluminous, smokeless and very hot flame. A common and popular use for charcoal is in stoves designed for outdoor cooking.

Coke is produced by the destructive distillation of bituminous coal. Like charcoal, it is an excellent fuel, being composed of almost pure carbon. When the volatile hydrocarbons have been driven from a lump of coal, the remaining lump of carbon has a honeycombed or spongy appearance. It also burns with a nonluminous, hot flame.

Methenamine, commonly known as hexamethylenetetramine or Urotropin, is a solid fuel for emergency use only. It is used most conveniently in the form of a 5-gr. tablet. When such a tablet is ignited, it burns with a nonluminous flame, and 1 tablet produces sufficient heat to bring 5 ml. of water to the boiling point. These tablets are useful to the physician for conducting bedside tests on urine, etc.

Liquid Fuels

Many liquids are flammable and are sources of intense heat. However, only a small number of liquids are economically practical for heating purposes. Those liquids which have widespread use as fuels are fuel oil, kerosene, gasoline and denatured alcohol.

Fuel oil has become an important source of heat, especially for space heating. It is obtained from crude petroleum oil by removing some of the more volatile constituents by distillation. When used in a special type of burner in which the oil is vaporized and mixed with air before being ignited, it is a very efficient fuel.

Kerosene, or **coal oil** as it commonly is known, has been used for many years for cooking and small-space heating purposes. Small, wick-type stoves for heating single rooms, for cooking and for other purposes long have been used. The kerosene is fed from the supply chamber by means of a wick, as in the kerosene lamp. These stoves frequently emit objectionable odors and soot due to improper regulation of the flame size in relation to the supply of air in the combustion chamber. Newer types of burners have eliminated the necessity of a wick. Kerosene under pressure is fed into these burners where it is vaporized and mixed with air before being ignited. This produces a nonluminous flame which utilizes the entire heat value of the kerosene, thus increasing its efficiency as a fuel.

Gasoline, also known as petrol or petroleum benzin, like kerosene is used in stoves for cooking and in special torches for spot heating, but is not employed in space heating. Gasoline is very volatile and highly flammable. These properties make it a dangerous fuel unless properly handled. Stoves which use gasoline as a fuel have a supply tank well removed from the flame. Gasoline under pressure is fed into the burner, where it is vaporized and mixed with air before being ignited, as in the newer kerosene stoves. Both gasoline and kerosene require a large quantity of oxygen for their complete combustion.

Denatured alcohol has limited use as a fuel in the laboratory. The spirit lamp is one of the oldest, yet the most commonly used, instruments for burning alcohol (Fig. 23). The lamp consists of a reservoir into which a wick extends for supplying alcohol by capillary attraction. The cap which fits securely over the burner serves to extinguish the flame and to prevent evaporation of alcohol when the lamp is not in use. Metal lamps can be carried in the physician's kit and are convenient in the clinical

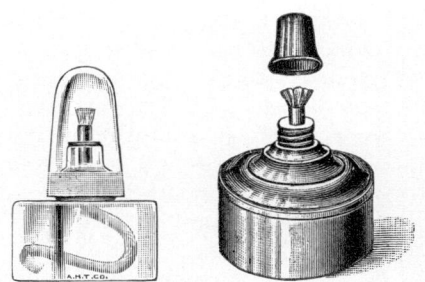

Fig. 23. Spirit lamps. *(Left)* Made of glass. *(Right)* Made of metal.

laboratory for heating small quantities of specimens.

Gas Fuels

Gases for heating purposes are too numerous to be discussed here in their entirety. Their use as illuminants preceded their use as fuel by many years, chiefly because no burner had been discovered in which they could be utilized without producing a smoky flame.

Coal gas, obtained by the destructive distillation of bituminous coal, is the oldest in respect to its term of use. For many years, it was employed only for illuminating houses, factories, city streets, etc. Illuminating gases are mixtures of methane, ethane, carbon dioxide, carbon monoxide, hydrogen, oxygen, nitrogen and an illuminant which gives the flame added candle power. A small amount of sulfur compounds is usually present to provide an odor by which leakage in the delivery system can be detected.

Natural gas is obtained from the interior of the earth, where it exists in vast quantities. Unlike coal gas, it has very little odor and must be mixed with sulfur compounds or other odorous materials so that leakage can be detected. Both natural and coal gases are systemic poisons, due to the presence of carbon monoxide.

Natural gas was first used as an illuminant in New York in 1824. In recent years, burners have been developed with which the gas can be burned with a nonluminous, hot flame. Pipe lines from sources in the petroleum fields to distant cities have made the gas available for cooking, space heating and many other purposes. Enormous quantities of the gas are distributed in pressure tanks, making it available even to outlying farm communities for cooking purposes.

Acetylene is obtainable in pressure tanks and is used principally in industry for welding and other operations requiring the intense, localized heat of a blast flame.

Propane, butane and other hydrocarbon gases are also available in cylinders for use as fuel.

All the above gases must be mixed with a large quantity of air before being ignited in order to secure a nonsmoky flame. Special burners having mixing chambers have been developed and have given these gases a respected place as sources of heat.

ELECTRICITY

Electricity rapidly has gained a place of importance as a source of heat during the past half century. Improvements in electric heating units have tended to minimize heat loss by radiation and to concentrate the heat. These developments, along with the production of accurate and dependable thermostatic controls and lower rates for electricity, have created an extensive demand for electric heating. Since there is no flame present, the use of electricity provides a cleaner source of heat than any other. It has the advantage over the gases in that there is no danger from poisoning or explosions due to flaws in the delivery system or through carelessness or accident in the use of burners.

Heat produced by an electric current can be explained by the friction theory previously mentioned. When a current of electricity is passed through a metal having a high resistance to its flow, the particles of the metal or conductor are set in vigorous motion, the velocity of which is proportional to the amount of current applied. As the particles vibrate, heat results, and, as this heat increases, the particles become incandescent. The production of light from wires heated to incandescence was one of the earliest uses of electricity.

The amount of heat developed for a given time when a current of electricity is passed through a conductor is directly proportional to the resistance of the conductor and to the square of the current. Therefore, in order to utilize electricity efficiently for heating, the heating element must have a high resistance to the flow of the current. Research has resulted in conductors which emit an intense degree of heat and are long-lived even though subjected to air and to subsequent vaporization and oxidation.

FUEL VALUES

At one time, the choice of fuel was largely a question of availability. However, improvements in transportation, the development of pipeline systems and better heating appliances, the discovery of new fuel beds and other advances have made it possible for a consumer to choose a fuel on the basis of cost, efficiency and convenience. The heating capacity of fuels is usually stated in British Thermal Units (B.T.U.) per ton, cord, gallon or 100 cu. ft., according to the physical state of the fuel. A British Thermal Unit is the amount of heat required to raise the temperature of 1 lb. of water from 60° to 61° F. at sea level. Two calories are also used—the *small calorie* is the amount of heat required to raise the temperature of 1 Gm. of water 1° C.; the *large calorie* is the amount of heat required to raise the temperature of 1 Kg. of water 1° C. and is equal to 3.96 B.T.U.

In choosing between coals, a comparison should be made between the cost and the B.T.U. rating of the coals. It might be found that a coal cheap in price is actually costly to use on the basis of its heat content.

MEASUREMENT OF HEAT

The sensations of "hot" and "cold" are the result of the development of our sensory organs and their responses to heat energy. However, these organs measure only a *qualitative* degree of heat. Arbitrary instruments for the quantitative measurement of heat were developed about 3 centuries ago. The measured degree of heat was then referred to as temperature and the instruments used in the measurements were called thermometers. Today, thermometers or temperature indicators have been developed in numerous modifications to fulfill special conditions of usage.

The simplest and the most common of all is the liquid thermometer (Fig. 24). In its construction, use is made of the property of expansion and contraction of a liquid when it is subjected to various degrees of heat. Mercury excels all other liquids for this purpose; alcohol is next in preference. Mercury is particularly suitable because of its high boiling point, 356.9° C., and its low solidifying point, —39° C. The mercury thermometer is more accurate than the alcohol thermometer, but is more difficult to read because of the small capillary required. It expands at approximately one sixth the rate of alcohol. Since the mercury capillary is so small, these thermometers often are constructed with a special reflecting or magnifying background to permit easier reading. The background may be built into the stem of the thermometer or it may consist of a separate strip of milk-white glass which is sealed to the thermometer at a fixed position. The scale appears on the background rather than on the thermometer and both are encased in a glass tube for protection. Figure 24 illustrates 2 types of thermometers commonly used in the laboratory.

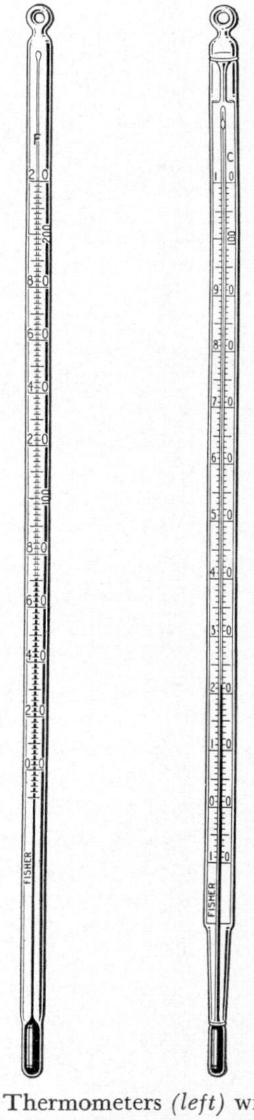

THERMOMETER SCALES

Many temperature scales have been proposed within the last 3 centuries. However, on any scale, it first is necessary to define 2 fixed points. The greatest differences in the scales which have been proposed have been in the choice of these fixed points. Isaac Newton (1642–1727) proposed a scale on which the temperature of ice was taken as the lower point and the temperature of blood as the upper point on the scale. Some years later, it was said that the temperature of freezing ice was variable because water could be supercooled below its freezing point. Consequently, Gabriel Daniel Fahrenheit (1686–1736) constructed a thermometer on which the zero reading was the temperature produced by a mixture of ice, water and an excess of salt. Fahrenheit believed that this was the lowest temperature possible to attain, and that, by using this as the zero point, minus readings would be eliminated. He retained blood temperature as the upper limit and divided the interval into 96°. This scale, the **Fahrenheit scale,** is still used predominantly among English-speaking peoples. On this scale, the freezing point of water falls at 32° and the boiling point at 212° (Fig. 25).

Anders Celsius (1701-1744) proposed a scale on which the freezing and the boiling points of water were chosen as the limits. These points were designated as 0° and 100°, respectively. This is now known as the **Centigrade scale** and is used universally in scientific works.

The scale introduced by René A. F.

FIG. 24. Thermometers *(left)* with scale on tube and *(right)* with built-in scale.

Réaumur (1683-1757), used largely in central Europe, defines the freezing point as 0°, but fixes the boiling point of water at 80°.

A fourth scale of temperature used by the physicist and the chemist in determining certain values is the **Kelvin or absolute scale.** This scale was proposed as a result of observations on the behavior of gases. It can be demonstrated that the volume of a gas decreases $\frac{1}{273}$ of its volume at 0° C. and 760 mm. pressure for each degree lowering in temperature. This direct relationship between volume and temperature lowering cannot be shown beyond conditions under which gases liquefy, but it is assumed that, at $-273°$ C., gases will have minimum volume and no further thermal motion will be possible. This is known as absolute zero. Since the temperature interval on the absolute and the Centigrade scales is the same, absolute degrees can be calculated from the simple formula:

$$A.° = C.° + 273°$$

Figure 25 shows the relationship between the Fahrenheit and the Centigrade scales

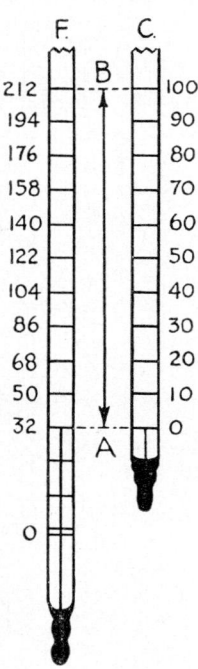

Fig. 25. Fahrenheit and Centigrade scales.

which are dealt with most commonly in pharmaceutical practice. Using the range between the freezing and the boiling points of pure water, it is seen that the distance is divided into 100° on the Centigrade and 180° on the Fahrenheit scale. Therefore, within this span on the thermometers, 1° C. is equal to 1.8° F. However, temperature readings on either scale are taken in respect to the number of degrees below or above zero; thus 32° must be added to the 180° F. between A and B in order to obtain the total reading from the Fahrenheit zero point. Substituting these values into the conversion formula, $(C.° \times 1.8) + 32$, we have $(100° C. \times 1.8) + 32$ or 212° F. If we wish to convert Fahrenheit degrees to Centigrade degrees, the algebraic order of calculation is reversed and we find that

$$F.° - 32 \div 1.8$$

or

$$\frac{F.° - 32}{1.8} = \frac{212° - 32}{1.8}$$
$$= 100° C.$$

A second method for expressing these conversions from one system to the other is represented as follows:

$$C.° = \tfrac{5}{9}(F.° - 32)$$
$$F.° = \tfrac{9}{5}C.° + 32$$

Special Thermometers

Clinical Thermometers. The clinical thermometer is so constructed that the mercury column will remain at the **maximum** height reached until it is lowered by force. This feature is accomplished by constricting the capillary immediately above the mercury reservoir or bulb so that mercury will not flow through except when force is applied. Thus, when the thermometer bulb is placed under the tongue or into the rectum, heat expands the mercury, forcing it through the constriction and up the scale. The mercury is forced back into the bulb by grasping the top of the thermometer and swinging it sharply through a downward arch. Most clinical thermometers register between 92° and 108° F. and must be "shaken down" to at least 95° before being used to determine body temperature.

Gas Thermometers. When a gas is heated, it expands $\frac{1}{273}$ of its volume at 0° C. and 760 mm. pressure for each degree of temperature raise. If expansion of the gas is prevented by using a closed vessel, the pressure within the vessel will increase in direct proportion to the increase in temperature. Any instrument which will register temperature in respect to the pressure produced is called a gas thermometer. This type of thermometer is more accurate than any other; however, it is too difficult to use for ordinary purposes.

Resistance Thermometers. When a current of electricity is passed through a conductor, the resistance to the flow of current is dependent on the temperature of the metal. Coils of various metals and alloys have been prepared and their resistance calibrated at various temperatures. When such a coil is placed in the center of a fermentation tank, a grain bin or a drying oven, or in other positions of difficult accessibility, and connected with an outside current, resistance to the flow of current is found to differ as the temperature around the coil changes. By referring the resistance readings to a chart, the corresponding temperature changes can be found. This type of thermometer can be used through a range of temperatures from very low to around 1,000° C.

Pyrometers: THERMOCOUPLE PYROMETERS. These are used to determine the temperature in ovens, furnaces and other chambers where the temperature may be as high as 2,500° F. The thermocouple operates on the principle that, when 2 wires of different metals are connected at both ends, an electric current will be developed if the 2 terminal couplings are not at the same temperature. The amount of current developed is proportional to the temperature difference and can be measured on a potentiometer.

OPTICAL PYROMETERS. These are used to determine the temperature of any hot object that glows. They contain a filament that glows with an intensity which varies with the amount of current passing through it. The current is adjusted until the glow of the filament blends with the glow of the object being viewed. The temperature can be determined from the amount of current passing through the calibrated filament or read directly on the modern instrument.

Several other types of special thermometers are in common use. Thermostats for controlling home and industrial heating are examples.

REGULATION AND DISTRIBUTION OF HEAT

NECESSITY FOR REGULATING AND DISTRIBUTING HEAT

In many processes used by the pharmacist, regulation of the quantity and the distribution of heat is essential to the safety and the success of the process. To illustrate, in the evaporation of an aqueous extraction of a vegetable drug, the directions may specify a temperature not to exceed 100° C. in order that the products to be obtained will not be destroyed. In this instance, evaporation over water will ensure that the temperature in the evaporating vessel will not exceed 100° C. If the extract were evaporated over direct heat, a temperature higher than 100° C. would be possible due to the elevation of the boiling point of the water present by the dissolved substances. Again, direct heat might become more intense at certain spots on the dish and possibly cause charring of some of the organic material present in the solution.

When glassware or porcelain ware is to be used in heating water, the heat applied should be distributed over the bottom of the vessel to prevent its being shattered by strains caused by localized heating and uneven expansion. These vessels should be protected by placing a piece of asbestos, plate metal or wire screen over the flame so that the heat transmitted will be distributed uniformly over a larger area.

METHODS OF REGULATING AND DISTRIBUTING HEAT

Various types of baths are used to distribute heat over a wide range of temperatures.

Sand Baths. These are any conveniently shaped vessel in which dry, fine sand can be heated. The vessel must be constructed of metal or other material which will withstand high temperatures. The vessel to be heated is placed on a thin bed of sand, then more sand is added until it extends well up

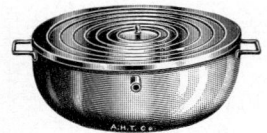

Fig. 26. Water bath.

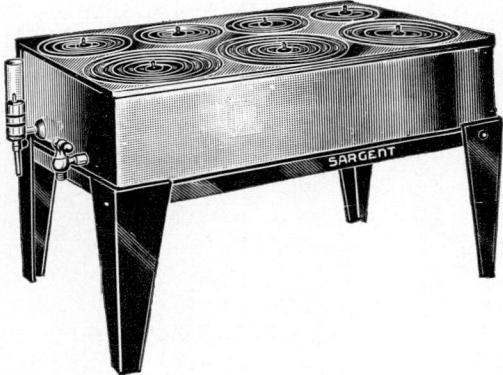

Fig. 27. Constant-level water bath.

on the sides of the vessel so that heat will be transmitted to a large area on the vessel. When heat is applied to the bath, it is transmitted throughout the sand bed so that no localization on the bottom of the vessel is possible. To a large degree, this prevents "bumping" in the solution being evaporated and decreases the danger of breaking glassware by uneven expansion. Bumping in liquids being evaporated is produced by the inability of small vapor bubbles forming at the bottom of the liquid to rise to the surface. The bubbles increase in size until their pressure is sufficient to carry them to the surface with great velocity. On reaching the surface of the liquid, they burst with great vigor and create splashing. Heating the sides as well as the bottom of the vessel assists in preventing bumping by decreasing the viscosity of the uppermost liquid and thus providing easier passage for the small bubbles which form at the bottom.

The sand bath can be used for operations requiring very moderate to extremely high temperatures.

Oil Baths. These can be used where a temperature of approximately 250° C. is not to be exceeded. Mineral oil commonly is used for this purpose since some vegetable oils begin to decompose at about 175° C. Of the vegetable oils, cottonseed oil is the most desirable since its decomposition temperature is quite high. When it is desirable to keep the oil in the bath between usages, the addition of a small amount of paraffin or wax will produce a semisolid at room temperature and thereby prevent spilling.

Glycerin Baths. These can be used up to a temperature of 250° C., after which the glycerin begins to decompose into acrolein, a product with a very disagreeable odor.

Water Baths. These are the most used of all baths where a temperature of 100° C. or below is desirable. Baths of this type vary in size and shape to satisfy the many needs of the laboratory worker. The usual form is a circular, tinned-copper bowl with a lid composed of several concentric, removable rings. These rings are removed to permit a maximum surface of the heated vessel being exposed to the heat. For operations requiring long periods of steam heating, the constant-level water bath is preferred since it requires no attention once it is regulated. Figures 26 and 27 illustrate these baths in sizes ordinarily found in the laboratory. Much larger and more elaborate baths are available for large-scale operations.

Constant-Temperature Baths. In these baths, the temperature can be maintained within a fraction of a degree. They are used in bringing about certain chemical

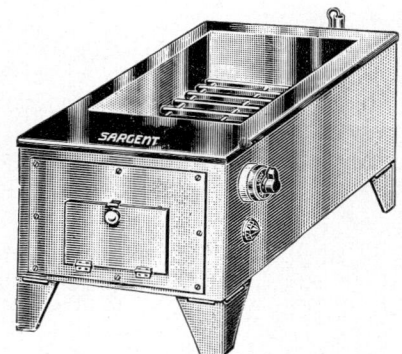

Fig. 28. Constant-temperature bath.

reactions which require heating at a specific temperature for a prolonged period of time; for determining the solubility of substances at a fixed temperature; for evaporation and drying when temperature control must be exercised. Figure 28 shows a constant-temperature bath which is insulated heavily to prevent rapid loss of heat by radiation. It is heated electrically, controlled thermostatically and provided with a constant liquid-level control.

Salt-Water Baths. These can be used when temperatures substantially over 100° C. are necessary and where other liquid baths are undesirable. When a non-volatile solute is dissolved in water, the boiling point of the water is elevated in direct proportion to the number of solute particles present in the solution. The boiling points of saturated solutions of a few common salts are given below.

Saturated Solution	Boiling Point
Sodium chloride	108.6°C.
Sodium nitrate	121.0
Sodium acetate	124.6
Potassium chloride	108.5
Potassium nitrate	115.9
Potassium acetate	169.0
Calcium nitrate	151.0
Calcium chloride	179.0

Steam Baths. Although the water baths previously discussed are actually steam baths, this term usually is applied to baths employing steam under pressure. This type of bath is used very widely in industry due to its convenience and safety for both short and prolonged operations.

When steam is brought in contact with an object at normal atmospheric pressure, it will transmit a temperature of 100° C. As the pressure is increased, a higher degree of heat is attained. To illustrate, steam has a temperature of 100° C. under normal pressure, which is 14.7 lb. per square inch. If the pressure is increased to 100 lb. per square inch, the temperature is increased to about 160° C. Such steam is said to be "superheated." Steam under pressure is used not only in evaporating liquids but also in supplying the necessary heat for many manufacturing processes.

If a steam bath which is connected permanently with the steam supply (Fig. 29, *top*) is not available, such a bath for temporary use can be provided by connecting the steam supply to the side tube of an ordinary water bath by means of a rubber tube.

A convenient steam bath for many purposes is shown in Figure 29, *bottom*. Being funnel-shaped, it will accommodate vessels ranging in size from a liter flask to an evaporating pan several inches in diameter.

The foregoing steam baths utilize live steam for their operation, permitting the steam to be discharged into the room. Evaporating pans, mixing and cooking tanks and various other types of manufacturing equipment which employ either free-flowing steam or steam under pressure also are used extensively. This equipment is jacketed with heavy metal which will

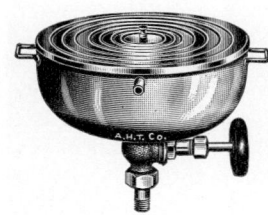

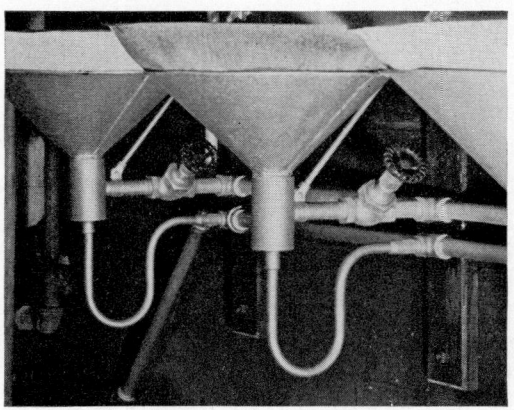

Fig. 29. *(Top)* Steam bath for permanent connection with a steam supply. *(Bottom)* Funnel-shaped steam bath.

withstand a pressure of several pounds per square inch. The jacket bears steam inlet and outlet valves and a safety valve which

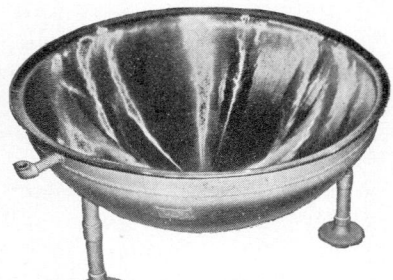

FIG. 30. Pfaudler evaporating pan.

prevents the maximum rated pressure being exceeded. Much of the equipment is porcelain- or glass-lined to prevent contamination of the products processed in them. The contents are heated by passing steam through the jacket or by closing the outlet valve and causing steam pressure to form, thus increasing the temperature. Since the contents are heated from the sides as well as the bottom of the apparatus, evaporation is very rapid.

Figure 30 illustrates a jacketed evaporating pan widely used by manufacturers for concentrating aqueous solutions. A jacketed tank suitable for preparing soaps by the saponification of vegetable oils, for cooking foods and for many other operations where continued heating is required is shown in Figure 31. Another very useful steam-heating device is the steam coil. The coil is immersed in the material to be heated so that no heat is lost by radiation since it is transmitted entirely to the surrounding material.

An extremely important use for steam under pressure is in the operation of an **autoclave** for sterilizing pharmaceutical preparations, surgical instruments, clothing, etc. The autoclave is constructed much the same as the jacketed kettle, except that the inner chamber can be closed hermetically during the heating period and controlled steam pressure can be maintained in the inner chamber as well as in the jacket. Autoclaves are operated under definite correlation between pressure and temperature.

The use of steam under pressure has some noteworthy advantages over the free-flowing steam: (1) a higher temperature can be attained; (2) steam is conserved since none is lost into the atmosphere; (3) moisture produced by condensation of the steam is drained off through the sewerage system.

APPLICATIONS OF HEAT

For many pharmaceutical operations, the degree of heat applied is extremely important to the success of the operation. In preparing some materials, a high degree of heat may cause decomposition and discoloration. Other operations require strong, direct heat in order that certain materials will be destroyed, leaving those which have their composition only modified or unaltered at the temperature applied. The concentration of solutions, the drying of both organic and inorganic products, the separation and the purification of volatile substances, the preparation of solutions and a large number of other processes require controlled heat.

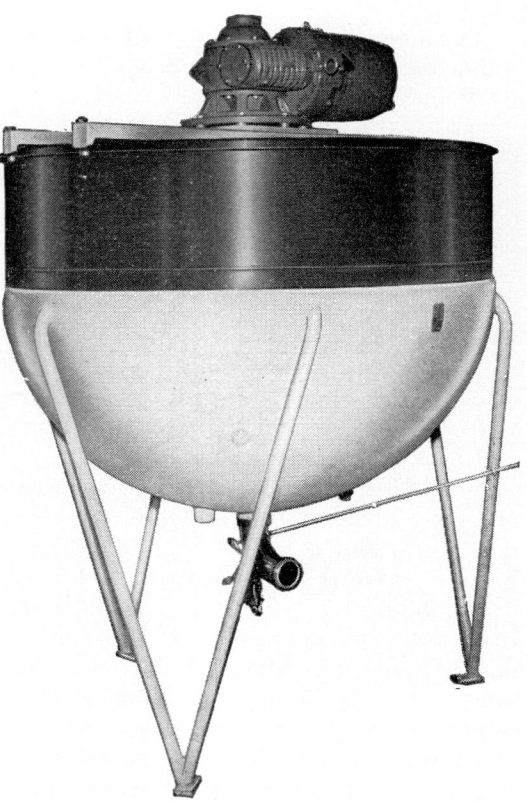

FIG. 31. Steam cooking kettle.

The pharmaceutical processes for which heat is required can be divided into 2 general groups: (1) those processes in which a chemical change results and (2) those in which only a physical change is produced. The first group can be divided further into processes in which only inorganic or organic materials are heated.

PROCESSES INVOLVING CHEMICAL CHANGES

Inorganic Materials

Calcination. This is the process of strongly heating an inorganic carbonate or hydroxide in an open vessel to expel carbon dioxide or water, leaving only the metallic oxide. The process received its name through the heating of limestone ($CaCO_3$) to form quicklime (CaO). However, calcination is now used in the preparation of other oxides in the *U.S.P.* The oxides formed frequently are termed "calcined," as illustrated by the name calcined magnesia for magnesium oxide.

Enormous quantities of quicklime and other metallic oxides are made commercially. In the pharmacist's laboratory, where calcination is used principally in analyses, porcelain, graphite, clay, platinum and other types of crucibles are employed. The porcelain evaporating dish also is used often when a relatively large quantity of material is to be heated. Platinum crucibles are preferred for some calcinations, but they are extremely costly and are damaged by lead salts, hypophosphites, potassium hydroxide and sulfides.

Ignition. The heating of an inorganic substance at a high temperature until all the volatile material is driven off is called ignition. Although ignition is used usually by the analyst to expel the last traces of moisture or other volatile material from a solid, the process is used also to determine the amount of inorganic material in a plant or animal tissue or in a metallic salt of an organic acid. Since materials which are ignited often contain destructible organic matter, the gases evolved may become ignited by the extreme heat applied.

The term ignition as it is used here must not be confused with the ignition of fuels, in which use the word means to "set on fire" or to "kindle."

Since ignitions are carried on over direct, blast heat, special supports or triangles are

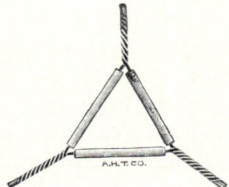

Fig. 32. Triangle of wire protected by fire clay, used as a support when applying heat.

required to hold the crucibles. A typical triangle of clay-pipe covered wire is illustrated in Figure 32.

Deflagration. This process is seldom, if ever, used by the pharmacist. It is the process of heating an inorganic substance which yields oxygen. The heating is accompanied by a crackling sound as oxygen escapes. Small amounts of material usually are heated on a platinum foil. The process can be used by the metallurgist for obtaining pure metals from metallic oxides. Thus, if ferric oxide is heated with aluminum, metallic iron and aluminum oxide are formed, the reaction proceeding with almost explosive violence.

Organic Materials

Carbonization. This is the process of heating a dry organic substance, in the absence of air, until all the volatile materials have been driven out and only carbon remains in the retort.

The production of charcoal from plant and animal tissue is a typical example of the process.

Incineration. The process of strongly heating organic material in the presence of air until all the carbon has been consumed and only an ash remains is called incineration. The ash is composed primarily of inorganic compounds. The muffle furnace (Fig. 33) is used for incinerating small amounts of materials in the laboratory. The muffle, or removable inner chamber, is heated electrically. The outside walls are insulated heavily against loss of heat by radiation since temperatures as high as 1,600° C. are employed not uncommonly.

Incineration is used in the pharmaceutical industry for determining the ash content of various plant and animal drugs as a step in their identification and analysis.

Torrefaction, or roasting, is the process of heating organic material, in the presence of air, and at temperature that will produce no carbonization, in order to modify or destroy some of the original constituents. This process has many applications in diverse fields. Medicinal rhubarb, in the dry unroasted form, contains 2 types of active principles: those which are cathartic and those which are astringent in action. When the drug is roasted, the principles responsible for the cathartic effect are destroyed, while the astringent principles which provide the usefulness of rhubarb in the treatment of diarrheas are unaffected.

The bark of cascara sagrada contains an enzyme which must be destroyed before the bark can be used for medicinal preparations. In order to provide for proper drying, the U.S.P. states that the bark should be collected at least one year prior to use. The same enzyme destruction can be obtained by heating the bark for a few hours at 100° C.

When coffee is roasted, certain components of the bean are altered, giving rise to the characteristic flavor, color and aroma. At the same time, the caffeine content remains unchanged.

The roasting of meats and other foods is an everyday application of torrefaction.

PROCESSES INVOLVING PHYSICAL CHANGES

In many processes, the application of heat produces no chemical change. Instead, only a temporary change in the physical state results from an elevation in the temperature. When the temperature is lowered, the materials assume their original physical characteristics. These processes are designated as fusion and vaporization.

Fusion. The process of liquefying a substance by the application of heat only is called fusion. In the preparation of ointments, pastes, plasters and other pharmaceutical products, the base or dispersing medium for the medicinal agent may be composed of petrolatum, beeswax, wool fat and other fatty or oily ingredients. These must be melted or liquefied together in order that a uniform and homogeneous mixture can be obtained before the medicinal agent is incorporated. The packaging of fats, waxes, some chemicals and many other products is facilitated best if they are first liquefied by heating and then poured into the stock containers.

In the metallurgical industries, pure metals are fused together to make the numerous alloys for industrial use.

Vaporization. This is the process whereby solids or liquids are transformed to the gaseous or vapor state. It was stated previously that all matter is composed of particles which are in constant motion, and that the sphere of their motion is dependent on the force of attraction between the particles (known as cohesion), the size of the particles and the position of the particles within the substance.

If we consider an open vessel containing a liquid and visualize a layer of molecules at the center of the liquid, it can be assumed that, no matter in which direction any one molecule moves, it is so surrounded by other molecules that its path of motion is limited. However, if a layer of molecules on the surface is selected, it is

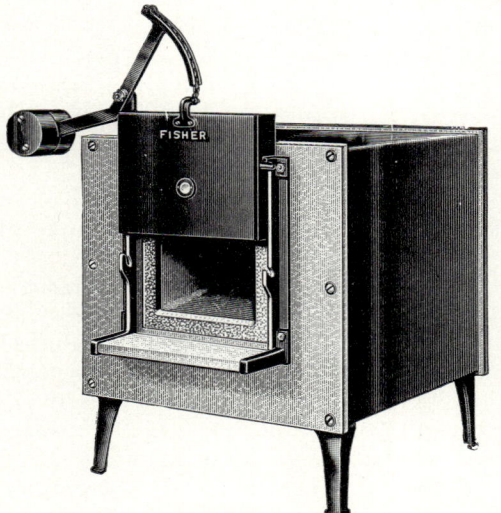

Fig. 33. Muffle furnace.

observed that, under ordinary conditions, the area above the molecules is occupied sparsely as compared with all other areas into which the molecules can move.

Once a molecule is in the air, it may collide with other molecules present and be forced back into the liquid surface or it may be forced farther into the air and be lost to the liquid. Any substance which, on being exposed to the air, will lose molecules as vapor particles is "volatile." Many liquids and solids possess internal forces of sufficient strength that they lose no molecules from the surface at ordinary or elevated temperatures. These are called "nonvolatile" substances.

In between the extremes of highly volatile and nonvolatile there is a continuous gradation of substances.

The ease or the difficulty with which liquids or solids will give up vapor molecules provides a means of classifying them as very volatile, volatile, slightly volatile or nonvolatile products.

VAPORIZATION

Vaporization Below the Boiling Point

The rate of vaporization below the boiling point varies from one substance to another according to the cohesional forces present. However, if a single liquid is considered, it is found that several factors influence its rate of vaporization.

Figure 34 shows a cylinder fitted with a piston which can be secured in a fixed position or permitted to move by virtue of forces exerted upon it. It is assumed that the weight of the piston is counterbalanced perfectly so that it will move only when outside forces act on its surface. When a layer of water is placed in the cylinder and the piston is fixed in a position above the surface of the liquid, water molecules enter the area above the liquid and create a pressure on the piston by their vibrations against it. Some of the molecules which escape from the surface of the water are forced back; however, the number leaving exceeds those returning, so the pressure exerted on the piston gradually increases. In a short time, the pressure will become constant, which indicates that an equilibrium has been reached between the molecules escaping from and returning to the surface of the liquid. The experiment shows that, as the number of vapor particles above a liquid increases, the rate of vaporization of the liquid decreases until an equilibrium is reached between the liquid and its vapor.

If, after equilibrium has been reached at a given temperature, the temperature is elevated by progressive intervals, it will be found that the pressure on the piston will have increased each time in proportion to the temperature elevation. This means that added heat gives the liquid particles greater velocity which enables them to escape from the surface more rapidly. Since pressure on the piston is in direct proportion to the number of vapor particles vibrating against it, an increase in pressure is to be expected.

That vaporization takes place at low temperatures, as well as at ordinary or elevated temperatures, is illustrated by a phenomenon which we observe but give little cognizance to during the winter months. For example, when a wet cloth is hung out of doors during freezing weather, the water freezes very quickly. If left for a few hours, the cloth will have dried, due to the slow vaporization of the ice. On a sunny day, the drying process is more rapid since heat from the sun increases the rate at which the ice vaporizes.

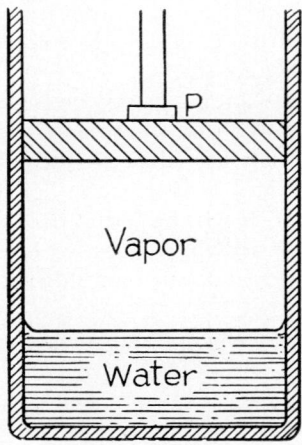

Fig. 34. Vaporization cylinder with piston.

When the above observations are applied to actual practice, we find that vaporization of liquids is much more rapid in a dry, warm room than in a room in which the atmosphere is moist and cold.

The rate at which a liquid will vaporize from an open dish is dependent also on the amount of liquid surface exposed to the atmosphere. Since vapor particles escape only from the surface of a liquid which is not boiling, it follows that the surface area has a direct relationship to the rate of vaporization. Therefore, it is best to use a shallow, flaring vessel such as an evaporating dish rather than one which is deep and narrow in diameter; flasks with sides converging at the top are distinctly to be avoided.

In summary, the rate of vaporization below the boiling point of a substance is: (1) inversely proportional to the atmospheric pressure, (2) directly proportional to the temperature and (3) directly proportional to the surface exposed to the atmosphere.

Vaporization at the Boiling Point

The rate of vaporization at the boiling point is influenced by: (1) the amount of surface exposed to the air, (2) the amount of surface exposed to the heat, (3) the depth of the liquid and (4) the quantity of heat delivered to the liquid, all other factors being equal. The larger the area exposed to heat, the greater will be the number of vapor bubbles that can be produced and the rate of evaporation will increase accordingly. Let us consider 2 vessels having the same internal diameter but with the bottom of one corrugated so that its surface is twice that of the other (Fig. 35). If both vessels are filled to the same level with water and heated to the boiling point of the water, it will be found that the water in the vessel with a corrugated bottom will be vaporized in about one half the time as that in the other.

When water is placed in a vessel and heated to the boiling point, the temperature will be 100° C. If the flame is adjusted so that the heat delivered to the water is just sufficient to maintain this temperature, vaporization will proceed at a uniform rate. When the flame size is increased so that the

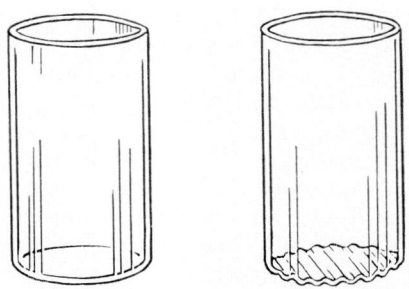

Fig. 35. *(Left)* Plain vessel. *(Right)* Vessel with corrugated bottom.

quantity of heat delivered to the water is greater, the rate of boiling is increased although the temperature of boiling remains the same. Since the quantity of heat is increased, more vapor bubbles are formed and rise to the surface than previously, thus expelling more vapor per unit of time.

Deep, narrow columns of liquid decrease the rate of evaporation at the boiling temperature. As vapor bubbles form on the bottom, they are retarded in their upward progress by the weight of the liquid, the increased area of cohesional forces which they must overcome and the differences in temperature toward the surface of the liquid, all of which may cause the bubbles to burst before reaching the surface. When a deep column of liquid has been heated until boiling is attained at the bottom, it will be observed that only very large vapor bubbles are able to reach the surface. Since it requires more time for large vapor bubbles to form than for small ones, the rate of vaporization is decreased very noticeably.

Effect of Stirring on the Rate of Vaporization

Stirring a liquid at any temperature tends to weaken the inherent internal forces which act to prevent the escape of vapor particles. The surface of the liquid exposed to the air is increased by the ripples produced. Externally, the motion of stirring produces air currents which assist in carrying the escaped vapor away from the liquid surface, making it easier for more vapor to escape.

is shown in Figure 40, *left*. A large test tube about 2 inches longer than the thermometer to be used is fitted with a 2-hole stopper. Insert a thermometer in one perforation so that the bulb is about 1 inch from the liquid surface and none of the scale is visible on the upper end. Place a bent glass tube in the second perforation and, if the vapor is to be recovered, connect this tube to a condenser. When the liquid is heated, the hot vapors warm the entire length of the thermometer and the mercury can expand uniformly through the capillary.

If a long tube is not available for this instrument, a second instrument can be improvised, using an ordinary flask. Since much of the thermometer extends outside the flask, it must be protected from air currents, as shown in Figure 40, *right*. A small flask is fitted with a cork stopper through which a glass tube about 12 mm. in diameter has been inserted. The tube should extend into the flask about 1 inch and above the flask far enough completely to enclose the thermometer. A thermometer is then suspended inside the tube by a piece of fine wire so that the bulb is about 1 inch above the liquid. When the liquid is boiled, hot vapors pass upward through the tube and warm the thermometer so that the mercury will expand uniformly in the capillary.

These 2 instruments are sufficiently accurate for routine laboratory work, but they are not to be used in determining boiling points for official data. Precise methods for determining this physical property are described in the *U.S.P.* Because few commercially available substances are sufficiently pure to have an exact boiling point, the *U.S.P.* uses the terminology "Boiling or Distilling Range or Temperature," and the procedures are established accordingly.

MELTING POINT

The melting point of a solid is the temperature at which it is in equilibrium with its liquid. Ordinary variations in atmospheric pressure have no effect on the melting point. However, if the melting point is determined under a pressure far removed from 1 atmosphere, a corresponding correction must be made.

The melting point of a substance is a criterion of its purity since the presence of an impurity lowers its melting point. This physical constant is of particular value in the purification of chemicals by crystallization, especially if the identity of the compound is unkown. Crystallization should be repeated until 2 successive melting points are equal, which indicates that all foreign materials have been eliminated. It is also a rapid method for checking the purity of substances purchased, for which an official melting point is recorded.

The official method for determining the melting range or temperature not only of crystalline, pulverizable solids, but also of fats, waxes, paraffin, fatty acids, etc., is described in the *U.S.P.* Five procedures are described for use with different classes of materials.

HUMIDITY

Humidity refers to the amount of moisture in the atmosphere. ABSOLUTE HUMIDITY is the actual weight of water contained in a unit volume of atmosphere. RELATIVE HUMIDITY is the ratio between the amount of moisture actually present in a unit volume of atmosphere at a given temperature to the amount that would be present under saturated conditions. Therefore, relative humidity always is expressed in per cent. For example, if 1 cu. ft. of air contains 6 gr. of moisture and is capable of containing 10 gr. at the same temperature, the relative humidity is 60 per cent.

Dew Point. When the atmosphere is completely saturated at a given temperature, it has reached the dew point. At this point, a slight drop in temperature causes condensation of a portion of the moisture.

Hygrometers. Instruments that measure relative humidity are called hygrometers. One type of hygrometer is shown in Figure 41. This is known as the WET AND DRY BULB PSYCHROMETER. The water reservoir in the center is connected with one thermometer bulb by means of a wick which is kept moist. As water evaporates from the wick, heat is absorbed from the bulb, causing a lowering of the thermometer reading. The second thermometer records the atmospheric temperature.

A relative humidity chart is supplied with each instrument and is used in the following manner. Differences in reading between the dry and the wet thermometers

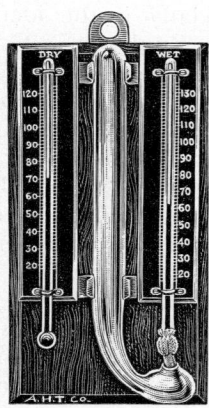

FIG. 41. Wet and dry bulb psychrometer.

are shown along the horizontal axis and air-temperature readings on the vertical axis. Relative humidity is indicated by a number at the intersection of the respective co-ordinates. For example, if the dry-bulb temperature is 100° and the wet-bulb temperature is 90°, the difference is 10°. This figure is located on the horizontal axis, and 100° is located on the vertical axis. By following the co-ordinates to their intersection, the number 68 is arrived at, which is the relative humidity.

The SLING PSYCHROMETER (Fig. 42) is a dry and wet bulb psychrometer which is whirled, thereby providing differences in the thermometer readings in a short time. The instrument is whirled until 2 successive readings correspond. The readings then are applied to the chart as described above.

The HAIR HYGROMETER is operated by means of a human hair, which expands and contracts with changes in humidity.

DISTILLATION

Distillation is the process of vaporization of a liquid accompanied by condensation. The fact that the vapors are condensed and the liquid is recovered differentiates distillation from evaporation. Condensation is the process of removing heat from a vapor in sufficient amount that a liquid or a solid is produced.

Distilling Apparatus. One of the oldest types of stills known is the alembic, in which the vapor is condensed in a chamber immediately above the liquid being heated. This type of still rarely is used at present, being replaced by the more efficient retort type in which condensation is produced in an instrument separated from the heating chamber.

Glass distilling apparatus is used almost exclusively in experimental laboratories. This provides a means of observing all changes produced in the process and eliminates the possibility of the contamination of products by contact with metallic equipment. All distillation units are composed of 3 chambers, each of which may be modified to meet the requirements of the quantity and the character of the material to be distilled and the space available for the unit. The 3 chambers are: (1) the vaporizing chamber, (2) the condensing chamber and (3) the receiver. A distillation assembly applicable for small-scale operations is illustrated in Figure 43.

As the liquid is vaporized, the hot vapors are forced into the condenser, where they are cooled and liquefied. As the hot vapor passes into the neck of the flask, it bathes

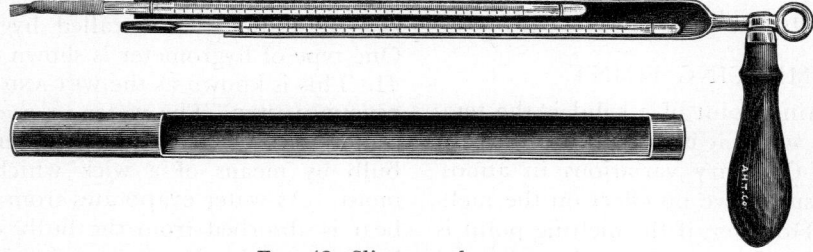

FIG. 42. Sling psychrometer.

the thermometer so that the temperature at which it leaves the flask can be observed. An adapter, which directs the flow of distillate into the receiver, may or may not be required, according to the type of receiver used. Adapters of various shapes can be purchased. However, very good ones can be made in the laboratory from broken inner tubes from condensers.

When an adapter is not used, the receiver must be placed in a position which permits the distillate to flow into it without undue exposure to air. Any flask or bottle placed so that the lower end of the condenser is well within the neck can serve as a receiver. Unless there is proper placement of the receiver, the distillate may become contaminated with dust and soluble gases or an appreciable amount may be lost by evaporation.

If the distillate is quite volatile, as in the case of ether, special measures must be taken to prevent loss by evaporation. The adapter tube should enter the flask through a 2-holed stopper, the second perforation being left open to permit air to escape from the receiver as the liquid enters. The receiver also should be placed in a cold mixture to reduce the vapor pressure of the distillate. Figure 44 shows a second distilling flask being used as a receiver to minimize evaporation and contamination of the distillate.

Condensers are manufactured in shapes and sizes which fulfill the requirements of the ordinary laboratory or a manufacturer of enormous quantities of distillates. The metal condenser shown in Figure 45 is a miniature example of condensers employed in large plants. Water enters the funnel-

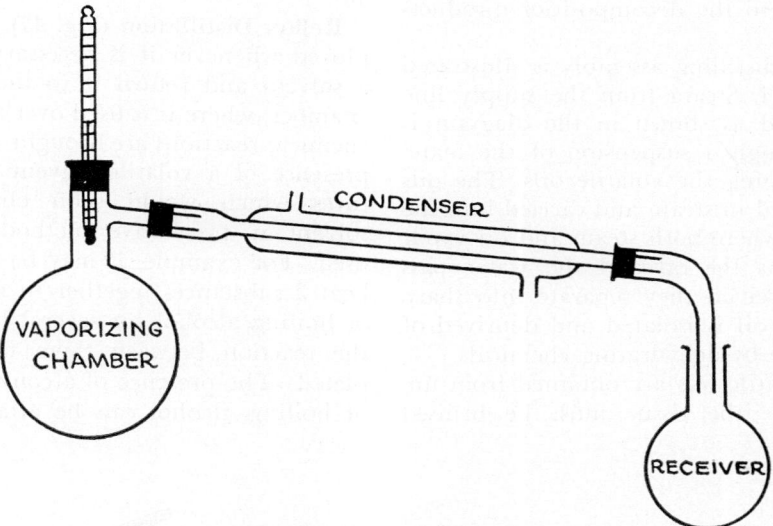

Fig. 43. Distilling assembly.

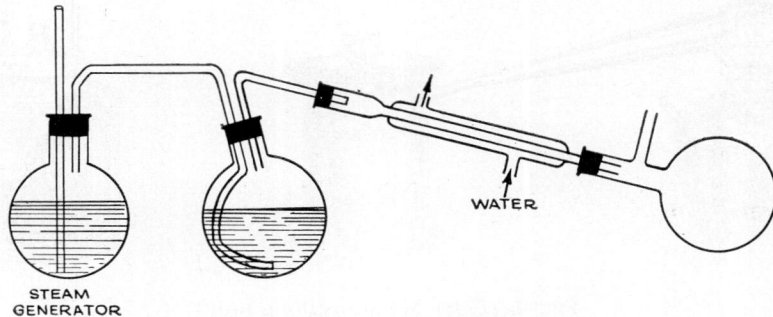

Fig. 44. Steam distillation assembly.

topped tube and is conveyed to the bottom of the vessel. A constant level of cooling liquid is maintained by an overflow pipe which is attached to the inside of the container and emerges at the bottom. The block-tin coil provides a long cooling surface so that no vapors escape condensation. If the distillate is extremely volatile, a mixture of ice, water and salt can be used in the jacket.

Steam Distillation. Of special interest to the pharmacist because it is used in obtaining volatile oils from cellular or resinous plant sources is steam distillation. The process also is used by chemists for separating certain products from reaction mixtures.

Steam distillation is essential in obtaining volatile oils since they contain constituents which are harmed at high temperatures and develop "empyreumatic or burnt odors" due to the decomposition products formed.

A steam distilling assembly is illustrated in Figure 44. Steam from the supply line or generated as shown in the diagram is passed through a suspension of the materials containing the volatile oils. The oils are vaporized in steam and carried into the condenser, where both steam and oil vapor condense. As the oil and the water pass into the receiver, they separate into sharp layers. The oil is isolated and deprived of all moisture by dehydrating chemicals.

Since volatile oils are obtained from undried tissue, the tissue must be bruised thoroughly before being subjected to steam distillation in order to break or weaken the cell walls to assist in rapid and thorough extraction of the oil.

When steam is to be generated in a vessel as shown, a safety tube should be extended to the bottom of the generator to prevent liquid being siphoned into the generator from the vaporizing chamber when the heat is removed and vapor pressure is decreased in the generator.

The aqueous mixture in the vaporizing chamber must be heated to the boiling point of water to prevent condensation of the steam as it passes through the material. By proper regulation of the heat, the liquid level in this chamber can be kept uniform even though steam is passed through it for several hours.

A small copper still used for distilling volatile oils with steam is shown in Figure 46.

Reflux Distillation (Fig. 47). This is employed whenever it is necessary to recover a solvent and return it to the vaporizing chamber, where it is used over again. Many chemical reactions are brought about in the presence of a volatile solvent at temperatures which would soon eliminate the solvent if preventive methods were not used. For example, it may be necessary to heat 2 substances together in the presence of boiling alcohol for several hours before the reaction between them will be completed. The presence of a constant volume of boiling alcohol can be attained by at-

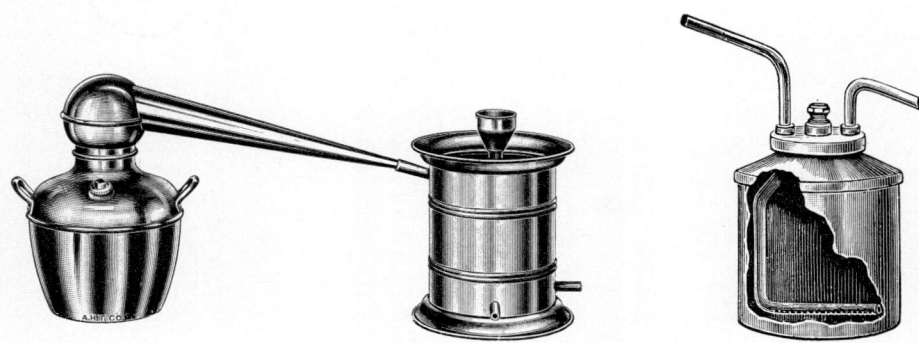

Fig. 45. *(Left)* Metal distilling unit.
Fig. 46. *(Right)* Copper still.

taching a condenser to the reaction flask at an angle which will return the condensed alcohol to the flask as shown.

Another application of reflux distillation is illustrated in the extraction of drugs by use of the Soxhlet apparatus (Fig. 48). This consists of a vaporizing chamber V, an extraction chamber E and a condenser C. The drug is placed in a porous extraction thimble which is inserted into the extraction chamber. The appropriate solvent is placed in flask V, after which the 3 chambers are assembled as shown in Figure 48. As the solvent is vaporized, it passes upward through the large outside tube on the extraction chamber and into the condenser, where it is liquefied and delivered to the surface of the drug in the thimble. As the level of the solvent rises in the extraction chamber, it also rises in the small outside tube until it overflows and runs into the vaporizing chamber, siphoning the solution from chamber E. This solution contains extractive principles from the drug which are retained in the lower flask, while the solvent is again vaporized and forced through another cycle.

This process is used in the analysis of vegetable drugs for alkaloidal content and is advantageous because only a small amount of solvent is required for completely extracting the drug sample.

Fractional Distillation. This is used to separate mixtures, the components of which have different boiling points. The process has many industrial applications. In the petroleum industry, crude oil is separated into groups of products which distil within specific temperature ranges. When coal tar is distilled fractionally, it is separated into light oils, middle or carbolic oils, heavy or creosote oils, anthracene oils and other oils, according to their distilling temperature. When a mixture of 2 or more volatile liquids is heated, both liquids will vaporize—not at the same rate, but at a rate corresponding to their boiling points. It can be stated roughly that when a mixture of 1 molecular weight each of ether, boiling point 35° C., and alcohol, boiling point 78° C., is heated to a certain distilling temperature, ether will vaporize twice as fast as the alcohol and the vapor over the liquid will contain 67 molecular or mole per cent of ether and 33 mole per cent of alcohol, whereas the original liquid contained 50 mole per cent of each. The above percentage conditions will prevail only momentarily

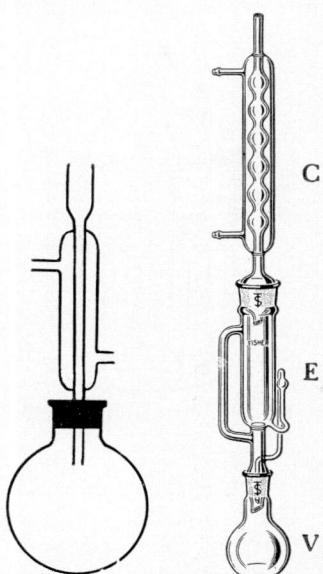

FIG. 47 *(Left)*. Reflux distillation assembly.

FIG. 48 *(Right)*. Soxhlet extraction apparatus.

due to constant changes in the ratio of ether and alcohol in the distilling flask, but they serve to illustrate the principle involved.

As the temperature of distillation of a mixture changes sharply, the receiver must be changed in order to obtain fractions of distillate containing an increasingly larger percentage of the least volatile substance. The first fraction is now distilled alone. It boils at a lower temperature than the original liquid because it has a higher percentage of low boiling component. When the temperature of boiling of fraction 1 has risen to the minimum boiling point of fraction 2, the latter is poured into the flask with the remainder of fraction 1 and distillation continued. This procedure is repeated until all the fractions from the original liquid mixture have been redistilled. The fractions of distillate obtained are subjected to a third redistillation whereby pure liquids ordinarily are obtained. Occasionally, a fourth distillation may be warranted.

When fractional and vacuum distillations are combined in one operation, as is often the case, a special receiver such as

when the pump is stopped. The vacuum must be released to prevent water being forced into the receiver from the pump by atmospheric pressure, unless the pump is equipped with a valve which prevents this back-flow.

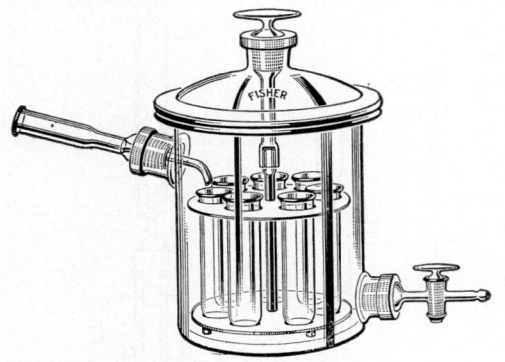

Fig. 49. Bruehl receiver.

that shown in Figure 49 has the advantage of permitting fractionation without interruption. The various fractions are collected in tubes that are mounted on a support which is rotated by means of the stopcock in the lid tubulature.

Vacuum Distillation. Some liquids cannot be boiled under ordinary atmospheric pressure since they decompose before a boiling temperature is reached. If the pressure above these liquids is decreased sufficiently, they can be made to boil and distil without decomposition. Figure 50 shows a laboratory set-up for vacuum distillation.

The tube extending into the distilling chamber provides for releasing the vacuum

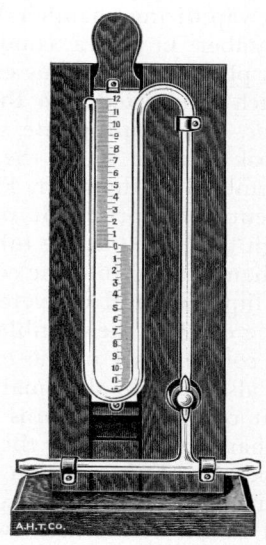

Fig. 51. Manometer.

For vacuum distillations, wherein a record of the exact pressure of boiling is required, a manometer (Fig. 51) is connected into the series between the receiver and the pump.

Destructive Distillation. As it is employed today, destructive distillation is synonymous with carbonization. It is the heating of dry organic substances, without access to air, to drive off the volatile con-

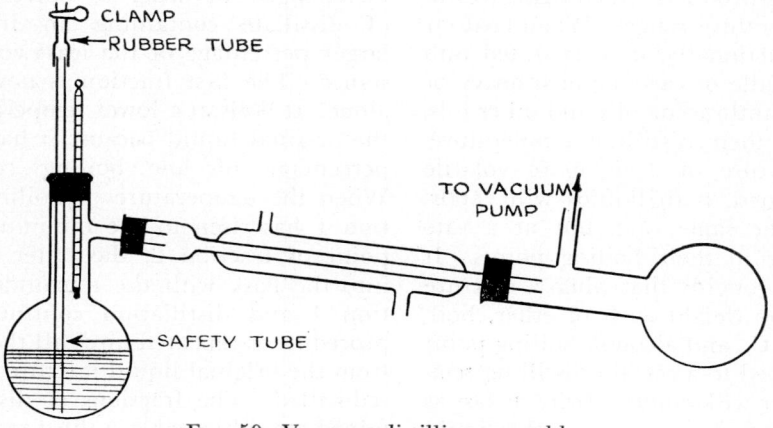

Fig. 50. Vacuum distilling assembly.

stituents. The object sought is primarily the volatile material, although the carbon remaining at the conclusion of the process often is utilized. At an earlier date, coal was distilled or carbonized destructively to obtain coke and the luminous gases which were evolved. The liquid obtained was useless and constituted a disposal problem as its highly important constituents had not been discovered. Today, the liquid is of primary concern as it is the parent substance for hundreds of pharmaceutical and other industrial products.

Pine wood is distilled destructively in order to obtain pine tar and wood charcoal, which have many practical uses.

Destructive distillation is always carried on in metallic instruments because of the high temperatures involved, which would fuse glass, and because of the difficulty in removing the residue after distillation, in which case glass retorts would be shattered.

Registration of Stills

Treasury Department regulations state that "any still, worm or condenser, of whatever size or capacity, with the exception of retorts for production of wood alcohol, and glass laboratory stills of trivial capacity" must be registered with the department. This regulation is effective irrespective of the repeal of the Eighteenth Amendment. Applications for the purchase of the above must be made to the Commissioner of Internal Revenue.

SUBLIMATION

When vaporization and condensation are applied to a volatile solid, the process is called sublimation. This process has one objective—the purification of volatile solids from less or nonvolatile solids. The solids may be natural mixtures or mixtures resulting from a chemical reaction.

Sulfur is forced from the interior of the earth by the use of superheated steam which melts the sulfur and carries it to the surface, where the hot mixture cools and separates as solid sulfur and water. The water escapes, leaving huge piles of impure sulfur, which must be sent to the refineries for purification. Here the crude sulfur is sublimed, leaving behind the impurities which are not volatile. Other materials which commonly are found in the drugstore and which are purified by sublimation are iodine, mercury bichloride, naphthalene (moth balls), ammonium chloride, camphor, etc. When the process is repeated several times, sublimates of a very high degree of purity are obtained. These contain from a negligible amount to no impurities and are referred to as "analytical" or "reagent" chemicals.

A common illustration of sublimation can be seen ordinarily in the menthol stock bottle, especially when it is nearly empty. Menthol is vaporized at room temperature and condenses on the sides of the container in beautiful long needles.

LYOPHILIZATION

Lyophilization, also known as "freeze-drying" or "drying by sublimation," is the removal of water from products while in the frozen state at extremely low pressures. The process is applied to products that are thermolabile or contain components that would be affected adversely if the usual heat-drying methods were applied. Widespread application of the process is seen in the drying of certain antibiotics such as penicillin, products containing thermolabile proteins, blood serum and plasma, certain biologicals, bacterial cultures and a growing list of other products. Lyophilization is advantageous in that, for a given product, certain of the following objectives can be attained:

1. The low temperature employed prevents chemical change in the thermolabile substances being dried. The product consequently retains its original chemical composition, therapeutic activity, odor, flavor or other inherent properties. When properly packaged and stored, many products that have been dried from the frozen state can be kept for long periods of time without deterioration.

2. A minimal loss of volatile constituents is attained. For example, when a fruit juice is lyophilized, so little of the volatile flavoring constituents is lost that the true odor and flavor are regenerated when the resultant powder is properly combined with water and aerated.

3. Blood plasma and other products which tend to foam when dried by the usual heat processes can be dried by lyophilization without encountering this difficulty.

4. The dried residue is spongy in structure, which contributes to the rapidity with which it can be dissolved in water. For example, ordinary gelatin is dissolved rather slowly even by boiling water, whereas spongy gelatin produced by freeze-drying is rapidly soluble in cold water.

5. The tendency to coagulate when certain products are concentrated by evaporation is greatly diminished.

6. The growth of micro-organisms and enzymatic changes are prevented by the application of freeze-drying. The dried product is also devoid of these processes since the moisture content is below the optimum required for their functioning.

7. The low temperatures required in lyophilization prevent oxidation of substances that are highly susceptible to being oxidized.

Except for modifications that are required in lyophilizing certain products, the process is carried out in the following manner. The liquid to be dried is placed in a chamber having a capacity much greater than that required for the liquid. The liquid is frozen quickly by placing the chamber in a bath in which temperatures as low as $-78°$ C. can be attained. During the freezing process, the chamber is rotated to produce a thin film of frozen material on the inner periphery. This reduces the depth of the frozen layer and subsequently reduces the time required to sublime the ice from the mixture. This chamber is then connected with a condenser of very large volume which, in turn, is connected to an exhaust pump capable of reducing the pressure to 0.01 to 0.05 mm. of mercury. The condensing chamber is immersed in a bath in which temperatures as low as $-78°$ C. are producible. During the initial drying process, the chamber containing the frozen mass may be surrounded by air or a low-temperature bath in accordance with the requirements of the product being dried. In no case should the temperature in this compartment be permitted to rise above $-5°$ C. Some products must be kept at temperatures much lower than $-5°$ C. to prevent changes in their thermolabile constituents. At the high vacuum required, ice is sublimed from the surface of the frozen mass and collected in the condensing chamber until the water content of the solids is reduced to 0.5 per cent or less.

In the secondary stage of drying, the solid is subjected to as high a temperature as permissible, further to reduce the moisture content as quickly as possible. The temperature at this point is contingent upon the stability of the solid and may range as high as 80° C.

Modifications of the above process include the Chryochem process, in which the water vapor is absorbed by strong dehydrating agents rather than being collected as an ice film on the inner periphery of the condenser. The Adtevac process utilizes a special vacuum pump in which the water vapor is entrapped in the oil of the pump and subsequently removed from the oil by a centrifuge which is a component part of the pump assembly.

DESICCATION

Desiccation is the process of removing water from substances at low or moderate temperatures.

Many substances contain moisture which is not a chemical part of their composition, but is held to or in the substance by mechanical means. All living tissue contains such moisture which is necessary to life in that it provides a means of transporting food and wastes within the plant or animal. It also provides elasticity to the tissues. This loosely held water is known as hygroscopic water and must not be confused with chemically held water, known as water of crystallization.

The process of desiccation has 3 purposes: preservation, reduction of bulk and weight and facilitation of comminution.

Preservation. Plant and animal tissue is subject to spoilage by the action of bacteria and molds which decompose the sugars, the fats and the other components of the tissues. However, these organisms cannot thrive except in the presence of an optimum amount of water. Therefore, vegetable and animal products will keep indefinitely if the moisture is reduced below the minimum required for the growth and the activity of micro-organisms. Vegetable drugs, including leaves, stems, barks and roots, and animal drugs, of which desiccated glands and stomach tissue are representatives, are thus preserved for long periods. In the field of foods, science is providing means for desiccating many products in such a manner that the fresh flavor is little impaired.

Reduction of Bulk and Weight. The reduction of bulk and weight has great economic importance. Hydrated products owe a great portion of both weight and bulk to water. Consequently, they require greater space for shipping and storing and the cost of transporting them is excessive. One example will illustrate the economic importance of drying materials for shipment. A case containing 36 dozen eggs requires 2.5 cu. ft. of space. When dried, the eggs require 0.38 cu. ft. of space and the weight of the powder is about one fiftieth of the weight of the fresh eggs.

Facilitation of Comminution. Tissues which are deprived of their moisture become brittle and are reduced easily to a fine state. The presence of water lends elasticity to the tissues, which then resist any crushing action, and they only become torn into coarse shreds or flattened.

Desiccation can be accomplished at room temperature by spreading the materials in a thin layer where air can circulate over and through them. Many materials will become dry or desiccated if exposed to air even at temperatures below zero. However, it is usually expedient to assist the natural processes of drying in order to conserve time and, in many instances, to prevent the spoilage which will occur during a slow drying process. Some common methods for hastening desiccation are elevating the temperature slightly, circulating warmed air through or around the materials, reducing the atmospheric pressure in the desiccating chamber, and centrifuging. Some operations utilize combinations of these methods to great advantage.

Large amounts of material can be desiccated by placing them in screen-bottomed trays in a large warmed room through which warmed air is circulated. This method is adaptable for desiccating crops of vegetable drugs such as leaves and barks of plants. For smaller quantities of materials such as are used in laboratory analyses and other experimental procedures, small drying closets are of practical value. The oven of an ordinary stove, used with the door open to permit circulation of air, is used commonly in drying many substances in the home. An excellent drying closet for rapidly drying small amounts of materials is shown in Figure 52. This consists of a drying chamber in which the materials to be dried are placed. The other compartment contains a fan and a heating coil. As air is drawn in, it is warmed and forced through the drying chamber. Since the temperature of drying can be controlled, no damage can result to the drug.

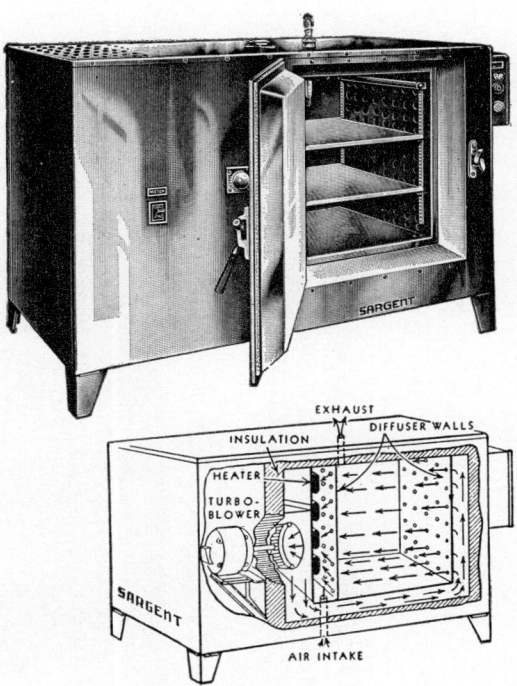

Fig. 52. Drying closet.

Figure 53 shows a commonly used laboratory oven which is controlled thermostatically. Circulation through the oven is by gravity and can be controlled by vents in the top. Once regulated, the oven will operate indefinitely without attention.

Occasionally, it is necessary to deprive a substance of traces of moisture which is difficult or impractical to remove by the foregoing processes. This can be done by use of

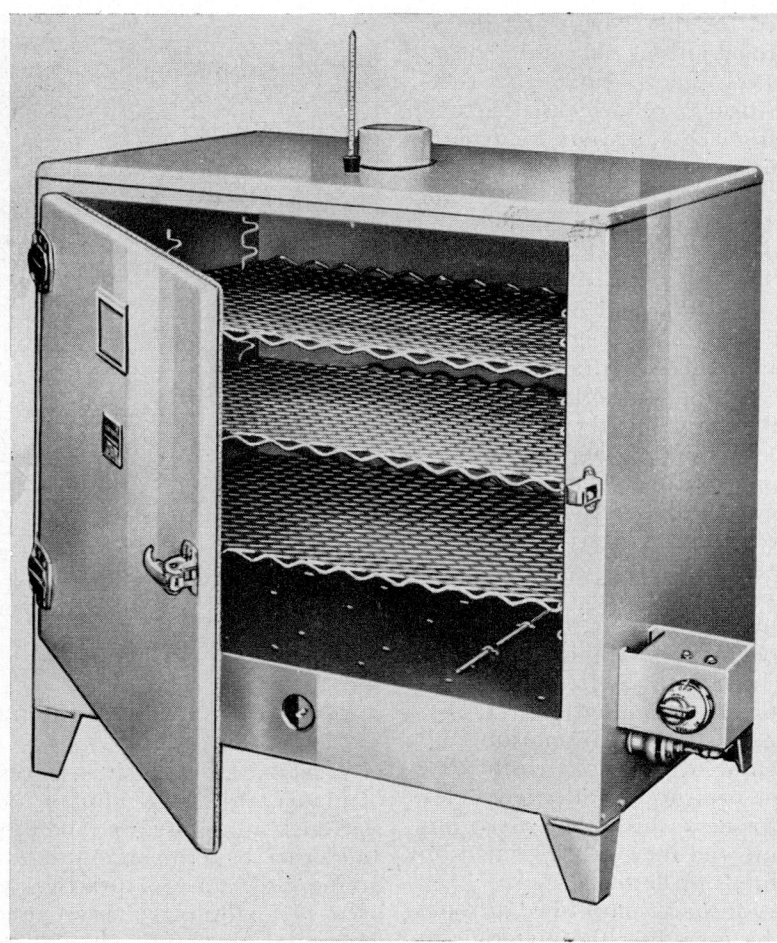

Fig. 53. Gas-heated hot-air sterilizer. Hot-air sterilizers are available in various sizes and may be electrically heated.

the desiccator. This vessel consists of 2 compartments, the lower for the drying agent and the upper for the substance to be dried. The 2 compartments are separated by a screen or a porcelain plate as shown (Fig. 54, *top*). The lid and the flange are ground to provide an air-tight seal. A substance having a great affinity for water is placed in the lower chamber. Chemicals commonly employed for this purpose are soda lime, sulfuric acid, phosphoric acid, phosphorus pentachloride, calcium chloride, etc. When the material to be dried is placed in the upper chamber, moisture slowly leaves it and is absorbed by the drying agent. After standing for several hours, all the moisture will have become absorbed by the drying agent.

Figure 54, *bottom*, shows a desiccator with a tube through which air can be pumped from the desiccator, thus accelerating the rate of drying.

Centrifuges. The basket centrifuge (Fig. 55) can be used not only in the laboratory to separate solids from adhering liquids but also on a larger scale to dehydrate many articles of commerce. The inner basket containing the materials to be desiccated is revolved at a great speed, which forces the liquid portion through the pores of the basket into the outer chamber, from which it drains through the side spout.

EXSICCATION

Exsiccation is the process of removing all water from certain chemicals; this process

Exsiccation 51

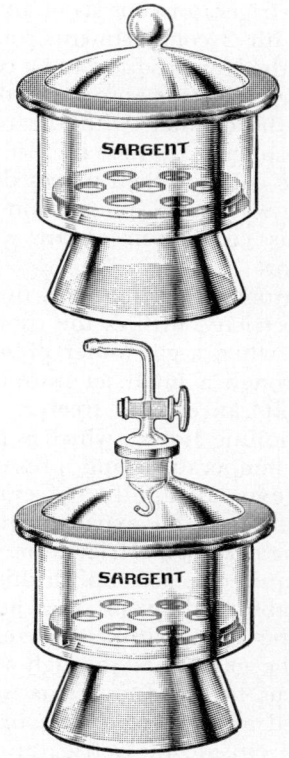

Fig. 54. (*Top*) Desiccator.
(*Bottom*) Tubulated desiccator.

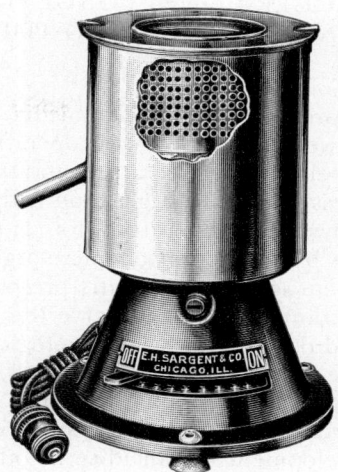

Fig. 55. Basket centrifuge.

is accomplished by the use of strong heat.

The objects of the process are twofold: (1) to reduce bulk and (2) to obtain a definite composition.

In the process of desiccation, the principal object is to remove hygroscopic water. For many substances, only hygroscopic water is present and the resulting desiccated product is entirely free of water. However, many substances possess an additional quantity of water which is a part of their crystalline structure and is held chemically. This is known as water of crystallization. For example, sodium sulfate appears as large, colorless, transparent crystals or granules having the composition $Na_2SO_4 \cdot 10H_2O$. The water is necessary for the formation of characteristic crystals or granules of sodium sulfate and, when this water is lost, only a white powder remains.

Another example will differentiate more clearly between hygroscopic water and water of crystallization. An alum has the empirical formula $M.M'(SO_4)_2 \cdot 12H_2O$, where M is a univalent metallic ion and M' a trivalent metallic ion. When an alum is crystallized, the crystals are moist from adhering water, which can be removed by desiccation. However, the 12 molecules of water held chemically within the crystal cannot be removed except by the application of strong heat.

Efflorescence. A few chemicals contain water of crystallization which is held much less firmly than the water in an alum. These gradually give up their water to the air, causing the crystal structure to be destroyed. This process is known as efflorescence. Sodium sulfate $Na_2SO_4 \cdot 10H_2O$, ferrous sulfate $FeSO_4 \cdot 7H_2O$ and magnesium sulfate $MgSO_4 \cdot 7H_2O$ all effloresce when exposed to air. Once efflorescence has begun, the composition of the remaining salt remains uncertain until the salt becomes anhydrous. Therefore, for many salts which effloresce readily, only the anhydrous form offers a definite percentage composition.

Deliquescence. In contrast with efflorescence, some compounds absorb moisture from the air even to the extent of becoming liquefied. These compounds are said to be deliquescent. Sodium hydroxide, potassium hydroxide, phenol, ephedrine and calcium chloride are among the many that possess this property.

REFRIGERATION, CONGEALING POINT AND FREEZING POINT

REFRIGERATION

The processes discussed immediately preceding were concerned with operations requiring elevated temperatures to attain the objectives sought. Refrigeration is the process of lowering temperatures to: (1) prevent spoilage by the action of micro-organisms; (2) prevent separation of fatty preparations, such as ointments; (3) preserve the activity of glandular products and biologicals; (4) promote the formation of crystals, which may not form at room temperature; (5) control certain chemical reactions; (6) defer the development of rancidity in oils, especially those which are to be administered internally, and for other purposes.

The prevention of spoilage by the action of micro-organisms is a universal economic and sanitary problem. Many animal and vegetable products are attacked readily by these organisms, which render the products unfit for their intended purposes.

The souring of milk products, fermentations in fruit, vegetable and syrupy products, the putrefying of meats and many other spoilages are familiar and commonplace. Besides these, the pharmacist must guard against spoilage in items commonly stocked for use in the prevention and the cure of diseases. Ointments improperly refrigerated may soften or liquefy to the extent that the active substances will separate, leaving part of the ointment depleted of activity while other parts become overactive. Ointments containing volatile constituents may lose them by evaporation if not properly stored. Many biologic products are dependable for administration for their dated period, if kept properly refrigerated, but, if stored at room temperature, they lose their dependability long before the expiration date.

Cod-liver oil and other vitamin-containing products remain palatable and therapeutically active much longer if stored in a cool place.

Many more examples of loss of activity, dependability and identity due to lack of proper storage can be cited almost at random.

Refrigerators can be divided into 2 types. The ice refrigerator consists of an insulated cabinet with 2 compartments, one for ice and the other for products to be cooled. As the ice melts, heat is absorbed from the interior of the cabinet, with the result that the atmosphere around the ice becomes cold. The cold air then moves downward, displacing warm air. This action results in continuous circulation of air within the refrigerator.

The automatic refrigerator, operated by gas or electricity, utilizes the cooling effect produced when a gas under pressure is released through a small jet into a chamber in which it can expand freely.

A low-boiling liquid, which is gaseous at ordinary temperature and pressure, is allowed to expand rapidly and evaporate as it passes through an expansion valve into the cooling coils of a refrigerator. The heat energy required to accomplish this evaporation is absorbed from the atmosphere around the coils within the refrigerated space. The gas passes through these coils and returns to the compressor where it is compressed and gives off heat in the coils which are outside the refrigerator. Under pressure and with cooling, the gas becomes liquefied and is ready to pass through the expansion valve and begin another cycle. The circulation of the refrigerant by the compressor is under the control of a thermostat so that the temperature within the refrigerator can be maintained within very narrow limits.

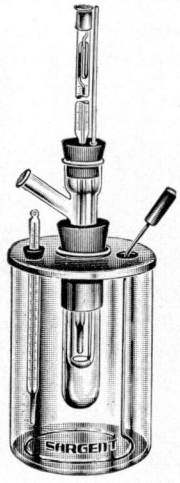

FIG. 56. Freezing-point apparatus.

Congealing Point

The congealing point or range is the temperature or range of temperatures at which a liquid or a melted solid becomes a solid. This property is used to determine the desired consistency of bases for ointments and similar products; also to determine the purity of some volatile oils which contain substances that separate when the temperature is reduced. The official method for determining congealing range or temperature is described in the *U.S.P.*

Freezing Point

The freezing point of a liquid is the temperature at which the liquid exists in equilibrium with its solid. It is analogous with the melting point of a solid. If the temperature is lowered below the freezing point, particles of solid will separate.

The freezing point of a pure liquid is valuable for determining its purity since any soluble adulterant will lower its freezing point. Use is made of the latter fact in determining the molecular weight of certain substances.

Method of Determining Freezing Points. The apparatus shown in Figure 56 is used for determining the freezing points of pure liquids, solutions and liquid mixtures. The cooling jar consists of a glass vessel with a metal clamp-down lid. An air-jacket tube passes through an opening in the lid and is held in place by a stopper. The freezing-point tube, furnished with a side tube for the introduction of solid pellets, is supported at the top of the air jacket by a second stopper. A metal stirrer provides for a uniform temperature in the cooling bath. The freezing tube also is provided with a stirrer to maintain a uniform temperature in the liquid to be frozen. The air space between the 2 tubes ensures a slow and uniform cooling of the freezing tube.

Many articles distributed by the pharmacist may be rendered unfit for sale if subjected to freezing temperatures. Typical of these products are the various liquid and solid emulsions containing a relatively large percentage of water. Freezing destroys the emulsion, causing the components to separate.

TABLE 3. FREEZING POINTS OF ETHYLENE GLYCOL-WATER MIXTURES

Per Cent Ethylene Glycol		Freezing Point	
By Weight	By Volume	0° C.	0° F.
10	9.2	— 3.6	25.6
20	18.3	— 7.9	17.8
30	28.0	—14.0	6.8
40	37.8	—22.3	— 8.2
50	47.8	—33.8	—28.8
60	58.1	—49.3	—56.7

* Lange's Handbook of Chemistry.

The freezing point of a liquid mixture is of practical significance in many respects. An almost universal example of this is found in mixtures used in the cooling systems of combustion engines which are operated under subzero conditions. Table 3 gives the freezing points of various mixtures of water and ethylene glycol, a permanent antifreeze now used in enormous quantities.

BIBLIOGRAPHY

Cook, E. F., and Martin, E. W.: Remington's Practice of Pharmacy, ed. 11, pp. 92–126, Easton, Pa., Mack, 1956.

Findlay, A.: Practical Physical Chemistry, ed. 7, pp. 119–120, 130–133, New York, Longmans, 1941.

Flosdorf, E. W.: Freeze Drying, New York, Reinhold, 1949.

Hickman, K. C. D.: High vacuum distillation, Ind. Eng. Chem. **40:**16–17, 1948.

Kremers, E., and Urdang, G.: History of Pharmacy, ed. 2, Philadelphia, Lippincott, 1951.

Mellor, J. W.: Modern Inorganic Chemistry, pp. 12–43, 381–391, New York, Longmans, 1951.

Millard, E. B.: Physical Chemistry for Colleges, ed. 7, pp. 126–136, 225–231, New York, McGraw-Hill, 1953.

Stewart, O. M., and Gingrich, N. S.: Physics, pp. 235–244, New York, Ginn, 1950.

Taylor, H. S., and Taylor, H. A.: Elementary Physical Chemistry, ed. 3, pp. 1–11, 73–78, 216–218, New York, Van Nostrand, 1942.

United States Pharmacopeia, Sixteenth Revision, Easton, Pa., Mack, 1960.

WILLIAM REESE LLOYD, Ph.D.

Director of Product Development, Texas Pharmacal Company
Formerly Professor of Pharmacy, College of Pharmacy,
University of Texas

4

Purification and Clarification

PRELIMINARY SURVEY
STANDARDS AND TESTS
STATES OF MATTER
SEPARATION OF GASES
SEPARATION OF A GAS FROM A LIQUID

SEPARATION OF LIQUIDS
SEPARATION OF A LIQUID AND A SOLID
SEPARATION OF SOLIDS
CLARIFICATION

PRELIMINARY SURVEY

Pharmaceutical preparations and the medicinal substances used in the compounding of prescriptions invariably contain some impurities. These may be due to the presence of impurities in the starting materials or to by-products of the chemical reactions involved in their preparation.

Purification is the process of removing foreign material from a substance, either from a single chemical compound or from a mixture. The necessity for purification is dependent on the possible pharmacologic action of the impurities and the difficulty of removing them. An impurity which is difficult to remove, but which has no deleterious effect on the efficacy or the palatability of the preparation, would not necessarily be removed. However, great pains would be exerted to remove an impurity which was toxic or which decreased the stability or the palatability of the preparation. Salt naturally contains magnesium chloride, which is not removed. However, the removal of arsenic is very necessary.

In modern pharmacy, purification is carried out almost entirely by the manufacturing pharmacist. However, a clear understanding of the technics involved is an important part of the scientific training of the professional pharmacist. It is also necessary that he be able to carry out these processes when the usual channels of supply temporarily become disrupted.

In the early days of pharmacy, the purification processes occupied a major part of the apothecary's time. Chemical science owes much of its present-day knowledge to discoveries made by the apothecary in his attempts to purify his products. Such valuable tools as fractional and steam distillation had their beginnings and much of their development in the isolation and the purification of volatile oils by the apothecary.

STANDARDS AND TESTS

GENERAL

Standards of purity for official medicinal substances and for substances used in the preparation and the testing of official preparations are prescribed in the *U.S.P.* and the *N.F.* For many unofficial drugs, the *N.N.D.* of the American Medical Association sets the standards. These requirements are the most important for the pharmacist. However, other standards are set for chemical substances used for various industrial and scientific purposes. The American Chemical Society, the Association of Official Agricultural Chemists and many other scientific and industrial organizations set specifications for various chemicals used in their work.

Various grades of chemicals are available for different purposes. Each manufacturer produces chemicals in several grades to meet various specifications. The usual grades, in addition to the medicinal, are:

crude, an unrefined grade suitable for some industrial purposes;
technical, an unrefined grade similar to the crude for use in technical processes where a high degree of purity is unnecessary;
purified, a grade which has been refined and for which no specifications have been set;
reagent, a highly purified grade suitable for most laboratory purposes;
analytical reagent, a highly purified grade suitable for use in analysis;
A.C.S. (American Chemical Society), a grade which meets the specifications set by the Committee on Analytical Reagents of the American Chemical Society;
C.P. (Chemically Pure), a grade containing a limited amount of impurities which may vary for different manufacturers.

Tests used for proof of purity depend on the character of the substance. Physical constants such as melting point, boiling point, specific gravity and refractive index are affected by the presence of slight amounts of impurities. The conformity of these constants to the established value for the pure substance, where applicable, is used as one criterion of purity in the official monographs.

Specific

Specific tests for impurities which may be present are included in the monographs for many official substances and preparations. In addition, the official assays specify methods for the quantitative determination of the active ingredients where such a procedure is available. For some products, biologic methods are used for the determination of the amount of active ingredients. The limits of amounts of the active ingredients for various preparations are specified in the monographs.

It should be remembered that no single test is a valid criterion for the purity of a substance, and each substance should conform to all tests and specifications in the official monograph.

The method of purification selected varies, depending on the amount of substance to be purified. Methods applicable to small-scale laboratory quantities may not be efficient or economical for the purification of large quantities on an industrial scale. Methods of both types are included here in the discussion of purification technics.

In its simplest form, purification consists of separating the components of a mixture. When 2 or more components of a mixture exist in different states, purification is a relatively simple process—e.g., the separation of a solid from a liquid by filtration. When the components of a mixture exist in the same state, purification consists of the change of one or the other of the substances into a different state in order to effect a separation—e.g., the separation of albumin from aqueous solution by converting the albumin into an insoluble form by heating. Methods of purification involve 2 steps: the conversion of the components of the mixture into different, distinct states, and the separation of these states. The first step is unnecessary when the impurities are already in a different state from the substance desired. Sometimes these 2 steps are separate and distinct, as in the conversion of albumin to the solid state by the application of heat, followed by the separation of these states by filtration. Often, the 2 steps merge into a single operation, as in the separation of a mixture of alcohol and water by distilling the alcohol from the water.

STATES OF MATTER

Matter exists in 3 states: the gaseous, the liquid and the solid. Theoretically, under the proper conditions, all substances are capable of existing in all 3 states.

The term *phase* refers to the physical state of the substance and to its identity. A system consisting of a single chemical substance in 2 different states is a 2-phase system—e.g., a mixture of water and ice. A system consisting of 2 different chemical entities in the same physical, homogeneous state is a 1-phase system—e.g., a solution of sodium chloride and water. A system consisting of 2 chemical entities (such as salt and water) is a *binary* system; and one of 3 chemical entities (such as a solution of salt, sugar and water) is a *ternary* system.

The *kinetic-molecular theory* postulates that all matter is composed of small particles, *molecules,* which are constantly in motion. These molecules are perfectly elastic, and exert a definite attractive force on each other. Each molecule has a definite mass, and the kinetic energy of the molecule is a function of the product of the mass of the molecule and its speed. When heat is absorbed, the kinetic energy of the molecule increases, and, since the mass is fixed, the speed of the molecule is increased.

The Gaseous State

In the gaseous state, the kinetic energy of the molecules is sufficient to overcome the attractive forces between the molecules. Each molecule is independent of the other molecules present except for changes in direction due to collisions between molecules. Since the molecules are perfectly elastic, no loss in energy results from these collisions. The distance between the molecules in the gaseous state is relatively large, making it possible to compress the gas into a smaller space. Since the molecules constantly are moving at a rapid rate, and since there are large spaces between the molecules, gases diffuse into each other and out of the container if an opening is provided. The speed of diffusion is inversely proportional to the square root of the mass or density of the gas.

The pressure exerted by a gas on the sides of the container is due to the impact of the rapidly moving molecules, and is a function of the mass and the speed of the molecules, since the force is equal to the product of the mass and the speed and to the frequency with which the impacts occur. If the kinetic energy is increased by the absorption of heat, the pressure must increase if the volume is kept constant, since both the force and the frequency of the impacts are increased. If the volume is increased sufficiently to lower the frequency of impacts to compensate for their increased force, the pressure remains a constant. Lowering the kinetic energy by lowering the temperature produces opposite effects. These relationships can be expressed mathematically by the combined laws of Boyle and Charles in the following form:

$$\frac{p_1 v_1}{T_1} = \frac{p_2 v_2}{T_2}$$

where p_1 and p_2 are the pressures of the gas, v_1 and v_2 are the volumes and T_1 and T_2 the absolute temperatures.

At the transition point between a gas and a liquid, the kinetic energy of the molecules of the gas is lowered, and heat is given off. The heat absorbed by 1 Gm. of a liquid changing to 1 Gm. of a gas at the same temperature is the *latent heat of vaporization,* and is equal to the heat lost by 1 Gm. of a gas changing to 1 Gm. of the liquid. This phenomenon accounts for the cooling effect of low-boiling-point liquids (such as ether) when placed on the skin. The liquid vaporizes at body temperature, absorbing heat from the skin and lowering the temperature.

The Liquid State

In the liquid state, the kinetic energy of the molecules is not sufficient to overcome the attractive forces between the molecules. The molecules are constantly in motion at a speed lower than in the gaseous state. Liquids flow and take on the shape of the container as does a gas, but do not expand to fill a container if the volume of the container is larger than that of the liquid. Liquids present a definite interface with gases and other liquids in which they are not soluble. In liquids, the space between the molecules is much less than in gases, so that liquids are compressible to only a slight degree.

Since the molecules of a liquid are constantly in motion, they leave the surface of the liquid at the interface between liquid and gas. This force is the *vapor tension* of the liquid, and is opposed by the downward pressure of the gas forcing the molecules back into the liquid. When the vapor tension is sufficient to overcome the pressure of the atmosphere above the liquid, the molecules of the liquid pass into the gaseous state with great rapidity, and the liquid is said to be boiling. The temperature at which this takes place is the *boiling point* of the liquid. The pressure exerted by the vapor above the liquid is the *vapor pressure*. If a liquid is placed in a closed vessel with a space above the liquid, molecules of the liquid leave the surface due to the vapor tension. As these molecules pass into the vapor phase, the vapor pressure above the liquid increases. This pressure opposes the vapor tension in the same way as does the pressure of the atmosphere. At the beginning, the vapor tension is greater than the vapor pressure, and more molecules leave the surface than return to it. The vapor above the liquid becomes richer in the molecules of the substance, and the rate of return to the surface increases. If these actions are allowed to go on long enough, the rate of return becomes as great as the rate of vaporization, and no further change in the concentration of the vapor occurs. When this situation has been achieved, the liquid is said to be at *equilibrium* with its vapor. It is to be remembered that this state is dynamic, and that as many molecules of gas return to the surface as molecules of liquid leave.

The Solid State

In the solid state, the molecules are moving at a comparatively slow speed, and are packed closely together, although there are definite spaces between the molecules. Solids are only slightly compressible. When a liquid changes to a solid, the kinetic energy decreases. The loss of heat when 1 Gm. of a liquid changes to 1 Gm. of a solid at the same temperature is the *latent heat of fusion*.

Although the kinetic-energy level of solids is low, every solid is thought to have a definite vapor tension, but frequently the value is so low that it cannot be measured with instruments now available. For certain substances, however, the vapor tension is appreciable, as with camphor.

A study of these facts shows that changes in state are a function of the kinetic energy of the substance. The kinetic-energy level of a substance can be altered by raising or lowering the temperature. Changes in state can be used effectively in the purification of substances used in pharmacy and in medicine. However, it is also necessary to take into consideration the chemical properties of the substances involved and the stability of the substance toward heat.

SEPARATION OF GASES

The removal of gaseous impurities from a gas is usually a simple process. The purification of gases containing gaseous impurities may be effected by conversion of either ingredient into the liquid or the solid phase. The usual methods are: condensation, solution, absorption by a liquid or a solid and adsorption by a solid.

Condensation. Gases can be converted into the liquid state by lowering the temperature, by increasing the pressure, or, as is common in actual practice, by combining the 2 methods. When the boiling points of 2 gases differ sufficiently, then separation in this way provides a simple and inexpensive method of purification. The liquefied substance is drawn off and separation thus is effected.

A modification of this method is used to obtain oxygen and nitrogen from air. The mixture of gases is first liquefied and the temperature allowed to rise slowly. The nitrogen, having the lower boiling point, evaporates first. When the residual liquid is almost pure oxygen, the gas coming off is condensed and pumped into cylinders. This process is essentially fractional distillation, and is applicable for mixtures of easily liquefied gases where a sufficient differential exists in the boiling points of the gases.

Solution. Gases may be separated by passing the mixed gases through a liquid in which the impurities are soluble, but in which the gas desired is insoluble. Water, dilute acids and dilute alkalis can be used alone or in combination to remove impurities from gases insoluble in water. Impurities which are soluble in water will dissolve, and acidic impurities will often form soluble reaction products in dilute alkali. Basic impurities may form soluble substances in dilute acids. An example of this method is the removal of water vapor by passing the gas through concentrated sulfuric acid.

Absorption by a Solid. Another method of separating gases is the conversion of a gaseous impurity into the solid phase by passing the mixture over a coarsely ground solid with which the impurity reacts to form a solid. Examples of this type of separation are the removal of carbon dioxide from a gas by soda lime or by Ascarite, a patented mixture of asbestos and sodium hydroxide, and the removal of water vapor by passing the gas over calcium chloride or over Dehydrite, a patented preparation of magnesium perchlorate trihydrate.

Adsorption by a Solid. Substances such as charcoal or silica gel which present enormous surface area because of large numbers of crevasses indenting the surface, exhibit a phenomenon known as adsorption. Molecules of gas are trapped in the crevasses and are held by forces which are not well understood. Various adsorbents exhibit different adsorptive powers for different gases, and purification may be obtained by the proper selection of adsorbent. Charcoal in its various forms, especially when it is treated chemically and physically to obtain high adsorptive qualities (activated charcoal, Norite, Nuchar) and silica gel are the most frequently used adsorbents. This method of separation can be used to obtain valuable by-products from waste gases, in water purification and in gas masks to remove poisonous gases.

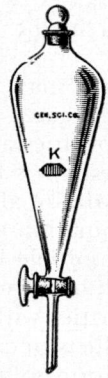

Fig. 57. Separatory funnel.

SEPARATION OF A GAS FROM A LIQUID

Gaseous impurities can be separated from liquids by reducing the solubility of the gas in the liquid by heat or aeration, or by adsorption.

Evaporation. The solubility of a gas in a liquid can be decreased by raising the temperature of the solution if its boiling point is sufficiently high, since the solubility of a gas decreases with an increase in temperature. This method is not applicable to liquids with low boiling points or to liquids which are decomposed by heat. Air can be expelled from water by boiling for a short time.

Aeration. A second method of separating a gas from a liquid is by aeration. If an insoluble gas is bubbled through the liquid, the gaseous impurities become entrapped in the bubbles of the insoluble gas and are thus removed. The purification of water by aeration is an example of this method.

Adsorption. Gaseous impurities may be adsorbed on the surface of adsorbents when the liquid is agitated with the adsorbent. This is one of the best and most frequently used methods of removing gaseous impurities.

SEPARATION OF LIQUIDS

IMMISCIBLE MIXTURES

Mutually insoluble (immiscible) liquids may be separated by allowing the mixture to stand until 2 distinct layers are formed. The lower layer is drawn off through an aperture near the bottom of the container, or the upper layer may be siphoned off or decanted. Complete separation is difficult to obtain by this method, as 2 completely insoluble liquids seldom are encountered. Most liquids dissolve in each other to some extent, so that further purification is usually necessary.

In the laboratory, the separatory funnel (Fig. 57) is generally used. The ground-glass stopcock at the bottom permits the removal of the lower layer. Care must be exercised to separate the 2 layers sharply.

One of the problems encountered in this type of separation is the formation of emulsions. Emulsions may be destroyed by the addition of electrolytes or alcohol.

SOLUBLE MIXTURES

Mixtures of soluble liquids can be separated by conversion of one liquid into the gaseous phase, by conversion of one liquid into the solid phase or by conversion of one liquid into an immiscible liquid phase. The first type of separation is the most valuable.

Conversion to a Gaseous Phase: EVAPORATION. When the vapor tension of a liquid impurity is considerably higher than the vapor tension of the desired liquid, purification can be effected by simple evaporation. This is accomplished by presenting as large a liquid surface as possible, since evaporation takes place only at the interface of the liquid with the atmosphere. The rate of evaporation can be increased by blowing a current of warm, dry air over the surface. Evaporation may be speeded by raising the temperature of the system if the desired liquid is stable toward heat. The liquid should be stirred to hasten the evaporation and to prevent scorching. The shallow porcelain evaporating dish of suitable volume is the preferred apparatus for small-scale evaporation (Fig. 58).

Evaporation Under Reduced Pressure. Substances which are labile toward heat can be evaporated rapidly at low temperatures by decreasing the pressure above the liquid. This method is applicable if the desired substance has a low vapor tension and does not evaporate. Elevated temperatures below the temperature at which the desired liquid decomposes may be used in conjunction with reduced-pressure evaporation. In this process, the mixture is placed in a large round-bottom flask, and the system evacuated by an aspirator or a vacuum pump. In using an aspirator, the lowest pressure obtainable is the aqueous tension of water at the prevailing temperature. In evaporating substances which might affect the mechanism of the vacuum pump, a trap to remove the offending vapors should be placed between the pump and the flask. This method is used to remove the excess of menstruum in concentrating fluidextracts which decompose at relatively low temperatures.

DISTILLATION. The process of vaporizing a liquid followed by condensation of the vapors obtained is distillation. Simple distillation is used to separate nonvolatile and volatile substances, especially the separation of such liquids. Actually, this means liquids whose vapor tensions are widely separated at the boiling point of the more volatile component. Since most liquids exert an appreciable vapor tension at ordinary temperatures, simple distillation does not always afford complete separation.

The process of distillation is carried out by placing the mixture in a distilling flask (Fig. 59) which is connected to a condenser which will liquefy the escaping vapors. The liquid is heated to the boiling point of the solution, and the vapors escaping into the condenser are converted into the liquid state and removed from the mixture.

Fractional Distillation. The process of separating the components of a mixture by distilling liquids at progressively increasing temperatures and collecting the distillate in

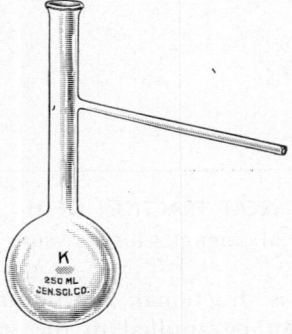

FIG. 59. Distilling flask.

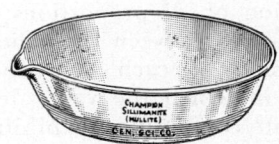

FIG. 58. Evaporating dish.

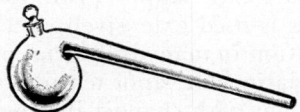

FIG. 60. Tubulated retort.

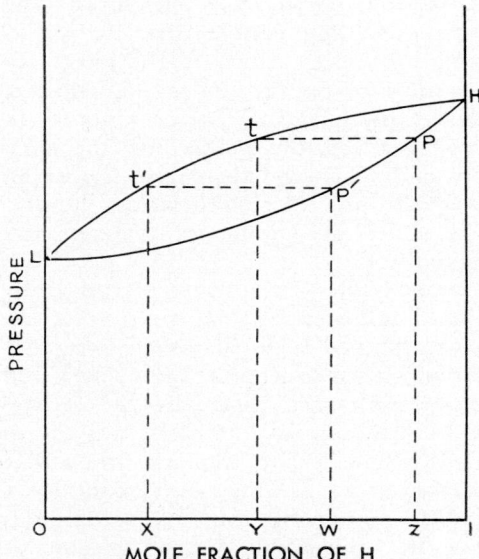

Fig. 61. Ideal vapor-pressure curve.

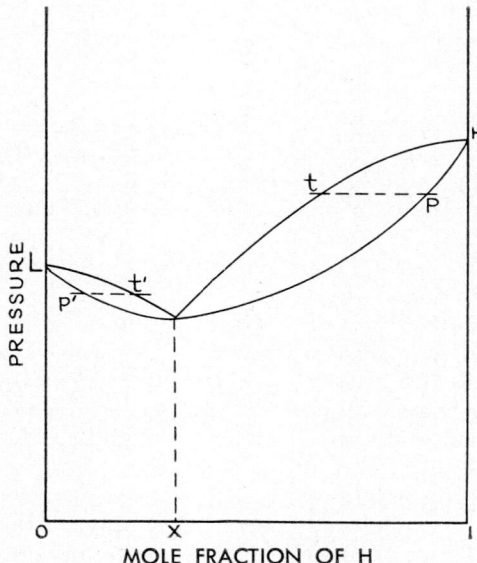

Fig. 63. Minimum vapor-pressure curve.

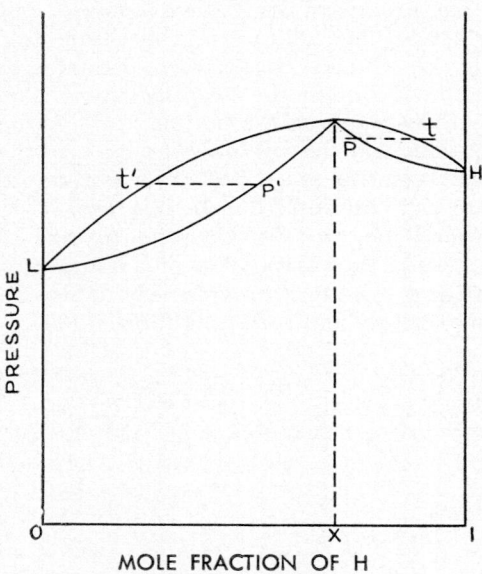

Fig. 62. Maximum vapor-pressure curve.

fractions is fractional distillation. This method can be applied to the separation of mixtures of volatile liquids more efficiently than can simple distillation, and the process is used extensively as a method of purification in many industrial processes.

The variations in vapor tension of binary liquid systems with changes in temperature differ according to the type of mixture formed. Binary liquid mixtures can be divided into 3 types: completely miscible, partially miscible and completely immiscible.

According to Henry's law, the vapor tension exerted by a volatile liquid in solution is proportional to its molecular concentration. It would be expected that the partial pressure of a volatile component of a liquid solution would be proportional to the mole fraction of the component present. However, it has been shown that this is true only when the components are similar in chemical structure—e.g., benzene and toluene. In most cases, considerable divergence from the value calculated from Henry's law is observed—e.g., methyl alcohol and benzene. It is thought that this divergence is due to the formation of molecular complexes.

The vapor tension of completely miscible systems at constant temperature exhibits 3 different types of behavior with changes in composition: *the ideal*, in which the vapor tension of all proportions of the 2 components lies between the values of the vapor tension of each component; *the minimum*, in which the vapor tension at some definite composition exhibits a minimum value below the vapor tension of either component; and *the maximum*, in which the vapor tension at some definite composition exhibits a maximum value above the vapor tension of either component.

It is possible to diagram the changes in vapor tension and vapor pressure with composition at constant temperature.

In Figure 61, the vapor tension and the vapor pressure of all possible mixtures of miscible liquids belonging to type I are shown. The line $Lt'tH$ indicates the composition of the liquid phase at changes in vapor tension from L to H, and the line $Lp'pH$ indicates the composition of the vapor phase in equilibrium with the liquid. Since the vapor above the liquid will contain more of the component having the higher vapor tension, the line $Lp'pH$ represents the vapor phase. In a mixture of the composition represented by Y, the vapor tension of the liquid will be t, and the composition of the vapor in equilibrium with the liquid will be the value represented by Z. If the mixture is allowed to evaporate at constant temperature, the liquid remaining becomes richer in L due to loss of the component having the higher vapor tension. When the vapor tension of the liquid reaches the value t', the liquid remaining will have the composition represented by X, and the vapor in equilibrium with it will have the composition W. Similar vapor-tension curves for maximum and minimum systems are shown in Figures 62 and 63.

The possibility of separating a binary system by distillation can be determined by an inspection of the boiling-point curve for the system. Such curves are shown in Figures 64, 65 and 66. These curves represent ideal, maximum and minimum boiling-point systems. In these curves, the boiling point of the mixture is plotted against the composition of the vapor and the liquid.

In Figure 64, L and H are the boiling points of 2 liquids; the line $Lt'tH$ indicates the composition of the liquid mixture boiling at temperatures between L and H, and the line $Lp'pH$ represents the composition of the vapor in equilibrium with the liquid at these temperatures. If a liquid of the composition represented by Y is distilled, it will boil at the temperature represented by t. The vapor will have the composition Z. If the distillation is carried out for some time, the liquid becomes poorer in the lower boiling component and the composition of the liquid will change between Y and O, while the boiling point of the liquid will increase along the line from t to L. If the distillation is carried out from t to t', the last part of the distillate will have the composition represented by X. The average composition of the fraction obtained by distilling between t and t' will be represented by U. If this portion is then subjected to redistillation, the first portion of the vapor will have the composition V. If this process is repeated several times, it can be seen that it will be possible to separate the mixture into pure L and H. This is the process of fractional distillation.

Figure 65 represents the boiling-point curve for binary systems having a maximum boiling point. The composition represented by X is the maximum boiling-point mixture where the compositions of the vapor and the liquid are the same and the mixture boils as if it were a single compound. If the mixture which boils at t is distilled, the vapor contains proportionally less H than the liquid so that the liquid becomes richer in H and the boiling point changes along the line LtM. When the boiling point reaches the value M, no further change takes place in the liquid, as both the liquid and the vapor have the same composition. Such a mixture can be fractionated into pure L, and the constant boiling mixture M. If a liquid boiling at t' is distilled, the vapors are proportionally richer in H than the liquid, and the liquid becomes poorer in H, the boiling point changing along the line $Ht'M$. When the boiling point reaches M, no further changes occur. Such a mixture can be fractionated into pure H and the constant boiling mixture M. The composition obtained at the constant boiling point is definite if the pressure at which the distillation takes place is constant. Constant boiling mixtures can be used to prepare standard solutions.

Minimum boiling-point mixtures are illustrated by Figure 66. These mixtures can be separated as discussed under maximum boiling-point systems. Alcohol and water form a minimum constant boiling mixture at 78.13° C. when the pressure is 760 mm. This mixture consists of 95.57 per cent alcohol by weight. Thus 95 per cent alcohol can be obtained by fractional distillation, but higher proportions of alcohol can be obtained only by removing the remaining 5 per cent of water by some other method. Theoretically, it would be possible to fractionate mixtures containing more than 95 per cent alcohol into pure alcohol and the constant boiling mixture. However, the difference in boiling points between pure alcohol and the constant boiling mixture is

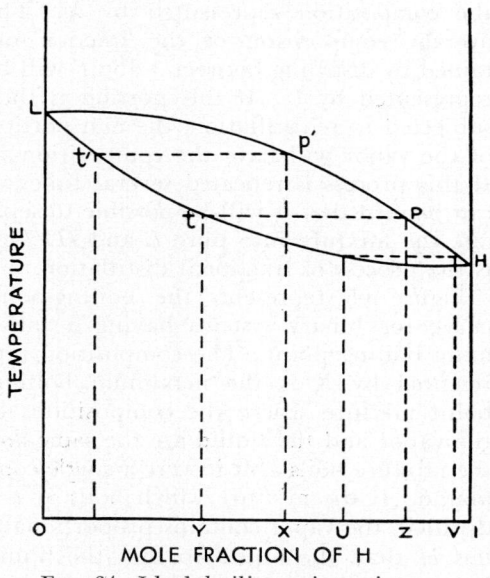

Fig. 64. Ideal boiling-point mixtures.

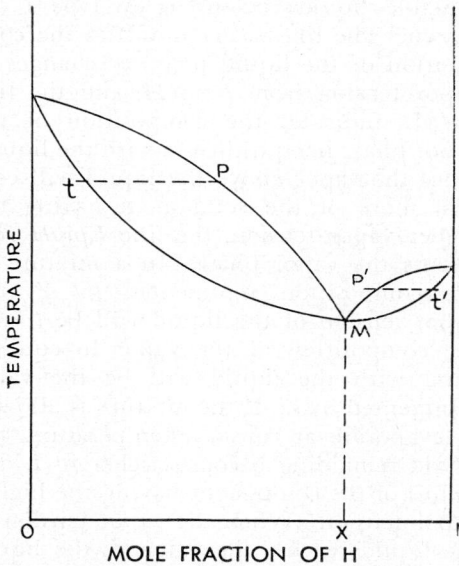

Fig. 66. Minimum boiling-point mixtures.

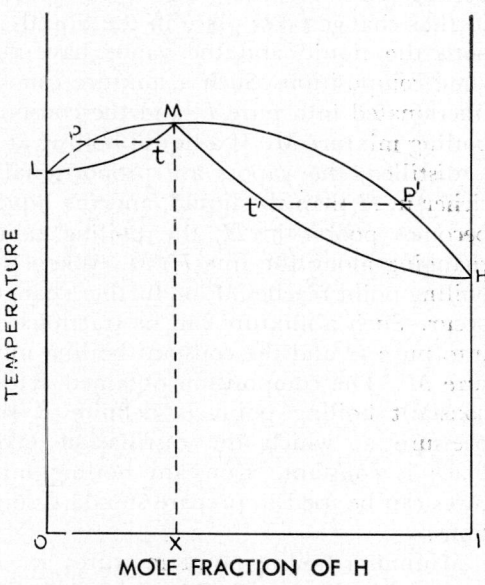

Fig. 65. Maximum boiling-point mixtures.

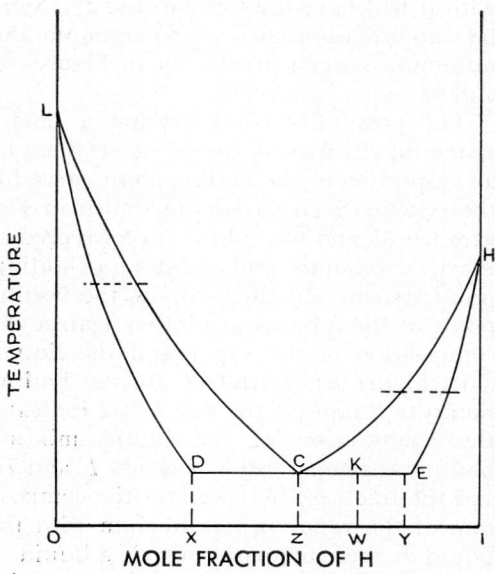

Fig. 67. Boiling-point curve for partially miscible systems.

so small that the separation is practically impossible.

The boiling-point curves for partially miscible systems are illustrated by Figure 67. In this type, 2 liquids form 2 layers consisting of a saturated solution of L in H and a saturated solution of H in L. In Figure 67, a mixture of the composition from O to X forms a single homogeneous phase, as will a mixture of the composition Y to 1. Mixtures of such composition can be fractionated into pure L and into pure H, as indicated by the curve. When 2 layers are formed, the 2 layers do not affect each other, their partial pressures being independent of the relative amounts of the 2 components present. If a mixture having the composition represented by W is distilled, the vapor will have the composition represented by Z. Since the distillate is richer in L than the liquid, the composition of the liquid will change along the line KEH. When the composition of the liquid reaches the value represented by Y, the mixture becomes homogeneous. Further distillation will result in the liquid becoming pure H. Distillation of a mixture of the composition between Z and X will result in the liquid's becoming richer in L and finally becoming pure L. An example of this type of mixture is water and butyl alcohol.

The boiling-point curves for immiscible systems will be discussed under "Steam Distillation," page 64.

This discussion of the behavior of binary systems illustrates the theory involved in fractional distillation. When the boiling-point curves for the systems are known, an inspection of the curve will be of value in predicting the efficiency of the separation by fractional distillation.

Fractional distillation can be applied in 2 ways: by successive fractionations of the distillate and by fractional condensation. The latter method consists of completely vaporizing the mixture and slowly condensing the vapor to obtain the component having the higher boiling point first. This method is not usually applied to the purification of liquid systems.

The practical application of fractional distillation is described in Chapter 3.

Fractionating Columns. The process of fractional distillation is long, difficult and expensive. To increase the efficiency of such separations, fractionating columns are used. A schematic representation of a fractionating column is shown in Figure 68.

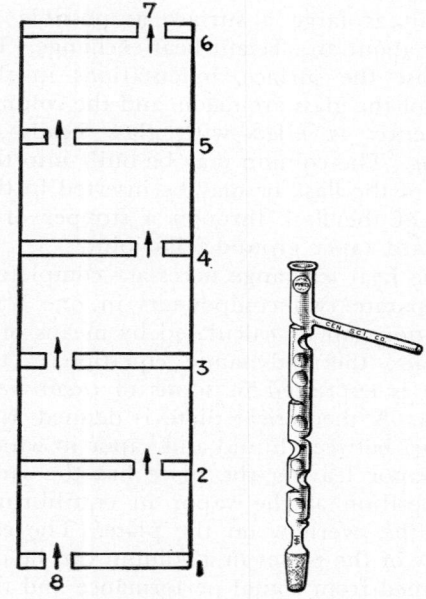

Fig. 68. Fractionating column.

The mixed vapors enter the column at *8*, and must follow the course indicated by the arrows. As the vapors ascend, the component having the higher boiling point condenses and accumulates on the surfaces of the plates *1, 2, 3,* etc. The vapor escaping from the last plate is almost completely free of the component having the higher boiling point. As fresh portions of vapor come in contact with the liquid on the plates, an exchange of heat takes place, the lower boiling component of the liquid being vaporized while the higher boiling component of the vapor is condensed. In this way, a more complete separation takes place during fractionation. This heat exchange in the column is an important factor of fractionation.

A similar method of obtaining a more complete separation is through the use of *scrubbers*. The scrubber is a liquid or a gas which selectively dissolves the higher boiling component and removes it from the vapor. The scrubbing liquid may be contained in a trap through which the vapor must pass, or it may be introduced at the top of the column and allowed to flow counter to the ascending vapors.

Fractionating columns for laboratory use take a variety of forms. Columns should present as large a surface as possible to bring about an efficient heat exchange. To increase the surface, indentations in the sides of the glass are made, and the column frequently is filled with glass beads or helices. The column may be built into the neck of the flask or may be inserted in the neck of the flask through a stopper or a standard taper ground-glass joint.

The heat exchange necessary completely to separate two components in one fractionation can be calculated by means of a complex thermodynamic equation. This value is expressed in terms of *theoretical plates*. A theoretical plate is defined as a contact between liquid and vapor in which the vapor leaving the plate has the same composition as the vapor in equilibrium with the overflow on the plate. The efficiency of the plates in a column can be determined from actual performance and the necessary length of column calculated. The performance of the column is dependent on its design and the character of the separation to be made. Data as to the performance of the column can be obtained from performance of similar designs for the same separation. From a consideration of the theoretical plates necessary and the column efficiency to be expected, the length of the column can be calculated with a fair degree of accuracy if the data used are dependable. Such calculations are of little importance in laboratory distillations but are of great importance in industrial purification.

The technic of fractional distillation using a fractionating column is essentially the same as that described for the separation of alcohol and water. However, the number of fractionations necessary is decreased due to the improved separation.

Steam Distillation. In a binary system of 2 immiscible liquids, the partial pressures of the components of the system are independent of their relative concentrations. The total vapor tension of such a system is the sum of the partial pressures of the components at the observed temperature. The boiling point of the system will be the temperature at which the sum of the partial pressures is equal to the prevailing pressure. The molar composition of the vapor will be proportional to the partial pressures of the components:

$$\frac{P_a}{P_b} = \frac{M_a}{M_b}$$

where P_a and P_b are the partial pressures of A and B at the boiling point of the system, and M_a and M_b are the moles of A and B in the vapor. A mixture of water and nitrobenzene boils at 99° C. The partial pressure of water at 99° C. is 733 mm. and that of nitrobenzene 27 mm. The ratio of moles of water to moles of nitrobenzene in the distillate will be:

$$\frac{733}{27} = \frac{M_w}{M_n} = \frac{27.15}{1}$$

This distillate will contain 27.15 moles of water to 1 mole of nitrobenzene. The ratio of the weights of water to nitrobenzene will be:

$$\frac{27.15 \times 18}{1 \times 123} = \frac{488}{123} = \frac{3.97}{1}$$

Thus, each 100 Gm. of distillate will contain 20.1 Gm. of nitrobenzene. These values are ideal and seldom are achieved in actual practice because of the partial solubility of the components. Distillations of immiscible binary systems can be used effectively in purification when the molecular weight of the component having the lower vapor pressure is considerably higher than that of the other component, and where the partial pressure of the higher boiling component is an appreciable value near the boiling point of the lower boiling component.

The process of steam distillation is an example of such a method. Steam is passed into a mixture of water and the substance to be purified. The steam raises the temperature of the system to the boiling point. The purified substance separates from the distillate and can be separated from the water by use of a solvent or by use of the separatory funnel, leaving the impurities in the still. Steam distillation also may be effected by directly heating a mixture of water and the substance to be purified, distillation taking place when the sum of the partial pressures of the water and the substance reaches atmospheric pressure.

With substances which do not steam distill under ordinary conditions, superheated steam sometimes will bring about distillation. In this process, steam is passed through a copper coil heated to a temperature of 115° to 130° C. This process is used in the purification of salicylic acid.

Steam distillation is used in the purification of volatile oils and in the purification of both liquids and solids which are unstable at the temperatures necessary to effect ordinary distillation.

Reduced-Pressure Distillation. The boiling point of a liquid is the temperature at which the vapor tension of the liquid equals the pressure above the liquid. If the pressure above the liquid is reduced, the temperature at which the liquid distills is lowered. If the liquid is unstable near its boiling point, it may be possible to purify it at lower temperatures by distillation under reduced pressure. The pressure can be reduced by means of an aspirator or vacuum pump. A description of a vacuum distillation is included in Chapter 3.

Molecular Distillation. Molecular distillation may be defined as a process of separation in which the distance traveled by the molecules in the vapor state from the evaporating surface to the condensing surface is less than the *mean free path* of the molecule. Molecules leave the surface of a liquid at a rate depending on the vapor tension of the liquid. The molecules travel in a straight line until they reach a surface, or until they strike another molecule which drives them back to the original surface. The distance traveled by a molecule before it strikes another molecule is its mean free path. This distance is dependent on the number of molecules in the atmosphere above the liquid. In molecular distillation, the system is evacuated to the point where the mean free path of the molecules of the evaporating liquid is greater than the distance between the evaporating and the condensing surfaces. In this process, the purification takes place at a temperature of about 100° below the boiling point of the liquid at a few mm. pressure. It is a valuable method for the purification of liquids and solids which decompose near their boiling points under the pressures usually attained in vacuum distillation—i.e., 1 to 10 mm. of mercury.

Two factors govern the application of molecular distillation: the distance between the evaporating and the condensing surfaces and the efficiency of the pump providing the vacuum. Distances of less than 1 cm. between the surfaces are impractical. For materials which require molecular distillation, pressures of 10^{-4} to 10^{-5} mm. are required. The development of the molecular still thus had to await the production of pumps capable of producing such vacua.

The limiting factor in the efficiency of a vacuum pump is the vapor tension of the pumping fluid at operating temperature. Since 1929, certain mineral oil fractions and organic esters which exhibit vapor tensions of the order of 10^{-5} to 10^{-6} mm. at room temperature have been produced. If the pump operates directly to the still, vapors coming from the distillation are carried into the pumping fluid, and may raise the vapor tension of the fluid, impairing the efficiency of the pump. To avoid this, the vapors from the still are condensed by passing them through a trap cooled by solid carbon dioxide or liquid air. In addition, it is necessary to *degas* the liquid before the distillation is started. This is accomplished by heating the material under low pressures until all the dissolved gases and volatile materials are removed.

The earliest molecular still was the *pot still*. This type consisted of 2 concentric vessels, the lower serving as an evaporating surface. The space between the 2 surfaces was evacuated and the distillation carried out by the application of heat. As no boiling took place, there was no mixing of the liquid, and the upper surface quickly was exhausted of the more volatile component. The distillate obtained later in the distillation was poorer in this component, while a large proportion of the more volatile component remained in the residue.

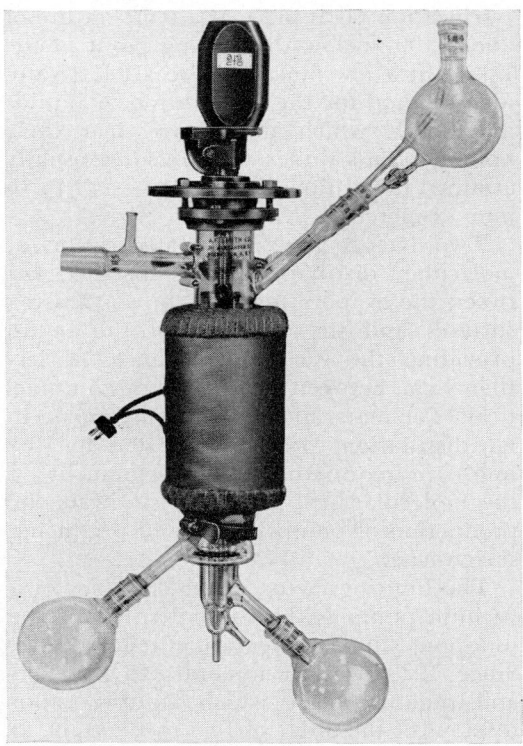

Fig. 69. The Rota-Film molecular still for separating compounds of high molecular weight. (Arthur F. Smith Co., Rochester, N. Y.)

The *falling-film still* is a later modification of the molecular still. It consists of a vertical evaporating surface containing hot oil heated by an electric coil, surrounded by a concentric, cooled condensing surface. The liquid to be purified is introduced at the top of the evaporating surface so that a thin film of liquid flows downward under the influence of gravity. The molecules leaving the surface of the film are condensed on the outer surface, approximately 1 cm. from the evaporating surface. The falling film is raised to the temperature required for only a short time so that little thermal decomposition occurs. Repeated passages of the liquid through the still result in a separation into the distillate of the more volatile component and a residue (Fig. 69). The *cyclic still* is similar to the falling-film type, but incorporates a pump to cycle the liquid through the still repeatedly.

Molecular distillation has been applied to numerous mixtures. It is used in the separation of various petroleum fractions and also in the purification of natural oils. Its most important application is in the preparation of high-vitamin concentrates from various fish-liver oils. It has proved to be of value in the purification of vegetable fats. Many vegetable oils contain natural antioxidants which are destroyed in the ordinary purification processes, rendering the purified product more susceptible to rancidity than the crude. These antioxidants survive molecular distillation, and oils purified by this process are more stable toward oxidation than fats purified by more conventional methods.

Molecular distillation requires specialized equipment for the production of the low pressures at which the distillations take place. It is therefore a relatively expensive method of purification, and is economical only when the purified product is of high value. However, it may be useful where vacuum or steam distillations are not applicable.

Conversion to a Solid. Soluble mixtures of liquids may be purified by changing one liquid phase into an insoluble solid phase. This may be accomplished by changes in temperature or by chemical reaction. The separation of the solid phase thus produced will be discussed under methods of separating liquids and solids.

CONVERSION BY LOWERING THE TEMPERATURE. Mixtures of liquids whose freezing points differ widely can be separated by lowering the temperature of the mixture. It is to be remembered that the freezing point of the mixture will be lower than the freezing point of the pure component having the higher freezing point. For solutions of nonelectrolytes, 1 gram-molecular weight of a liquid dissolved in 1,000 Gm. of water forms a solution which freezes at $-1.86°$ C. Thus a 50 per cent solution of water and ethyl alcohol by weight contains 1,000 Gm. of alcohol dissolved in 1,000 Gm. of water. This is 1,000/46 (molecular weight of ethyl alcohol) moles of alcohol, and the freezing point of the solution will be $0°$ C. $- 21.74 \times 1.86°$ C., or $-40.43°$ C. The solid which forms will be pure water, and a reasonably good separation will be obtained. Familiar examples of this phenomenon are the tormation of icebergs of pure water from sea water containing appreciable quantities of salt; and the concentration of weak alcoholic solutions by allowing the solutions to remain outdoors in extremely cold weather followed by the collection of the concentrated solution of alcohol, which does not freeze. The low temperatures required and the mechanical difficulties encountered limit the usefulness of this method of purification.

Low temperatures can be used to decrease the solubility of liquids, causing a separation. The 2 layers are then separated by use of the separatory funnel.

CONVERSION BY CHEMICAL REACTION. Some liquids form insoluble solids when they undergo chemical transformation. The use of this method of purification requires a thorough knowledge of the chemical and the physical properties of the components of the mixture and of the resulting compounds. If the substance desired forms an insoluble compound and the impurities do not, the pure substance may be precipitated from solution. Only if the original substance can be regenerated from the product formed will this method be of value. Salicylaldehyde and other liquid aldehydes form insoluble sodium bisulfite addition products and can be purified in this way. If the impurities form the insoluble product, the removal of the excess precipitant becomes of increasing importance unless the presence of the excess precipitant is not harmful. The preparation of absolute alcohol from 95 per cent alcohol by treatment with calcium oxide is an example of this method. The relatively insoluble calcium oxide reacts with the water to form insoluble calcium hydroxide.

A similar method, applied to the preparation of absolute alcohol, is the treatment of the solution with sufficient metallic sodium to react with the water present plus a slight excess. The excess reacts with alcohol to form sodium ethoxide. Since the affinity of water for sodium is greater than the affinity of the alcohol for sodium, all of the water will react to form sodium hydroxide, and the excess sodium is added to ensure the reaction of all the water. The sodium hydroxide and the sodium ethoxide formed are soluble to some extent in the alcohol, but are nonvolatile at the boiling point of alcohol, and absolute alcohol is obtained by distillation of the reaction mixture. This method is applied to the separation of solid substances as well as liquids from solution, but the principles are the same in either case. Factors which must be considered are: (1) the solubility of the product formed, (2) the effect of the precipitant on other components of the mixture and (3) the difficulty of removing the excess precipitant, if necessary.

Conversion to an Immiscible Liquid. Mixtures of soluble liquids may be separated by the formation of an insoluble liquid phase through the use of selective solvents or by a decrease in the solubility of one component.

EXTRACTION. The separation of 2 components by allowing one of the components to dissolve in a liquid which is immiscible with the solvent of the original solution is *extraction*. If a mixture of a liquid A in solution in liquid B is mixed with a liquid C in which A is soluble but in which B is insoluble, 2 layers will be formed. If the 2 layers are agitated so that complete contact is obtained by the 3 liquids, a state of equilibrium will be reached in which A will be distributed between B and C proportionally to its relative solubility in B and C. If the 2 layers are separated, a fresh portion of C added and the process repeated, a new equilibrium will be set up, more A dissolving in C. If this process is repeated several times, a large proportion of A can be removed from solution in B, but a complete separation cannot be achieved, as an inspection of the example given below will show. The ratio of the solubility of a liquid in 2 immiscible liquids is its *distribution* or *partition coefficient* between the 2 solvents. If 100 ml. of B dissolves 1 Gm. of A, and 100 ml. of C dissolves 5 Gm. of A, then the partition coefficient of A between C and B is 5.

An example will illustrate the process of extraction. If a 200 ml. portion of a 1 per cent solution of A in B is extracted with 100 ml. of C, A will be distributed between

C and B according to the following equation:

$$\frac{\frac{x}{100}}{\frac{2-x}{200}} = 5$$

where x is the amount of A dissolved in C. Solving this equation, x equals 1.428 Gm. of A removed by 100 ml. of C. If a second 100 ml. portion of C is added,

$$\frac{\frac{x}{100}}{\frac{0.572-x}{200}} = 5$$

and x is found to equal 0.409 Gm. of A removed, or a total of 1.837 Gm.

The number of extractions is more important than the volume of solvent used. If one portion of 200 ml. of C had been used in the above example,

$$\frac{\frac{x}{200}}{\frac{2-x}{200}} = 5$$

and x equals 1.667 Gm., 0.170 Gm. less than when the same volume of C was used in 2 divided portions.

Extractions may be applied in 2 ways. The extraction may be carried out in a separatory funnel, using fresh portions of solvent for each extraction. If the solvent used is lighter than the liquid to be extracted, and the substance to be dissolved is nonvolatile and stable at the boiling point of the solvent, a continuous extractor may be used. Such an extractor results in a saving of time and solvent.

The selection of the solvent depends on the partition coefficient, the ease of removal of the solvent following the extraction and the possibility of chemical reaction between the solvent and the materials to be extracted.

Extraction is a valuable method of removing liquids from aqueous solution when the substance is thermally labile at the boiling point of water, or where fractionation is not feasible. This method is also applicable to the separation of solids from solution.

SALTING-OUT EFFECT. The addition of a soluble salt to a solution of 2 liquids or a solid and a liquid can be used to decrease the solubility of the solute. The addition of sufficient sodium or calcium chloride to form a saturated aqueous solution of the salt will cause a slightly soluble liquid to separate from a saturated aqueous solution of the liquid. This effect is used to improve the separation of the distillate in steam distillation. It is also of value in the separation of solids from solution—e.g., the separation of sodium benzenesulfonate from aqueous solution.

SEPARATION OF A LIQUID AND A SOLID

The separation of a solid from a liquid is purely a mechanical process. When the impurities in a liquid are present in the solid phase, or when the impurities in a solid are in the liquid phase, purification consists merely of separating the 2 phases. If the impurities form a solution with the desired substance, a single-phase system results, and a change in phase becomes necessary to effect separation and purification.

Separation of Insoluble Mixtures

Decantation. The process of gently pouring off a supernatant liquid is decantation. While this method can be applied to the separation of 2 immiscible liquid phases, the separation is not sharp, so that decantation is limited to the separation of a liquid phase from a solid phase. Decantation is applied by allowing the suspended solid material to settle to the bottom of the container and gently pouring off the supernatant liquid without disturbing the settled materials. It is impossible to remove all of the liquid from the solid by this method. The last traces of liquid must be removed by evaporation. Decantation can be applied best by using a tall, cylindrical container which presents a relatively small cross section in proportion to its volume. This results in a longer column of supernatant liquid above the settled solid and facilitates the removal of larger quantities of liquid. The use of a glass rod to guide the flow of the liquid and to steady the hand of the operator is recommended. One end of the rod is placed along the lip of the container and the other is placed in the receiver.

Siphoning. The siphon is sometimes of value for removing large quantities of supernatant liquid from the settled solid. A glass tube bent to form an angle of about 60°, the arms of which are of unequal length, or a length of rubber tubing will serve as a siphon. The flow of liquid is started by applying gentle suction to the free end of the tube, or by filling the tube with liquid.

Another variation of this method is to insert a stopper into the neck of a flask containing the settled suspension, the stopper carrying a siphon tube and a rubber bulb for pumping air into the flask. The air pumped into the flask exerts a pressure on the surface of the liquid, forcing it through the siphon tube. In all forms of the siphon, the end of the tube should not extend too close to the settled solid, as the currents set up by the siphon may disturb the solid and necessitate waiting for the solid to subside.

A pipet may be used to withdraw a small amount of supernatant liquid from a settled solid. The tip of the pipet is placed just above the surface of the settled material, and the pipet filled by gentle suction so as not to disturb the precipitate.

Colation. The process of separating a liquid from a solid by passing the suspension through a porous material which allows the liquid to pass but which retains the solid is colation or straining. Colation is the term applied to the process using relatively coarse strainers such as wire sieves, muslin, wool, gauze and felt. The straining medium is placed on a wooden (tenaculum) or wire frame, in a funnel, or suspended from a wire collar in the form of a sleeve. The suspension is placed on the strainer, and the liquid which flows through is collected in a suitable container. The hard-rubber strainer, which is a 2-piece hard-rubber funnel fitted to hold a small piece of muslin or surgical gauze, is useful in small-scale operations. Colation is applicable in the separation of a coarsely divided solid and is faster than filtration.

Filtration. Filtration differs from colation only in the degree of fineness of the straining media. The most frequently used filtering media are filter paper, paper pulp, asbestos fibers, ground glass or glass wool, charcoal, porous stone, sand and glass cloth. In pharmacy, filter paper is the usual filter medium.

Filter paper is a porous, unsized paper of varying degrees of fineness and purity. Three types of filter paper are of importance in pharmacy. The gray filter paper containing some coloring material may be used in filtering drug products, but the desirability of using this paper is questionable. *Qualitative* filter paper in varying degrees of porosity is a white, highly purified paper suitable for most pharmaceutical uses. *Quantitative* filter paper, sometimes misnamed ashless, has been treated with acid, alkali, water and other solvents to dissolve most of the inorganic material. When ignited, this paper burns almost completely, leaving a negligible quantity of ash. It is used in gravimetric analysis for the collection of precipitates which are to be ignited.

Filter paper is used with a funnel in the usual filtering process. Various forms of funnels are available. The usual funnel is a glass cone attached to a stem of varying lengths. Funnels are made of glass, copper, hard rubber or tinned iron. In pharmaceutical purifications, the glass funnel is to be preferred even though it is more fragile. The inner surface of the bowl may be ribbed to afford a passage for the filtrate, thus speeding filtration. The analytical funnel has a long stem which aids in filtrations by exerting a slight suction effect when the stem is filled with liquid.

The Büchner funnel is a special type of funnel, usually made of glazed porcelain (Fig. 70). The perforated floor is covered by a circular piece of filter paper, and the funnel is used in conjunction with suction. This funnel is of value in the filtration of large quantities of organic compounds, and is available in a wide range of sizes. A new modification of the Büchner funnel has the suction flask as an integral part of the funnel.

The Gooch crucible (Fig. 71) is a small

porcelain crucible with a perforated floor similar to the Büchner funnel. The perforated bottom may be covered by a thin

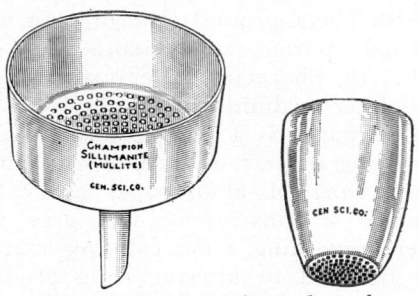

FIG. 70. *(Left)* Büchner funnel.
FIG. 71. *(Right)* Gooch crucible.

layer of purified asbestos fibers to serve as the filtering medium. This layer is built up before each filtration. The crucible is used in gravimetric analysis for the collection and the ignition of precipitates.

The fritted or sintered glass funnel is finding increased use in filtering operations. Such funnels are made of powdered Jena glass granules which are fused to the sides of a glass funnel to form a porous filtering medium. These funnels are made in the forms of the Büchner funnel and the Gooch crucible. This filter requires the use of suction. The filter can be cleaned by drawing an acid or some other solvent through the filter, but this sometimes does not remove all traces of the material filtered out.

The patented Alundum crucible of porous aluminum silicate is a useful piece of filtering apparatus. It withstands high heat and can be used for the collection of various precipitates which are to be ignited without using any other filtering medium.

Bacterial filters are filters which prevent the passage of bacteria and other suspended material. Unglazed porcelain, diatomaceous earth and asbestos are the usual filtering media in these filters.

There are several methods of folding filter paper for use with the conical funnel. The simplest method is to fold the circular paper along one diameter, and to make a second fold at right angles to the first so as to divide the circle into quarters. The paper is then opened to form a cone of 3 thicknesses of paper on one side and one on the other. If the sides of the funnel make an angle of 60°, the cone will fit the funnel snugly and the liquid which passes through the filter will form an uninterrupted column in the stem. Frequently, the funnel is not exactly 60°. In this case, the second fold is made slightly less than even with the edge. By experimentation, the fold can be made so that the cone fits the funnel snugly. If a small piece is torn away at the longer side near the top, the filter can be adjusted more easily.

The above method of folding a filter is the quickest and the simplest. The disadvantages in this fold are that the filtration is not even, because of the uneven thickness of the filtering media and the slowness of filtration. Faster filtration is obtained by use of the quadruplet filter, or the plaited or fluted filter.

The quadruplet filter is so named because 4 folds are made. The first fold is made to divide the paper into halves, as in the first method. The paper is opened, and a fold made at right angles to the first on the same side of the paper. The third fold is made $22\frac{1}{2}°$ from one of the first two folds, and on the opposite side of the paper. This can be done best by first matching two adjacent creases from the first two folds, and making a short crease near the circumference of the paper. This divides the quadrant into two 45° segments. The halving procedure is repeated to form two $22\frac{1}{2}°$ segments. The third fold is then made at this point, and the fourth fold made at right angles to the third on the same side of the paper. When the filter is opened, it will be possible to form a cone which presents a more even filtering surface than the usual fold.

The plaited or fluted filter is called the *pharmaceutical filter* since it is used frequently by the pharmacist. Only one thickness of paper is presented to the filtering liquid, and filtration is rapid. Various methods of folding these filters are used, but only one will be presented here. The first two folds are made in the same way as in the first method. The outside edges of the two outer quadrants formed are folded back against the adjacent edge.

This divides the paper into 8 equal segments. The outside quarter of half of the paper is next bisected by bringing the outer edge up to the adjacent fold and the paper creased. The fold used as the base for the last fold is now brought up against the center fold and a new crease made. This will divide one half of the paper into 8 equal segments. If the center fold is now reversed, and the remaining half of the paper treated in the same manner, a plaited filter of 16 segments will be obtained. A plaited filter of 32 segments can be made if the paper is large enough, by repeating the above process with each of the original 4 segments. In folding the plaited filter, it is important that the creases should not be made to the center, as this will weaken the filter at this point. Plaited filters can be purchased ready for use.

The addition of insoluble absorbent powders to the liquid before filtration aids in the clarification of fine suspensions. The powder added should be completely insoluble, and should not adsorb soluble materials intended to remain in solution. Talc, kieselguhr, paper pulp and silica can be used in most cases, but the use of fuller's earth, bentonite, charcoal or magnesium carbonate may affect the quality of the preparation. Fuller's earth, bentonite and charcoal may adsorb substances from solution, while chalk and magnesium carbonate are not completely insoluble and may react with the substances in solution. The use of these filtering aids must be governed by the character of the liquid to be filtered.

The collection of the insoluble material in the pores of the filter media increases the efficiency of the filtration. In many instances, if filtration is not complete at first, the filtrate may be clear after filtration has proceeded for a while. If the cloudy liquid from the early part of the filtration is again passed through the filter, the filtration may be carried out without resort to filtering aids. The same effect may lower the speed of filtration when large quantities of solids are filtered out. In this case, the suspension may be filtered in 2 portions.

Special modifications of the filtration process are used to facilitate the filtration of large quantities of suspensions, or to filter suspensions which filter slowly.

CONTINUOUS FILTRATION (Fig. 72). Sometimes continuous filtration is used for large quantities. This method is applicable when only a small quantity of solid material is

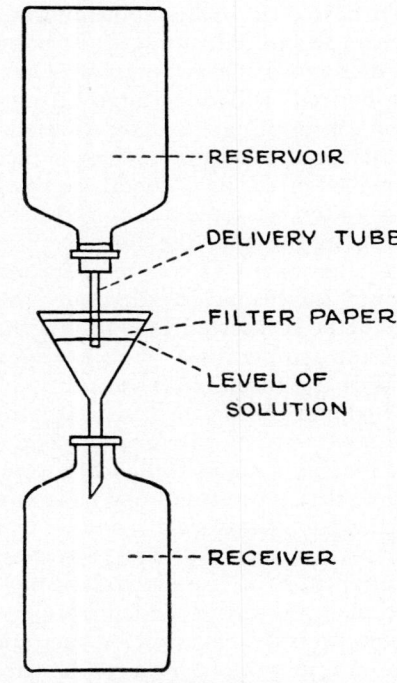

FIG. 72. Continuous filtration.

present. The suspension is placed in a bottle which contains a stopper and a tube of sufficient bore to carry the material which settles from the suspension. The bottle is inverted over the funnel and supported by an iron ring. The length of the tube is adjusted to the desired level of the liquid in the funnel. When the level of the liquid in the funnel reaches the end of the tube, liquid will not flow from the bottle. When the level in the funnel falls below the end of the delivery tube, air will pass into the bottle, forcing the liquid out until the level of the liquid in the funnel again covers the end of the delivery tube. If the amount of sludge formed in the suspension is not so large as to clog the delivery tube, and if the level of the liquid in the funnel and the bore of the delivery tube are adjusted properly, satisfactory continuous filtration will take place. This apparatus is better adapted to continuous washing in which no sludge forms in the reservoir.

Hot Filtration. In some instances, it is of value to filter a suspension at an elevated temperature. If the substance to be purified is soluble in hot solution and the impurities are not, filtration of the hot mixture will remove the impurities. The substance desired will precipitate from the solution on cooling. Special funnels are available for this purpose. One of these is a funnel inserted in a metal jacket containing water or some other liquid with provision for heating the liquid. The filtration takes place at the temperature of the liquid in the jacket. In some cases, a thermometer is inserted for the determination of the temperature. Another method is to insert the funnel into a conical coil of iron or copper tubing through which steam is circulated. An improvised method consists of placing a metal funnel in a ring gas burner so that the funnel may be heated to any desired temperature.

Suction Filtration. The filtration of large quantities of liquids containing suspended material can be made under suction or under pressure. Suction or vacuum filtration on a laboratory scale can be effected by use of an aspirator or suction pump. The funnel is inserted into a stopper which is then inserted into the neck of a suction flask. The suction flask is a heavy-walled glass Erlenmeyer flask carrying an outlet tube at the top of the conical section of the flask (Fig. 73). This outlet tube is connected to the aspirator by heavy-walled rubber suction tubing. When the aspirator is turned on, the air is exhausted from the flask, and the suction produced pulls the liquid through the pores of the filter. Suction filtration is carried out using a Büchner funnel, a Gooch crucible, a sintered or Alundum crucible or some other funnel providing a support for the filtering media. A conical funnel may be used with suction filtration, but the paper may rupture at the apex of the filter cone. This may be avoided by supporting the tip of the filter cone with a piece of parchment paper properly folded, or by one of the commercial supports supplied for this purpose. It is advisable to use a trap between the aspirator and the suction flask to prevent contaminating the filtrate if water is drawn back into the flask when the water pressure in the line changes.

Pressure Filtration. In laboratory purification, pressure filtration seldom is used, but it is used in most industrial purifications. Many designs of pressure filters are available, using a wide variety of filtering media. The suspension is introduced into the filter press under pressure, and rapid filtration takes place. Filter presses are available in a variety of sizes from small laboratory models up to immense industrial models for the filtration of large quantities of suspensions.

Centrifugation. The use of the centrifuge affords a rapid method for separating fine suspensions. A centrifuge is a machine which rotates at a high speed. The suspension is placed in a centrifuge cup or tube which fits into a bracket at the ends of the arms of the centrifuge. The brackets are fitted in such a way that when the centrifuge is in operation, the tubes are rotated rapidly in a horizontal position. When the centrifuge is operating at high speeds, the heavier particles are forced to the bottom of the tube by the intense centrifugal forces generated.

Centrifuges differ in type, size, operating speeds and motive powers. Small laboratory models and some older designs are operated by hand, using gears to increase the speed of the rotary motion, but newer models are operated by electric motors suitably geared to produce high speeds. The centrifuges operating at higher speeds exert considerably more force than those operating at

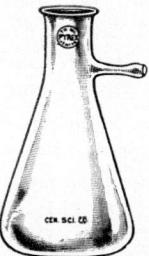

Fig. 73. Filter or suction flask.

lower speeds, and are useful for the separation of finely divided suspensions.

Care should be used to balance the centrifuge before use. If the weights at each end of the arms of the centrifuge are not balanced properly, intense vibratory forces are set up which may break the tubes or the centrifuge. The suspension may be divided into 2 or 4 equal portions and each portion placed in a tube or cup. Another method is to balance the cup containing the suspension with a cup containing an equal weight of water.

Serious injuries may result from contact with the rapidly rotating cups. In using centrifuges which have a protective housing, the housing should not be opened until the centrifuge has come to rest. Some small centrifuges are made with a protected conical rotating head in which the centrifuge tubes are inserted. Injuries from the rotating cups are less frequent with this type of centrifuge.

Care should be exercised to prevent the centrifuge from slowing down too rapidly, as the residue may be stirred up if the deceleration of the rotating cups is too abrupt. With centrifuges equipped with a brake, the brake should be applied slowly and evenly.

After centrifuging the suspension, the clear supernatant liquid is removed by decanting or siphoning.

SEPARATION OF SOLUBLE MIXTURES

Single-phase systems of a liquid and a solid are of 3 types: (1) an apparently single-phase solid system in which water has been absorbed, such as moist salt or a fresh drug; (2) a solid containing a liquid held by loose chemical union, such as water or alcohol of crystallization; and (3) a liquid system containing a dissolved solid.

Conversion to a Vapor. The first two types are purified, when necessary, by conversion of the liquid into the vapor phase. The processes of desiccation and exsiccation are used for these separations. For many pharmaceutical purposes, small amounts of water are not harmful and it is not necessary to remove such water. In other cases, this water is objectionable and must be removed. As an example, in the preparation of syrups, the control of the concentration of sugar is necessary to stabilize the syrup. It is desirable to remove any moisture in the sugar to simplify obtaining the proper concentration of sugar in the finished syrup.

DESICCATION. Desiccation is the process of removing water from a substance by vaporization at relatively low temperatures. Desiccation is used to dry solid chemical compounds and mixtures, and to dry crude drugs. The term applies specifically to the removal of water, but the methods can be used for the removal of other volatile liquids.

Desiccation can be carried out by placing the material on an evaporating dish, a tray or a watch glass, and heating the material in an oven or over a water bath. The desiccation should be carried out at the lowest possible temperature to avoid decomposition. The process is speeded by passing a current of warm, dry air over the surface of the material. The speed of desiccation is dependent on the area of surface presented, so that the substance to be dried should be spread out in a thin layer.

Desiccation at reduced pressure results in a more rapid desiccation at lower temperatures. Electrically heated ovens which can be evacuated are available for this purpose. Reduced pressure hastens the speed of the vaporization and makes it possible to carry out the process at a lower temperature. In using electric ovens, care should be exercised to make sure that all combustible liquids are removed before the sample is placed in the oven, as a spark may ignite the vapors.

The Aberhalden type of drying apparatus is useful for the desiccation of material in small amounts. This apparatus uses phosphorus pentoxide or calcium chloride as an absorbent, and the desiccation is carried out at the boiling point of the liquid used by allowing the vapors of the boiling liquid to bathe the compartment containing the sample.

The desiccation of crude drugs may be carried out when speed is unnecessary by spreading the drug in a warm, dry room. Satisfactory desiccation can be effected in this manner, but provision must be made to prevent the accumulation of dust.

Desiccated chemicals absorb moisture very rapidly. They should be stored in tightly stoppered containers. The desiccator

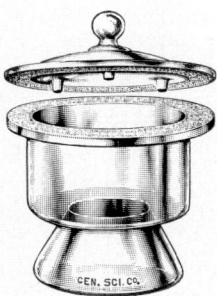

Fig. 74. Desiccator.

is a useful container for the storage of highly hygroscopic materials (Fig. 74). The desiccator is charged with calcium chloride, lime, sulfuric acid, phosphorus pentoxide or Dehydrite in the lower section, and a perforated porcelain disk placed in the top section to serve as a floor. The dry substance is placed in the top section, and the desiccator closed with a tight lid. The dehydrating material absorbs moisture from the atmosphere in the desiccator, so that the material in the upper section is kept dry.

Exsiccation. Exsiccation is the process of removing water of crystallization from a hydrated salt by the application of strong heat. The process is carried out by placing the material in an evaporating dish, and applying heat by means of a direct flame or a sand bath. Heat is applied slowly at first to prevent fusion of the hydrated salt. The hydrated salt is unstable at high temperatures, and the water of crystallization is given off. In many cases, the salt dissolves in this water, and at this point, the heat is increased to vaporize the water. The exsiccated salt is highly hygroscopic, and must be stored carefully.

Separation of Components of Solutions

The purification of liquid systems containing dissolved solids can be effected by changing the liquid phase into the vapor phase, by changing either phase into an immiscible liquid phase and by changing the soluble substance into an insoluble solid phase.

Conversion to Vapor Phase. The liquid phase may be converted into the vapor phase by evaporation, by simple distillation under normal or reduced pressure or by fractional distillation if the solid is also volatile.

Steam distillation can be used to separate a partially volatile solid or liquid from a liquid or solid which is not volatile with steam.

Solids dissolved in a liquid can be separated from the liquid by extraction with an immiscible solvent.

Conversion to a Solid. Numerous methods are available for the conversion of a soluble solid into an insoluble solid. One of the most useful is through chemical reaction or precipitation. The principles discussed under the separation of soluble liquid states apply to the separation of a solid from solution.

Common Ion Effect. The common ion effect can be used to decrease the solubility of a slightly soluble compound, effecting a more complete separation of the substance to be purified. The addition of sodium chloride, sodium sulfate, etc., will decrease the solubility of chlorides, sulfates, etc., in the solutions.

Chromatographic Adsorption. The terms *chromatography, chromatographic adsorption* and *chromatographic analysis* are applied to a group of procedures based on partition of a solute between two immiscible solvents supported on an immovable solid phase and on selective adsorption of a solute on the surface of a solid particle. The terms are also applied to methods in which an ion exchange resin is used as the immobile phase, but in such cases, a chemical reaction probably occurs as well as adsorption and partition. In the earliest applications of these methods, they were applied to colored solutes, which accounts for the terminology *chromo-*, but the principles are equally applicable to colorless solutes. However, the original nomenclature has persisted.

The three basic types of chromatography are: (1) partition; (2) adsorption and (3) ion exchange. Various supportive and adsorptive materials are used. When finely divided solids such as silica gel, alumina, sucrose, charcoal, etc., are used, the solid is packed into a cylindrical column, and the method is referred to as *column chromatography*. Filter paper can also be used as a support for the immobile liquid, in which case, the method is known as *paper chromatography*.

The theoretical bases for chromatography are complex. In the earlier stages of the development of the methods, they were primarily empirical. More recent work has led to considerable elucidation of the underlying principles of chromatography, and its applications have been extended widely until it has become an extremely useful research tool.

Although chromatographic methods are of greatest usefulness on a micro- or a semimicro-scale, in some cases good separation of relatively large quantities of materials can be effected. When significantly different responses to partition and adsorption are present in the components of a mixture, a practical separation or purification can be obtained by chromatography.

Ion Exchange. The process of ion exchange is a method of purification in which a soluble ion can be removed from a solvent, usually water. This method is widely used in the purification of water for pharmaceutical and industrial purposes, but is applicable to other types of purification such as the removal of ionizable impurities from aqueous solutions of nonionizable substances.

Ion exchange is discussed in Chapter 9.

Electrolysis. To purify solutions of electrolytes and to obtain the component elements in a pure state, electrolysis can be used. If an electric current is applied to a solution of an electrolyte, the charged ions migrate to the electrode of opposite charge, and the charge on the ion is neutralized. This results in the precipitation of the neutral radical. Electrolysis of a solution of copper sulfate results in the formation of free copper and sulfuric acid; a solution of sodium chloride results in the formation of gaseous chlorine, hydrogen and sodium hydroxide, the less active hydrogen ions from the ionization of water being liberated in preference to the more active sodium. Electrolysis finds wide application in purification and manufacturing processes.

SEPARATION OF COLLOIDS

The separation of colloidal suspensions can be effected in several ways. These methods are applicable to the separation of 2 solids, one of which is crystalloidal and one of which is colloidal.

Dialysis. If a semipermeable membrane is inserted between a solution containing both a colloid and a crystalloid and pure water, the membrane will allow the passage of the solvent and the crystalloid but not the colloid. The crystalloid will pass through the membrane until the concentration of the crystalloid is the same on both sides of the membrane. By employing sufficient quantities of water, an essentially complete separation can be effected by dialysis. The extraction of sugar from sugar beets by dialysis through the cell membrane illustrates this process.

Precipitation by Electrolytes. Colloidal suspensions can be destroyed by the addition of electrolytes which neutralize the charge on the particles, resulting in precipitation of the colloid.

Electric Methods. When a colloidal suspension is formed, the colloidal particles assume a definite charge, the liquid taking the opposite charge. If a colloidal suspension is placed in a cup separated from a dilute solution of an electrolyte by a semipermeable membrane, and a potential difference applied, the solvent will migrate toward the electrode of opposite charge. This process is known as *electro-endosmosis*.

Cataphoresis. This is the phenomenon observed when a potential difference is applied to a colloidal solution. The charged particles move toward the electrode of opposite charge, thus effecting a partial separation.

SEPARATION OF SOLIDS

The separation of 2 or more solid substances can be effected by converting one phase into a gaseous or a liquid phase.

Conversion to the Vapor Phase

Simple and fractional distillation at ordinary or reduced pressure can be employed in the purification of solids which are stable at their boiling points under the pressure employed. In addition, steam and molecular distillation can be applied to mixtures of volatile solids.

Sublimation. The process of converting a solid into the vapor phase and the condensation of the vapor back into the solid phase without the formation of an intervening liquid phase is sublimation. This process is used extensively in pharmacy for the purification of substances having a high vapor tension, and for the separation of volatile solids from nonvolatile solids or liquids. Sublimation can be carried out by heating the substance in an evaporating dish surmounted by a funnel to serve as a condenser above the dish. A perforated filter paper placed over the dish will allow the vapors to pass through but will prevent the sublimed solid falling back into the mixture. Sublimation can be carried out under reduced pressure. The process can be applied to the separation of volatile solids from solution in nonvolatile liquids. Iodine, benzoic acid, camphor and many other pharmaceuticals are purified by sublimation.

Pseudosublimation. A new method for the purification of benzoic acid and other substances consists of heating the impure solid until it liquefies, but below its boiling point. A blast of air is blown across the surface of the melted solid, carrying the vapors into a condensation chamber where the vapors solidify, the nonvolatile impurities being removed.

Conversion to the Liquid Phase

Mixtures of solids can be purified by the introduction of a liquid phase in which one solid is soluble and in which the other components are insoluble.

Washing. The process of dissolving out a soluble substance from an insoluble solid is washing or lotion. It can be carried out by adding the proper solvent to the mixture contained in a suitable container. The mixture is stirred and allowed to subside, and the supernatant liquid removed. This process is repeated until all the soluble material is removed. Washing is carried out until the wash liquid fails to give a test for the soluble salts.

Washing may be carried out on a filter. The wash liquid is added to the solid and filtered. When the liquid has drained completely, a new portion of solvent is added, and the process repeated until complete.

As with extraction, the number of washings is more important than the volume of solution used. The volume of liquid retained by the solid after draining (l), the volume of wash liquid used (w), and the concentration of the salt in the liquid held by the solid (s) are involved in determining the efficiency of washing. The weight of soluble material held by the solid is the product of the volume and the concentration of the liquid retained, ls. If wash liquid is added, the total volume of liquid is ($w + l$) and the concentration becomes:

$$s_1 = \frac{ls}{(w + l)} \quad (1)$$

Assuming that the same volume of wash liquid is used and that the same volume of solution is retained by the residue, the concentration of the solution after the second washing is:

$$s_2 = \frac{ls_1}{(w + l)} \quad (2)$$

If the value for s_1 from (1) is substituted in (2), the concentration s_2 becomes:

$$s_2 = \frac{l\left[\dfrac{ls}{w + l}\right]}{w + l}$$

When simplified, this equation becomes:

$$s_2 = \left[\frac{l}{w + l}\right]^2 s$$

which, in its general form, may be written:

$$s_n = \left[\frac{l}{w + l}\right]^n s$$

The application of this equation to a specific example will illustrate the advantage of several washings over 1 washing using the same total volume of wash liquid. If a residue which holds 1 ml. of wash liquid containing 0.1 Gm. of soluble material is washed with 5 portions of 5 ml. each, the concentration of the wash solution adhering to the solid will be:

$$s_5 = \left[\frac{1}{5+1}\right]^5 \times 0.1 = 0.000013 \text{ Gm./ml.}$$

If the residue is washed with one 25 ml. portion, the concentration after 1 washing will be:

$$s_1 = \left[\frac{1}{25+1}\right]^1 \times 0.1 = 0.00385 \text{ Gm./ml.}$$

The amount of material left in the residue after one washing of 25 ml. is about 300 times as much as after 5 washings of 5 ml. each. These calculations assume that the quantity of wash liquid used in each washing is sufficient to dissolve all the soluble material present, and are based entirely on the amount of liquid retained by the residue.

Washing always results in some loss of the less soluble substance, as some of the residue is dissolved with each washing. For this reason, washing should not be carried farther than is necessary to remove all of the impurities. Continuous washing may be effected by using the apparatus described under continuous filtration (p. 71).

Extraction. The process of removing a soluble component from a crude drug by extraction with a solvent is used for the isolation and the purification of plant substances. Extraction is discussed in detail in Chapter 8.

CRYSTALLIZATION

Mixtures of solids may be separated by crystallization, if the material desired is soluble. Substances which crystallize can be purified by this process. Each crystalline chemical compound crystallizes in a definite, pure form which is constant within definite limits. Impurities hinder the formation of crystals and do not enter into the crystal form. However, impurities may be adsorbed on the surface of the crystals.

The success of crystallization depends primarily on the selection of the proper solvent. Water, alcohol, pyridine and dioxane are valuable solvents for crystallization, although almost all liquids are used. A solvent is chosen in which the substance is soluble when hot but almost insoluble when cold, and in which the impurities are soluble in both the hot and the cold solvent. A sufficient amount of the hot solvent to dissolve the sample is added and the mixture filtered to remove insoluble impurities. If the substance is desired in fine crystals, the liquid is cooled rapidly, but if large crystals are desired, the liquid is cooled slowly. When cool, the crystals precipitate in a relatively pure state and are filtered off. The liquid should not be evaporated, as the impurities will also remain after evaporation.

Occasionally, a supersaturated solution is formed when the solution is cooled. Precipitation can be brought about by scratching the side of the vessel to produce a rough spot for crystallization to start, or by adding a pure crystal of the substance sought (seeding). Sometimes, merely jarring the container or inserting a stirring rod will cause crystallization to take place.

If large quantities of impurities are present, an appreciable quantity may be adsorbed on the surface of the crystals. Repeated recrystallizations using fresh portions of the solvent, each reducing the amount of impurities, may be necessary.

The liquid remaining after filtration (mother liquor) invariably contains some of the desired substance in solution. Several crops of crystals of lower purity may be obtained by partially evaporating the mother liquor. However, in many cases it is difficult to purify these crystals sufficiently to obtain an acceptable product.

Fractional Crystallization. This process is valuable when the components of a solid mixture exhibit wide differences in solubility toward a solvent. The mixture is dissolved in the smallest amount of the hot solvent possible, and the solution allowed to cool. The first crop of crystals obtained will be the almost pure substance least soluble in the solvent. The mother liquor is evaporated to a lesser volume, and a second crop of crystals obtained. This process is repeated several times to obtain a number of fractions, the last fraction being a fairly pure sample of the substance of highest solubility. Further purification can be obtained by separate recrystallizations.

Miscellaneous Methods

A special method of purification is through the use of biologic methods. Essentially, this method consists of introducing an organism which reacts with one component of a mixture but not with the other. The organism is allowed to destroy or use up one of the components, leaving the other components unaffected. These methods are applicable when none of the components of the mixture is antagonistic toward the organism. An example of this method is the separation of the *d-* and the *l-* forms of amyl alcohol by *Penicillium glaucum*.

Sterilization is a special type of purification involving the destruction of bacteria. It is discussed in Chapter 12.

CLARIFICATION

Clarification is a special type of purification process for the removal of finely divided suspended material from liquid preparations.

The general methods of clarification are: (1) by facilitating the settling of the solid material; (2) by adding an insoluble substance to entrap the finely divided solid material; and (3) by fermentation.

Facilitation of Settling. The separation of finely divided particles from a liquid can be facilitated by decreasing the viscosity of the liquid so that the particles rise or fall, depending on their specific gravity. The viscosity may be decreased by heating the liquid, or by adding alcohol or some liquid of lower viscosity. The separated particles may be removed by skimming, by decantation or by filtration of the precipitated material.

The simplest and the least expensive method of clarification is to allow the liquid to stand until the particles have settled out.

Precipitation. The use of solid materials to trap the suspended particles may be applicable. A solution of albumin is added to the liquid and mixed well. If the solution is heated, the albumin is coagulated, entrapping the solid particles. The coagulated albumin rises to the top, carrying the impurities, and may be skimmed off the liquid.

Gelatin may be added to solutions containing tannins with the formation of a precipitate of gelatin tannate which entraps the particles. The solution is then strained or filtered to remove the suspended material. Milk may be added to suspensions containing acids. The acid precipitates the casein, entrapping the suspended particles.

Purified paper pulp can be used in the same way. The pulped paper entraps the particles, and the solution is filtered to remove the suspended material.

In all these methods, an agent should be selected which does not react with any of the components of the solution which are a part of the preparation.

Fermentation. Fermentation is of value in the clarification of certain solutions such as fruit juices and wines. The suspended material is insoluble in the alcohol produced, and settles out and can be removed by filtration.

BIBLIOGRAPHY

Brimley, R. C., and Barrett, F. C.: Practical Chromatography, New York, Reinhold, 1953.

Carney, T. P.: Laboratory Fractional Distillation, New York, Macmillan, 1949.

Daniels, F. C., and Alberty, R. A.: Physical Chemistry, New York, Wiley, 1955.

Dickey, G. D., and Byrden, C. L.: Theory and Practice of Filtration, New York, Reinhold, 1946.

Gatterman and Wieland: Laboratory Methods of Organic Chemistry, London, Macmillan, 1938.

Kirschbaum, E.: Distillation and Rectification, English translation by Wulfinghoff, Brooklyn, Chem. Pub. Co., 1948.

Lederer, E.: Chromatography, ed. 2, Amsterdam, New York, Elsevier, 1957.

Riegel, E. R.: Industrial Chemistry, ed. 5, New York, Reinhold, 1949.

Robinson, and Gilliland: The Elements of Fractional Distillation, New York, McGraw-Hill, 1950.

Zechmeister, L., and Cholnoky, L.: Principles and Practice of Chromatography, English translation from the 2nd edition by A. L. Bacharach and F. A. Robinson, New York, Wiley, 1951.

JAMES WILSON JONES, PH.D.
Professor of Pharmacy, College of Pharmacy, State University of Iowa

5

Physical and Chemical Subdivision of Drugs

COMMINUTION
PRECIPITATION

GRANULATION
SEPARATION OF PARTICLE SIZES

COMMINUTION

Comminution is the process of reducing the particle size of vegetable, animal or chemical drugs by a physical process. The objects of the process are threefold: (1) to increase the rate of solution of solids, (2) to increase the ease and the thoroughness of extraction of animal and vegetable drugs and (3) to obtain a uniform powder or mixture of powders for the purpose of preparing medicinal solids in the most desirable form for administration.

Rate of Solution. In the first instance, it must be remembered that comminution does not increase the solubility of a solid. With few exceptions, only the rate of solution is affected. The increase in the rate of solution can be explained in the following manner. Consider that a crystal of copper sulfate is composed of a definite pattern in which the cupric and the sulfate ions are arranged in a lattice, and that these ions can escape only from the surface of the crystal. If the crystal is a perfect cube, the edges of which are 1 inch in length, the total surface exposed to the action of the solvent is 6 square inches. By subdividing the cube into 1,000 cubes, each of which is one tenth inch along all edges, the total surface exposed is 60 square inches. Therefore, 10 times as many ions are exposed to the solvent from the 1,000 cubes as from the single cube and solution should proceed 10 times as rapidly.

Extraction. Many compounds of medicinal value are stored within the cells of plants. In the early history of medicine, many herbs were gathered, cured and administered in the form of crude powders, in which case the extractive materials were utilized therapeutically in part or entirely as the drug passed along the alimentary tract. As progress has been made in biologic and pharmacologic studies, it has been demonstrated that more desirable effects and more dependable results can be obtained when the extractive material is separated from plant and animal tissues and administered in a standardized form. Many drugs from the plant and the animal kingdoms are now isolated and purified before being administered. This eliminates undesired action due to other products in the extractive material and helps to provide a more accurate standardization and dosage of the specific compounds.

The cells of plants which contain these soluble principles vary in their compactness, cellular tissue and other properties, and these variations affect extraction. If the cells are grouped loosely and are encased in easily permeated walls, coarse pieces can be extracted rapidly and thoroughly. However, when the cells are grouped compactly and are encased in walls which are permeated by a solvent only with difficulty, the drug must be subdivided finely to facilitate thorough extraction.

Reduction to Powder. There are many medicinal agents which are administered internally or externally in the solid form, either alone or admixed with other solids. Compressed tablets, pills, capsules, powders, ointments, lotions and liniments are examples of preparations in which solids are employed. In order to ensure uniformity, to eliminate grittiness and, in general, to prepare products which are attractive, the solids must be reduced to powders and thoroughly mixed with or incorporated into the companion ingredients.

METHODS OF COMMINUTION

The comminution of animal and vegetable drugs presents problems which are not encountered in the production of fine chemical particles. The latter can be produced by a crushing action or by controlled precipitation. The crushing or the grinding of large aggregates of chemicals is facilitated by the absence of connective tissues and by the brittle rigidity of their particles. Animal and vegetable tissues are composed of groups of specialized cells bound together by tough connective and supporting fibers which resist subdivision. Although the anhydrous tissues are brittle and can be pulverized by rubbing or pounding in apparatus adapted to the reduction of chemical particles, these methods are not adapted to the powdering of large quantities of drugs. Therefore, apparatus and methods especially suited to the comminution of each class must be employed.

Cutting, Slicing and Chopping. These methods are employed on friable animal and plant drugs which need not be pulverized in order to be treated effectively with solvents for the extraction of their desirable principles. Any sharp cutting instrument such as a knife or a strong pair of scissors can be used to reduce thin barks, leaves, twigs or fine roots to the desired particle size. Leaves can be cut with an instrument composed of several disks mounted in fixed positions on an axle. Cutting is effected by rolling the instrument over a thin bed of leaves and exerting pressure on the handles as the cutter is rolled, exactly as is done in rolling out pastry dough with a rolling-pin.

The Wiley mill (Fig. 77) can be used for cutting large quantities of drugs by properly adjusting the knives and using the proper mesh of screen, through which the cut drug must fall.

Chopping is accomplished best by a long, sharp blade or group of blades attached to a common handle by means of a rigid frame. The drug is spread out on a smooth, soft surface which will not injure the blades and chopped until the desired degree of subdivision has been attained.

Rasping or Grating. Rasping or grating has very few pharmaceutical applications. One common example of its use in the practice of pharmacy is the grating of cocoa butter preparatory to making suppositories by hand or by the compression method. The ordinary household grater often is used for grating drug materials, although, for large amounts of material, rotary graters are preferred since they are more rapid and easier to operate.

Contusion or Bruising. This procedure is applied to fresh drugs in order to break down their supporting structure and render them more easily extracted. For example, when an essential oil is to be steam distilled from undried leaves, the leaves should be bruised thoroughly prior to distillation in order to ensure rapid and complete extraction of the oil.

Contusion must be brought about in an instrument which can withstand sharp blows. The instrument should be constructed of brass or any of the iron alloys which are durable. The contusion mortar must have a thick, flat base which permits it to be solidly supported and provides against breakage by the sharp blows dealt with the pestle.

The process of contusion is probably the oldest method for reducing substances to a fine state. It was used by the ancients for reducing grains to meal and flour for use as food. The instruments were often crude, being fashioned from stone or hollowed wood.

Pulverization by Intervention. The process of reducing substances to a fine state by the assistance of a second substance which easily can be removed at the end of the process is called pulverization by intervention. For example, camphor cannot be pulverized if triturated alone in a mortar. However, if the camphor is sprayed lightly with alcohol, ether, chloroform or some other volatile solvent, it easily can be reduced to a powder. When pulverization is complete, the camphor is spread out in a thin layer to permit the liquid to evaporate spontaneously. Gold leaf easily is reduced to a powder when it is triturated in the presence of potassium sulfate. The latter can be removed by the addition of water. Paper pulp can be triturated to a powder if a strong alkali such as sodium hydroxide is added. The alkali is removed with water, after which the powdered pulp is dried spontaneously or by the application of heat.

Trituration. The process of reducing the size of particles by rubbing them in a mortar with a pestle is called trituration. The process is characterized by a crushing and mixing effect as the pestle is plied under pressure in a circular movement.

Mortars and pestles are constructed of various types of materials. Those made of Wedgwood ware or glass are best suited for ordinary pharmaceutical operations. These properly are known as trituration mortars since they are fragile and must not be subjected to blows in the process of pulverization. The grinding action of these instruments is provided by their roughened surfaces. Wedgwood-ware mortars are porous and stain easily, but they are preferred to other types because of their durability.

Iron mortars and pestles are used when it is necessary to crush large aggregates of very hard materials. These substances must be dealt sharp blows before they will disintegrate. For example, fused masses of resinous material such as benzoin can be reduced to particle sizes more suitable for handling if they are chilled thoroughly and pounded in an iron mortar. Care must be exercised in the use of iron utensils since many products are rendered unfit for use by contact with iron. Mortars to be used for such vigorous service must be supported solidly to increase the efficiency of each blow dealt and to prevent breakage due to strains.

Levigation. This is the process of reducing the particle size of a solid by first forming a mass of the solid with a liquid, then grinding the mixture in a mortar with a pestle or on a slab with a spatula or muller, as in smoothing a small amount of an ointment. A muller is a flat-surfaced instrument shaped much like a collar button. A circular or figure-eight path of movement on the slab with the muller is used in grinding.

In the preparation of many ointments, powdered medicinal agents are incorporated into a fatty base in a state of subdivision that renders the powders invisible to the naked eye. For the most part, these powders cannot be reduced to the required particle size prior to their being incorporated into the base. When the powders are made into a concentrated paste with a portion of the fatty material, they can be reduced to extremely fine particles with little difficulty. The fatty base tends to hold the particles in position so that they can be crushed by the rubbing process. Zinc oxide can be reduced to an extremely fine state by levigation if it is made into a paste with light mineral oil.

Grinding. Grinding is as ancient as the use of grain foods by man. Although grinding to coarse particles and subsequent pulverization of coarse to fine particles was once the function of the housewife or the merchant, both processes now are performed at specialized milling centers. Whereas the druggist of former days comminuted his own crude drugs, these are now purchased as standardized powders ready for compounding. However, the possibility of acquiring commercially ground or pulverized drugs does not obviate the necessity for the pharmacist to be thoroughly familiar with the processes used. Lack of this knowledge indicates lack of familiarity with drug properties and may contribute to the improper storing and compounding of such drugs.

Drugs that are to be powdered finely must be dried thoroughly to destroy the elasticity of the tissues and to ensure the maximum capacity to be shattered. When

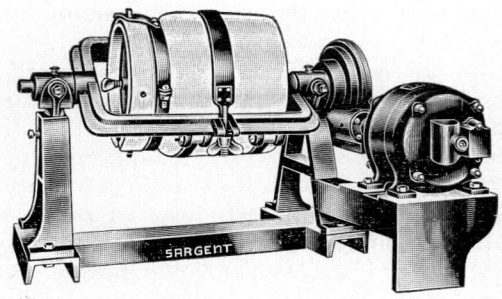

Fig. 75. Ball mill.

coarse particles are satisfactory, the drying need not be so thorough even though the coarse powder may be dried further before being stored. Those drugs which contain volatile constituents may be rendered unfit for use if subjected to dehydration. Spicy and odorous drugs (like clove, cinnamon, nutmeg, the various mint leaves) contain volatile oils which impart flavor and therapeutic significance to a host of pharmaceutical and food products. As in all vaporization processes, due to the enormous increase in the amount of surface produced the volatile constituents are lost from the surface of the drug and may escape almost completely in a very short time if the drug is reduced to minute particles.

MECHANICAL AIDS IN COMMINUTION

Burrstone Mill. One of the oldest of all mills is the burrstone mill. It was used by the founders of our country to grind the cereal grains which were used for food. Since the stone used in these mills must be very hard and the best has to be imported from France, steel burrs largely have replaced stone burrs at the present time. Burrstone mills operate by revolving either the lower or the upper burr against the other. The grinding surfaces must coincide perfectly in order that grinding will ensue over the entire area. Each burr bears a series of fine grooves or troughs, radiating from the center to the periphery, which provide passage for the powder to the outer edge of the burrs, where it falls into a receiver. The powder is forced outwardly by the centrifugal forces produced by the revolving burr. Fineness of the powder is regulated by adjusting the distance between the burr surfaces. The material to be ground is fed into the mill through an opening in the center of the upper burr. Steel burr mills operate along the same principles as burrstone mills and are more durable.

Ball Mill. The ball mill (Fig. 75) is composed of a porcelain or a glass jar provided with a cover which can be sealed tightly. The material to be comminuted is placed in the jar along with several steel, flint or porcelain balls. The jar is then fitted to a rotating machine and rotated at the desired rate until pulverization is complete. As the jar revolves, the enclosed material is pulverized by the balls as they fall. The ball mill finds extensive use in producing fine powders, in mixing powders, in incorporating medicinal agents into bases for external or internal application and in many other functions. It provides a satisfactory means of intimately mixing minute quantities of pure vitamins in special dietary foods used in biochemical research. It also finds use in homogeneously incorporating extremely active medicinal agents with certain diluents in order to attain accuracy in the amount administered.

Chaser Mill. The chaser mill consists of 2 thick disks of granite or other stone connected by a short axle which is rotated by a shaft attached perpendicularly to the center of the axle. The disks rest on a stone base which is surrounded by a curb to hold the coarse particles of the material being ground. A scraper in front of each disk keeps the material on the base continually in the path of the disks. As the disks are rotated, they appear to be chasing each other, hence the name for the mill. Grinding is produced by a crushing and skidding action much the same as that produced when an automobile skids on a dirt road when rounding a curve at high speed.

Roller Mill. The roller mill consists of 2 steel rollers bearing sharp corrugations which extend the full length of the rollers in long spirals. When viewed in cross section, the rollers have the appearance of a circular saw. The rollers rotate in the same direction but at different speeds so that the action of the mill is a combination of crushing and ripping.

Comminution

Mead Disintegrator. The Mead disintegrator (Fig. 76) operates at an exceedingly high speed and pulverizes a dry drug by throwing it against sharp steel screens until the drug is sufficiently fine to pass through the perforations. One type of screen is constructed of square steel bars between which the drug passes when it has been beaten to fine particles. Screens such as shown are employed when a very fine powder is demanded; they consist of hundreds of sharp-edged pyramids which provide a large cutting area. Each pyramid bears a perforation at its apex through which the powder must pass. The drug is fed into the mill through a hopper on the side. It is picked up by the beaters attached to the steel disk and thrown at a terrific speed against the screen, which faces about two thirds of the perimeter of the disk.

Bogardus Mill. The Bogardus mill consists of 2 horizontal plates bearing concentrically arranged, sharp-edged corrugations. The center of the lower plate does not coincide with the center of the upper plate so that, when the former revolves, it throws the drug at an angle against the sharp edges, which slice the drug to fine particles. Drugs that are not absolutely dry can be ground effectively in this mill.

Wiley Mill. The Wiley mill (Fig. 77) is efficient in comminuting both friable and fibrous drugs. It operates without elevating the temperature and consequently causes little loss of volatile material from the drug. It contains a revolving element carrying blades made of tool steel. These knives move with a shearing effect against knives mounted in the enclosing compartment. As the revolving element rotates, the drug is carried over a screen, through which it

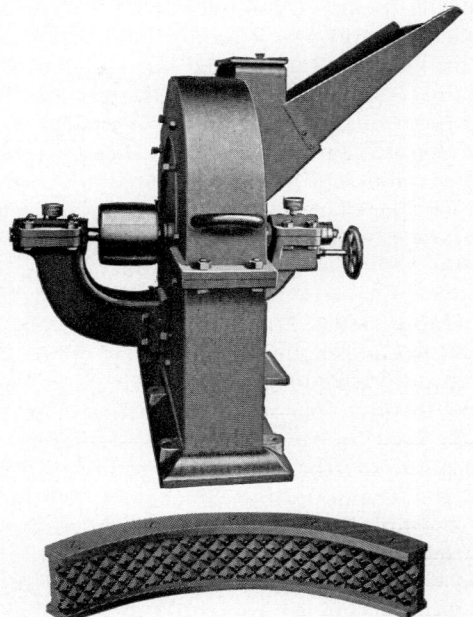

FIG. 76. Mead disintegrator. The illustration at the bottom shows a grinding surface.

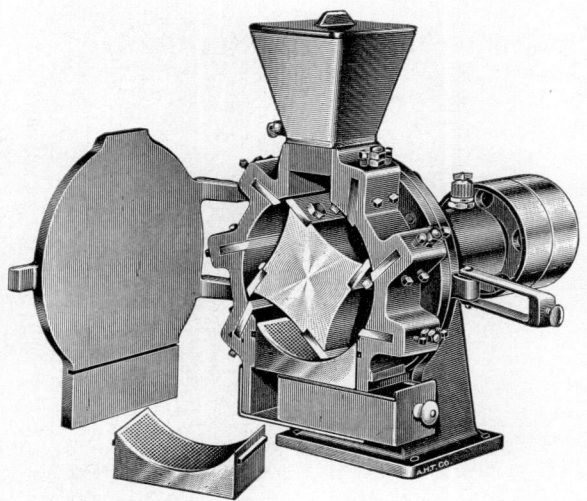

FIG. 77. Wiley mill.

passes into a receiving compartment when it has been sliced sufficiently fine. Therefore, the degree of fineness is determined by the mesh of the sieve through which the drug must pass.

Fitzpatrick Mills. These mills are available in more than 200 styles and combinations for comminuting many types of materials, chopping, emulsifying, mixing, dispersing solids in oily or other media, and for many other processing operations. They are constructed of noncorrosive metal or alloys, which prevents metallic contamination in the products being processed. Figure 78 shows a Model D Comminuting Machine and the comminuting chamber. This machine can be used for comminuting plant or chemical materials, wet or dry granulations, dispersion of powder mixtures, milling ointments, and other purposes. Some models are water-jacketed to permit processing of certain materials at low temperature without loss of volatile constituents. An example is the pulverizing of spices which contain volatile oils.

Hand Mills. Hand mills are now little used in the practice of pharmacy. They are employed primarily in the private laboratory for grinding small quantities of materials used in research work. It rarely is necessary for the pharmacist to mill a drug in the compounding of a stock product. These mills are found most often in trade outlets where coffee is freshly ground for the customer. Figure 79 illustrates a type of mill employed for this purpose. It is capable of reducing any dry vegetable material to a coarse powder. The grinding

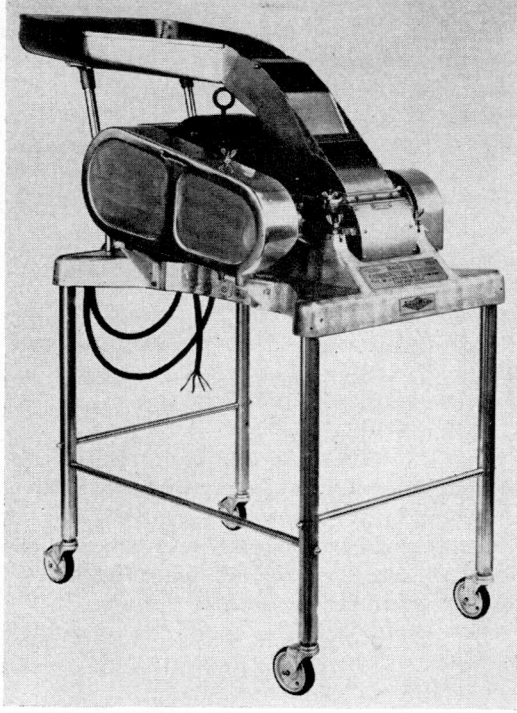

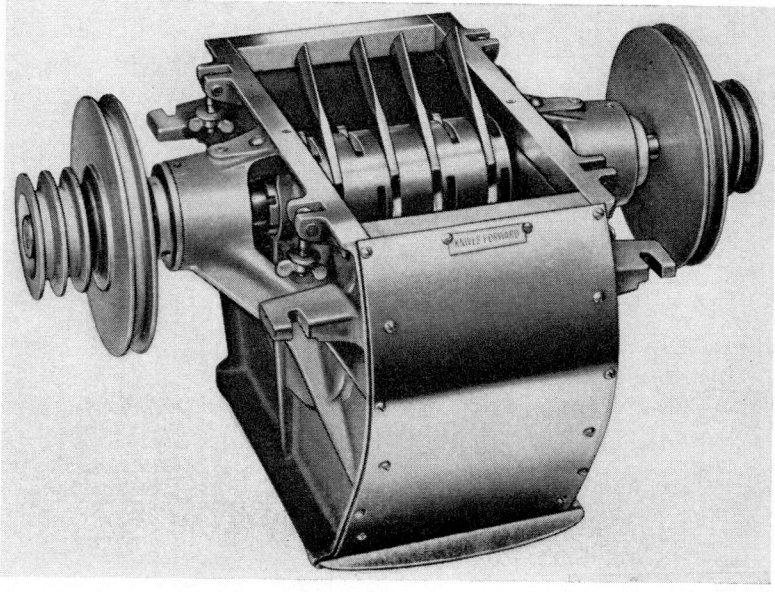

FIG. 78. Fitzpatrick Model D comminuting machine. (*Top*) Machine as assembled ready for use. (*Bottom*) Comminuting chamber.

plates stand vertically and can be adjusted to grind to different degrees of fineness.

PRECIPITATION

Precipitation is the formation of solid particles in a previously clear solution by a physical or chemical process. The objectives of precipitation are as follows: (1) to obtain chemicals in a fine, uniform state without the application of grinding, (2) to purify chemicals and (3) to make qualitative and quantitative tests for certain substances in a solution.

Chemicals to be used for therapeutic administration must be reduced to fine particles to facilitate their best method of administration. In order to obtain fine particles of a chemical, the process of precipitation is superior to grinding in that purification can be attained simultaneously. The grinding of a chemical provides no means of purification except by garbling or hand-picking coarse mixtures of solids. Also, grinding results in particles of heterogeneous rather than uniform sizes and shapes, which fact in itself renders even pure substances undesirable for some forms of administration. However, many compounds do not form precipitates sufficiently fine for the preparation of certain pharmaceutical products. This is especially true of solids to be used in ointments. In such cases, the solids must be reduced further in particle size by trituration or other suitable crushing procedures.

Precipitation as a means of purifying chemicals is used to provide products free from impurities which contribute nothing or may interfere with the usefulness of the chemicals. In qualitative analysis, the formation of precipitates by the addition of reagents to a clear solution indicates the presence of specific ions in the original solution. Observation of the color, the type and the quantity of the precipitate further aids in the identification of the ions and in estimating to what extent they are present.

Precipitation by Heating. Heating a solution containing albuminous material causes the albumins to be coagulated into large aggregates which can be removed by filtration. This phenomenon can be demonstrated by heating a dilute solution of egg albumin in water, whereupon the albumin will be coagulated to white, flocculent particles. Heating also causes precipitation of certain inorganic salts from their solutions. Hard water contains calcium and/or magnesium bicarbonate. Heating causes these bicarbonates to decompose to normal carbonates, carbon dioxide and water. The carbonates precipitate and gradually separate from the liquid. This fact is evidenced by the scale which collects in hot-water systems, in teakettles and in water baths in which hard water is heated. Heating Calcium Hydroxide Solution, U.S.P., produces a precipitate by decreasing the solubility of calcium hydroxide.

Precipitation by Cooling. Cooling a supersaturated solution causes separation of the dissolved material. A supersaturated solution is one in which the solute is present in an amount greater than its true

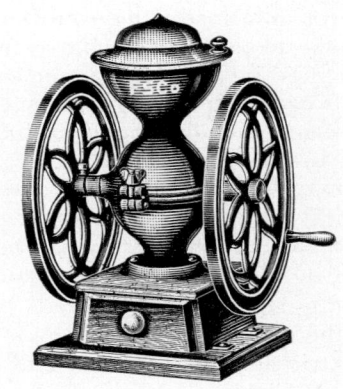

Fig. 79. Hand mill.

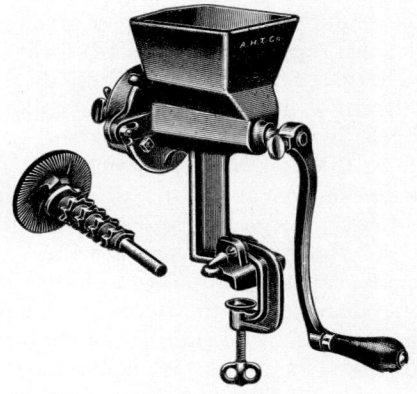

Fig. 80. Rotary grater.

solubility at a given temperature. This condition can be achieved by making a saturated solution at a given temperature, then cooling the solution a few degrees. Supersaturated solutions of certain salts sometimes fail to form precipitates as expected when they are cooled. This phenomenon often is encountered with salts capable of crystallizing with several molecules of water of crystallization, as does sodium sulfate $Na_2SO_4 \cdot 10H_2O$, sodium carbonate $Na_2CO_3 \cdot 10H_2O$ and ammonium alum $NH_4Al(SO_4)_2 \cdot 12H_2O$. If water is saturated with sodium sulfate at 30° C., the excess of solid removed and the solution allowed to cool without agitation in a covered vessel to exclude dust, often no precipitate will form when room temperature has been reached. Such abnormal solutions can be kept indefinitely if left undisturbed.

Crystallization. Crystallization in solutions such as described above can be effected by several means.

DISTURBANCE OF THE SOLUTION. A slight disturbance of the solution may cause crystals to form throughout the entire solution, with an accompanying evolution of heat.

SEEDING OR INOCULATION. Crystals also will start forming if a tiny fragment of the salt is laid on the surface of the solution. This process is called seeding or inoculation and provides a nucleus on which crystals can form. Most solutions require seeding with a fragment of the solute present; however, crystals will form in some solutions if a particle of dust, powdered glass or almost any minute particle is added to provide a nucleus.

ADDITION OF A LIQUID with which the solvent is miscible in all proportions, but in which the solute is insoluble, often will cause precipitation of a solute from its solution. For example, when absolute alcohol is added to a saturated aqueous sucrose solution, the sucrose will precipitate from the solution. Certain organic compounds can be precipitated from their aqueous solutions if the aqueous phase is saturated with sodium chloride. This process is known as "salting out."

CHEMICAL REACTIONS. Chemical reactions often result in the formation of precipitates. This fact is utilized in the synthesis and the analysis of many compounds. For instance, when a solution of barium chloride is added to a solution containing sulfate ions, barium sulfate is precipitated as a white solid. The reaction is represented empirically as follows:

$$BaCl_2 + Na_2SO_4 \rightarrow BaSO_4 + 2NaCl$$

Since barium sulfate precipitates quantitatively, this reaction can be used to determine the amount of barium or sulfate in an unknown.

The above equation represents the reaction between 2 nonvolatile, solid solutes to form 2 new compounds. Solids may also separate from a solution upon the introduction of a gas. The sulfides of some metals are precipitated when hydrogen sulfide is passed into a solution of their chlorides under certain conditions of acidity or alkalinity. The introduction of ammonia solution or other alkaline solutions will cause a few metals to precipitate as hydroxides. Metallic instruments cannot be used in preparing solutions containing copper sulfate because metallic copper will deposit on the instruments.

EXPOSURE TO LIGHT. This will cause some compounds to decompose and precipitate. A solution of silver proteinate, when exposed to light, will decompose gradually and liberate silver, which deposits on the sides of the container.

Iso-electric Point. An important property of colloidal particles is the fact that they generally bear an electric charge with respect to their surrounding medium. It can be demonstrated that, for a given colloidal solution, the particles all bear the same charge. For example, when an electric current is passed through a colloidal solution, the dispersed particles will accumulate at the pole of opposite charge. The movement of the charged particles, induced by an electric current, is known as cataphoresis. As the particles come within the sphere of electric charge around the pole, they are deprived of their charge and flocculation results. The stability of the original colloidal solution is dependent on the electric charge borne by the dispersed particles. These particles are in vigorous motion, but, as they approach each other, adhesion of the particles is prevented by a repelling electric sphere surrounding each particle. As the amount of charge on each particle is diminished by an electric current, the sphere of electric repulsion also is diminished until it is destroyed entirely and the particles are free to adhere to each other and to flocculate. The charge on colloidal particles also can be destroyed by the addition of a strong electrolyte, by mixing 2 colloidal solutions in which the particles are oppositely charged or by adjusting the acidity or the alkalinity (pH) of the solution. The point at which colloidal particles are deprived of their charge and flocculation occurs is called the iso-electric point.

TYPES OF PRECIPITATES

Crystalline Precipitates. Those solids which assume a characteristic, geometric pattern when they separate from their solutions are called crystalline precipitates. The ions of the compounds arrange themselves in a definite pattern so that many compounds can be identified by their crystal structure.

Amorphous Precipitates. Those precipitates in which the ions do not arrange themselves in a definite pattern and, therefore, form no characteristic or differentiable masses, are called amorphous precipitates. They may have a gummy or resinous appearance. In some instances, amorphous precipitates gradually will become crystalline if permitted to stand several days. This phenomenon is known as *devitrification*.

Light Precipitates. Light precipitates usually are produced from cold, dilute solutions. These solids are flaky and bulky and settle very slowly in water. Ordinarily, they are difficult to wash free of impurities. The large flakes may curl and form pockets or tubes which hold a portion of the mother liquor containing the impurities. They also may form agglomerates. Both tubes and agglomerates are difficult to destroy so that the entrapped solution of impurities can be liberated. They require vigorous agitation with several portions of wash liquid before they are freed entirely of contamination.

Heavy Precipitates. Heavy precipitates are produced from hot, concentrated solutions. They usually are fine and granular and settle to the bottom of the container very rapidly. Due to the fineness of the particles, these precipitates are washed free of impurities easily and rapidly.

COLLECTION OF PRECIPITATES

The method of collecting precipitates is dependent largely on the amount to be collected and the objective of the procedure. Small amounts of solids obtained in analytical procedures should be collected on the smallest filter paper possible, using an ordinary funnel if filtration is rapid or a Büchner funnel and vacuum filtration if filtration is slow, as in the case of gelatinous solids. Large batches of solids which are difficult to filter may be separated qualitatively from their mother liquor by colation or straining. The strained liquid then can be filtered to recover the last traces of solid material.

WASHING PRECIPITATES

The washing of precipitates involves 2 important considerations. The wash liquid must be one in which the impurities are readily soluble and in which the solid being washed is insoluble. The wash liquid may consist of pure water, dilute acid solutions, dilute alkali solutions, or any of the host of organic solvents. The following methods are employed in washing precipitates.

Lotion or Displacement Washing. This is a convenient method for washing large amounts of solids. The solid material is transferred to a filter or a strainer in such a manner that it is packed evenly to ensure uniform flow of the wash liquid through it. If the wash liquid is not to be recovered, it can be directed to the sink by means of a piece of rubber tubing. A constant and uniform flow of wash liquid can be provided by supporting an inverted bottle filled with the liquid in a position such that the neck of the bottle is a short distance above the surface of the solid. Flow of the liquid is controlled by atmospheric pressure, keeping the surface of the solids covered as long as liquid remains in the bottle. This method requires little attention and is efficient if the precipitate has an even firmness throughout to prevent channeling of the liquid through it.

Decantation. This is recommended whenever its use is possible. By this method, the solids are agitated vigorously with the wash liquid in a capacious container. After the solids have separated completely, the supernatant liquid is poured off as closely as possible without losing any of the precipitate. When the precipitate is disturbed easily during decantation, the liquid should be poured through a filter in order to avoid any loss of solid. This step is of further importance in the quantitative analysis of certain compounds wherein the precipitates are washed by decantation. Decantation is especially recommended for washing light precipitates which form tubes and, in general, give up their impurities with difficulty. Strong agitation assists in breaking up the aggregates to liberate the entrapped impurities. This method is not suited to the washing of precipitates which do not settle quickly and completely to the bottom of the container.

Siphoning. Siphons are used to convey a liquid from a high to a low level when some intermediate obstacle prevents its natural flow. A simple siphon can be prepared by bending a glass tube at an acute angle so that one arm is longer than the other. To illustrate the direction of flow from the tube, turn the ends upward and fill it with water. Place a finger over the end of the long arm and turn the tube to a siphoning position. When the finger is removed, all the water will escape through the long arm due to a combination of gravitational and vacuum effects. If the short arm of the tube is immersed in a liquid before permitting liquid to flow in the filled siphon, the flow of liquid will continue until the entire body of water has been removed from the vessel or the level of liquid in the receiving vessel becomes equal to that in the first vessel.

When removing the supernatant liquid from a solid, the solid sometimes is disturbed and drawn into the siphon by the liquid current set up at the mouth of the siphon. This can be remedied if the end of the arm above the solid is bent upward so that the liquid must first pass downward in the tube rather than rise directly in it.

There are several ways in which siphons can be started. All depend on the tendency of a liquid to flow from a high to a low level if permitted to do so. A simple method, where the supernatant liquid to be removed is aqueous and additional water is not objectionable, has been described above. When objections to this method are met, a siphon can be started as follows:

Pass the short arm of the siphon through a 2-holed stopper which fits tightly into the neck of the container from which the liquid is to be removed. Through the second perforation of the stopper insert a piece of glass tubing. Blowing through the latter tube creates additional pressure on the surface of the liquid, forcing it upward and through the siphon.

The vacuum method for filling a siphon has several modifications. A long rubber tube can be attached to the long arm of a siphon and the liquid drawn into the siphon by suction. When the siphon is filled, the rubber tube can be removed and the liquid will flow in a steady stream. This method is objectionable in transferring corrosive or otherwise dangerous liquids and, therefore, is not used commonly. A much better method is to pass the long arm of the siphon through a 2-holed stopper which fits tightly into the neck of the receiving vessel. Withdraw air from the receiving vessel through the second perforation in the stopper. As air pressure is decreased in this vessel, the liquid is forced into the siphon by atmospheric pressure and will flow as long as the 2 liquid levels are unequal. Once a siphon has started to flow, it is permitted to operate without the aid of an outside stimulus.

Siphons cannot operate unassisted if the upward-moving column exceeds approximately 33 feet in height. This fact is explained as follows: 1 atmosphere of pressure supports a column of mercury 76 cm. or 29.92 inches high at sea level. Since mercury is 13.456 times as heavy as water, a column of water 13.456 × 29.92 or 402.6 inches (33.55 ft.) high would be supported.

GRANULATION

Granulation is the production of fine crystals by disturbed crystallization. This can be effected by preparing a solution of a pure substance, evaporating the solution until a pellicle or film begins to form on the surface of the liquid, then stirring the mixture vigorously as it is cooled rapidly. Stirring prevents separation of the solute in a single mass, but rather as a fine, granular aggregation. Since granular salts are coarse, they can be washed conveniently in a funnel on a pledget of cotton.

SEPARATION OF PARTICLE SIZES

After drugs or chemicals have been comminuted or otherwise reduced in particle size, often they are separated into powders of standardized size specifications. Plant drugs, such as leaves, contain circulatory ducts which resist pulverization. Since these tissues are devoid of active constituents, they may be separated from the active portion of the drug without loss of medicinal value. It has been mentioned previously that drugs which are to be extracted with solvents require a degree of fineness according to their structural characteristics. In the process of comminution, a drug cannot be reduced to particles of identical size. A portion of the drug is reduced to a fine powder while much of it still remains as coarse material. Further comminution continues to reduce all the states of aggregation present, with the possible result that some of the drug will be too fine for practical use. In order to avoid this possibility, the drug should be alternately ground and sifted. This not only eliminates the portion that is sufficiently fine, but also, through reduction of the bulk, makes comminution of the remaining drug more rapid.

High-speed mills are provided with screens through which the drug passes when it has been reduced to the proper size.

The following processes are used to separate or grade powders according to their particle size.

Elutriation. This process is better known as water-sifting. It can be used to separate nonhydrating, inorganic powders which have been prepared by levigation or other processes. The levigated paste or dry powder is placed in an elutriating apparatus and highly diluted with water. The mixture is stirred thoroughly to distribute the solid throughout the liquid. When the mixture comes to rest, the solid remains suspended or completely settles out according to its state of subdivision. The very fine portion of the powder will remain suspended temporarily near the surface of the mixture and can be obtained by drawing off the suspension and evaporating it to dryness. An elutriating jar with outlets for withdrawing the mixture at various levels is illustrated in Figure 81. Powders much finer than could be obtained by the use of sieves can be separated by elutriation.

Garbling. This is the process of separating solids by "hand picking" the particles which are not desired in a mixture. This method of separation has very little pharmaceutical use except in sorting crude drugs to remove contaminants such as leaves, twigs, stones, etc.

Sifting. Sifting of materials has 2 purposes: (1) to separate solid particles into particles of approximately equal size and (2) to mix 2 or more fine powders intimately. As has been stated, plant drugs often contain structures which resist pulverization and contain little or no active material. These coarse particles often are separated from the fine, active portion of

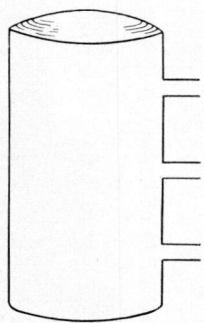

FIG. 81. Diagram of an elutriator showing outlets at different levels.

the drug by sifting. The separated inactive portion is called gruffs or tailings and is either discarded or used as a diluent for the active powder if the necessity arises.

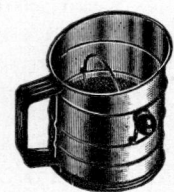

FIG. 82. Hand sifter.

Separation of the inert portion of the drug necessitates an adjustment in the dosage, especially if the drug contains a very active principle, since most of the active ingredient will be found in the decreased amount of powder.

One of the most familiar of all sieves is the one used in the home for sifting flour (Fig. 82). In this type of sieve, an agitator is revolved by means of an outside crank. The agitator scrapes and cleans the screen as it revolves and serves to disintegrate lumps of the material being sifted. Intimate mixtures of powders can be prepared by passing them through the sieve several times.

Figure 83 shows a group of sieves attached to a mechanical agitator. Powder is placed in the uppermost sieve, and agitation is continued until little or no powder passes from one sieve to another. When the sieves are of different degrees of fineness, the apparatus can be used to separate a powder into its various states of division. It also can be used to mix intimately 2 or more powders, if the sieves are of the same mesh.

Sieves are available in crude and standard forms. The crude forms are those used on farms, in kitchens, in pastry shops and in trades which do not require standardi-

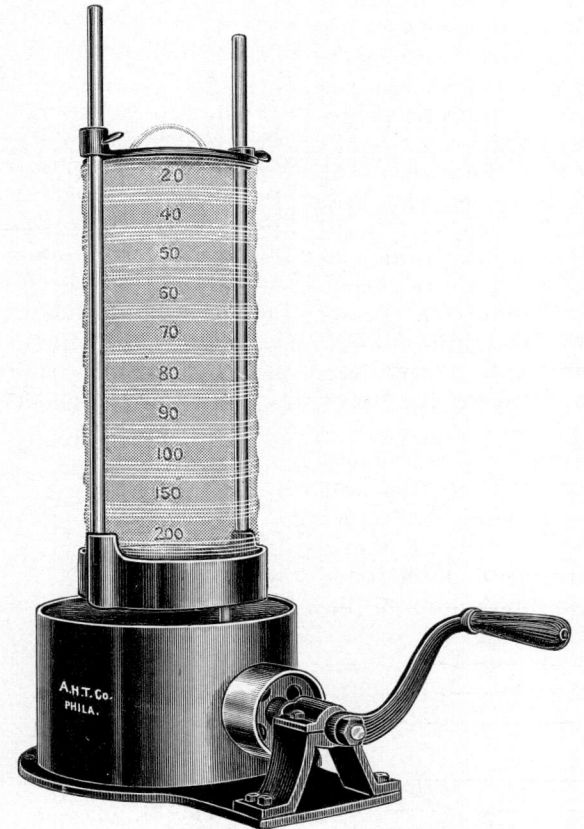

FIG. 83. A group of sieves and a mechanical agitator.

zation of powders. However, in describing pharmaceutical powders, a precise range of particle size is understood, and standard sieves have come into use to produce such powders. Sieves for pharmaceutical testing must be of cloth woven of bronze, brass or other suitable wire which will not be attacked by the materials to be sifted. The wire should not be plated or coated since the materials used for such treatment might become dislodged and contaminate the otherwise pure powders. Complete standardization of sieve and screen specifications has been effected by the National Bureau of Standards, so that not only the sieve number is given but also the area of free space and the size of the wire are specified. The sieve number in the N.B.S. series corresponds approximately to the number of openings per linear inch. This designation also has been adopted for standard screens.

SIZES OF POWDERS. Powders are designated by a number which refers to the size of sieve through which they will pass. In order to distinguish between powders in the various states of subdivision, the following specifications have been adopted for animal and plant drugs.

A very coarse powder, No. 8, must all pass through a No. 8 sieve and not more than 20 per cent through a No. 60 sieve.

A coarse powder, No. 20, must all pass through a No. 20 sieve and not more than 40 per cent through a No. 60 sieve.

A moderately coarse powder, No. 40, must all pass through a No. 40 sieve and not more than 40 per cent through a No. 80 sieve.

A fine powder, No. 60, must all pass through a No. 60 sieve and not more than 40 per cent through a No. 100 sieve.

A very fine powder, No. 80, must all pass through a No. 80 sieve. There is no limit as to how much finer this powder may be.

Due to the absence of connective tissues, chemicals are reduced to fine powders more readily by crushing than are animal and plant drugs. For this reason, the fineness of chemicals is indicated as follows:

A coarse powder, No. 20, must all pass through a No. 20 sieve and not more than 60 per cent through a No. 40 sieve.

A moderately coarse powder, No. 40, must all pass through a No. 40 sieve and not more than 60 per cent through a No. 60 sieve.

A fine powder, No. 80, must all pass through a No. 80 sieve.

A very fine powder, No. 120, must all pass through a No. 120 sieve.

In the case of the last 2 powders, no limit of fineness is affixed. From this fact, it is possible that a very fine powder also could be called a fine powder, while the opposite is not true.

Blowing or Air Sifting. Powders also can be separated into their particle fractions by blowing or air sifting. When a current of air is passed into the base of a tower containing a powder, the lighter particles of powder will be carried toward the top of the tower, while the coarser particles will remain nearer the bottom. The fine powder is then withdrawn into a settling room, where it is collected. This method is used to obtain extremely fine, "air-floated" powders to be used in the manufacture of cosmetics. It is also used to separate zinc oxide from its impurities after calamine is roasted. Calamine ore and coal are ground together and roasted in a furnace. The vapors are blown up through a large tower, permitting the heavier particles such as iron oxide to settle toward the bottom. The zinc oxide in the upper reaches of the tower is then blown into a room where it settles.

BIBLIOGRAPHY

Burlage, H. M., Burt, J. B., Lee, C. O., and Rising, L. W.: Introduction to Pharmacy, ed. 3, pp. 496–526, New York, McGraw-Hill, 1954.

Cook, E. F., and Martin, E. W.: Remington's Practice of Pharmacy, ed. 11, pp. 127–142, 226–232, Easton, Pa., Mack, 1956.

Jenkins, G. L., Christian, J. E., and Hager, G. P.: Quantitative Pharmaceutical Chemistry, ed. 5, pp. 31–65, 139–153, New York, McGraw-Hill, 1957.

United States Pharmacopeia, Sixteenth Revision, pp. 931–932, Easton, Pa., Mack, 1960.

KARL JOHN GOLDNER, Ph.D.
Professor of Pharmacy, University of Tennessee

6

Solutions

GENERAL CONSIDERATIONS
FACTORS AFFECTING SOLUBILITY
EFFECT OF OTHER SUBSTANCES ON SOLUBILITY
EXPRESSION OF SOLUBILITY
PERCENTAGE SOLUTIONS
SOLUTIONS OF LIQUIDS IN LIQUIDS

SOLUTIONS OF GASES IN LIQUIDS
SOLVENTS FOR PHARMACEUTICAL USE
PROPERTIES OF SOLUTIONS
DETERMINATION OF pH
BUFFER SOLUTIONS

GENERAL CONSIDERATIONS

A *dispersion* is a mixture produced by subdividing 1 material and scattering its particles throughout another. When bismuth subnitrate is mixed with water and the mixture allowed to stand, the salt gradually settles to the bottom of the container. Such a dispersion, in which the particles are large enough to be seen with the naked eye or with the aid of an ordinary microscope, is called a *suspension*.

If the dispersed particles are so small that they cannot be seen under the microscope but are still large in comparison with ordinary molecules, the mixture is called a *colloidal dispersion,* or *colloidal solution*. A knowledge of the properties of colloidal dispersions is essential for an understanding of biologic processes; this subject will be dealt with in a later chapter.

When the dispersed particles are so small that they consist of molecules or ions, the dispersion is a molecular dispersion, commonly called a *solution*. A solution may be defined as a mixture of 2 or more substances that is homogeneous by all tests and yet whose composition and properties are capable of being varied by imperceptible degrees, within certain limits of composition. For example, a solution of sugar in water may be varied from a very weak solution, whose sweetness scarcely can be tasted, to a very thick syrup.

Although solutions may be liquid, gaseous or solid, discussion will be confined to liquid solutions in which the dissolved substance may be liquid, gaseous or solid. This limitation is made because only liquid solutions are of particular importance in the manufacture of pharmaceuticals.

In a liquid solution of a solid or a gas, the liquid is termed the *solvent* and the other component the *solute*. When dealing with 2 liquids, the distinction is arbitrary. For example, water and alcohol mix in all proportions, and solutions might vary from practically pure water to practically pure alcohol. In this case, the component which is present in the larger amount usually is designated as the solvent.

If a small amount of a soluble salt is dissolved in water and the solvent is capable of dissolving more of the solute, the solution is said to be *unsaturated*. If the amount of solute is increased, a time will be reached when no more of the solute can be dissolved, except by changing the temperature. Such a solution is said to be *saturated*. At this point, molecules leave the surface of the solid and become dispersed throughout the solvent exactly as fast as other molecules of the same kind return from the liquid and become reattached to the solid. The solid is then in equilibrium with the solution, since solution and redeposition do not cease at this point but merely continue to balance each other. This can be shown by hanging an irregular crystal in a saturated solution of the same substance. It will neither increase nor decrease in weight, but it will improve its form, by the dissolving of material from certain faces and edges and the redeposition at others.

FACTORS AFFECTING SOLUBILITY

Supersaturation. When a saturated solution is in contact with excess solute and the temperature is raised, ordinarily more of the salt will dissolve. If such a solution is then filtered and cooled to the original temperature, it often will retain all the extra material that it dissolved at the higher temperature. Therefore, the solution now is supersaturated. A supersaturated solution often can be kept indefinitely, if it is kept protected from dust and evaporation. Crystallization can be induced by shaking the vessel vigorously, by scratching the sides of the vessel or by adding a fragment of the solute. Sodium thiosulfate and potassium acetate are examples of substances which readily form supersaturated solutions.

Solubility vs. Rate of Solution. A distinction should be made between solubility and rate of solution. An increase in the rate of solution does not mean an increase in the amount of solute which will dissolve. The rate of solution is dependent on the particle size of the substance to be dissolved and on agitation and temperature. Since solution takes place at the surface of the solid, an increase in the surface will result in an increased rate of solution. It is for this reason that we commonly grind crystals in a mortar before attempting to dissolve them. It also explains why pharmacists prefer to purchase salts in the granular rather than the crystalline form.

Circulatory Displacement. As a solid dissolves, it becomes surrounded by a saturated solution, and the rate of solution is decreased greatly. The common procedure to bring fresh or unsaturated solvent to the solid is to stir the liquid. Another process which is used for the same purpose is called circulatory displacement (Fig. 84). The solid is suspended in a bag or placed on a shelf near the surface of the solvent and, as it dissolves, forms a solution which is denser than the solvent. This solution consequently sinks, and fresh solvent rises, creating a circulation and thereby increasing the rate of solution. Circulatory displacement commonly is used in chemical factories, because shaking several tons of a mixture is out of the question, and stirring is prohibitive in cost. The material may be dissolved in a surprisingly short time and without any labor.

Heating Liquids. Heating a liquid also causes solution to take place more rapidly by increasing the frequency with which solvent molecules collide with the surface of the dissolving material. With increased molecular motion, diffusion increases, hastening the removal of the material just dissolved and tending to maintain a condition of unsaturation around the solid.

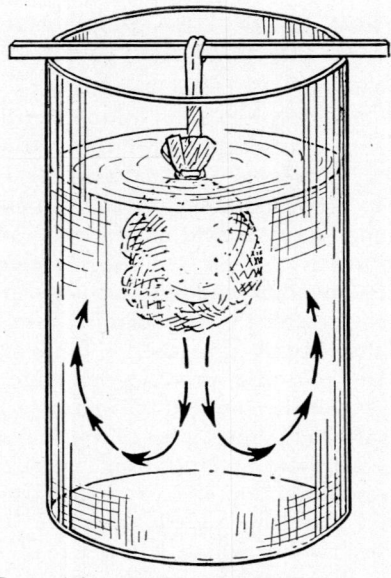

Fig. 84. Circulatory displacement.

Increase in Temperature. With most solids, an increase in temperature not only speeds up the process of solution but also increases the total weight dissolved. If a saturated solution in equilibrium with excess solute is heated, a change takes place which will absorb heat and thereby tend to restore the original conditions. Since the dissolving of a solid to form a liquid involves a change from the solid to the liquid state, which is an endothermic process, the application of heat will cause more of the solute to go into solution. Sometimes a chemical reaction, such as hydration, takes place between the solute and the solvent, with the evolution of heat (exothermic process). This heat may be greater than the heat of solution, and the temperature will rise. This is true for sodium and potassium hydroxides in which the heat evolved may be sufficient to cause the water to boil. However, when sodium or potassium hydroxide is dissolved in an almost saturated solution, the process is endothermic, and it is found that these substances are more soluble at higher temperatures. A few substances which give off heat during solution are more soluble in cold than in hot water. Some calcium compounds belong to this group. Thus, calcium hydroxide is soluble to the extent of 0.17 Gm. per 100 ml. of water at 15° but only 0.14 Gm. at 25° C.

EFFECT OF OTHER SUBSTANCES ON SOLUBILITY

In general, a saturated solution is capable of dissolving another solute, but at the same time the solubility of the first solute is either increased or decreased. It is difficult to predict the behavior of nonelectrolytes and very soluble electrolytes. When the solute is a slightly soluble electrolyte and the substance added furnishes an ion already present in the saturated solution, the solubility is decreased. This follows from the solubility-product principle. Advantage of this common-ion effect is taken in qualitative and quantitative analysis, where complete precipitation is desired.

The common-ion effect is complicated by the fact that the added substance always furnishes an ion which is not already present in the solution. These attract oppositely charged ions in the crystal lattice and assist in bringing them into solution. Thereby the solubility of the original substance is increased. This "electrostatic effect" is most pronounced when doubly or triply charged ions are present in the solution or are added. It may be great enough to more than compensate for the common-ion effect.

The solubility-product principle holds for aqueous solutions of slightly soluble salts, provided that the concentration of added salt is not too great. For example, a dilute solution of sodium chloride decreases the solubility of silver chloride, but larger concentration of sodium chloride causes an increase in solubility. It is still true that

$$[Ag^+][Cl^-] = S$$

but another equilibrium also has been established in the solution:

$$Ag^+ + 2Cl^- \rightarrow AgCl_2^-$$

As the concentration of chloride ions is increased, the concentration of the complex chloroargentate ion, $AgCl_2^-$, also is increased. This results in a removal of simple ions from solution, and more of the solid dissolves until a new condition of equilibrium is reached. This is an example of the complex-ion effect.

In pharmacy, mercuric iodide frequently is dissolved by the addition of a soluble iodide, such as potassium iodide. A complex ion is formed:

$$Hg^{++} + 4I^- \rightarrow HgI_4^=$$

The equation for this reaction often is written:

$$HgI_2 + 2KI \rightarrow K_2HgI_4$$

The solubility of iodine in a solution of a soluble iodide is explained by the tendency of halogen atoms to share electrons, forming a covalent bond. They form diatomic molecules, such as I_2, and also interhalogen molecules, such as ICl and BrCl. The large radius of the iodine atom probably is responsible for its forming the triiodide ion, I_3^-. As a result, iodine dissolves freely in solutions of soluble iodides, forming a dark brown solution.

$$I_2 + I^- \rightarrow I_3^-$$

Several official preparations, among them strong iodine solution and iodine tincture, are made by the use of this principle.

EXPRESSION OF SOLUBILITY

The solubility of a substance may be expressed as the number of grams required to saturate 100 Gm. of water. The solubility curves for several common substances are shown. The solubility, expressed in grams of the anhydrous compound in 100 Gm. of water, is plotted as ordinate and the temperature as abscissa. Note that the solubility of sodium chloride is almost unaffected by changes in temperature.

The solubility of a substance may be expressed in several ways:

1. As in Figure 85, that is, the number of grams of solute that will dissolve in 100 Gm. of solvent.

2. **The U.S.P. and the N.F. Method.** These books of standards give the number of milliliters of solvent required to dissolve 1 Gm. of solute. For example, it is stated that "One Gm. of Sucrose dissolves in 0.5 ml. of water and 170 ml. of alcohol. It dissolves in slightly more than 0.2 ml. of boiling water and is insoluble in chloroform and in ether." Such statements are not intended as physical constants for the determination of identity or purity but are included for the information of the pharmacist when preparing and dispensing medicines.

3. **Percentage of Solute, by Weight.** This method gives the number of grams of solute in 100 Gm. of a saturated solution.

4. **Percentage of Solute, Weight in Volume.** This method gives the number of grams of solute in 100 ml. of a saturated solution.

5. **Molar Solubility.** This method uses the number of moles of solute which are contained in 1 liter of a saturated solution. This may be calculated by dividing the number of grams of solute in a liter of a saturated solution by the molecular weight of the solute.

6. **General Terms.** Where the exact solubility is not known, descriptive terms are applied in the *U.S.P.* and the *N.F.* These terms and their meanings are given in Table 4.

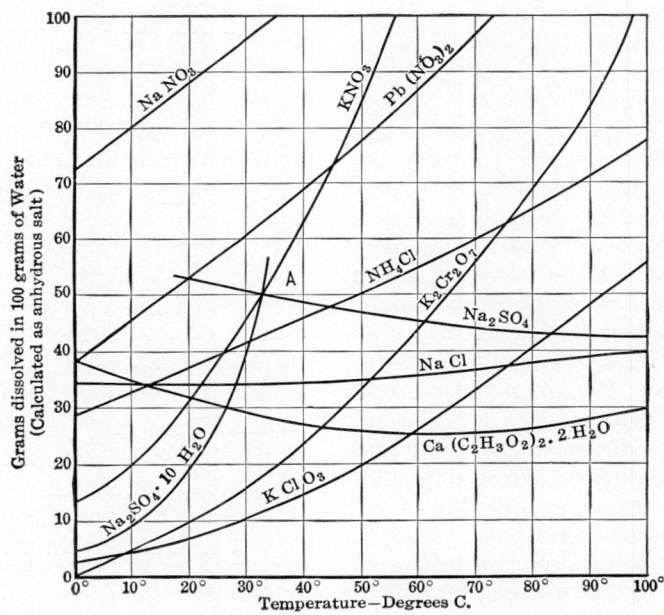

FIG. 85. Solubility curves. (Deming, H. G.: Fundamental Chemistry, New York, Wiley)

TABLE 4. GENERAL TERMS USED TO EXPRESS SOLUBILITY

Descriptive Terms	Relative Quantity of Solvent for 1 Part of Solute
Very soluble	Less than 1 part
Freely soluble	From 1 to 10 parts
Soluble	From 10 to 30 parts
Sparingly soluble	From 30 to 100 parts
Slightly soluble	From 100 to 1,000 parts
Very slightly soluble	From 1,000 to 10,000 parts
Practically insoluble	More than 10,000 parts

7. Solubility Product. The solubility of very slightly soluble salts may be expressed in terms of their respective solubility products. Thus, a saturated solution of silver chloride will contain 1.5 mg. per liter, or 1.1×10^{-5} moles. Being completely ionized, it will yield 1.1×10^{-5} moles of silver ions and an equal number of moles of chloride ions. The solubility product is, therefore, $(1.1 \times 10^{-5})(1.1 \times 10^{-5})$, or 1.2×10^{-10}.

Determination of Solubility. The solubility of a solid can be found by preparing a saturated solution and determining by analysis the quantity of the solute in a definite weight of solution. The solvent and an excess of solid are placed in a test tube equipped with a motor-driven, glass spiral stirrer. The tube is immersed in a constant-temperature bath, and the contents are stirred vigorously for several hours. After this time, the stirrer is removed, the tube is stoppered and the excess solid is allowed to settle. A portion of the clear supernatant liquid is removed and weighed accurately. This portion is evaporated to dryness on a water bath and finally heated to constant weight in an oven. The weight of the residue is then determined.

From the weight of the sample taken and the weight of the residue, the solubility of the substance, in grams per 100 Gm. of solvent, can be calculated easily. For example, a portion of a saturated solution of potassium bromide, at 25° C., weighed 6.830 Gm. and yielded a residue of 2.732 Gm. The amount of water in the solution would be 6.830 − 2.732 or 4.098 Gm. The weight of potassium bromide that will dissolve in 100 Gm. of water would then be 2.732 (100 ÷ 4.098) or 66.7 Gm.

In the determination, particular attention must be paid to the following:

1. The solvent and the solute must be pure, since impurities in either will affect the solubility.

2. The temperature must be kept constant, since the solubility of many substances varies markedly with the temperature.

3. The dissolving substance should be in a fine state of subdivision to hasten solution.

4. Stirring must be adequate.

5. An additional determination must be made after a longer period of stirring to make certain that saturation had been accomplished.

PERCENTAGE SOLUTIONS

The subject of percentage solutions is an important one to the pharmacist because he frequently is called upon to prepare such solutions on prescription. Percentage means parts per 100 parts, and, for a true percentage solution, the parts involved must be of the same kind. However, the term "percentage" commonly is applied to a solution which contains a certain number of grams of an active constituent in 100 ml. of solution. The *U.S.P.* defines the various kinds of percentage solutions as follows:

"Per cent 'weight in weight' *(w/w)* expresses the number of Gm. of a constituent in 100 Gm. of solution.

"Per cent 'weight in volume' *(w/v)* expresses the number of Gm. of a constituent in 100 ml. of solution and is used in prescription practice regardless of whether water or another liquid is the solvent.

"Per cent 'volume in volume' *(v/v)* expresses the number of ml. of a constituent in 100 ml. of solution."

There formerly existed some controversy as to whether solutions of solids should be prepared weight in weight or weight in volume, and, consequently, there was lack of uniformity in the preparation of percentage solutions. While there is little difference in the strength of solutions prepared by these

2 methods when the concentration is below 5 per cent, above this percentage there is an appreciable difference. For uniformity, the *U.S.P.* now states that, for solutions of solids in liquids, weight in volume solutions are to be prepared, unless otherwise specified in the prescription. These not only are prepared more easily but also are in accord with our customary method of making liquid preparations to a definite volume. Since a dose of a liquid preparation is invariably measured, the amount of solute in a dose is calculated more easily. Solutions of liquids in liquids are to be prepared volume in volume and solutions of gases in liquids, weight in volume.

Solids in Liquids. In the preparation of w/v solutions, calculations in the metric system are very simple. The number of milliliters required is multiplied by the per cent, expressed as a decimal fraction. For example, 60 ml. of a 5 per cent solution would require 60×0.05, or 3.0 Gm. of the active ingredient. This amount is dissolved in enough solvent to make 60 ml. The same quantity of active ingredient is used regardless of the specific gravity of the solvent used.

If the prescription is written in the apothecaries' system, the same procedure can be followed by multiplying the weight of a fluidounce of water (455 gr.) by the number of fluidounces and by the per cent, again expressed as a decimal fraction. For example, 4 fluidounces of a 10 per cent solution would require $455 \times 4 \times 0.10$, or 182 gr. of active ingredient. The *U.S.P.* suggests the following method. Since 4.5 gr. of active ingredient will make 1 fluidounce of a 1 per cent solution, the figure 4.5 is to be multiplied by the number of fluidounces and by the per cent, now expressed as a whole number. The above solution would then require $4.5 \times 4 \times 10$, or 180 gr. of active ingredient.

Another commonly used method, which has the disadvantage of a change from one system to another but has the advantage of simplicity, is to replace the fluidounces by milliliters, i.e., instead of making 4 fluidounces, to make 120 ml., a quantity very slightly more. By this method, $120 \times$ 0.10, or 12 Gm. of active ingredient will be used and enough solvent to make 120 ml.

It is difficult to prepare a definite volume of a percentage solution by weight, since ordinarily neither the volume occupied by the solute nor the specific gravity of the finished solution is known. Therefore, it becomes necessary to take as much solvent as is desired of finished solution and add enough of the active ingredient to make the required percentage. For example, if one were to prepare 500 ml. of a 10 per cent solution by weight of potassium iodide, one would take 500 ml. of water and add enough potassium iodide until it was 10 per cent of the total weight. The water used would now be $100 - 10$, or 90 per cent of the total. The amount of potassium iodide could be calculated according to the following proportion:

$$10 : 90 :: x : 500$$

$$x = 55.6$$

Therefore, 55.6 Gm. of potassium iodide would be dissolved in 500 ml. of water. The volume of the finished solution would be greater than 500 ml., and the excess solution then would be either furnished the customer, discarded or kept in stock, depending on circumstances and the cost and the stability of the preparation.

If some solvent other than water is used, the volume, in milliliters, must be multiplied by the specific gravity of the solvent. For example, if it is desired to prepare 240 ml. of a 2 per cent solution, by weight, of salicylic acid in alcohol, the specific gravity of which is 0.82, the amount of salicylic acid to be added to 240 ml. of alcohol would be calculated as follows:

$$240 \times 0.82 = 196.8 \text{ Gm. of alcohol.}$$

$$2 : 98 :: x : 196.8$$

$$x = 4.0 \text{ Gm. of salicylic acid.}$$

Liquids in Liquids. Percentage solutions of liquids are prepared volume in volume. A 5 per cent solution of acetone in water contains 5 ml. of acetone in 100 ml. of solution. To calculate the quantity of active ingredient needed to make a particular solution, the number of milliliters required is multiplied by the per cent, expressed as a decimal fraction. Thus, 250 ml. of a 5 per cent solution of acetone would require 250 × 0.05, or 12.5 ml. of acetone. When the quantity desired is given in the apothecaries' system, the number of minims of solution desired is first calculated and then multiplied by the per cent, expressed as a decimal fraction. Thus, 8 fluidounces of a 5 per cent solution of acetone would require 480 × 8 × 0.05, or 192 minims of acetone. Since 4.8 minims will make 1 fluidounce of a 1 per cent solution, the same result can be obtained by multiplying 4.8 by the number of fluidounces and by the per cent, now expressed as a whole number. Thus, 4.8 × 8 × 5 = 192 minims.

The concentration of dilute solutions of solids commonly is expressed, not in terms of percentage, but in terms of the number of milliliters which will contain 1 Gm. of the active ingredient. A 1 in 1,000 solution, abbreviated 1-1,000 or 1:1,000, would then contain 1 Gm. of active ingredient in 1,000 ml. of solution. The number of grams needed to make a solution of this kind is found by dividing the number of milliliters required by the number of milliliters which will contain 1 Gm. of the active ingredient. Thus, 500 ml. of a 1:1,000 solution of mercury bichloride will require 500 ÷ 1,000, or 0.5 Gm. of mercury bichloride, to be dissolved in enough water to make 500 ml. When the desired quantity is given in the apothecaries' system, the weight of that quantity of water is calculated first and then this is divided by the number of grains which are to contain 1 gr. of active ingredient. Thus, 16 fluidounces of a 1:1,000 solution of mercury bichloride would require (455 × 16) ÷ 1,000, or 7.3 gr. of mercury bichloride, to be dissolved in enough water to make 16 fluidounces.

SOLUTIONS OF LIQUIDS IN LIQUIDS

When 2 liquids, such as alcohol and water, are mixed, they form 1 homogeneous liquid, regardless of the proportions in which each is taken. Such pairs of liquids are said to be miscible in all proportions. Other pairs of liquids, such as ether and water, dissolve in each other to a definite, limited extent. When such liquids are mixed, they soon separate into 2 layers, the lighter, on top, being a solution of water in ether, and the heavier, beneath, a solution of ether in water. Such pairs of liquids are said to be immiscible.

Although molecules are electrically neutral, the positive and the negative charges in the molecules are not always distributed symmetrically. The result is that molecules of some substances are polar —that is, they behave as though they had a positive and a negative pole. Of course, there are relative degrees of polarity. Polar molecules in a liquid are attracted to each other and tend to form chains, in which they are arranged positive pole to negative pole. These chains are constantly being broken and reformed, due to molecular motion. We should expect polar molecules to be attracted to polar molecules of other substances and not to nonpolar molecules. Therefore, polar substances (such as water) should dissolve solutes composed of polar molecules and should be miscible with other polar liquids. When mixed with nonpolar liquids, the polar molecules pull together and, in effect, squeeze out the nonpolar molecules. The molecules of a nonpolar liquid possess a slight gravitational attraction for one another, and so nonpolar liquids, in general, are miscible with other nonpolar liquids. Examples of polar liquids are: water, methyl and ethyl alcohols and liquid ammonia. Nonpolar liquids include many organic solvents, such as the petroleum hydrocarbons, carbon tetrachloride, benzene, toluene, etc.

SOLUTIONS OF GASES IN LIQUIDS

A gas can be dissolved by bubbling it through a liquid or by confining the liquid and the gas in a vessel. Some gases are very soluble, others are not. The molecules of the gases that are condensed with difficulty are nearly nonpolar and attract one another very slightly. Therefore, they do not attract water molecules and so are but slightly soluble. Such gases include nitrogen, oxygen, hydrogen and helium. For example, oxygen dissolves to the extent of about 3 per cent, by volume.

The molecules of the more readily condensable gases are somewhat polar and attract one another more strongly. They also attract solvent molecules and so are soluble to the extent of several hundred per cent, by volume. Such gases include carbon dioxide, sulfur dioxide and nitrogen monoxide, which react to some extent with water to form carbonic acid, sulfurous acid, etc. The molecules of some readily condensable gases, such as ammonia and hydrogen chloride, are so polar that they react extensively with water. Such gases are very soluble and dissolve to the extent of several thousand per cent, by volume.

The solubility (by weight) of a gas is very nearly proportional to the pressure, provided that the gas is only slightly soluble. This is the law of Henry, which applies to slightly soluble gases but less accurately to the moderately soluble gases and not at all to the readily soluble gases. These react chemically with the water, and, therefore, their solubility is increased only slightly by increased pressure.

The solubility of a gas in a liquid decreases as the temperature is raised. For example, carbon dioxide is twice as soluble at $0°$ as it is at $20°C$. It is for this reason that we cool solutions of gases before opening the container and releasing the pressure. Supersaturated solutions of gases are common. Carbonated beverages are supersaturated solutions, as may be shown by shaking an open bottle. Copious effervescence takes place, and the gas leaves the solution until it becomes merely saturated at the given temperature and atmospheric pressure.

SOLVENTS FOR PHARMACEUTICAL USE

The statement has been made that "like dissolves like." That is, a substance is most soluble in the solvents to which it is related chemically. However, the choice of a solvent for pharmaceutical use is narrowed by other considerations, among which are the toxicity, the volatility and the flammability of the solvent, as well as the stability of the solution.

Water. The most universally used solvent is water. Not only is it available in unlimited quantities, but also it has a wide range of usefulness. It is the best solvent for most inorganic salts and, in addition, it dissolves many organic compounds. Many plant constituents, such as sugars, gums, tannins and albuminous substances, are extracted by water.

Alcohol is the next most useful solvent. It dissolves many organic substances, both synthetic and natural, including important plant constituents, such as resins, and volatile oils, alkaloids, glycosides and neutral principles. It has an advantage over water in that solutions in alcohol are not subject to deterioration through the growth of micro-organisms. It often is used diluted with water in the preparation of tinctures, fluidextracts, etc. Such hydroalcoholic liquids have the advantage of conserving alcohol and, at the same time, dissolving active principles and leaving behind most of the inactive plant constituents, the so-called extractive matter. Alcohol is flammable and volatile and boils at $78°C$.

Dehydrated alcohol (absolute alcohol) contains not less than 99 per cent by weight of C_2H_5OH. Being practically free from water, it has a greater range of solvent power. For example, it is miscible with paraffin hydrocarbons, and in some countries it is added to gasoline as a motor fuel. Its chief use in pharmacy is in research and analytical work and in the preparation of synthetic organic medicinals.

Isopropyl alcohol, $(CH_3)_2CHOH$, boils at $82.4°C$. and has solvent properties similar to those of ethyl alcohol. Like ethyl alcohol, it has germicidal and disinfectant properties. Being anhydrous, it may be used to advantage in keeping hypodermic needles and other metallic instruments which are prone to rust in ethyl alcohol. It is used as a rubbing alcohol and in liniments, skin lotions, cosmetics, hair tonics, etc. It should not be taken internally, owing to its toxic nature. It was admitted to *N.F. IX.*

Glycerin (glycerol, $CH_2OH \cdot CHOH \cdot CH_2OH$) is obtained by the saponification of fats or from propylene, a product of petroleum. It is miscible with both water and alcohol but not with chloroform or ether, or with fixed oils, despite the fact that it is prepared from them. It is an excellent solvent for tannins, phenol and boric acid.

Preparations in which glycerin is the solvent are called glycerites. While tannins are very soluble in water, they tend to agglomerate and precipitate on standing. The addition of glycerin to such solutions prevents this precipitation and keeps the preparation clear. Wild cherry syrup is an example of a preparation in which this principle is used. In its concentrated form, glycerin acts as a preservative. It frequently is used in ear drops because it softens wax but does not become rancid as do the vegetable oils.

Propylene glycol, $CH_3 \cdot CHOH \cdot CH_2OH$, is a clear, colorless, practically odorless, viscous liquid with a slightly acrid taste. It is miscible with water and alcohol in all proportions, and is soluble in ether, acetone and chloroform. It will dissolve many essential oils but is immiscible with fixed oils. When exposed to moist air, it absorbs moisture. It has a wide range of usefulness as a solvent, dissolving such substances as sulfonamides, local anesthetics, antiseptics, vitamins A and D, sex hormones and phenothiazine. The toxicity of propylene glycol is about the same as the toxicity of glycerin, and permission was given for the wartime substitution of propylene glycol for glycerin in a number of elixirs and solutions and in some other miscellaneous preparations.

Polyethylene glycol 400 is represented by the formula $HOCH_2(CH_2OCH_2)nCH_2OH$, where n varies from 8 to 10. It is a clear, colorless, viscous liquid. It is a very versatile solvent, dissolving water-soluble organic compounds and many which are insoluble in water, such as acetylsalicylic acid, ethyl aminobenzoate and theophylline. Feeding experiments have shown it to be nontoxic in the amounts in which it would be used.

Ethyl oxide (solvent ether, $C_2H_5 \cdot C_2H_5$) is soluble to the extent of 1 volume in 12 volumes of water. It is miscible with alcohol, benzene, chloroform, petroleum benzin, and with fixed and volatile oils. It is highly volatile and boils at 35°C. It is flammable, and, when its vapor is mixed with air, it may explode violently upon ignition. It dissolves oils, fats, resins and many alkaloids. It may be used to extract oleoresins from aspidium, capsicum and ginger. Although pyroxylin is insoluble in either ethyl oxide or alcohol alone, it may be dissolved in a mixture of 3 volumes of ethyl oxide and 1 of alcohol to form collodion.

Petroleum benzin (purified benzin) is a purified distillate from petroleum and consists of hydrocarbons, chiefly of the methane series. It is immiscible with water but miscible with dehydrated alcohol, ether, chloroform, benzene and with most fixed and volatile oils. It distills between 35° and 80°C. It is highly flammable, and its vapor, when mixed with air and ignited, may explode. Its chief use in pharmacy is for the removal of objectionable waxes and fats from ergot and strophanthus before extracting the active principles with alcohol or a hydroalcoholic menstruum.

Acetone (dimethyl ketone, $CH_3 \cdot CO \cdot CH_3$) is miscible with water, alcohol, ether, chloroform and most volatile oils. It boils at about 56°C. and volatilizes even at low temperatures. While it is flammable, there is not the danger of explosion that there is with ether, and so it has been used in preparing oleoresins, despite its higher cost.

Chloroform, $CHCl_3$, is soluble to the extent of about 0.5 per cent in water. It is miscible with alcohol, ether, benzene, petroleum benzin, and with fixed and volatile oils. It is nonflammable, but its vapor is decomposed by a naked flame, producing noxious gases. It is a solvent for many alkaloids and is used in alkaloidal assaying. It has also been used as a solvent for phosphorus in phosphorus pills. A solution of coal tar in chloroform was official in the N.F., and chloroform can be used to remove coal tar from utensils as well as from the skin.

Carbon tetrachloride, CCl_4, is only very slightly soluble in water but is miscible with the common organic solvents. It distills between 76° and 78°C. It dissolves fats and oils and commonly is sold in drugstores as a spot remover. It has the advantage over petroleum benzin in being nonflammable.

Benzene, C_6H_6, is obtained from coal tar. It boils at 80.6°C., and congeals at 5.4°C. It is immiscible with water but miscible with the common organic solvents. Its chief pharmaceutical use is not as a solvent but as the starting point in the synthesis of many organic medicinals.

Carbon disulfide, CS_2, boils between 46° and 47°C. It is immiscible with water but very soluble in common organic solvents. It is an excellent solvent for rubber and sulfur, but its flammability, disagreeable odor and toxicity have limited its use greatly.

Modern Solvents. Before World War I, there were only about a dozen industrial solvents of any importance. Since that time, there has been a remarkable growth in the solvent industry. Hundreds of organic solvents have been developed for industrial and commercial purposes and, of these, about 300 are now being produced on an industrial scale. The main sources of these substances are petroleum, coal tar, forest and agricultural products. Compounds which occur naturally are modified or converted to entirely new substances by physical and chemical processes. Chemically, they include a great variety of organic compounds, ranging from hydrocarbons through alcohols, esters, ethers and acids to the newly developed nitroparaffins. They find their main applications in the lacquer, the paint, the varnish and the textile industries. Some are used in the preparation of synthetic rubber and in the rapidly growing field of plastics. While many are used in the synthesis of organic medicinals, few are used as solvents by the pharmacist. In the field of cosmetics, we find Carbitol used as a glycerin substitute, and morpholine, the ethanol and propanol amines, and amines derived from the nitroparaffins used as emulsifying agents, in combination with fatty acids.[1]

PROPERTIES OF SOLUTIONS

Several properties of solutions are related because the change in properties is dependent on the number of molecules in solution in a given volume. These properties, which are dependent on the number of molecules and not on their kind, are called colligative and include lowering vapor pressure, raising osmotic pressure, raising boiling point and lowering freezing point.

The molecules of a liquid are in constant motion, and, if the liquid is in an open vessel, some of the molecules will leave the surface of the liquid and enter the gaseous state. This results in evaporation. However, if the vessel is closed, the air above the liquid eventually will become saturated with vapor, and a state of equilibrium is reached wherein molecules leave the surface of the liquid at the same rate at which they re-enter. The pressure exerted by the vapor above the liquid is a constant at a given temperature and is called the vapor pressure. The vapor pressure depends on the nature of the liquid (that is, its volatility) and on the temperature. Raising the temperature causes an increase in vapor pressure; lowering the temperature decreases it.

The vapor pressure of the solvent in a solution is lower than the vapor pressure of the pure solvent. This may be explained by the fact that the concentration of the solvent in a solution is lower than in the pure solvent. In the pure solvent, all of the molecules at the surface are volatile, while, in a solution, some of the molecules at the surface are not volatile. Therefore, the vapor pressure will be lowered in proportion to the concentration of the solute molecules. In addition, the molecules of the solvent and the solute must attract each other for solution to take place. This attraction also would reduce the tendency of the molecules of the solvent to escape as vapor.

Raoult's law states that the vapor pressure of the solvent in a dilute solution is proportional to its mole-faction. The mole-fraction of solvent may be found by dividing the number of moles of solvent by the total number of moles of solvent plus moles of solute. In a solution containing 1 mole (342 Gm.) of sugar in 99 moles (1,782 Gm.) of water, the mole-fraction of the solvent is 0.99, and the vapor pressure of the solution is 0.99 of the vapor pressure of pure water. However, one component modifies the properties of the other, and so, even in

---

[1] Space limitations prevent discussion of the individual solvents, and so the student is referred to *Industrial Solvents* by Ibert Mellan, Reinhold Publishing Co., New York, 1950, and to the excellent articles in the October, 1943, issue of *Industrial and Engineering Chemistry*, Industrial Edition.

this moderately concentrated solution, Raoult's law does not hold exactly.

Since the depression of the vapor pressure depends on the number of molecules of solute in solution, the molecular weight of a nonvolatile substance may be determined by vapor-pressure measurements. This method is not used frequently because accurate measurements are experimentally difficult and time-consuming.

Diffusion in Solution. Just as molecules in a gaseous system diffuse until the mixture becomes homogeneous, so do the molecules of a solute move about, although much more slowly, until the composition of the solution is uniform. This may be demonstrated by placing a crystal of potassium permanganate in water. The crystal will be seen to dissolve, and the area around the crystal becomes purple. This purple color gradually spreads until the entire solution becomes a uniform purplish tint. The molecules of the solute must be in rapid motion, although their rate of dispersion is much slower than in the case of gases because of the close packing of the solvent molecules with which they continually are colliding.

Osmosis and Osmotic Pressure. When 2 solutions are separated by a semipermeable membrane which allows solvent molecules to pass freely but prevents or impedes solute molecules, there is a flow of solvent toward the more dense side. This phenomenon is called osmosis and ordinarily occurs with aqueous solutions. In such cases, the solvent is water and this continues to flow unless a pressure is exerted on the solution sufficient to prevent the flow or until the densities of the 2 solutions become equal. The pressure which is needed to prevent the flow of solvent through the semipermeable membrane is called osmotic pressure. It varies with character and concentration of the solute and the temperature. Various substances can be used as semipermeable membranes. Among these are parchment paper, cellophane, collodion film and animal membranes, such as bladder.

The osmotic pressure may be demonstrated by fastening a semipermeable membrane securely to the large end of a thistle tube (Fig. 86). The chamber is filled with an aqueous solution of sugar, or other suitable solute, and immersed in purified water. The water enters the chamber by osmosis, and the level of the liquid gradually rises in the glass tube until a definite hydrostatic pressure is established, provided that the membrane is truly impermeable to the solute.

To explain this phenomenon, consider that the molecules of water in the pure water outside the chamber and the molecules of water and of sugar inside the chamber are in constant motion. When they strike the membrane, water molecules have an opportunity to pass through, but sugar molecules do not. The concentration of water molecules in pure water is higher than the concentration of water molecules in the solution, and, therefore, more water molecules will enter the chamber than will leave, and the level of the liquid inside the tube must rise. Equilibrium will be reached, and the level of the liquid inside the tube will cease to rise when the hydrostatic pressure becomes great enough effectively to oppose the entrance of water from the pure solvent and to assist the exit of water from the solution inside the chamber. The sugar molecules are not concerned directly, as their function is merely to reduce the concentration of water molecules inside the chamber. Any solute, to which the membrane is impermeable, will give the same

Colligative Properties

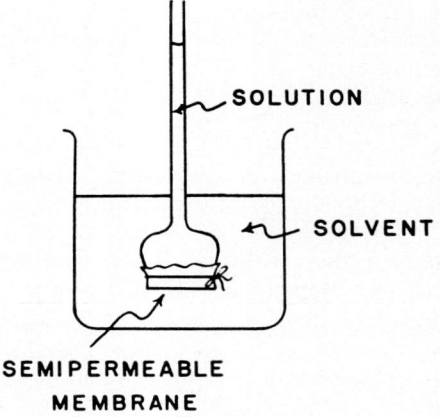

FIG. 86. Apparatus for demonstrating osmosis.

are compared, and the pH value of the solution thus determined. For details of the colorimetric method, see *U.S.P. XVI*.

With buffer solutions differing by 0.1 pH units, the experimental error can be reduced to about 0.02 pH. The method is most satisfactory when applied to clear, colorless solutions. It gives fairly good results in the case of slightly turbid or slightly colored solutions if the turbidity or the color is compensated for by placing a tube containing the unknown solution without indicator behind the buffer solution containing indicator and a tube of purified water behind the unknown containing indicator.

Potentiometric Determination of pH. The potentiometric determination of pH depends on the measurement of the difference of potential set up between 2 electrodes immersed in the solution to be tested. The measuring electrode assumes a potential dependent on the pH value of the solution, while the reference electrode, which is used as the standard, assumes a constant potential.

For general laboratory and for pharmaceutical manufacturing work, the glass electrode commonly is used. Its use depends on the measurement of the difference of potential between solutions of different pH which are separated by a very thin glass membrane. Several types of pH meters with glass electrodes are on the market. These are simple to use and to read. The scale is graduated in pH units so that the pH can be read directly, and no calculations are necessary. The glass electrode may be used in the presence of oxidizing or reducing agents, or proteins. The solutions may be colored, turbid or colloidal, and only small amounts of liquid are required. A special glass electrode has been developed which, with proper care, can be used to measure pH values as high as 13.5 with only very small corrections.

Figure 87 shows a pH meter with glass electrode. Other electrodes can be used for various pH and electrometric measurements.

BUFFER SOLUTIONS

In the preceding section, it was mentioned that pH determinations could be made colorimetrically by adding an indicator to the solution to be tested and comparing the resulting color with the colors of a series of solutions of known pH, containing the same indicator. How can these solutions of definite pH be prepared? Suppose it is desired to prepare a solution with a pH of 4.7. The log of the corresponding hydrogen ion concentration would be $-5.0 + 0.3$, and the hydrogen ion concentration is, therefore, 2×10^{-5}. As hydrochloric acid is a strong acid, the problem could be solved by diluting a standardized solution of acid to a normality of 0.00002. However, it would be extremely difficult to prepare such a solution with accuracy. The carbon dioxide of the water, a trace of alkali from the glass container or impurities in the air would affect the pH of such a dilute solution to a great extent, and, even though the solution had the proper pH when prepared, it would not be stable.

To prevent such changes, buffer solutions are prepared. These are resistant to changes of hydrogen ion concentration. In general, buffer solutions of pH less than 7 are prepared from known quantities of a weak acid and a salt of that acid. Solutions of pH greater than 7 are prepared from a weak alkali and a salt of that alkali.

Let us represent the ionization of acetic acid, a weak acid, as an equilibrium:

$$HC_2H_3O_2 \rightleftharpoons H^+ + C_2H_3O_2^-$$

By adding a quantity of sodium acetate, which is a strong electrolyte, a large excess of acetate ions is furnished. By the law of mass action, the equilibrium would be displaced to the left, decreasing the hydrogen ion concentration and increasing the concentration of acid molecules. If we now add a small amount of an acid or alkali, the hydrogen ion concentration of the solution is altered, but not nearly so much as it would be if we had not previously added the excess of acetate. If an acid is added, hydrogen ions tend to combine with the previously added acetate ions and pass into reserve as nonionized acetic acid molecules. If, on the other hand, an alkali is added, the reserve acetic acid is drawn upon to help neutralize it. Therefore, the change in hydrogen ion concentration is less than it would have been had there been present only acid and no salt.

The ability of a buffer to resist changes in pH upon the addition of either acid or alkali is called the buffer capacity or buffer action. A maximum buffer action is observed in a mixture containing equivalent concentrations of the weak acid and its salt or the weak base and its salt. Buffer solutions may be diluted with considerable quantities of water without causing an appreciable change in pH. However, dilution does decrease the buffer capacity of such a solution. In practice, buffer solutions generally are used with a total concentration of acid and salt of the order of 0.05 to 0.1 normal. By varying the ratio of a particular acid to its salt, stable buffers can be prepared which have a range of approximately 2 pH units.

There are many examples of buffer solutions in nature—in fact, all of the processes of life in both animals and plants take place in solutions which are buffered to the particular hydrogen ion concentration most suitable for the chemical changes taking place within the organism. The juices of most of the fruits and the vegetables have a definite, though slight, acidity. Milk is buffered to a slight alkalinity and, therefore, remains uncurdled for a longer time, even though bacteria have changed some of its milk sugar to lactic acid. Blood has a definite, very faint alkalinity at pH 7.4, which it maintains with the greatest precision.

U.S.P. XVI gives complete directions for the preparation of standard buffer solutions. These solutions have a range from pH 1.2 to 10.0, in intervals of 0.1 or 0.2 pH unit.

BIBLIOGRAPHY

Babor, J. A., and Lehrman, A.: Basic College Chemistry, 2nd Ed., New York, Crowell, 1953.

Deming, H. G.: Fundamental Chemistry, New York, Wiley, 1947.

Dole, M.: The Glass Electrode, New York, Wiley, 1946.

Kolthoff, I. M., and Furman, N. H.: Potentiometric Titrations, New York, Wiley, 1946.

MELVIN F. W. DUNKER, Ph.D.
Professor of Pharmaceutical Chemistry, Wayne State University

7

Colloids, Emulsions and Suspensions

GENERAL CONSIDERATIONS
COLLOIDS
   HISTORY
   THE COLLOIDAL STATE
   PREPARATION OF COLLOIDAL DISPERSIONS
   PROPERTIES OF COLLOIDAL DISPERSIONS
   PRECIPITATION OF COLLOIDS
   LYOPHILIC COLLOIDS
   PROTECTION
   GELS
   AEROSOLS
   ADSORPTION
   SURFACE FILMS—SURFACE-ACTIVE AGENTS
   FOAMS

EMULSIONS
   FORMATION AND STABILITY
   EMULSIFYING AGENTS
   RECOGNIZING TYPES OF EMULSIONS
   PREPARATION OF EMULSIONS
   CREAMING
   CRACKING OR DE-EMULSIFICATION
   EFFECT OF ELECTROLYTES ON EMULSION STABILITY
   TRANSPARENT AND CHROMATIC EMULSIONS
SUSPENSIONS
APPLICATIONS

GENERAL CONSIDERATIONS

Colloids, emulsions and suspensions represent types of dispersion systems in which the substance scattered or dispersed through the medium is found in discrete particles which may be many times the size of ordinary molecules or ions. The particles of suspensions are quite coarse and usually settle rapidly. Colloids and emulsions contain particles which, because of special properties attendant on their tremendous surface area, usually do not settle readily. A discussion of these 2 classes of dispersions forms the major portion of this chapter.

While the use of materials containing colloidally dispersed particles extends back for centuries, recognition of the peculiar and distinctive behavior of such materials began a little over a century ago. In the past several decades, the properties associated with substances in the colloidal state have been investigated widely, and the field of colloid chemistry has become one of the sciences bridging the gaps between the biologic and the physical sciences. Present-day industrial processes (such as the various catalytic syntheses of chemicals, the production of synthetic rubber and the grading and the separation of ores by the flotation process, to mention only a few) depend on the principles governing substances with very large surface areas. The field of pharmacy is included among the sciences that draw upon the basic principles applying to colloidally dispersed matter. The *U.S.P.*, the *N.F.* and the *N.N.D.* describe many preparations which are examples of material in the colloidal state or are dispersed by colloidal materials. An understanding of some of the basic principles of colloid chemistry should lead to more intelligent handling of these materials in the dispensing of prescriptions involving these and other substances in the colloidal state.

COLLOIDS

HISTORY

The gelatin in Chinese ink or in paints, the glue used in veneering woods and colloidal gold used as a medicament or a dye represent some of the examples of materials of a colloidal nature used by early peoples. While such colloidal substances had been known and used for a long time and while descriptions of the preparation of some colloidal dispersions had appeared in the literature, it was Thomas Graham (1805–1869) who first recognized the special properties of highly dispersed materials and clearly stated many of the principles of colloid chemistry. For this reason, he commonly is regarded as the father of colloid chemistry.

Among the contributions of Graham are the recognition of the adsorption of ions from solution by solids, the easy diffusibility of crystalloids as compared with the slow diffusibility of other materials such as proteins or gums which he called *colloids* (from the Greek *kolla* meaning glue and *oid* meaning like), the passage of crystalline substances through animal skin membranes (semipermeable membranes) and the introduction of many of the terms still used in this field. In spite of the many remarkable contributions of Graham, the phenomena of colloid chemistry as a separate field of study were largely neglected. In 1903, only 23 papers or patents dealing with colloid principles appeared in the entire world chemical literature. In this year, the names of several investigators who have become recognized as outstanding contributors to the field appeared. Colloid chemistry in the past half century has grown rapidly so that texts now appear which are devoted to restricted areas of colloid science.

Von Weimarn, a Russian scientist, presented conclusive evidence that there is no sharp boundary between the crystalloids and the colloids. In 1903, Zsigmondy invented the ultramicroscope (Fig. 88), which, for the first time, permitted the observation of colloidal particles. In 1907, Wolfgang Ostwald showed that a *colloidal dispersion* was a system consisting of one or more substances in a very finely divided state dispersed or scattered through another substance. Combining this concept with that of the three states of matter, Ostwald was the first to point out the theoretically possible types of colloidal systems.

Of special interest to pharmacists is the development of colloidal preparations containing silver or silver compounds for use as antiseptics. Prior to 1895, silver caseinate containing 4.2 per cent silver was introduced into medicine under the name Argonin, and ethylenediamine silver nitrate was introduced under the name Argentamine. In 1897, Credé described the preparation known as Collargol, and Neisser brought

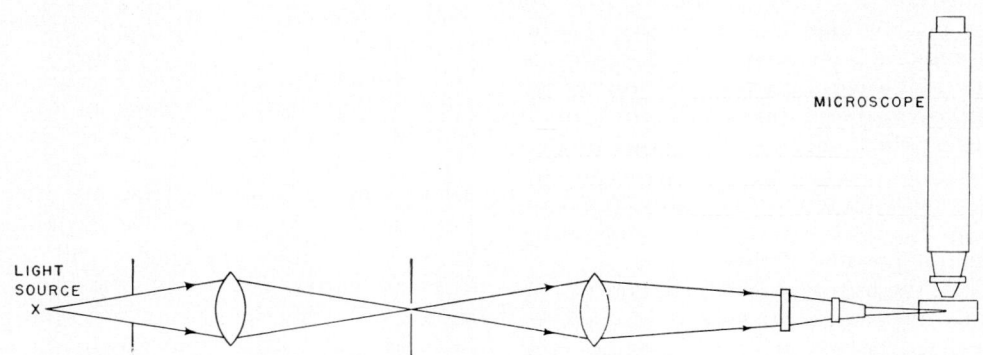

Fig. 88. Early type of Zsigmondy ultramicroscope. The sol is placed in the small black chamber below the microscope and at the focal point of the light-lens system. (After Ward, A. G.: Colloids, Their Properties and Applications, New York, Interscience)

out Protargol (8.3% silver albumin "salt"). Engelmann began the first large-scale commercial production of a colloidal silver preparation and became the first technical chemist dealing with colloids. From this beginning have come similar preparations for pharmaceutical use.

THE COLLOIDAL STATE

With the fundamentals well established, scientific articles in the field of colloid chemistry since 1910 have increased enormously, both in journals of chemistry and in journals devoted exclusively to this field. Much material on the theoretical aspects of systems with large surface areas has been published and is reviewed in texts on colloid chemistry, a partial list of which will be found in the Bibliography at the end of the chapter. Some of the general considerations of colloidal systems will now be taken up.

The colloidal state may be thought of as a state of matter analogous to the gaseous, the liquid or the solid states, in which the degree of subdivision is such that the large surface area with its associated forces produces a special type of behavior. When one substance is dispersed or scattered throughout another, the properties of the resulting mixture depend, to some degree at least, on the size of the dispersed particles. If the dispersed particles are in the ionic or molecular state, the mixture appears to be homogeneous, both physically and chemically, and may be considered to be a true solution. The true solutions are discussed in Chapter 6.

When a mixture of 2 or more substances is not uniform throughout, it is spoken of as a *heterogeneous system*. Each of the homogeneous, physically distinct and mechanically separable types of matter in such a system is called a *phase*. When the dispersed (finely divided) phase is not very soluble in the dispersing (continuous) medium and is divided into particles of such size that they scatter light and would readily settle out if not stabilized (sand in water), the mixture is referred to as a *suspension*. The grains of sand represent one phase, and water is the other phase of this 2-phase heterogeneous system.

The rate of settling of a suspension will depend on such factors as the size and the density of the particles, the density and the viscosity of the dispersing medium, the presence of some third substance which changes the viscosity of the dispersing medium or alters the interfacial tension, thereby retarding settling, and others. Thus sand of a given fineness and density will settle more rapidly in pure water than in water whose viscosity is increased by the solution of large amounts of sugar (syrup), or of glycerin. However, if all other factors are kept constant, the rate of settling of a given sample of a powder will depend only on the size of the particles. The large particles which expose a relatively smaller surface per unit of weight than the finer particles will settle out more rapidly, leaving the finer particles suspended. If these slowly settling finer particles could be subdivided repeatedly, they eventually should approach molecules in size and the heterogeneous mixture should approach more nearly a true solution in properties. Before reaching the state of subdivision found in true solutions, there should be a stage at which the particles would be fine enough to have a very slow settling rate, and the mixture should appear homogeneous to the *eye*. Such a heterogeneous system may be considered as an example of a *colloidal dispersion*. It may be pointed out that the term "colloidal solution" is not strictly applicable and represents a loose use of the word "solution." These systems will be designated as colloidal dispersions.

The precipitation from solution of substances in the ionic or molecular state is a common practice in qualitative and quantitative analysis. This represents the coalescence of many particles to form a coarse, rapidly settling particle. It would appear that, by the selection of the proper conditions, the growth of the particles could be controlled in such a way as to produce a typical colloidal dispersion. These theoretical considerations can be proved in the laboratory, and colloidal dispersions may be produced in this way; in fact, the accidental production of such colloidal dispersions may result in errors in quantitative gravimetric procedures. For example, the precipitation of silver chloride in dilute solution in the cold frequently will lead to the formation of some colloidal dispersion. A significant amount of the silver chloride would pass through the filter.

As the size of the particle is decreased slowly, gradual changes in properties of the material occur. Whether particles of a given size suspended in a medium are classed as a suspension or a colloidal dispersion depends on the properties of the mixture. It should be emphasized that *there are no sharp transitions from solutions to colloidal dispersions to suspensions,* and that the boundaries of the systems overlap. However, as a matter of convenience, it has been customary to define the colloidal range or zone in terms of the size of the particles of the dispersed phase. Wolfgang Ostwald was the first to propose such an arbitrary set of boundaries, but others have suggested different values for the zones. Ostwald's values are shown in Table 5, the dimensions referring to diameters of the particles considered to approximate spheres. With respect to inorganic and many organic substances, particles of colloidal size would consist of aggregates of molecules. On the other hand, single molecules of some proteins and of some organic polymers will fall in the colloidal range.

Under the highest magnification obtainable and the best conditions of lighting, the smallest particle visible under the ordinary microscope is one with a diameter of about 130 mμ or 1.3×10^{-5} cm. From Table 5 it may be seen that the largest particle falling in the colloidal range according to Ostwald may be visible under the ordinary microscope under favorable conditions. A better idea of these sizes may be obtained by comparison with other objects. The human red blood cell has an average diameter of about 7,200 mμ or 7.2 μ. The diameter of the hydrogen molecule is about 0.1 mμ, which is one tenth the diameter of the particles at the lower end of the colloidal range. Perhaps these values may be compared better still if they are converted to distances which we are more accustomed to measuring. If the diameter of the hydrogen molecule is taken as 1 mm., the smallest colloidal particle would then have a diameter of 1 cm. and the largest a diameter of 500 cm. or 5 m. On this scale, the red blood cells have a diameter of about 72 m.

Particles of such small sizes as those in the colloidal range expose enormous surfaces to the dispersion medium when compared with the surface of an equal volume of larger particles. For simplicity in calculation, consider the surface of a cube in

TABLE 5. CLASSIFICATION OF DISPERSE SYSTEMS (OSTWALD)*

Type	Range of Particle Size†	Characteristics
Coarse dispersion	>0.5 μ or >5 $\times$ 10^{-5} cm.	Particles do not run through a paper filter, do not diffuse and do not pass through a dialyzing membrane; are microscopically visible.
Colloidal dispersion	0.5 μ to 1.0 mμ or 5 $\times$ 10^{-5} to 1 $\times$ 10^{-7} cm.	Particles run through a filter paper but not an ultrafilter; are not resolved in an ordinary microscope but usually are recognizable in the ultramicroscope; diffuse and pass through a dialyzing membrane very slowly, if at all.
Molecular dispersion, solution	<1 mμ or <1 $\times$ 10^{-7} cm	Particles pass through both a filter paper and an ultrafilter; are not visible in the microscope or the ultramicroscope; diffuse and pass through dialyzing membranes quite rapidly.

* Ostwald: Kuhn's "Kolloid chemisches Taschenbuch," Leipzig, 11 (1935) *through* Weiser, H. B.: Colloid Chemistry, ed. 2, New York, Wiley, 1949.

† A micron, μ, is a unit of length and is defined as one thousandth of a millimeter or 10^{-3} mm. A millimicron, mμ, is one thousandth of a micron or 10^{-6} mm.

redispersion of the colloid occurs. Many of the artificially prepared colloidal dispersions (although not all) are lyophobic sols, as for example, gold sols and arsenous sulfide sols.

The methods used to prepare colloidal dispersions may be classified according to Svedberg into 2 main groups: the *condensation methods* and the *dispersion methods*.

Condensation Methods

The condensation methods depend on the preparation of a molecularly dispersed, supersaturated solution of the substance under conditions which lead to the formation of many fine particles. This may be achieved by altering the conditions of solution or by chemical reaction.

Changed Conditions of Solution. One of the simplest of the condensation methods is changing the conditions of solution such as temperature or solvent. For example, when a solution of rosin or sulfur in alcohol is poured slowly into water with stirring, a precipitate forms, some of which is in colloidal dispersion.

Reduction methods are quite general. The salts of the noble metals, such as gold, silver and platinum, are reduced easily to give colloidal dispersions. Usually neutral or slightly alkaline solutions are treated with any of a wide range of reducing agents such as pyrogallol, formaldehyde, hydrazine, phosphorus and others. Colloidal dispersions of gold are prepared quite easily and were among the earliest to be made. They vary considerably in color, depending on the reducing agents chosen and other conditions of preparation, from red sols which have very small particles to purple sols which have larger particles.

Carey-Lea produced relatively concentrated sols of silver which, though not pure, were quite stable and were largely reversible after precipitation by alcohol or by electrolytes or after drying. These unusually stable metal sols were prepared by reducing solutions of silver nitrate with ferrous sulfate in the presence of the strongly adsorbed sodium citrate. Mild Silver Protein, N.F. is defined as "silver rendered colloidal by the presence of, or combination with, protein." It is largely a reversible colloid.

Oxidation methods may be used as a means of causing particles to grow by condensation. When cold solutions of hydrogen sulfide and sulfur dioxide are mixed, the sulfide ion is oxidized, the sulfur dioxide is reduced and the sulfur formed is in colloidal dispersion. The equation may be written as $2H_2S + SO_2 \rightarrow 3S + 2H_2O$.

Hydrolysis of the salts of weak bases or weak acids will lead to the production of hydroxides of the metals or to hydrated oxides. For example, pouring a solution of ferric chloride into a large volume of boiling water is a simple way of obtaining a beautiful bright red sol of hydrated ferric oxide. If a solution of ferric chloride is dialyzed against distilled water, a sol of hydrated ferric oxide is obtained. Likewise, sols of aluminum oxide or chromium oxide and many others may be obtained by suitably controlling the hydrolysis procedure. Iron and Ammonium Acetate Solution (Basham's Mixture), N.F., X, owes its color in part to hydrated ferric oxide or to basic ferric acetate in colloidal dispersion, stabilized to some extent by glycerin, sugar and some excess acetic acid, and in part to complex acetates. The iron scale salts such as iron and ammonium citrate, iron citrate, iron pyrophosphate and ferric phosphate have been reported to be partly colloidal[1] while iron and potassium tartrate, iron and ammonium tartrate and iron glycerophosphate were reported to be entirely colloidal. Aluminum Hydroxide Gel, U.S.P., is largely hydrated aluminum oxide in colloidal dispersion.

Double decomposition reactions may produce colloidal dispersions under the proper conditions. If, for example, hydrogen sulfide is passed into solutions of arsenous acid or mercuric cyanide, colloidal arsenous sulfide or mercuric sulfide easily can be obtained. If such factors as speed of mixing, concentration of solution and temperature are controlled carefully, it should be possible to produce colloidal dispersions of nearly all water-insoluble salts. The addition of substances which will be strongly adsorbed, such as other colloids, sugar or glycerin, often is effective in preventing the coagulation from going beyond the colloidal range to produce a precipitate.

The Bredig arc method consists of sparking electrodes of the material to be dispersed under the surface of water containing a trace of electrolyte. Either alternating or direct current may be used. The method first was regarded as a forcible tearing apart of the electrodes, producing colloidal particles. However, Svedberg has suggested that the intense heat of the electric arc results in vaporization of the metal and that the colloidal particles are formed by condensation of the vapor.

Dispersion Methods

The dispersion methods involve the disintegration of large particles until the resulting material displays colloidal properties. As before, there must be some control over the process to prevent "overshooting" the colloidal range.

Grinding or crushing large masses down to particles in the colloidal range is not efficient, and the results are not uniform. The method has the additional disadvantage that the grinding of very fine powders is accompanied by the danger of dust explosions. A few sols have been prepared in this way. The so-called colloid mills may be used for soft materials but they will not disintegrate hard materials into particles of colloidal dimensions.

Peptization. The greater dispersion of solid particles may be brought about by peptization. Graham suggested this term to indicate the analogy to the dispersing effect of the digestive juices, and pepsin in particular, on the proteins. The term is applied generally to the dispersion of gelatinous masses to colloidal dispersions and is thought to result from adsorption of a solvent, of ions or of a nonelectrolyte on the solid. For example, if freshly precipitated ferric hydroxide is treated with a few drops of dilute hydrochloric acid, or with a few drops of ferric chloride solution, a clear red sol is obtained. Gelatin adsorbs water and readily is peptized to a colloidal dispersion. Mixed solvents sometimes peptize a solid more readily than either solvent alone. For example, Collodion, U.S.P., is a preparation in which cellulose nitrate has been peptized by a mixture of ether and alcohol.

Washing out the electrolytes formed during a reaction sometimes disperses a precipitate. A precipitate of silver chloride, if subjected to prolonged washing with distilled water, slowly passes into the colloidal state. This fact must be kept in mind in quantitative analytical procedures. Most freshly precipitated hydrous oxide gels are peptized to a certain extent by washing. Therefore, it is common practice in analytical chemistry to wash certain precipitates with a solution of ammonium nitrate or other suitable electrolyte to prevent peptization.

Since 1930, the exposure of substances to supersonic or ultrasonic waves (high-frequency sound waves) has been employed to produce colloidal dispersions, emulsions and suspensions. This method is useful for liquids, for solids of low strength and for the redispersion of fresh precipitates. Silver sols have been produced in this way. However, ultrasonic irradiation may induce undesirable chemical changes in the components of the system.

PROPERTIES OF COLLOIDAL DISPERSIONS

The recognition or the differentiation of colloidal dispersions from the true solutions is based on the properties of colloids. Those properties which lend themselves most easily to use in distinguishing colloids may be grouped into 3 classes: optical differences, size difference phenomena and the solution laws.

Optical Differences

Turbidity. The simplest of the optical differences is the appearance of turbidity to transmitted light. A true solution does not scatter light and, therefore, it appears clear, whereas a colloidal dispersion contains opaque particles which scatter light and consequently it appears turbid. However, not all colloidal dispersions are turbid. Colloidal gold dispersions or hydrated ferric oxide sols appear clear to the unaided eye.

Tyndall Effect. This is observed when a colloidal dispersion is examined at right angles to a strong beam of light. (Fig. 90). The particles of clear sols become visible under these conditions.* Faraday first employed this phenomenon in 1857 to demonstrate the presence of particles of suspended matter in gold sols. In 1869 and the following years, Tyndall investigated the phenomenon extensively, especially for smokes, and this behavior has since become known as the Tyndall effect. When colloidal dispersions are observed, a diffuse band of scattered light marks the passage of the beam of light through the dispersion. The light emerging from the dispersion is partly polarized and may have a color, depending on the particle size of the disperse phase. It must be remembered that water is not always optically void, that is, free of particles which scatter light, and likewise that some salt solutions and concentrated solutions of some sugars, such as dextrose, also scatter light under these conditions.

Ultramicroscopy. As has been mentioned before, the ordinary microscope may enable one to see some of the larger colloidal particles. However, it was not until Zsigmondy developed the ultramicroscope that the particles of colloidal dispersions could be generally observed. Basically, the Tyndall phenomenon is involved. The ultramicroscope employs a regular microscope to magnify and make visible the tiny flashes of light reflected from the individual particles. The colloidal dispersion is illuminated by a strong beam of light at right angles to the direction of observation against a black background (Fig. 88) in such a way that only the light reflected by the particles as they move through the beam of light is observed. It is also possible with the proper equipment to illuminate the colloidal dispersion in the line of observation (coaxial illumination). It

---

* This behavior may be compared with a more common observation. In an evenly lighted room, the dust particles floating in the air are not visible. However, in a room illuminated by only a narrow slit of light, the dust particles become visible by means of the flashes of light they reflect as they turn in the air. Similarly, the particles in colloidal dispersions become visible when strongly illuminated on one side only.

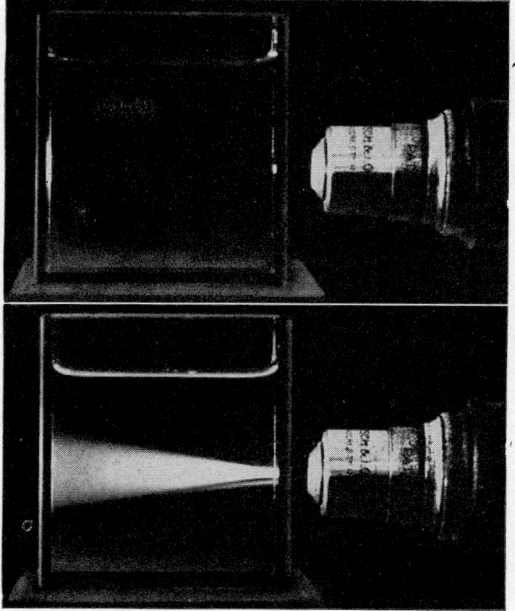

Fig. 90. (*Top*) A true solution does not reflect a beam of light directed through it. (*Bottom*) Reflection of the light beam reveals the presence of collodial particles. (From Atlas Surface Active Agents, Wilmington, Del., Atlas Powder Co.)

should be remembered that the actual particles are not observed but only the light which is reflected, refracted and scattered by the solid phase.

This scattering of light by suspended finely divided particles is applied also in quantitative analysis. The *nephelometer* is an instrument which measures the intensity of scattered light and so permits the quantitative estimation of a very small amount of precipitate which cannot conveniently be removed and weighed.

Electron Microscopy. In the last several decades, the development of the electron microscope has made possible the extension of visibility down to the lower limits of the colloidal range (see Table 5). The range of the electron microscope is from 10 μ to about 3 mμ. With this instrument it has become possible to determine the size of colloidal particles more accurately and to observe the shape of the particles. Gold sols have been found to consist of triangular, hexagonal, rhombic and tetragonal crystals.

Vanadium pentoxide sols contain fine rods; iron hydroxide sols appear as strongly oriented blunt rods; and tungsten oxide particles appear as neat rectangles.

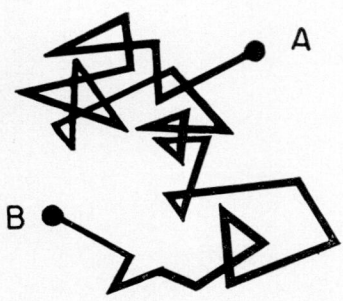

FIG. 91. Brownian movement. The path of a particle, beginning at *A* and ending at *B,* as projected in the focal plane of the microscope.

Brownian Movement. While studying pollen grains in 1827, the English botanist, Robert Brown, was the first to report the observation of the zigzag, random motion of particles suspended in a liquid. The motion is caused by a bombardment of the particles by molecules of the dispersion medium and is referred to as *brownian movement* (Fig. 91). Particles above 4 μ in diameter do not show brownian movement. The speed of the particles increases as they become smaller. The rapid brownian movement of colloidal particles is observed readily under the ultramicroscope.

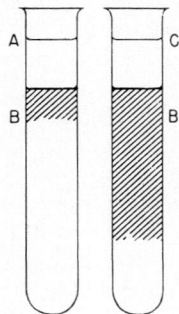

FIG. 92. Rate of diffusion in agar. Tubes containing agar gel *B,* on which is superimposed a colored sol *A,* or a solution of a colored ion *C.* The extent of diffusion is indicated by the shaded areas.

SIZE DIFFERENCES

The differentiation of colloidal dispersions from true solutions on the basis of the larger particle size in the colloidal dispersions may be made under the proper conditions. For example, Graham was able to show that the *rates of diffusion* (Fig. 92) of substances varied inversely with the sizes of their particles. Therefore, ions and molecules should diffuse quite rapidly as compared with colloidal particles. If a colored colloidal dispersion and a solution containing colored ions are poured into separate tubes containing agar gel, the more rapid diffusion of the colored molecules or ions as compared with that of the colloidal particles can be observed.

In a somewhat similar manner, if a sieve or a screen of the proper pore size were available, the larger particles of colloids should be held back, whereas molecules or ions would pass through freely. Such a filter is known as a semipermeable membrane. Substances such as glucose, urea and sodium chloride pass through the capillaries of the membrane by a simple diffusion process. Graham applied the technic of *dialysis* to colloids, a process in which the colloidal material admixed with ionic or molecular material is separated from pure water by means of a semipermeable membrane. Graham employed animal membranes, but parchment paper, sausage casings, cellophane, collodion sacs and other materials may be used. The process may be illustrated on a grossly exaggerated scale by Figure 93. The electrolyte and the water pass through the membrane freely in both directions until equilibrium is established between the rates of passage in each

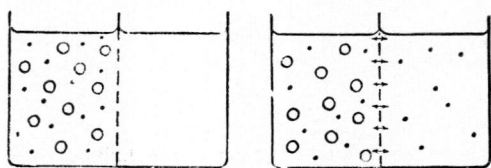

FIG. 93. Diffusion of electrolytes through a semipermeable membrane. (*Left*) At start. (*Right*) At equilibrium. Circles represent colloid particles; dots represent electrolyte particles; line in center represents semipermeable membrane.

direction, whereas the colloid particles do not pass through the membrane. This failure on the part of colloids to pass a semipermeable membrane is partially responsible for the fact that ions and simple molecules readily pass from the blood serum to tissue fluids, whereas the proteins and other colloidal serum components remain within the capillary system. This fact permits the use of specially purified dispersions of acacia or gelatin or sterile dispersions of the synthetic polymers dextran or polyvinylpyrrolidone as blood substitutes to maintain blood volume (Gelatine Solution, Special Intravenous; Dextran, N.N.D., 1960). Similarly, the artificial kidney depends on the dialysis of the simple molecules of body waste materials through the semipermeable membrane of the system and the retention of the colloids and the blood cells.

Various factors hasten the process of dialysis, such as frequent or continuous change of the water outside the membrane to remove the electrolytes, an increase in temperature if the colloid is not thermolabile (i.e., destroyed by heat) or the application of an electric current to attract the ions of the electrolyte (Fig. 94). This latter modification is referred to as *electrodialysis*. Dialysis also may be accelerated by forcing the liquid and the molecularly or ionically dispersed material through the membrane under pressure. This was called *ultrafiltration* by Bechhold. A satisfactory ultrafilter is obtained if filter paper is impregnated with collodion or with a solution of gelatin followed by hardening with formaldehyde. Many types of clay filters are available with pores sufficiently small to hold back colloidal particles. Among the better known is the Berkefeld filter widely used in bacteriology and in the pharmaceutical industry for the sterilization of solutions. The use of ultrafilters of graded size has been employed in the determination of the average particle size of colloidal dispersions.

The process of dialysis is useful in the purification of colloidal dispersions. While much of the free electrolyte may be removed from a hydrophobic sol, Graham pointed out that a certain amount must remain for stability to be retained.

The *ultracentrifuge,* which produces forces many times stronger than those of the conventional centrifuge, may be used to estimate the sizes and the masses of colloidal particles by determining the migration velocity in the centrifuge operating at steady conditions. This has been applied particularly in estimating the molecular weight of proteins.

Other methods of estimating size are based on the diffraction of x-rays, the use of the electron microscope and particle counting devices combined with the ultramicroscope.

DEVIATIONS FROM SOLUTION LAWS

Some of the fundamental laws governing solutions are considered in Chapter 6. It will be recalled that the solution of a compound in a solvent leads to a lowering of the freezing point of the solvent, a rise in the boiling point and a lowering of the vapor pressure. All of these effects are dependent on the total number of particles of solute in a given amount of solvent. Since colloidal particles are large in comparison with ions or molecules, the dispersion of a given weight of substance in the colloidal state has many less particles than the same weight in the molecular or ionic form. Consequently, colloidal dispersions

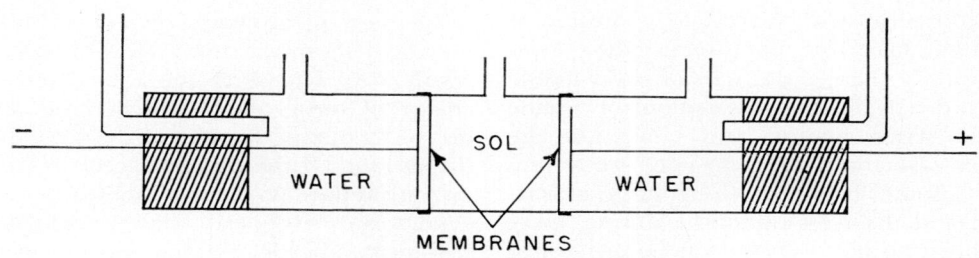

FIG. 94. Simple electrodialysis set-up.

generally have only a slight effect on the freezing and the boiling points of solvents or on the osmotic pressure, as compared with molecularly or ionically dispersed material, and this fact may be used to recognize colloidal dispersions.

Electric Properties

Colloidally dispersed particles bear a charge, and the electric properties of colloids are related to this charge. The colloidal dispersions may be classified on the basis of the charge on the particles into positive colloids (the hydrous oxides of metals, basic dyes, etc.) and the negative colloids (hydrous oxides of nonmetals, dispersions of noble metals, sulfides, sulfur, gums, resins, etc.). Such hydrophilic sols as proteins, agar and the like differ in that stable sols may be obtained in which the charge on the particles may be positive or negative or lacking entirely. In the latter case, the effect on the stability of the sol of the layers of adsorbed solvent is usually greater than that of the charge on the particles.

Several ideas have been proposed as to the origin of this charge on the particles. The theory of colloidal ions assumes that a number of ions are associated with an aggregate of molecules to produce the colloidal particle. Helmholtz proposed the double-layer concept for the arrangement of charges, each layer being mono-ionic. Later, this idea was extended to include diffuse layers rather than single layers of ions. Freundlich and others have advanced the idea of the preferential adsorption of ions by the colloidal particles, depending on chemical similarity and abundance of the particular ions around the colloidal particle when it is formed. For example, adding a dilute solution of silver nitrate drop by drop with stirring to a solution of a slight excess of potassium iodide gives negatively charged particles of silver iodide resulting from the adsorption of iodide ions. These iodide ions constitute the inner layer, and the associated potassium ions (some held by electrostatic attraction and the remainder in a diffuse, more mobile coating) represent the outer layer of the Helmholtz double layer. The iodide

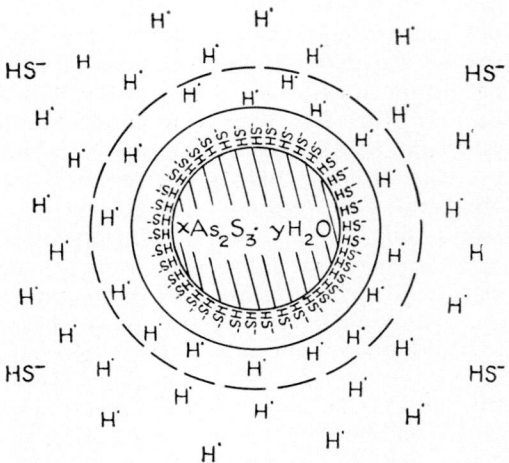

Fig. 95. Colloid particle of arsenic trisulfide stabilized by HS^- ions. The hydrogen ions within the broken circle are held by electrostatic attraction; those outside are free. The HS^- ions impart a negative charge to the particle. (After Weiser, H. B.: J. Phys. Chem. 36:2811)

ions are held more firmly and impart the negative charge, so that, in a suitable electric field, the charged particle moves to the positive pole. The aggregate of silver iodide and the entire double layer is known as the colloidal particle. On the other hand, if a dilute solution of potassium iodide is added slowly to a slight excess of a solution of silver nitrate, the particles will be charged positively as the result of the adsorption of silver ions in the inner layer. The diagrammatic sketch in Figure 95 was suggested by Weiser as an illustration of a particle of arsenic trisulfide sol stabilized by hydrogen sulfide. A predominating factor in the stabilizing effect of the ionic layer seems to be the energy required to bring particles together against the action of their electric fields.

The **sign of the charge** on a given colloid may be determined in a variety of ways. If a colloid of known charge is on hand, the charge of the given colloid may be determined by mixing samples of the 2 colloidal dispersions. If the charges are of like sign, no precipitation occurs; whereas, if the charges are of opposite sign, a precipitate will form. The electron microscope has permitted the examination of such precipitates. When a negative hydrosol of vanadium pentoxide is precipitated by a positive dialyzed sol of ferric hydroxide or a positive sol of silver iodide, the particles of positive sol adhere to the rods of vanadium pentoxide uniformly along the length. However, the precipitation may be complicated by other factors, such as the presence of precipitating ions as impurities in one of the sols, the interaction of the stabilizing ions of the respective sols, and the like. Another very simple method is based on the following: when a strip of filter paper is in contact with water, it assumes a negative charge. Thus, if a strip of dry filter paper is dipped into a negative hydrosol, no precipitation occurs and the sol rises in the filter paper. On the other hand, a positive sol will precipitate in the paper as a result of the neutralization of the charge by the negatively charged paper, and only water rises in the paper. If suitable equipment is available, an electric current may be passed through the sol. The colloidal particles will then migrate or be drawn toward the electrode of opposite charge and repelled from the electrode of the same charge. (See Fig. 96.)

PRECIPITATION OF COLLOIDS

When colloidal dispersions settle out in macroscopic particles, the process is referred to as *flocculation* or *coagulation*. Faraday showed that colloidal dispersions were sensitive to impurities. For example, a weakly hydrated positive colloid is caused to coagulate or flocculate by the addition of a solution containing negatively charged ions. The Schulze-Hardy rule states that a colloid particle is precipitated or coagulated by ions of opposite charge; and the higher the valence of the precipitating ion, the greater the precipitating power. Within limits, the precipitating power of ions varies with the concentration of the sol. Obviously, this will apply only when there is no interfering chemical reaction between the added ion and the protecting ion or sol. The addition of electrolytes seems to allow the particles of colloid to cohere rather than to rebound when they collide. This phenomenon is also explained on the basis of preferential adsorption of ions resulting in a neutralization of the charges on the particles, allowing them to coagulate. The emulsoids or hydrophilic colloids are surrounded by a protecting layer of solvent and are not nearly so sensitive to electrolyte precipitation. On the other hand, the addition of nonelectrolytes either may stabilize or may sensitize the sol toward precipitation by ions.

The precipitation of a colloidal dispersion by another sol of opposite charge has been mentioned previously. The mutual coagulation of hydrophobic sols has been shown to be totally dependent on the magnitude of the charge on the particles, and is at its maximum when the total charges of the two colloids are equal. Mutual coagulation also may occur between hydrophobic and hydrophilic sols. Other conditions which may lead to partial or complete precipitation of colloidal particles are: addition of an immiscible liquid, passage of an electric current, vigorous shaking, boiling, freezing and the passage of ultrasonic waves. Ultraviolet light and roentgen rays often

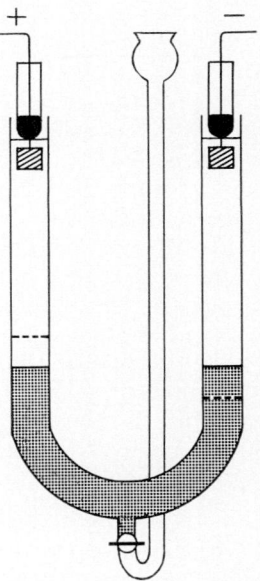

Fig. 96. Burton's cataphoresis apparatus. The sol (stippled portion) is shown moving toward the positive pole (broken lines indicate new boundaries). (After Burton: Phil. Mag. (6), 11:436)

have been found to sensitize sols to electrolyte precipitation.

LYOPHILIC COLLOIDS

Much of what has been said about colloids in the previous pages has been based on studies of lyophobic colloids. Nearly all naturally occurring colloidal dispersions are lyophilic and generally are considered as being composed of highly solvated particles. The adjective *lyophilic* (i.e., solvent-loving) is applied to a substance which, upon dispersion, shows an attraction or affinity for the dispersion medium, swelling as it passes into colloidal dispersion. More specific terms (such as hydrophilic, alcoholophilic, etc.) may be used to denote the solvent attracted. The terms *reversible, stable* and *emulsoid* sometimes are applied to such materials. These sols are usually stable to small concentrations of electrolytes (hence the term stable), generally will redisperse after drying at ordinary temperatures (hence the term reversible) and, being highly solvated particles, may be looked upon as liquid particles (emulsoids). Examples: gelatin and other proteins, plant gums (acacia, tragacanth), colloidal silicic acid.

The lyophilic colloidal dispersions may be turbid, do not diffuse through a membrane and exhibit many other properties of the lyophobic colloids. However, they are much more stable to electrolyte precipitation, possibly because of the protecting layer of adsorbed solvent. Many lyophilic sols are stable to drying and will redisperse completely in water, as, for example, the proteins, the soaps and the gums. The surface tension of the lyophilic sols may be nearly the same as that of the medium (starch, silicic acid) or may be considerably lowered as is the case with protein or soap sols and usually changes with the age of the sol. The lyophilic sols generally are much more viscous than the medium alone, as contrasted with the lyophobic sols. Concentrated sols often gel. The higher viscosity is associated with the swelling of the particles as they become more and more solvated, increasing the volume of the disperse phase. The lyophilic sols are not so sensitive to electric currents as are the lyophobic sols. The lyophilic sols often have a refractive index only slightly different from that of the medium and sometimes give only a slight Tyndall cone. The coagulation of certain protein sols by heat is well known, especially, for example, the heat coagulation of egg white. The coagulation appears to involve 3 distinct processes: a generally nonreversible denaturation, a reversible flocculation and a nonreversible coagulation.

The hydrogen ion concentration is a factor in the stability, particularly of the protein sols. Proteins in "solution" behave as amphoteric substances and produce either anions or cations, depending on the hydrogen ion concentration. As this is varied, a point of minimum concentration of protein ions is reached at which both anions and cations are present in equal numbers. This is referred to as the "iso-electric point." Colloidal particles at the iso-electric point do not migrate in an electric field and have a minimum stability. Maximum precipitation of proteins is obtained at the iso-electric point, and the "solutions" exhibit minimum viscosity, minimum osmotic pressure and minimum optical rotation. Since the iso-electric point for the proteins varies, it may be used to advantage in the precipitation of individual proteins by electrolytes from a mixture of proteins. The precipitated protein may then be washed free of electrolyte and redispersed.

A variety of hydrophilic colloids of natural and synthetic origin are used as bulk laxatives, utilizing their emollient coating and lubricating effect as well as their water-retaining properties. Methylcellulose of the U.S.P., especially the high gel grade, is superior to the natural hydrophilic colloids in water-retaining power.[2]

At present, no correlations have been found between the hydrophilic properties and the laxative action of plant gums, colloidal clays and cellulose derivatives.[3]

PROTECTION

Lyophilic and lyophobic colloids often affect the stability of one another, depending on the relative amounts present. Thus, when a hydrophilic sol such as gelatin is added to a gold sol, the gold sol may be coagulated and precipitated. Sometimes 2 types of sols may be mixed without any apparent effect, but the sensitivity to electrolytes may be increased. Other times it is found that the mixture is more resistant to coagulation by electrolytes, and the hydrophobic sol is "protected" by the hydrophilic sol. Protection generally occurs when the lyophilic sol is in excess and neutral or charged with the same sign as the lyophobic sol. The stabilizing action of these protecting colloids probably results from their adsorption on the surface of the lyophobic colloidal particle. However, it should be pointed out that true solutions may be protectors, and, as examples, the citrates and the tartrates may be cited. Ferric Ammonium Citrate of the N.F. seems to produce colloidal dispersions, the hydrated ferric oxide probably being protected by the citrates.

Imferon is a recently introduced proprietary preparation consisting of a colloidal dispersion of ferric hydroxide in complex with partially hydrolyzed dextran.

Zsigmondy investigated the idea of protective colloids and was able to show that different substances varied in their ability to protect other colloidal dispersions. Zsigmondy also developed a measure for the protective power in the "Gold Number" which is defined as the number of milligrams of protective substance which just fails to prevent the change of color from red to violet in 10 ml. of a pure red gold sol (0.05 to 0.06 Gm. gold/liter) upon the addition of 1 ml. of 10 per cent sodium chloride solution. It has been found possible to differentiate normal spinal fluid from the spinal fluid of patients suffering from spinal meningitis or syphilis, on the basis of its protective power for gold sols. A striking difference has been noted in the protective power of the serum of cancer patients for a Congo red sol as compared with the protective power of normal serum.

Protected sols of silver or silver salts are used quite commonly in pharmacy for the antiseptic action of the silver without the corrosive or the protein-precipitating properties associated with the water-soluble salts. Such preparations are, for example, Mild Silver Protein, N.F. XI., and Strong Silver Protein and Colloidal Silver Iodide of the N.F. X.

In the presence of protective colloids, large crystals generally do not form. For example, gelatin is often used in ice cream to give it a smooth feeling by preventing the growth of large crystals of ice, which impart grittiness. The concept of protective colloids has been found useful in those patients who develop kidney stones. The parenteral administration of hyaluronidase causes an increase in the urinary colloids which serves to reduce the tendency toward the formation of large stones which would be difficult to pass.[4]

In a system in which the colloid is protected, any changes resulting in a coagulation of the protector upset the equilibrium and result in separation of the colloid.

GELS

Definition. Gels are somewhat difficult to define; consequently, there is considerable difference of opinion as to what constitutes a gel. The rapid precipitation of a highly insoluble material which adsorbs water strongly usually results in a gelatinous precipitate, leaving a clear supernatant liquid, as, for example, the precipitation of ferric hydroxide or aluminum hydroxide. A uniform precipitation throughout the entire solution with the formation of a somewhat rigid but plastic mass in which all or nearly all of the liquid is enclosed by the precipitate may be termed a *jelly*. Mixing of the materials must be complete, and the separation of the gelatinous material must take place slowly and uniformly enough to permit the formation of a good gel structure. Gels have a few of the properties of solids in that they retain their shape, cohere and show strains when subjected to a stress. Like the sols, the gels may be grouped as hydrophilic, alcoholophilic, hydrophobic, etc.

Classification. Gels have been classified as *heat-reversible* (examples: gelatin, soap) if, upon warming, they liquefy and reset on cooling, and *heat-irreversible* (example: silica gel in water) if they do not reset. Freundlich has suggested the terms *elastic* and *nonelastic* for the same classes of gels. For example, gelatin continually shrinks to scales on drying and when moistened swells and returns to colloidal dispersion (elastic), whereas silica gel shrinks uniformly to a limiting volume,* after which little change in volume occurs on further drying or upon wetting (nonelastic). In many cases gels can be liquefied by shaking or other mechanical action, but they return to the gel state more or less rapidly after the mechanical disturbance has ceased. This is referred to as *thixotropy* (changing by touch). The principle has been applied in the use of drilling muds used in sinking oil wells, in the dripless paints presently on the market and in a few pharmaceuticals.

Structure. There is a division of opinion on the structure of gels, some postulating more or less definite structures and others being able to find no definite arrangement. The honeycomb or network theory visualizes the internal phase as a network of walls enclosing spaces in which the external phase or liquid is trapped. Soap jellies show a definite fibrillar arrangement and on setting are supposed to swell and hydrate, thereby holding the dispersing medium. In a more recent theory, the particles of the internal phase are thought of as elongated solvated particles which are able to link together in chains and 3-dimensional meshworks which entrap the free liquid remaining after the formation of the solvated hulls around the particles. Agar gel seems to have a tangled lattice structure made up of nonspherical molecules. In solutions of macromolecular substances, the macromolecules, frequently elongated, may link together to form a homogeneous 1-phase system; or the macromolecules may partially orient themselves at junction points to result in partial crystallization.

The shape of the colloid particle has a bearing on gelation. Colloids known to have particles spheroid in shape set to gels with difficulty. The more asymmetric the particles, the lower the concentration at which gel formation may occur. Fibrillar colloidal particles generally may be expected to give gels easily, but there are notable exceptions to this.

---

* Limiting volume is that point beyond which there is no further change in volume.

The swelling of a gel is accompanied by the development of both heat and pressure. In general, the presence of nonelectrolytes does not affect swelling, whereas electrolytes have a definite influence on swelling. The swelling of proteins is at a minimum at the iso-electric point but is increased considerably by either acids or bases. The effect of neutral salts on the swelling of gels is variable. Hofmeister observed that, in general, the anions are more effective than the cations in causing an increased swelling of gels. He arranged them in the order of decreasing effect as follows: $CNS^- > I^- > Br^- > NO_3^- > ClO_3^- > Cl^-$. Some, such as sulfate, tartrate and citrate, cause shrinkage. This order of ions is known as the *Hofmeister* or *lyotropic series*.

Freshly formed gels undergo changes in properties referred to as aging. A fresh hydrous oxide gel is highly hydrous, adsorbs ions readily and is peptized easily. On standing, it slowly becomes less hydrous and the other properties mentioned recede also. Sometimes the gel exudes liquid as it shrinks. Graham first noticed this and referred to it as *syneresis*.

In very dilute gels, the rate of diffusion may not differ much from that in pure water. In the more concentrated rigid gels, diffusion takes place much more slowly. In this way, the production of insoluble crystalline materials may be slowed down and larger and better formed crystals grown. The reactions in gels or jellies sometimes lead to the formation of rhythmic bands or rings of precipitated material instead of large crystals. These are known as *Liesegang rings*.

AEROSOLS

The term *aerosol* applies to lyophobic colloidal systems, the external phase of which is a gas or a mixture of gases and the internal phase a solid or a liquid. When the internal phase consists of liquid particles sufficiently small to remain suspended, the resulting colloidal system is referred to as a cloud, a fog or a mist. When the internal phase consists of solid particles, the resulting colloidal system is referred to as a smoke.

On the whole, the aerosols are less stable

systems than the hydrosols. The density and the viscosity of gases are low and offer little resistance to motion of the particles, particularly the settling out of the more dense solid or liquid particles. In addition, the particles of dispersed liquid evaporate and disappear if the liquid has a high vapor pressure, or may agglomerate and settle out.

Like the lyosols (dispersions in liquids), the aerosols may be prepared by both condensation and dispersion methods. Any substance readily vaporized should form a mist. The formation of a cloud or a mist by the condensation of vapors requires a slight supersaturation and the presence of suitable nuclei upon which the condensation can occur. These nuclei may be carriers of electricity such as α or β rays and ions, or dust and smoke particles. Mists show the Tyndall phenomenon and brownian movement and bear charges.

Various devices are available for the mechanical dispersion of liquid particles. The ordinary atomizer is an example of a liquid dispersion device but the particles produced are usually rather large in diameter. By suitable modification, smaller droplet sizes can be obtained, but the size of the droplets is generally more variable than that produced by the condensation method.

The idea of air-borne pathogens grew, then declined between 1910 and 1930, but again grew with the spread of psittacosis. The spread of epidemics of virus infections such as influenza, measles and chickenpox may result from the evaporation of droplets of nasal secretions leaving nuclei which are or become air-borne.

The eminent Lord Lister, the man generally given credit for the application of antiseptics to surgical operations, was the first to suggest the sterilization of the air in the operating room by spraying antiseptic materials around the room. Since the devices used produced only coarse particles which settled rapidly, the method was relatively ineffective. Since 1940, there has been an awakened interest in the possibility of disinfecting the atmosphere in confined areas. Using improved devices for dispersing the particles, propylene glycol containing 10 per cent hexylresorcinol and 0.05 per cent sulfonated lorol (a wetting agent) was found to be an effective disinfectant.[5] The particle size must be below 1 μ for the material to give the desired action. The results of controlled tests[6] in an experimental chamber and in a schoolroom show that the glycols do not destroy the airborne bacteria but simply increase the rate of fall of the organisms. Further, the glycol does not condense on dust-borne organisms and, therefore, does not carry them down.

Hand-size aerosol dispensers containing compressed Freon gas, a very concentrated pyrethrum extract and some sesame oil, were introduced for the protection of Armed Forces overseas personnel from malaria mosquitoes. Aerosol dispensers containing solutions of DDT are available for home use.

Aerosols produced from a variety of therapeutic agents have been useful in the treatment of respiratory conditions.[7] Aerosols have been recommended as carriers for atropine or drugs for the treatment of asthma, and devices are available which force very finely powdered penicillin into the lungs for the treatment of respiratory infections. Nebulized epinephrine will exhibit the bronchodilating effect without a systemic effect on circulation when administered in this way. For maximum safety and effectiveness, it appears that the particle sizes dispensed by the nebulizer should range between 0.5 and 2.0 microns.[8] The enzyme dornase may be used to thin out viscous bronchial secretions or necrotic accumulations. The increasing number of therapeutic products becoming available as aerosols include antibiotics, local anesthetics, burn treatments, vitamin preparations and dermatologic products, including poison oak and ivy treatments. A wide variety of cosmetic products are being packaged in this way also.

Smokes contain solid particles dispersed in a gas, and, when the particle size is sufficiently small, these aerosols show the same properties mentioned for the clouds or the mists. Smokes may be produced by the condensation of vapors as, for example, when hydrogen chloride gas and ammonia gas are allowed to react, producing ammonium chloride. The powdering of many solids leads to dispersions of the very fine particles in air. These dispersions sometimes have been the cause of serious dust explosions around grinding equipment. The air around cities generally contains a considerable amount of finely divided solids, as a result of combustion of fuels in homes, industries and automobiles, and has been implicated as a contributing factor to the development of cancer, especially respiratory forms.

The combination of certain geographic and weather conditions with relatively high concentrations of combustion products in the air has resulted in the smogs at Donora, Pennsylvania and in the Los Angeles area in California. One phase of chemical warfare is the artificial production of smokes to hide movements of men and equipment or to signal information. Miners are often subjected to the inhalation of smokes, some of which have been found to produce serious lung disturbances (silicosis, anthracosis).

Various devices have been suggested and used for the *flocculation* of aerosols such as high-frequency sound waves or a high-tension electric field. The Cottrell precipitator is an arrangement for coagulating particles by means of a high-tension electric discharge and is used to some extent in industry to flocculate smokes. The increasing adoption of smoke-control ordinances will stimulate the application of this and other devices for the flocculation of aerosols discharged by industry.

ADSORPTION

Adsorption occurs when no chemical reaction is expected and may be defined as the concentration of a substance, irrespective of its state, on the surface of a liquid or a solid with which it is in contact. The substance being adsorbed is called the *adsorbate*, and the substance on which it is adsorbed is called the *adsorbent*. Adsorption differs from *absorption* in that adsorption (a sucking to) is a surface phenomenon, whereas absorption is an actual penetration of the molecules of the substance being taken up between those of the absorbent. The adsorptive power of carbon in the form of coal, vegetable or animal charcoal was recognized, studied and demonstrated by the pharmacists Scheele, Lowitz, Figuier and Hagen in the 18th and 19th centuries. During adsorption, the concentration of the substance being adsorbed, the adsorbate, changes rapidly and a dynamic equilibrium is soon set up between the concentration of the adsorbate in the original phase and on the adsorbent.

An attempt to explain the mechanism of adsorption has led to a number of theories which are reviewed in detail in texts devoted to colloid chemistry. It is more or less generally accepted that the adsorbed layer is not monomolecular but is composed of many layers of molecules arranged in such a fashion that the packing of molecules is tightest immediately on the surface of the adsorbent and looser the greater the distance from the surface of the adsorbent. The arrangement of adsorbed molecules on the surface of the adsorbent then would be somewhat analogous to the arrangement of adsorbed ions on the colloidal particle diagrammed in Figure 95.

Adsorption is one of the important properties displayed by colloidal dispersions, although it is by no means limited to materials in the colloidal state. Any substance in the liquid or the solid state may be an adsorbent. There are then 6 theoretically possible, simple adsorption systems (that is, a gas, a liquid or a solid adsorbed on liquid or solid substances). There may be combinations of these when, for example, adsorption takes place from a solution. It is likely that both solute and solvent will be adsorbed, although preferential adsorption of one or the other is not only possible but also well recognized. When increasing the concentration of the solute results in a lowering of surface tension, the solute is largely adsorbed and concentrates at the surface or interface, leaving the solution relatively less concentrated. The process is referred to as *positive adsorption*. On the other hand, if the solute results in an increase in surface tension, the solvent is adsorbed selectively and tends to increase at the surface or interface. *Negative adsorption* occurs, and the solution becomes more concentrated with respect to solute.

One of the most general statements

which may be made with respect to adsorption is that it is selective and specific, depending on the nature of both adsorbent and adsorbate. A good illustration of this statement is the behavior of charcoal. It has varying adsorptive power for different substances, and charcoal obtained from different sources or prepared by different methods will have a varying adsorptive capacity for a given substance. The degree of adsorption varies with conditions involving both the adsorbent and the adsorbate.

Most of the adsorbents which have been studied are solids. Little is known of the actual nature of the surfaces of these materials, and it is not possible to measure accurately the specific surface (ratio of surface to volume) of the adsorbent. Sometimes amorphous forms of a given substance are better adsorbents than the crystalline form, and sometimes the reverse is true.

From a study of adsorbents, it is found that charcoal has an adsorptive power greater than that of most other substances. The use of charcoal for the adsorption of poison gases was developed rapidly during World War I. The charcoal must be very active and must be prepared carefully to provide as large a surface as possible. The strong adsorption of gases by activated charcoal may be employed to produce low pressures within sealed containers, and the selective adsorption of gases may be utilized in the separation of the components of a gaseous mixture. An activated charcoal is official in the *N.F.*, and its adsorptive power is tested by means of its ability to remove the dye methylene blue and the alkaloid strychnine (as the sulfate) from aqueous solutions. It was introduced into medicine with the idea that its adsorptive capacity would be evident, removing gases and other materials, thereby relieving gastric distress. This objective has not been attained in practice, since it has been shown that the adsorptive capacity of charcoal is diminished greatly in the presence of gastric contents. On the other hand, there is evidence that, besides adsorbing bacteria and toxins, charcoal may adsorb other components of the intestinal content such as trypsin, tryptophan and carotene, and therefore may impair the nutrition of the patient. Charcoal is employed effectively in the concentration of penicillin from the culture broth in the course of the manufacture of penicillin.

Aluminum oxide (alumina) has been found to be a good adsorbent for water, carbon dioxide and alcohol, while the great capacity of silica gel for organic vapors can be used in the recovery of benzene from coke plants, and the recovery of other solvents such as alcohol, ether and acetone. The administration of aluminum hydroxide gel to control nausea may be detrimental during therapy with Aureomycin Hydrochloride and Terramycin Hydrochloride since both are adsorbed significantly. Anticholinergic drugs are also adsorbed appreciably and counteracted.[9] On the other hand, it has not been possible to show any correlation between the activity of an antibiotic and its adsorption by resistant and nonresistant bacteria.

Bentonite, a clay derived from volcanic ash, is composed of hydrated aluminum silicate; it is mined in South Dakota, Wyoming and California. It was official for the first time in *U.S.P. XII*. It is a good adsorbent and will take up water to form a swollen, sticky, gelatinous mass 10 to 30 times the original volume of the dry bentonite. The official requirements specify a minimal amount of swelling equivalent to about the lower limit mentioned above. It has been shown that it also undergoes swelling in ethyl, propyl, butyl and isoamyl alcohols, benzene, acetone and paraffin oil.[10] It is used medicinally largely as a suspending or emulsifying agent and has a wide variety of industrial uses in cosmetics, horticultural sprays, insecticides, soaps, etc.

Other industrially important applications of the adsorption of liquids are found in the adsorption of lubricants and adhesives on the surfaces to be lubricated or cemented together, in the manufacture and the application of paints, and in agriculture in the wetting of soils and the spreading of sprays and insecticides on the leaves of plants.

The adsorption of ions on colloidal particles is considered to be one of the factors governing the stability of lyophobic colloidal dispersions. The adsorption of ions by the particles of a precipitate is pointed out in texts on quantitative analysis as a source of error in certain types of procedures. Likewise, the adsorptive capacity of filter paper for ions or of glass surfaces for thiamine and similar substances at low concentrations may be a source of error in analytical procedures unless suitable precautions are observed.

John Uri Lloyd, a pharmacist and manufacturer of pharmaceuticals in Cincinnati, published many papers in the field of colloid chemistry and discovered the peculiar adsorptive property of a hydrous aluminum silicate (Lloyd's reagent) for alkaloids. With it, alkaloids can be removed readily from acid solution and concentrated, improving the methods of preparation of alkaloids. Other clays have since been found useful as adsorbents for alkaloids.

Another example of the application of adsorption on solids which has been put to spectacular use in recent years in the separation of mixtures of plant pigments and in the separation and the purification of hormones and vitamins is the *chromatograph*, first developed by the Russian botanist Tswett in 1906. The increasing use of the method dates from about 1931, when Kuhn and co-workers used it in preparative studies on the carotenoids and through its agency were able to separate the isomeric carotenes. A solution containing a mixture of solutes is passed through a column of adsorbent packed in a suitable glass tube constricted at the lower end. A variety of solvents may be used, depending on the nature and the solubility of both the solute and the adsorbent. It is sometimes advantageous to prepare the column with layers of 2 or more adsorbents. The selection of solvent and adsorbent is largely empirical. As the solution passes down through the column, the most actively adsorbed substance or substances are deposited near the top of the column, the less adsorbed near the bottom; the unadsorbed substances pass through the column with the effluent. The zones of adsorbate may be made sharper by passing some of the pure solvent through the column. The moist column of adsorbent is pushed out of the tube and, if the zones are colored, may be cut into segments along the boundaries and the components dissolved out of the sections of adsorbent with another solvent. Several ingenious methods have been developed to permit the accurate sectioning of columns containing adsorbed colorless substances. If these modifications fail, the column is sectioned arbitrarily, or a process of fractional elution is employed. Chromatography has been applied in a wide variety of research problems such as the determination of homogeneity of substances, the comparison of substances thought to be identical, the concentration of materials present in very dilute solution and the determination of molecular structure.

The use of the chromatograph has been suggested as a means of detecting the presence of materials such as glycosides, alkaloids and vitamins, and also for the detection of the adulteration of pharmaceutical preparations, such as tinctures, etc. The process has been modified further by the adsorption of 1 or 2 drops of a liquid galenical preparation or a solution of a solid galenical on a flat layer of adsorbent on a slide and observation of the concentric zones under a microscope. Adsorption of substances on filter paper strips, sheets or disks has been developed extensively as a means of separating and identifying very small amounts of materials in fairly complex mixtures. Some official assays involve chromatographic separation of the desired component of the mixture prior to its determination, as is the case in the assay of Digitoxin preparations and sulfonamide mixtures (N.F.). Laboratory devices for producing deionized water represent another application of the process of chromatography.

Bacteria have been shown to adsorb hydrogen ions in varying degree, depending on the species, and it is suggested that the toxic or disinfecting character of certain electrolytes seems to be associated with the adsorbability of the cation. The adsorption of germicides on micro-organisms has been shown to depend on the electric charge and is independent of chemical composition.

Modern theories of contact catalysis are

based on the phenomenon of adsorption, and this represents one of the most important applications of adsorption.

SURFACE FILMS—SURFACE-ACTIVE AGENTS

The formation of surface films is dependent on adsorption of a substance at a surface. The Langmuir theory may be presented in the following way. If a small amount of a pure saturated hydrocarbon or a mixture of saturated hydrocarbons is placed on pure water, it remains in a globule resembling a lens in shape, it has no effect on the surface tension of the surrounding water, and the water does not cover over the lens. However, if a small amount of a substance such as stearic acid or stearyl alcohol which contains a long hydrocarbon chain with a carboxyl or hydroxyl group at one end is placed on pure water, there is an almost instantaneous spreading over the surface of the water. The carboxyl group or the hydroxyl group has a solubilizing effect on this end of the molecule. The remainder of the molecule exhibits the insolubility in water characteristic of a hydrocarbon, and the stearic acid is prevented from being dispersed evenly as a true solution in water. Therefore, it spreads on the surface as a film, the carboxyl groups being submerged in the water, and the hydrocarbon radicals sticking up into the air above the surface (Fig. 97). The spreading of the stearic acid film may be observed readily if most of the surface of the water is coated with a thin layer of talc. When a drop of stearic acid solution is placed in the clear area, the boundary of the talc is pushed back immediately in all directions as the film spreads.

Substances which, like stearic acid, will spread on water, with a consequent lowering of surface tension, are spoken of as *surface-active substances*. They are made up of a nonpolar or hydrocarbon chain and a polar grouping (any of the oxygen-containing groups, the nitrogen- and sulfur-containing groups and unsaturated linkages). For accumulation of the substance at the surface, the hydrocarbon chain must be sufficiently long so that the strong mutual attraction of the water molecules will force the nonpolar hydrocarbon portion out to the surface.

A new concept of surface films based on an analysis of x-ray diffraction patterns of foams and films indicates that the surface film is composed of a hydrous gel structure. Water oriented in an icelike structure makes up the principal portion of the film and serves as a linkage to promote the cohesion of the unit cells of surface-active agents.

The study of the accumulation of such substances at the surface and the behavior of such surfaces has been applied to the determination of the cross-sectional area of molecules and the length of molecules, and to supplement the proof of the structure of some types of complicated molecules in the field of steroids and triterpene derivatives. By the proper manipulation, oriented layers of metal salts of palmitic and other fatty acids can be deposited upon clean glass to give a surface which prevents the reflection of light.

Substances which do not alter the surface tension of the solvent by more than a few per cent in molar concentration are termed *surface-inactive substances*. Electrolytes such as salts of short-chain aliphatic acids and bases, and nonelectrolytes such as sucrose and glycerin, are surface-inactive.

Surface-active agents frequently are useful as wetting agents and detergents. An illustration of the results of a surface-active agent in promoting wetting and spreading

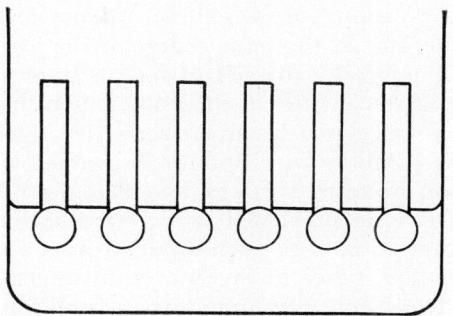

Fig. 97. Orientation of stearic acid molecules at the surface of water. The circular end represents the carboxyl group and the rectangular portion the hydrocarbon chain.

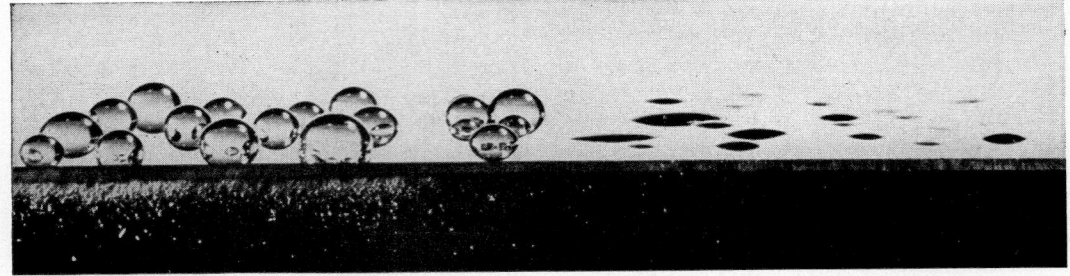

Fig. 98. Illustrating the effect of a surface-active agent on the spreading properties of a liquid. At the left are globules of water standing on the waxed surface of a pane of glass. (Parallel lines across the bottom of the photograph are the edges of the pane.) At the right are water globules to which a surface-active agent has been added, on the same surface. Note how the water spreads out in a thin film. (From Atlas Surface-Active Agents, Wilmington, Del., Atlas Powder Co.)

is shown in Figure 98. The preferential wetting of substances is applied in many fields, such as the manufacture or the processing of leather and textiles, and in the application of solders, paints, varnishes and insecticides. Caryl and Ericks[11] have set up 4 qualifications of a good wetting agent as follows:

1. High wetting power even in very low concentrations.
2. Stability in the dry form and in solutions, especially in acid solutions where soap cannot be used.
3. Solubility in water and organic solvents, especially in nonpolar solvents.
4. Resistance to hard water.

These properties can be attained by properly selecting and balancing a hydrophobic group with a hydrophilic group which is not hydrolyzed easily and gives the compound solubility in water without depriving it of solubility in the organic solvent.*

Caryl and Ericks have classified wetting agents as shown in Table 7, where R is a fatty alkyl group and R' a primary or secondary nonfatty alkyl group and Ar is aromatic.

* A tabulation of surface-active agents commercially available in 1939 may be found in Ind. Eng. Chem. **31**:66, and a list of more than 200 agents available in 1943 is given in Ind. Eng. Chem. **35**: 126. Agents for use in insecticides are listed in U.S. Dept. Agr. Bur. Entomol. Plant Quarantine E-607, Oct. 1943, while a list of agents of possible value in hydrophilic ointment bases is given in Bull. Nat. Form. Com. **10**:173, and in Pharm. J. **164**:265.

Gershenfeld[12] has classified the wetting agents into 3 groups: (1) *anionic* or *anion-active agents* in which the lipophilic (fat-loving) group is a portion of the negative ion (attracted to the anode in an electric field), such as the sulfonated alcohols, amides and esters, the alkylarylsulfonates, the alkylarylether sulfonates, salts of the bile acids and the soaps; (2) the *cationic* or *cation-active agents* in which the lipophilic group is a portion of the positive ion such as the quaternary ammonium salts, cetyl pyridinium chloride, alkyl substituted pyridinium or ammonium chlorides, bromides or iodides and others; and (3) *nonionic agents,* such as the Carbowaxes (polyethylene glycols), Tweens and Sapamines.

The bactericidal action of surface-active agents has been investigated and found to be dependent on the chemical structure and the hydrophilic-hydrophobic balance of the molecule, on the ionic charge of the hydrophobic group, the pH of the medium and the characteristics of the micro-organisms.[13] It is suggested that surface-active agents may combine with oppositely charged sites upon bacterial surfaces, and that the process can be prevented or reversed through competition with such substances as phosphatides, other detergents, or hydrogen or hydroxyl ions. In some cases, adsorption of small amounts of agent leads to irreversible damage to the cell membrane. All cationic detergents (quaternary ammonium compounds, lauryl esters of amino acid hydrochlorides, Zephiran and Emulsols) in-

Table 7. Classification of Wetting Agents

Group	Type	Formula	Description	Relative Wetting Power of the Best of Each Type as Marketed, in Per Cent
A	1	RCOONa	Soaps	..
	2	RSO$_4$Na	Fatty alcohol sulfates	23
	3	RCON—C$_2$H$_4$SO$_4$Na | H	Sulfated fatty acid amides	5
		RCOOC$_2$H$_4$SO$_4$Na	Sulfated fatty acid esters	6
B	1	H | R$'_2$C—SO$_4$Na	Secondary alcohol sulfates	25
	2	R'—OOC—CH$_2$ | R'—OOC—C—SO$_4$Na | H	Sulfated esters of higher alcohols and dibasic acids	Not marketed
	3	R'—Ar—SO$_3$Na	Alkylarylsulfonates	6
	4	R'—OOC—CH$_2$ | R'—OOC—C—SO$_3$Na | H	Sulfonated esters of alcohols and dibasic acids	100
C			Miscellaneous	24

hibit bacterial metabolism, some at concentrations of 1 to 30,000. The cationic detergents act best at an alkaline pH and the anionic at an acid pH. The cationic agents as a group exhibit marked bactericidal effects on gram-positive organisms and a somewhat less-pronounced action on gram-negative organisms. The anionic detergents [cetylsulfate sodium, myristyl sulfate sodium, Duponol L. S. (oleyl sulfate), Tergitol-8, etc.], are germicidal only against the gram-positive organisms and are considerably less effective than the cationic compounds.

The addition of chemicals commonly employed as wetting agents is variously reported to potentiate the bactericidal or bacteriostatic effectiveness of antiseptics or to be without effect on the activity of other antiseptics.[14] Nonionic and anionic surfactants did not interfere with the antibacterial activity of 4 antibiotics commonly used topically.[15] The presence of nonionic and anionic wetting agents in ointments produces little enhancement or even a diminution in the fungistatic effectiveness of various antiseptics.[16]

In a study of 9 selected surface-active agents for use in ointment bases,[17] the ionic surface-active agents Trigamine Stearate (similar to triethanolamine stearate), sulfonated hydrogenated castor oil, Cationic Agent D (essentially the stearylamine salt of the stearyl amide of ethyl phosphoric acid), and Triton K-60 (cetyl dimethyl benzyl ammonium chloride) were found to be irritating to the human skin; while the nonionic surface-active agents, the Carbowaxes 4,000 and 1,500 (mixtures of polyethylene glycols), glyceryl laurate, Tween 60 (a polyoxyalkylene derivative of sorbitan monostearate) and Arlacel B (mannitan mono-oleate) were found to be nonirritating. On the other hand, many surface-active agents will penetrate the mucosa of the eye, producing lesions when applied as ophthalmic ointments. This toxic effect was greatest with the cationic agents and least with the nonionic agents.[18]

Dilute solutions of surface-active agents in water can disperse appreciable amounts of dyes, hydrocarbons and other substances that are notoriously insoluble in water to produce true colloidal dispersions. There are on the market clear stable dispersions of the oil-soluble vitamins A and D which are miscible with water and aqueous fluids (Water-Miscible Vitamin A Solution, U.S.P., Vi-Syneral and others). To explain the phenomenon, it has been proposed that the collidal surfactants orient themselves in such a manner that the polar groups are exposed to the water, while the hydrophobic groups are in contact. The resulting structure is referred to as a *micelle*. It is then assumed that the normally water insoluble substance "dissolves" in the hydrophobic portion of the micelle and is carried into apparent solution in water.

Surface-active agents and emulsifiers have come into extensive use in the commercial processing of foods, although the practice has been questioned in some cases by the Food and Drug Administration. The widespread use of surface-active agents for home cleaning purposes has resulted in alterations in the treatment of sewage because of the foam stabilizing and the dispersing properties of surface-active agents.

FOAMS

Foams consist of disperse systems in which a gas or a vapor is enclosed in a film of the liquid dispersion medium. Liquids with a low surface tension and a low vapor pressure, while at the same time having a high surface viscosity, will foam easily. Consequently, those substances which, when dissolved in a liquid, result in a lowering of the surface tension and concentration at the interface, tend to increase foaming. The tougher the liquid film around the gas bubble becomes, the more stable is the froth. It will be recalled that such substances as soaps, saponins, hydrophilic colloids (for example, proteins) accumulate in the surface and, consequently, are expected to favor foam formation. Any material which increases the tenacity or the viscosity of the film as, for example, finely divided solids (i.e., coagulated protein in milk foam, finely ground ores in the flotation process) will increase the permanence of the foam. The systems represent dynamic equilibria and are comparatively unstable.

The dispersion of gas in the foam is relatively coarse and for the most part does not approach colloidal dimensions. The justification for including these systems along with colloids is the fact that the films may be of colloidal dimensions (lamellar difform systems) or may exhibit colloidal properties. The thickness of the films surrounding the bubbles influences the color of the light reflected from the surface of the bubble. The films around the gas bubbles of a foam are formed by the approach to each other of 2 already formed liquid surfaces. In the case of pure liquids, there is no resistance when these surfaces approach, and they merge without the formation of a froth. With solutions of soluble salts, there is a difference in the concentration of the salt in the surface layer and the body of the liquid, and when the layer of liquid between the films becomes thin, there is a resistance to mixing (Fig. 99). With many simple salts, the film is not very viscous, and the froth is not stable unless finely divided solid is present. In the case of solutions of surface-active materials, there is formed a more tenacious film, mixing does not occur,

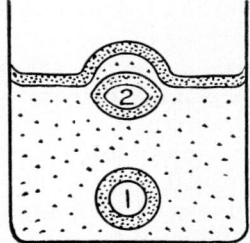

Fig. 99. Bubble under surface film. The bubble forms at *1* and is shown at *2* just below the surface. The relative concentration in the film and the body of liquid is indicated by the closeness of the dots (positive adsorption). (After Foulk, C. W.: Ind. Eng. Chem. 23:1283)

the concentrations in the film and the body of the liquid remain different, and the film persists, giving a more permanent foam.

Foams may be both desirable and undesirable, depending on the purpose for which the mixture is to be used. The hydrophilic colloids easily give foams, and in the transfer of large volumes of protein solutions this can be a disadvantage. For example, foams are undesirable in steam boilers, in distillation processes, in evaporations and during the deep culture production of antibiotics. On the other hand, a fairly stable foam is desirable in sodas and beer, the foam of either being stabilized by proteins. The copious foaming of saponins is responsible for the froth on root beer. The albumin of egg white produces a thick rigid foam (meringue). Soap lather aids in carrying away the solid particles from soiled material. The separation of valuable ores from inert material by the flotation process depends on the formation of a foam by blowing air through water containing surface-active substances, the fine ore particles collecting in and tending to stabilize the froth.

When the foam from a sterile gelatin solution, with or without added thrombin, is dried at low temperature and pressure, an absorbable hemostatic sponge (solid foam) is obtained. Absorbable Gelatin Sponge is now a *U.S.P.* product. Stable foams are effective in extinguishing small, confined fires.

The destruction of foams is of some importance in laboratory operations as well as in industrial operations. Foams of the less-persistent films can be broken by the addition of materials which give very weak films, as, for example, ether and the higher alcohols (heptyl, octyl or nonyl alcohols). Capryl Alcohol, (a U.S.P. reagent), is used for this purpose in laboratory testing. A current of cold air, by causing a condensation of vapors within the bubble, often will break up a foam. Castor oil has been effective in breaking up boiler foams.

EMULSIONS

INTRODUCTION

Several types of colloidally disperse systems have been discussed previously;

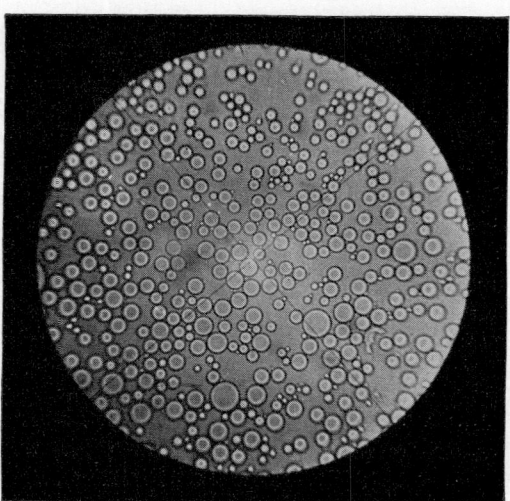

FIG. 100. A moderately concentrated emulsion of oil in water. The circles are the droplets of the internal or disperse phase (oil) in the external phase or dispersion medium (water.) (From Atlas Surface-Active Agents, Wilmington, Del., Atlas Powder Co.)

namely, solids in liquids (sols), gases in liquids (foams), liquids in gases (mists) and solids in gases (smokes). The dispersion of droplets of a liquid in a second liquid with which it is immiscible is referred to as an *emulsion*. The predominant size of the globules determines whether an emulsion belongs to the coarse or the colloidal system. In a very large number of the emulsions studied, the size of the droplets falls outside the usually accepted limits of the colloidal range, the droplets being visible under an ordinary microscope. However, emulsions are considered as colloidal systems since the third component generally necessary to stabilize the system, the emulsifying agent, either is distinctly colloidal or exhibits colloidal properties. The stable film is the lamellar type of difform system.

The liquid divided into small globules is called the *disperse, internal* or *discontinuous phase,* while the liquid in which the globules are scattered is called the *dispersion medium, external* or *continuous phase.* Both phases expose boundaries or surfaces to each other, the surface of the disperse phase being convex and that of the dispersion medium concave. (See Fig. 100.)

If one liquid is water and the other an oil or other liquid immiscible with water, then obviously 2 types of emulsions may be formed. The oil may be dispersed in the water to produce an oil-in-water (o/w) emulsion or the water may be dispersed in the oil, when a water-in-oil (w/o) emulsion is recognized. The nature and the behavior of the emulsifying agent probably are the main factors in determining the type of emulsion which will result. Since the substances which may serve as emulsifying agents are so widely different chemically and physically, *no one theory completely explains the formation of all emulsions.*

FORMATION AND STABILITY

A wide variety of ideas and theories have been proposed to account for the formation and the stability of emulsions. The large number of factors involved in the formation of emulsions and the determination of stability have resulted in considerable discussion in the literature. As a rule, only one or a very few systems or characteristics have been investigated at a time by an author.

In general, the formation of emulsions of a pure oil in water is limited to systems of very low oil content. About 2 per cent of oil seems to be the maximum amount which has been dispersed in water. In order to obtain more concentrated emulsions, a third substance, the emulsifying agent, is necessary. The manner in which this third substance alters the properties of the systems to produce stable emulsions forms the basis of many of the theories which have been proposed.

Surface and Interfacial Tension

When two liquids are in contact, each liquid has a tendency to maintain as small a surface as possible, as a result of its surface tension. *Surface tension* is a force which becomes evident near the surface of the liquid where the molecules are subjected to unequal attraction. As shown in Figure 101, the molecules of liquid at the surface are subjected to attractive forces (van der Waal's forces) acting on approximately one half of the surface as contrasted with the molecules within the body of the liquid which are attracted equally in all directions. As a result of the sideways and downward pull on the molecules in the surface layer, these surface molecules act as if they formed a tightly stretched but elastic skin over the surface of the liquid. The molecules which have escaped from the liquid into the space above the liquid exert practically no attractive force for the surface molecules. A liquid in contact with its vapor tends to contract so as to present a minimal surface in contact with its vapor. The Du Nouy tensiometer, being used as shown in Figure 102 to determine interfacial tension, also may be used to measure the force required to lift the ring through the liquid-vapor interface, namely, the surface tension.

The surface tension between the 2 liquid boundaries, or the force necessary to break the interface between 2 immiscible liquids, commonly is referred to as the *interfacial tension.* The numerical value of the interfacial tension generally lies between the surface tension of the 2 liquids. When a pair of immiscible liquids is shaken together, both liquids are broken up into small drops. The forces of surface tension tend to draw the liquids together so as to present as small a surface as possible, and the drops tend to coalesce. If there is present a third substance which tends to change the surface tension of the liquid having a high surface tension in such a way as to decrease the interfacial tension, the emulsion will be somewhat more stable. It has been shown that the interfacial tension is definitely a factor contributing to the stability of most emulsions, although there are cases where it seems to have little effect. While good emulsifying agents generally give solutions with lowered

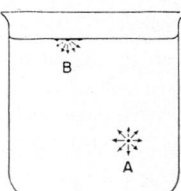

Fig. 101. Illustrating the unequal attractive forces on molecule *B* at the surface as contrasted with molecule *A* in the body of the liquid.

Formation and Stability 133

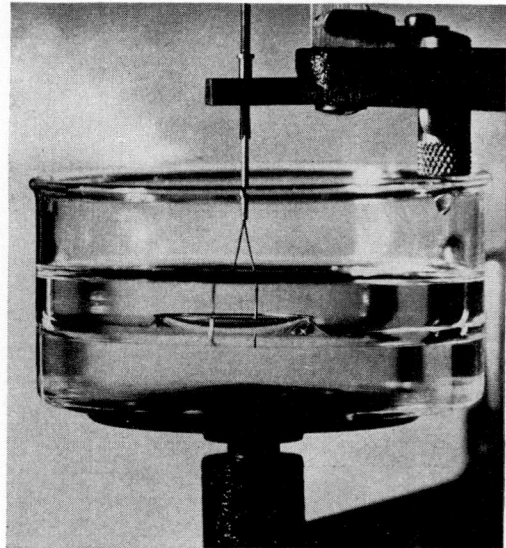

Fig. 102. Interfacial-tension measurement. Oil is layered over water, in which the ring is immersed. Measurements are made of the force required to lift the ring through the oil-water interface. (From Atlas Surface-Active Agents, Wilmington, Del., Atlas Powder Co.)

surface tensions, not all substances lowering the surface tension of a given liquid will produce good emulsions; also, emulsions may be produced without any appreciable effect on surface tension, as when finely divided insoluble solids stabilize emulsions. It is evident that surface tension is not the only factor involved in the formation and the stabilization of emulsions. It can be shown that, as a general rule, the stability of emulsions increases when the interfacial tension decreases.

VISCOSITY

The general opinion is that viscosity of the emulsion exerts a greater influence on its stability than on the process of emulsification. Viscosity aids emulsification only by increasing the resistance to the coalescence of the globules of the emulsion. The viscosity of an emulsion may be dependent on a variety of factors: the addition of an emulsifying agent may result in an increase in the viscosity of the dispersion medium, a very viscous oil may be the internal phase of the emulsion, the viscosity of an emulsion may increase because of temperature

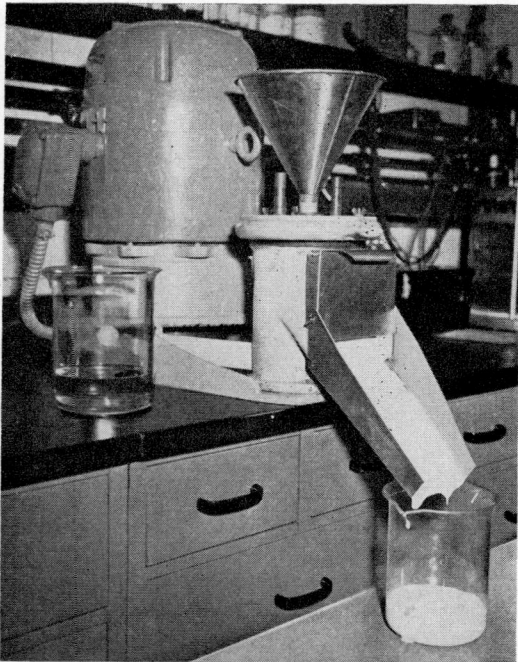

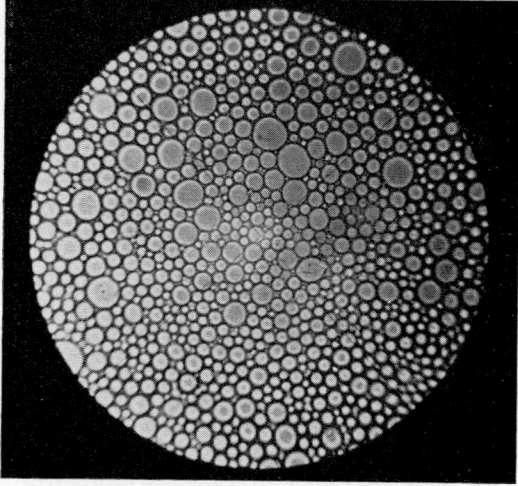

Fig. 103. (*Top*) Homogenizer. (*Bottom*) Shows nature of concentrated o/w emulsion which sticks to trough leading from homogenizer to receiver. (From Atlas Surface-Active Agents, Wilmington, Del., Atlas Powder Co.)

change or an increase in the number of globules, or a very concentrated emulsion may have been made. (See Fig. 103.) As a single factor, viscosity does not assure the production of stable emulsions since very viscous liquids (such as 50 % glycerin or a thick acacia solution) do not necessarily produce stable emulsions, while on the other hand, weak soap solutions which have low viscosity are very good emulsifying agents. However, substances which in solution have a high surface viscosity (such as saponin or albumin) produce more permanent emulsions. The viscosity of the emulsion may have an effect on the size of the globules of the dispersed phase and on the permanency of the emulsion as a result of a slowing of diffusion and a slowing of brownian movement, in this way tending to retard coalescence. A recent paper indicated that viscosity plays only a minor role in the gross stability of some emulsion systems.[19]

Hydration Theory

The Fischer hydration theory for the formation of emulsions postulates that emulsions can form only when the liquid which is to become the continuous phase is used in the formation of a hydrated compound of the emulsifying agent. Other points of the theory are that emulsifying agents vary in their capacity to produce emulsions in the same way in which they vary in the degree to which they are able to hydrate and that all of the water present should be combined with the emulsifying agent. Several objections have been raised to the theory on the basis that the small amounts of emulsifying agents sometimes necessary could hardly combine with all of the water present, that the theory is one-sided and does not consider the possibility of w/o emulsions and that emulsions can be stabilized by hydrophobic materials. Undoubtedly, the hydration of the emulsifier does play a part in the formation of certain emulsions, but the effect should not be overemphasized.

Adsorbed Films

Perhaps one of the more widely applicable theories of emulsion formation and stability is the theory of adsorbed films or film formation. While there has been much discussion on the nature of the film and its orientation, it generally is agreed that coalescence of the globules of the internal phase is retarded in a measure corresponding to the degree of film formation and the tenacity or the rigidity of the film. If an emulsion prepared with soap is diluted too greatly, the emulsion separates. The dilution may be increased if certain other colloids have been added previously. King[20] considers the strength and the compactness of the interfacial film as the most important factors favoring the stability of an emulsion. Most other factors are effective only insofar as they modify the properties of the film. One of the subsidiary factors in emulsion stability is the concentration of the emulsifying agent. The stability of an emulsion of moderately high oil concentration is affected seriously by the addition of electrolytes only if the amount of agent is insufficient to form a coherent film around the globule.

It has been possible to observe the film in some cases as in o/w emulsions in gelatin and in saponin solutions. The latter contain films of considerable rigidity so that the oil droplets may retain distorted shapes for a measurable period of time before the droplets become spherical. In the case of soap emulsions, Bancroft has suggested that the soap forms a third phase, separating the oil from the water, and that two surface tensions are involved in the formation of emulsions: the surface tension between the soap and the oil, and between the soap and the water. The side of the film that shows the higher surface tension becomes concave, and the phase (oil or water) on that side becomes the internal phase. This indicates that the nature of the emulsifying agent controls the type of emulsion formed. The soaps of monovalent metals are wetted more easily by water and, therefore, show a lower surface tension against water than against oil, and oil becomes the internal phase. In any event, the soap must concentrate at the oil-water interface. With the soaps it has been possible to show that the salts of the fatty acids below lauric acid are in molecular solution and act as poor emulsifying agents or not at all, whereas the salts beginning with laurates are partially or entirely colloidal and are good emulsifying agents. Many other emulsifiers are colloidal also, but some emulsions have been prepared without colloidally dispersed material.

ORIENTED WEDGE THEORY

Another idea which has been proposed to account for the soap emulsions is the so-called oriental wedge theory, suggested by Harkins, Hardy and Langmuir. According to this theory, when an emulsifier is com-

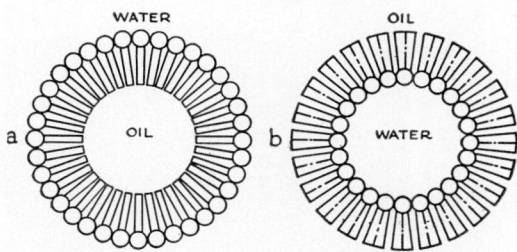

Fig. 104. The circles represent monovalent or divalent salt groups, the rectangles represent hydrocarbon radicals. (a) o/w emulsion; (b) w/o emulsion.

posed of a polar and a nonpolar portion and the 2 liquids to be emulsified differ in polarity, the molecules of the emulsifying agent will orient themselves at the interface between the 2 liquids in such a manner that the polar end of the emulsifier is attracted by the more polar liquid, the nonpolar end being repelled. This causes the molecules to line up in a more or less regular fashion, and, since the polar end in the case of a monovalent soap is considered to be larger in diameter than the hydrocarbon chain, the film would tend to be curved, enclosing the oil droplets as the internal phase. On the other hand, should the hydrocarbon end have the greater diameter, as when 2 hydrocarbon radicals are attached to a single divalent metal ion, the film would tend to curve so that the hydrocarbon radicals are to the outside and the water becomes the internal phase. These ideas are illustrated in Figure 104. Actual measurements of globule diameters and diameters of hydrocarbon radicals as well as the polar groups have shown that the dimensions are not sufficiently different to account for the differences of globule size, curvature of the interface or emulsion stability. However, there is evidence that the molecules of the emulsifier are oriented at the interface.

MIXED EMULSIFIERS

A more recent theory applies particularly to mixtures of emulsifiers. It was noticed that certain water-soluble surface-active agents would penetrate a water-insoluble film at the air-water interface but could be displaced by compression of the film. With other substances, a molecular complex seemed to form, in which case the film would withstand greater pressures than either component alone. If it is assumed that these facts would apply also at the water-oil interface, then it can be reasoned that such mixtures would produce a stronger film with greater resistance to rupture and would favor a more stable emulsion. The most favorable system develops when there is an oil-soluble material capable of forming a complex with an ionizable water soluble emulsifying agent. The ionizable substance provides surface charges which promote emulsion stability. Certain practical applications help to substantiate this idea. For example, the removal of mineral oil from wool can be promoted by adding oleyl alcohol to the detergent solution. A stable o/w emulsion forms as a result of closer packing of the molecules of the film. As with other theories, some data have been obtained which are contradictory to parts of the theory.

The viscosity of the oil phase may play a part in retarding the formation of emulsions with mixed emulsifiers or may account in part for inversion of the emulsion. This may result because the diffusion of the oil-soluble surface-active agents to the surface of the oil may be retarded by the high viscosity of the oil.

Concentrated emulsions stabilized with mixtures of aliphatic alcohols and sodium oleate produce thixotropic mixtures (see p. 122). The structure of the mixture traps the droplets of the internal phase and retards coalescence.[21]

SOLID EMULSIFIERS

The idea also has been advanced that the emulsifiers are in colloidal dispersion in the external phase and may represent a third phase in the same way as insoluble solid emulsifiers. Pickering has prepared emulsions of a petroleum oil in water with the aid of finely divided precipitated dry solids, such as lime, plaster of paris, chalk, silica or alumina. These were relatively unstable and were referred to as "quasi-emulsions." Moist basic sulfates of iron, copper, nickel and aluminum were more efficient agents for the formation of petroleum oil in water emulsions. He was able to show that the oil particles were coated with a film of solid particles. Hydrophilic solids such as bentonite, silica or alumina, which have a greater affinity for water than for oil, tend to promote o/w emulsions, whereas hydrophobic solids such as carbon black or graphite tend to promote w/o emulsions. For the solid to stabilize emulsions, it must concentrate in the interface, the particles must be very fine and the film elastic and continuous.

The information with respect to the formation of films surrounding the globules of the internal phase may be summarized as follows. To be good emulsifying agents, both hydrophilic and hydrophobic colloids, apparently soluble substances or finely divided solids must form a coherent film around the particles of the internal phase which film tends to prevent coalescence. The absorbed layer of emulsifier at the interface is subjected continually to several forces, of which the interfacial tension is perhaps the greatest. In order for the emulsion to become permanently stable, it is suggested that the interfacial film should assume the nature of a plastic solid which is better able to withstand the forces involved. The fact that some cases of increased stability have been found when the emulsion has stood quietly for an hour or so after formation leads to the suggestion that a rest period is necessary to allow the film to become uniformly distributed and to allow the establishment of an equilibrium.

Volume Effect

An effort has been made to relate emulsion stability and type to the volumes of immiscible liquids involved. Ostwald is responsible for calculations on the volume occupied by the internal phase. He assumed that the maximum packing (without distortion) of uniform spheres should lead to emulsions in which about 74 per cent of the volume would be occupied by the oil or internal phase. In reality, emulsions

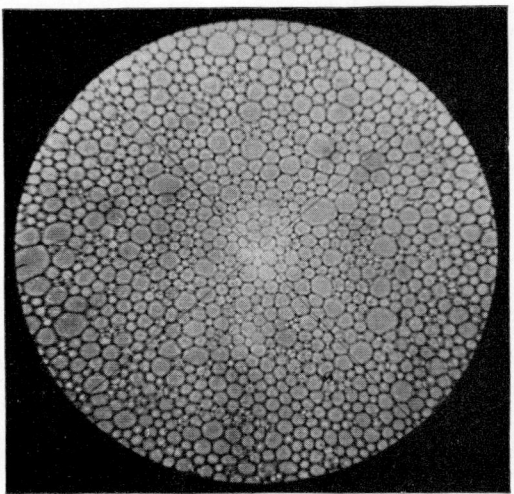

Fig. 105. Close packing in a concentrated o/w emulsion. Note the small globules packed in the spaces between the larger globules and the lack of clear areas of dispersion medium. (From Atlas Surface-Active Agents, Wilmington, Del., Atlas Powder Co.)

have been prepared with as much as 99 per cent of oil emulsified in 1 per cent of water. To explain such cases, it should be remembered that the globules usually are not of uniform size and that the smaller ones can pack in the interstices between the larger ones, and, secondly, that the spheres are not rigid but may flatten on packing or become nonspherical (Fig. 105). While some cases have been reported where the ratio of the phases apparently determined whether o/w or w/o emulsions were obtained, it is generally the nature of the emulsifier which determines the type of emulsion. Changing the volume ratio of the phases may result in inversion of the type. Over a narrow range of volume concentration of the disperse phase just prior to the inversion point, the viscosity of the emulsion system increases at a more rapid rate than at lower concentrations, after which it usually drops abruptly on inversion. With a given emulsifier, the point at which a volume inversion may occur is dependent on the concentration of emulsifier. However, there is often a limit to the amount of liquid which can be emulsified with a given emulsifying agent, and above this ratio the emulsion will break. The permanence of an emulsion cannot be predicted on the basis of volume relationship alone, but the volume relationship may be of help in determining the conditions for equilbrium in a permanent emulsion.

INVERSION

The inversion of the phases of an emulsion, that is, the conversion of an o/w to a w/o emulsion, or the reverse, may result under certain conditions. For the most part, the inversion studies have been made on emulsions stabilized by soap. Parsons and Wilson studied emulsions of Nujol in dilute sodium oleate solutions and stated that inversion upon the addition of salts of magnesium, calcium, barium, iron, etc., resulted from a chemical reaction destroying the film followed by a breaking of the emulsion when an equivalent amount of one of the salts was added. The polyvalent metallic soap formed then dissolved in the oil and re-established an emulsion of the other type as soon as an excess of polyvalent metal ion was present. Mineral oil emulsified with soap gave better emulsions with distilled water than when prepared with hard water. The effect of the hardness-imparting calcium ions could be largely nullified by chelating them with ethylenediamine tetraacetic acid.[22] Inversion of soap-stabilized emulsions of benzene has been demonstrated upon the addition of dry ammonium or sodium chloride, carbonate or sulfate: In this case, the salts apparently "dehydrate" the hydrophilic film to a point where its solvation is less than that of the hydrophobic part. Hatschek pointed out that in oil emulsions made with emulsifying agents other than soap (as, for example, acacia), the emulsion is not inverted as a result of the addition of divalent or trivalent electrolytes.

Clowes actually has followed the inversion of an o/w emulsion to a w/o emulsion under the microscope. The inversion may be followed also by observing changes in the conductivity of the emulsions. In general, it is difficult to draw a sharp line between the conditions suitable for the formation of one type of emulsion or the other, or for the inversion from one type to another.

ELECTRIC CHARGE

When one liquid is dispersed in another, the particles of the dispersed liquid have been found in nearly all cases to bear an electric charge. This charge appears to be one of the factors in the stability of emulsions, but the charge alone is insufficient to maintain stability except in very dilute and highly dispersed systems. The particles are surrounded by a diffuse double layer whose thickness is small compared with the diameter of the globules and whose repulsive effectiveness does not extend beyond the thickness of the double layer. The particles will move in an electric field, depending on their charges. It is suggested that the charge results from the preferential adsorption of ions from electrolytes present, from ions of the emulsifying agent, or from frictional contact.

The double layer of emulsions differs from the double layer on the particles of a colloidal dispersion in that the layer may exist on *both* sides of the interface. By measuring the potential in each phase and at the interface, certain facts may be observed. In the absence of surface-active agent, the smallest part of the double layer potential occurs in the outer aqueous phase. This leads to easy coalescence of the globules and poor stability. In the presence of surface-active agents, there is adsorption at the surface and a rearrangement of ions across the interface resulting in a large charge in the aqueous phase. A stable o/w emulsion can result. The addition of a large amount of electrolyte to the water phase reduces the effective radius of the diffuse double layer. The counterions move in among the surface ions, producing a thin layer of uniform potential. The net effect of this is variable and is dependent on the nature of the emulsifier. There is no doubt that an electric charge exists on the globules in emulsion systems, and this charge is one of the factors in the stability of the system.

The electric double layer is not held solely responsible for emulsion stability, although instances have been found in which the electric double layer is itself capable of imparting stability to concentrated emulsions without the aid of surface-active agents.

GLOBULE SIZE

The particle size may be a factor in determining the type, the permanence and the viscosity of an emulsion system. Since the size of the globules of the disperse phase is not uniform, it is necessary to estimate the average globule size. A variety of methods has been devised to arrive at an average globule size or at a particle size analysis.[23] In many instances, the diameters of a large number of globules have been measured under the microscope, and size-distribution curves have been plotted. The droplets may range from 0.25 μ to 25 μ in diameter. If the large proportion of droplets has diameters near 1 μ, the emulsion may be considered as fine, whereas droplet diameters in the range of 5 μ to 10 μ would indicate a coarse emulsion. Droplet diameters near 25 μ are indicative of incomplete emulsification or of beginning coalescence and separation. The droplets of the internal phase have a tendency to increase in size as a result of coalescence on aging, especially if the emulsifier film is incomplete. It has been found that in a reasonably stable emulsion of an oil in a soap solution, the size-distribution curve shows the presence of a large number of globules having a diameter of 1.0 μ to 1.5 μ, although some globules may be much larger than this. The presence of a large number of small-sized globules is associated with good stability, and particle size methods now are used commonly as a measure of emulsion stability. Passing the emulsion through a homogenizer produces a greater uniformity of globule size in the direction of smaller globules and generally enhances the stability of the emulsion.

EMULSIFYING AGENTS

As has been pointed out, emulsions of 2 pure immiscible liquids usually are stable only in low concentrations. In more concentrated emulsions, the globules collide because of brownian movement and motion resulting from density differences, and coalesce under the force of interfacial tension to settle out as a layer of liquid unless a third substance, the emulsifying agent, is added. So many substances are used as emulsifying agents that it is difficult to classify the materials in any systematic manner. For example, emulsifiers may be *carbohydrates* of variable composition (gums, dextrin, starches, pectin), *soaps* (amine, alkali metal, or alkaline earth salts of long-chain fatty acids), *proteins* (casein, albumin), *solids* (bentonite, kaolin), *quaternary salts* (the cationic wetting agents), *hydroxyalkylamine salts* (salts of triethanolamine, triisopropanolamine), *sulfonated and sulfated oils, long-chain alcohols* (lauryl or cetyl alcohol) and others. A more extensive listing is found in the chapter dealing with pharmaceutical emulsions (Chap. 15), and an expanded list of emulsifying agents appears in the book by Becher (see Bibliography). However, all of the materials must have one common property: namely, the ability to concentrate at the interface between the 2 immiscible liquids. The behavior of the resultant film determines to a large extent the type and the

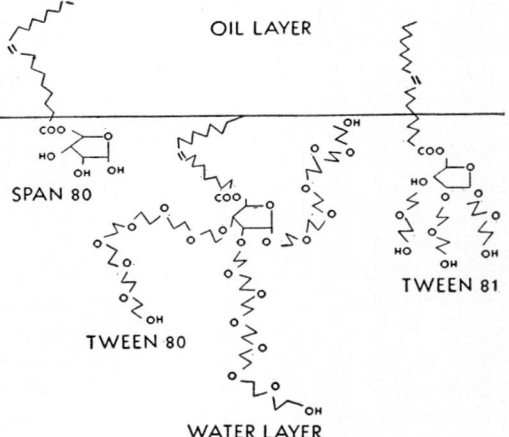

FIG. 106. (*Left*) The hexitan residue in Span 80 is not sufficiently water-loving (or hydrophilic) to draw the oil-loving (or lipophilic) oleic acid chain into the water layer. (*Center*) In this example, Tween 80, the accumulation of polyoxyethylene chains on the hexitan residue renders this part of the molecule sufficiently hydrophilic to drag the oleic acid chain completely into the water layer. (*Right*) Tween 81 is an intermediate type. (From Atlas Surface-Active Agents, Wilmington, Del., Atlas Powder Co.)

stability of the emulsion. The particles of the emulsifier must be wetted more strongly by one liquid than by the other and must form a coherent plastic film for good emulsion permanence.

The emulsion stabilizers are those substances which require much mechanical energy to achieve the proper globule size, whereas the true emulsifiers achieve the same result with a reduced amount of energy input. Because of the dual nature of the molecules, emulsifiers serve as ties between the oil and the water. By balancing the hydrophile and the lipophile portions of the molecule, the preferential solubility of the synthetic emulsifier can be adjusted in varying degrees for oil or water as conditions require. The balance between the strength of the hydrophilic and the lipophilic groups, or the polar nonpolar balance, is referred to as the HLB or Hydrophile-Lipophile Balance. The HLB permits the prediction of the type of behavior expected from the emulsifier or the combination of emulsifiers. The relative solubility of the emulsifier in the aqueous and the oil phases influences the character of the emulsion and, in part, determines the type of emulsion formed. The nonionic emulsifiers (Polyethylene Glycol 400 or 4,000, Spans, Tweens) depend chiefly on hydroxyl groups and ether linkages to provide hydrophilic character. (See Fig. 106.) The nonionic surface-active agents are neutral, versatile and nontoxic and give emulsions stable to freezing and to acid electrolytes.

Numerous studies have appeared in the literature over a long period dealing with the emulsifying capacity of various emulsifying agents and the stability of the resulting emulsions. As a general rule, the work of different authors is not strictly comparable because of variations in the factors involved, such as pH, concentration of phases, concentration of emulsifying agents, method of preparation and methods of evaluating stability. On the other hand, the wide variation in the nature of emulsifying agents makes it impossible to prepare all emulsions under the same conditions. King[24] studied o/w emulsions stabilized by agar, gelatin, acacia, tragacanth, egg yolk, lecithin, Irish moss and saponin by the size-frequency technic. Most of these agents formed emulsions considerably coarser but often more stable than soap-stabilized systems. High viscosity promotes stability of emulsions by minimizing creaming and coalescence due to kinetic impact.

A rather comprehensive study of emulsifying agents used pharmaceutically and suitable for preparations intended for internal administration was made by Münzel.[25] Only o/w emulsions of the following 6 oils were studied: olive oil, cod-liver oil, castor oil, light and heavy mineral oil and turpentine. As far as possible, all variables were maintained constant while preparing emulsions with acacia, tragacanth, agar, carrageen, malt extract, Tylose (methyl cellulose), saponin (purified quillaja saponin, Merck), casein and skim milk powder, egg yolk, egg white, gelatin, lecithin and Tegin (a mixture of sodium stearate, stearic acid, stearic acid esters of glycerin, water and glycerin). The emulsifiers were arranged in the following order of decreasing effectiveness for emulsifying olive oil: saponin, egg yolk, casein, acacia, Tegin, gelatin (pH of 1), lecithin, gelatin (pH of 3) and egg white. For liquid petrolatum, the series is egg yolk, lecithin, casein, acacia and saponin, while for turpentine it is saponin, casein, egg yolk and acacia. The dispersity of the emulsion with a given weight of mixed emulsifying agents falls between the degrees of dispersion obtained with the same weight of either agent alone under the same conditions. No synergistic action of emulsifiers could be shown. Münzel has also presented a series of papers on those agents particularly suitable for the preparation of washable ointment bases with single and complex mixed emulsifiers and has tried to correlate the results with theoretical considerations.[26] Husa[27] stated that mixtures of acacia and tragacanth were of no advantage in preparing emulsions of cod-liver oil, linseed oil or mineral oil in a mortar and pestle, but if the emulsions were passed through a hand homogenizer, there was less creaming than when acacia alone was used.

A comparison of the relative efficiencies of pectin, tragacanth, karaya and acacia,[28] for the emulsification of olive, cottonseed and mineral oils indicated that pectin and tragacanth gave more stable emulsions at a lower pH for olive oil, that pectin was better for cottonseed oil, and that pectin and karaya were better for mineral oil.

A number of the newer synthetic emulsifying agents are suggested and used in the preparation of shampoos and cosmetic creams, as, for example, the ethanolamines, the isopropanolamines and their salts; morpholine; glycerylmonostearates; lauryl, cetyl and stearyl alcohols, including the product Lanette Wax; partially phosphated stearyl and cetyl alcohols (Lanette Wax SX); sulfonated lauryl alcohol; cellulose esters; sodium alginate, and others. Solid emulsifiers have extensive industrial uses, and one of the more popular ones, bentonite, is now official as an emulsifying and suspending agent.

Attempts to evaluate emulsifier efficiency have been based on hydrophile-lipophile balance (see p. 139), on water number (for w/o emulsions), the ASTM "steam emulsion" test, the centrifugal test and others.

The efficiency of lipase in splitting fats in the intestinal tract is promoted by emulsification achieved partly by the bile salts under normal conditions. The intermediate diglycerides and monoglycerides resulting during hydrolysis of the fat appear to be more effective emulsifying agents than the bile salts, whereas the otherwise efficient phosphatides, Tween-80 and other commercial emulsifying agents, do not seem to influence the rate of hydrolysis in vivo.[29]

RECOGNIZING TYPES OF EMULSIONS

In the studies on emulsions, it often has been necessary to determine which liquid has become the internal phase. It is not always a simple matter to obtain positive information. Several methods have been proposed.

Drop-Dilution Test. Perhaps one of the simplest tests is the so-called drop-dilution test. This test depends on the idea that an emulsion may be diluted with the external phase but not with the internal phase. Thus an o/w emulsion will be readily miscible with, and will diffuse in, water but not oil. This idea was first proposed by Pickering and has been modified by others. For example, a drop of oil may be added to a drop of the emulsion on a slide under a microscope. If ready mixing occurs, the emulsion was of the w/o type. If the emulsion is not too opaque or colored, a drop of water or of the oil may be placed in the emulsion near the glass wall of the container. If the liquid added is the external phase, it will diffuse into the emulsion, giving a less opaque area, whereas, if it is the internal phase, it will rise or fall as a globule, depending on the density of the liquids.

Dye or Indicator Test. The appearance of a sample of emulsion is noted after the addition of a dye soluble in only one of the phases. Sudan III is oil-soluble and, if added to an o/w emulsion, will agglomerate around and enter the oil globules; whereas, if it is added to a w/o emulsion, it dissolves readily in the oil and diffuses, coloring the emulsion. Methylene blue, a water-soluble dye, may be used similarly. Other dyes have been recommended, and discussions of the relative dependability of the drop-dilution and the indicator methods have appeared.

Electric Conductance Test. The electric conductance test is dependent on the higher conductivity of water, particularly in the presence of electrolytes, than of oil, an electric insulator. Therefore, the w/o emulsions give lower conductivities than the o/w emulsions. The method has been used also to follow the breaking and the inversion of emulsions.

Other methods have been suggested to take advantage of the differences in surface tension and viscosity of o/w and w/o emulsions, but these are not suitable for rapid routine examination. Another method is based on the difference in refractivity of oil droplets and water droplets. The observations may be made under the microscope by suitable illumination and have the advantage of causing no changes in the emulsion. The fluorescence of oils under ultraviolet light, the filter paper wetting method and other lesser methods also have been employed.

PREPARATION OF EMULSIONS

The preparation of emulsions is dependent on methods of breaking up into small globules the liquid which is to become the internal phase. These globules must then be coated with a film of the emulsifying agent. The degree of dispersion obtained is the resultant of 2 forces: the formation of globules by the forces applied and the tendency of the globules to coalesce. The various factors in the formation and the stability of emulsions have an effect on the intensity of these forces. Using some emulsifiers, the order of mixing of the components may be varied, but in other cases a definite order must be followed.

Agitation by Hand

The simplest method of emulsification is manual agitation of the emulsion components in a suitable partially filled container. The container should not be full, otherwise there is not sufficient room for the development of the splashing and the breaking up of the internal phase into globules. It has been shown that intermittent shaking is preferable to continuous shaking in many cases. During the agitation, both phases are broken up into globules. Since the external phase of the final emulsion is to be continuous, the rest period allows it to coalesce and gives time for the globules of the internal phase to become enclosed in a film of emulsifier. It also has been shown that too violent agitation and agitation at a given intensity for too long a period tend to increase the size of the dispersed globules.

The mortar and pestle is another means of providing agitation of the emulsion components by hand. The particles of the internal phase produced by agitation generally are not of uniform size. For a description of the procedures customarily used in preparing emulsions by use of the mortar and pestle, see Chapter 15.

Mechanical Agitation

Mechanical agitation may be brought about on a small-scale or laboratory basis by means of equipment such as a mechanical shaker or high-speed electric stirrers with various paddle designs. Such factors as temperature and degree of agitation have a bearing on the final product, and it has been suggested that there is an optimum speed of rotation or degree of agitation for any given emulsion system in any piece of equipment. Prolonged agitation may result in increased size of the globules and even in complete separation of the emulsion in some cases. Cases in which the separation of commercially prepared emulsions has occurred as a result of vibrations during transportation by train or truck are well known.

Subjecting 2 immiscible liquids to ultrasonic waves provides another method of producing emulsions.[30] The use of ultrasonic equipment in the production of emulsions is increasing, especially in Europe.

The formation of emulsions of vegetable oils by means of ultrasonic waves indicates that frequency is important both in the formation of the emulsion and in determining the type of emulsion produced. It should also be noted that certain frequencies favor the breaking rather than the formation of emulsions. It is found that the stability of the emulsifying agent to ultrasonic waves is a factor in the choice of agent used.[31] For example, polyethylene glycol 400 monostearate, tragacanth and hard soap solutions showed significant losses in viscosity on exposure to ultrasonic waves, while solutions of acacia, sodium lauryl sulfate and polysorbate 80 showed no significant change. The best emulsification efficiency developed when the equipment was arranged so that the distance between the bottom of the chamber and the activating crystal was an exact number of half wave lengths. Decreasing the viscosity of the oil increased the ease of formation of emulsions. Emulsification of viscous oils improved with increased exposure time, possibly because of a decrease in viscosity as the temperature rose. Of several agents tried, hard soap, polyethylene glycol 400 monostearate and polysorbate 80 were best with acacia, sodium lauryl sulfate and tragacanth being decidedly less effective.

Large-Scale Emulsification

Mechanical agitation on a large scale is provided by a wide variety of machines. The equipment may be divided into several groups: the agitators, which include various types of mixing and stirring equipment, the colloid mill, centrifugal emulsifiers and homogenizers.

Mixing and Stirring Equipment. This equipment varies widely in the arrangement of the paddles or other devices used to produce rapid mixing and breaking up of the liquid to be emulsified. Many types of blades, paddles, arrangements of paddles and the like are patented, the agitators rotating at speeds of 200 r.p.m. up to 3,000 r.p.m., depending on the type and the area of the blade and other factors. Churn types of equipment are used also, in which 2 paddles rotate in opposite directions, or a single shaft carries paddles which pass between stationary baffles on the inside wall of the container. One of the disadvantages of these devices is the incorporation of air in varying amounts, which is sometimes objectionable, especially with materials sensitive to oxidation.

Colloid Mills. The colloid mills form a sharply defined class of emulsifying machines. Many of them were designed primarily for the preparation of special emulsions and later have been applied to emulsions in other fields. There are 2 main types of colloid mills: the *smooth-surface* mills and the *rough-surface* mills. The emulsion may pass through the mill by means of centrifugal force, or the surfaces may be so designed that there is no force which tends to make the material leave the surfaces other than the feeding in of new material. The 2 phases of the emulsion may be fed in simultaneously, or a coarse emulsion prepared in a mixer of some type may be fed in. There are 2 essential sections, a *rotor* operating at speeds of 1,000 to 20,000 r.p.m., and a *stator,* the emulsion passing between the faces of these two. The clearance between the 2 faces may not be constant all over the face and is adjustable down to 0.001 inch. The adsorption of fluid films leads to tremendous shearing forces at the surfaces. The mills may be provided with jackets for heating or cooling. The smooth surfaces may be in the form of disks, cones, cylinders and the like. The rough surfaces may be disks with radial grooving, they may bear meshing pins, or they may be truncated cones with rough surfaces.

Homogenizers. As has been pointed out, the emulsions prepared by the manual or mechanical mixing type of equipment contain globules which are not of uniform size. The homogenizers are so named because they reduce the limits between which the sizes of the globules fall, producing a more uniform dispersion, which does not cream and has a homogeneous appearance. The design of the homogenizers also varies widely. The liquids to be emulsified, or a coarse emulsion obtained from mixing equipment, are fed into a centrifugal head containing narrow spiral passages, slots or other types of openings through which the liquids pass with considerable force, producing shearing stresses which result in emulsification. The mixture may be forced through nozzles of varying design at high velocity and allowed to impinge on a flat surface, resulting in considerable dispersion of the globules. Sometimes the homogenization is carried out in 2 stages, the first being at a much higher pressure than the second. Small, hand-operated models are available for use by the dispensing pharmacist (Fig. 148).

CREAMING

Frequently, emulsions on standing undisturbed for a period of time will cream, that is, the globules of the internal phase rise to the top part of the container, producing a more concentrated emulsion in that region. The rate of creaming varies with such factors as temperature, difference in density between the 2 phases, viscosity of the emulsion and volume of the internal phase globules. An emulsion which has creamed has not necessarily broken and will be redispersed satisfactorily on agitation. The rise of the butterfat globules in milk is the most common example of creaming and, in fact, is the origin of the term. Obviously, if the internal phase is heavier than the external phase the product will sediment or "cream downward."

CRACKING OR DE-EMULSIFICATION

Some knowledge of the factors which destroy emulsions is desirable in order to avoid these conditions during the preparation of emulsions or to be able to destroy undesirable emulsions. The latter represents an important problem in the petroleum industry in particular since many crude oils contain w/o emulsions. As no fixed rules can be formulated for emulsification, no general rule can be stated for breaking emulsions, although there are certain conditions which have a tendency to be detrimental to emulsions.

The agents useful for the breaking of emulsions may be effective either because they destroy the emulsifying agent or because they remove the protective power of the agent by destroying the film surrounding the globules. Much of the literature dealing with breaking emulsions and with the compounds which may be used to break emulsions pertains to crude petroleum emulsions.

Chemical De-emulsification. This type of de-emulsification may be illustrated by the following examples. Substances may be added which take up water, as, for example, calcium chloride or unslaked lime. The use of concentrated solutions of salts which probably dehydrate the emulsifier film also has been found effective in some instances. Sometimes acids or bases are effective. Certain salts may be added which result in flocculation or precipitation of the substances forming the film. Substances which will react with any acids present to form a water-soluble soap may reverse the w/o emulsions. In general, substances with a strong tendency to reverse the type of emulsion may lead to de-emulsification. Some electrolytes of opposite sign may neutralize the charge on the particles and cause a separation of the emulsion. Some colloids and soaps may be used to bring about separation. A large number of commercial synthetic de-emulsifiers are covered by patents.

Physical Methods. Various physical changes sometimes lead to separation of emulsions. A rise in temperature results in changes in the specific gravity of both phases and in the viscosity of the oil and of the emulsion, increases the collisions of the globules and alters the emulsifying agent. Heat alone may lead to de-emulsification or may improve the effectiveness of other treatments. Likewise, freezing will produce changes in the emulsifying agent or, by freezing out the water, often results in a separation of the emulsion. However, some emulsions will re-form on thawing.

The incorporation of coarse-grained materials such as sand or glass may assist in the separation of water from crude oil emulsions. Dilution of the emulsion with an excess of the dispersed phase and agitation sometimes lead to a separation of the emulsion.

Filtration is a physical means frequently effective in breaking emulsions. The emulsion may be forced through some porous material under applied pressure or drawn through by reduced pressure on the receiver side. The process is not strictly comparable with filtration, which generally is applied to the removal of suspended solid matter from a liquid. During the filtration of emulsions, both phases pass through the pores of the filter medium, and the globules of the internal phase are caused to coalesce. If the filter is preferentially wetted by one phase, then the other phase may be retained on the filter.

The use of various processes for the application of an alternating current has been successful, particularly in w/o emulsions, such as petroleum emulsions. Many theories have been offered to account for the separation. A number of pieces of equipment have been developed and patented.

The slow separation of some emulsions on standing often can be hastened by centrifuging, particularly if there is an appreciable difference in the densities of the 2 liquids and the viscosity of the external phase is not high.

EFFECT OF ELECTROLYTES ON EMULSION STABILITY

The effect of electrolytes on the stability of emulsion systems seems to be dependent on the type of emulsifying agent. Sometimes a stabilizing effect is shown, and sometimes a breaking effect is noted. When the electrolyte reacts with the emulsifier, the emulsion may break or be inverted as already has been pointed out with respect to the inversion of soap-stabilized emulsions. The dehydration of hydrophilic emulsifier films by electrolytes has also been referred to under inversion.

A neutral electrolyte may produce coalescence of the internal phase as the result of adsorption by the film and neutralization of the charge on the globules. The more effective ions are those having a charge opposite to that on the particles, and their efficiency increases with increasing charge on the ions. In dilute solutions, hydrogen and hydroxyl ions produce effects out of proportion to their charge and concentration. Hydroxyl ions in low concentrations may stabilize an emulsion of negatively charged particles or coagulate an emulsion of positively charged globules. According to Hatschek, the electrolytes produce a discharge of emulsion globules when a sufficient percentage of electrolyte is present, and the discharged particles continue to show brownian movement, resulting in collisions and coalescence. When the particle size becomes large enough, the brownian movement ceases, and, if the densities of the phases are very similar and the viscosity high, further coalescence may not occur.

On the other hand, the presence of electrolytes may aid greatly in stabilizing emulsions of both types as a result of the production of a difference in potential between the disperse phase and the continuous phase. A difference of about 0.06 volt has been considered to give a fairly stable emulsion.

In studies by King and co-workers[32] on the effect of electrolytes on emulsions, the following results have been obtained. In concentrated o/w emulsions stabilized by sodium oleate, saponin, alumina or bentonite, the nature of the anion was found to be important and was determined by its position in the lyotropic series (see p. 122). The emulsions prepared with the colloidal agents soap and saponin were unaffected by sulfates but were broken by sodium iodide and potassium thiocyanate, whereas the reverse effect was noted on emulsions stabilized by the solids, alumina and bentonite. The hydrophobic thiocyanate and iodide ions caused a decrease in the particle size of the sol, which is detrimental to the colloidal soap and saponin but favorable to the solids. With high concentrations of emulsifying agent, the electric behavior of the emulsion bears an insignificant relation to stability. Certain electrolytes were found to stabilize emulsions of water in polar organic liquids over limited ranges of concentration. The potassium salts give emulsions of water in amyl alcohol in the following order of decreasing stability: thiocyanate, iodide, nitrate, bromide, chlorate, chloride and sulfate. There appeared to be no relation between electric charge and emulsion stability in the absence of chemical reaction for stabilized (emulsifying agent present) o/w emulsions.

TRANSPARENT AND CHROMATIC EMULSIONS

Very dilute emulsions may be practically clear in transmitted light. However, as the concentration of the internal phase is increased, the emulsion becomes more opaque, usually being milky white in appearance unless one or the other phase is colored. When the 2 liquids have the same index of refraction, the emulsions appear homogeneous and *transparent*. Some combinations of liquids which produce transparent emulsions are found in the journal and patent literature. If the 2 liquids have the same refractive index but different dispersive power for light, the emulsion shows one color by transmitted light and another when viewed from the side (reflected light). Such emulsions are called *chromatic* emulsions. Holmes and Cameron[33] and others have prepared a variety of such emulsions. For example, an emulsion of glycerin in a solution of pyroxylin in acetone was milky. As benzene was added in small portions with shaking, the refractive indices approached one another, the emulsion became transparent and appeared yellow when viewed from the side and blue by transmitted light. As more benzene was added, the yellow changed to pink and the blue to green.

SUSPENSIONS

The suspensions are heterogeneous systems containing coarsely dispersed material which settles out more or less rapidly, depending on a variety of factors. The rate of settling is dependent on such factors as density, size and shape of the particles, the density and the viscosity of the medium, temperature, convection or other factors leading to agitation and the like. It has been pointed out earlier that, all other factors being constant, the rate of settling of an insoluble powder varies with the particle size, the larger particles settling more rapidly. Hence, it is important from the standpoint of pharmaceutical elegance that substances to be suspended be in as fine a powder as possible. The density and/or the viscosity of a given medium may be increased by dissolving substances in it (glycerin or sugar in water), by dispersing colloidal or partly colloidal substances in it (agar, tragacanth, acacia in water) or by the presence of highly hydrous substances such as bentonite. All of the above-mentioned possibilities are illustrated in official preparations.

The viscosity of the liquid phase will set the lower limit of the viscosity of any dispersion in which it forms the continuous phase. The dispersion of a sufficient quantity of the second phase in the liquid will greatly modify the consistency and the viscosity of the system.

Flocculation resulting from aggregation of particles results in more rapid settling of suspensions to fairly high volumes, while deflocculated particles settle more slowly to relatively low volumes. Stokes' Law is an attempt to evaluate mathematically the settling of particles and is based on spherical particles falling in a homogeneous fluid medium.

$$V = \frac{2r^2 (s-s^1) g}{9n}$$

The mathematical representation of this can be simplified for an ideal system where the particles are settling under gravity in liquids of equal density and viscosity to $V = r^2K$, where V is the velocity of settling, r is the effective particle radius and K is a constant. Since the velocity of settling is related to r^2, it is apparent that flocculation will result in a large increase in settling velocity. These same considerations lead also to the conclusion that for suspensions to be reasonably stable and to permit uniform dosage, it is important that the material to be suspended be finely ground to begin with. It is obvious also that if the sedimented powder cakes, it will not be readily resuspended for subsequent doses and will settle very rapidly after efforts to suspend it. In a similar vein, suspensions in mixtures which are thixotropic (see p. 122) will have a low settling viscosity and a high sedimentation volume.

Any changes which lead to an increase in particle size of the suspended medicament will obviously increase the sedimentation rate and decrease the uniformity of dosage in a pharmaceutical preparation. Likewise, conditions which lead to precipitation or other change in the suspending agent will likewise increase the settling rate. A useful discussion of the major factors affecting the choice of suspending agents for pharmaceutical purposes may be found in a paper by Gerding and Sperandio.[34]

Comparisons have been made of the suspending capacity or activity of a variety of suspending agents. When the concentrations used were varied so that the liquid had the same viscosity within a narrow range, it was found that tragacanth, methylcellulose-15 cps., and Veegum-HV were the best suspending agents for bismuth subcarbonate.[35] Veegum-HV is also a good suspending agent for barium sulfate, kaolin, prepared chalk, calamine and zinc oxide.[36]

Attempts to evaluate or predict the stability of suspensions have met with variable success. Measurements of pH or viscosity of the suspension are not satisfactory, and measures of sedimentation rate or particle size indicate the suspending ability of the agent for the drug but do not predict whether agglomeration or caking will occur. The addition of dyes, preservatives and flavoring agents to a satisfactory basic formula may adversely affect the stability. By calculating the zeta potential from measurements of the conductance of the suspension, it is possible to predict the stability of the product and to indicate a critical potential, at which serious flocculation or other evidence of instability will appear.[37]

The dispersing agents currently available are useful in improving the stability of suspensions. On the other hand, mixtures of suspending agents may counteract each other. For example, bentonite and Veegum precipitate a variety of cationic surface-active agents.[38]

It is possible to prepare dispersions of solids by means of ultrasonic waves. The final particle side obtained is proportional to the initial size and the time of exposure up to a certain maximum time.[39] For example, starting from 200 mesh progesterone, maximum reduction of particle size occurred in 15 to 20 min., and further exposure had no effect. Beginning with a larger particle size of powder required a longer period of exposure. Increasing the intensity of the ultrasonic waves increased the dispersion. The inclusion of a surface-active agent in the suspending liquid is necessary to the production of a satisfactory dispersion. Increase in the temperature to approach the boiling point of the suspending liquid had an unfavorable effect on dispersion. Applying a pressure of one atmosphere on the suspending liquid during insonation gave better dispersions. The particle size of suspended bismuth subcarbonate, zinc oxide, sulfathiazole and penicillin G can be decreased by the application of ultrasonic energy. However, deterioration of the last two occurred.[40]

SOME APPLICATIONS OF COLLOIDS, EMULSIONS AND SUSPENSIONS IN PHARMACY

Throughout this chapter, a number of properties of colloids, emulsions and suspensions have been illustrated with official examples. Some of the broad groups of materials which are used in medicine and can be expected to have colloidal properties include the various blood derivatives, sera, toxins, vaccines, toxoids, the official plant gums, mucilages and pectins. A variety of cationic and nonionic surface-active agents are represented in official and N.N.D. products. A number of official products are suspensions stabilized by means of suitable nontoxic hydrophilic colloids or surface-active agents, or through the formation of emulsions.

All living matter contains protein material which is considered as being in colloidal dispersion. Colloids play an important role in soils and represent problems in the treatment of water for drinking purposes and in the treatment of sewage. The comparatively recent development of the frozen food industry must be concerned with the changes in the nature of the colloidal materials in foods resulting during freezing. Foods such as milk, butter and salad dressing are well-known examples of emulsions. In the manufacture of oleomargarine, the inclusion of the monoglycerides and the diglycerides not only provides for emulsification but also reduces the loss of water from the product.

The therapeutic value of some European mineral waters as they emerge from the natural springs has been correlated with the colloidal state of certain constituents of the waters. The usefulness of the synthetic blood extenders as blood substitutes in transfusions is dependent on the preparation of polymers such as dextran and periston (polyvinylpyrrolidone) with ranges of molecular size similar to those of blood proteins. These polymers are tolerated well and removed from the plasma only slowly.

REFERENCES

1. Loeser, D.: J. Am. Pharm. A. 18:124, 1929.
2. Monaco, A. L., and Dehner, E. J.: J. Am. Pharm. A. 44:237, 1955.
3. Lehman, A. L.: Modern Hosp. 64:98, 1945.
4. Butt, A. J., and Hauser, E. A.: Science 112:308, 1950.
5. Twort, C. C., et al.: J. Hyg. 40:253, 1932.
6. Nagy, R., and Mouromomseff, G.: Science 112:593, 1950.
7. Dautrebande, L.: Physiol. Rev. 32:214, 1951.
8. Munch, James C.: J. Am. Pharm. A. 44:208, 1955.
9. DiGangi, F. E., and Rogers, C. H.: J. Am. Pharm. A. 38:646, 1949; Paul, H. E., and Harrington, C. M.: J. Am.

Pharm. A. **41**:50, 1952; Grote, I. W., and Woods, M.: J. Am. Pharm. A. **42**: 319, 1953.
10. Cf. Bull. Soc. chim. **7**:943, 1940; also Ewing, C. O., Politi, F. W., and Schackelford, C. H.: J. Am. Pharm. A. **34**:134, 1945.
11. Caryl and Ericks: Ind. Eng. Chem. **31**: 44, 1939.
12. Gershenfeld, Louis: Am. J. Pharm. **113**: 215, 1941.
13. Baker, Z., et al.: J. Exper. Med. **73**:249, 1941.
14. Gershenfeld, L., and Witlin, B.: Am. J. Pharm. **113**:215, 1941; Tobie, W. C., and Orr, M. L.: J. Lab. & Clin. Med. **30**:741, 1945.
15. Barr, M., and Tice, L. F.: Am. J. of Pharm. **127**:260, 1955.
16. Bouchardy, M., and Mirimanoff, A.: Pharm. Acta Helv. **26**:69, 1951.
17. Dodd, M. C., et al.: J. Am. Pharm. A. **25**:38, 1926.
18. Draize, J. H., and Kelley, E. A.: Proc. Sci. Sect. Toilet Goods A. **17**:1, 1911.
19. Knoechel, E. L., and Wurster, D. E.: J. Am. Pharm. A. **48**:1, 1959.
20. King, A.: Trans. Faraday Soc. **37**:168, 1941.
21. Schulman, J. H., et al.: Proc. Roy. Soc. (London) **122B**:29, 46, 1937; **126B**: 356, 1938; Trans. Faraday Soc.: **36**: 651, 960, 1940; Kolloid-Z: **115**:67, 1949.
22. Marchisotto, R., Christian, J. E., and Sperandio, G. E.: J. Am. Pharm. A. (Pract. Ed.) **16**:613, 1955.
23. Cohan, L.: Ind. Eng. Chem., Anal. Ed. **12**:210, 1940.
24. King, A.: J. Soc. Chem. Ind. **59**:185, 1940.
25. Münzel, K.: Pharm. Acta. Helv. **18**:32-71, 99-199, 1943.
26. Münzel, K., and Ammann, R.: Pharm. Acta Helv. **29**:1, 91, 171, 1954.
27. Husa, W.: J. Am. Pharm. Assoc. **30**:171, 1941.
28. Lotzka, H., and Maclay, W. D.: Ind. Eng. Chem. **35**:1294, 1943.
29. Shoshkes, M., Geyer, R. P., and Stare, F. J.: Proc. Soc. Exper. Biol. & Med. **75**:680, 1950; Sager, C. A.: Biochem. Ztschr. **321**:44, 1950.
30. Sollner, K.: Chem. Eng. Progr. Symposium Series # 1, Ultrasonics **47**:30 reviews the colloidal effects of ultrasonics. See also: Alexander, J.: Colloid Chemistry Theoretical and Applied, V., pp. 337-373, New York, Reinhold, 1944.
31. Beal, H. M., and Skauen, D. M.: J. Am. Pharm. A. **44**:487, 490, 1955.
32. King, A. and coworkers: J. Chem. Soc. (London), 1513, 1940; Trans. Faraday Soc. **36**:241, 1940; Cheesman and King: Nature **141**:1099, 1938.
33. Holmes, H. N., and Cameron, D. H.: J. Am. Chem. Soc. **44**:72, 1922.
34. Gerding, P. W., and Sperandio, G. J.: J. Am. Pharm. A. (Pract. Ed.) **15**:356, 1954.
35. Lesshafft, Jr., C. T., and DeKay, H. G.: J. Am. Pharm. A. (Pract. Ed.) **15**:410, 1954.
36. Pienta, Jr., J. J., Marcus, A. D., and Benton, B. E.: J. Am. Pharm. A. **15**: 414, 1954.
37. Stanko, G. L., and DeKay, H. G.: J. Am. Pharm. A. **47**:104, 1958.
38. Nakashima, J. Y., and Miller, O. H.: J. Am. Pharm. A. (Pract. Ed.) **16**:496, 1955.
39. Misek, B., and Skauen, D. M.: J. Am. Pharm. A. **47**:32, 36, 1958.
40. Araujo, O. E., and Belcastro, P. E.: J. Am. Pharm. A. **47**:309, 1958.

BIBLIOGRAPHY

Alexander, A. E., and Johnson, P.: Colloid Science, Vol. I, London, Oxford University Press, 1949.

Alexander, Jerome: Colloid Chemistry, Principles and Applications, ed. 4, New York, Van Nostrand, 1937.

Becher, Paul: Emulsions: Theory and Practice, New York, Reinhold, 1957.

Berkman, Sophia and Egloff, Gustav: Emulsions and Foams, New York, Reinhold, 1941.

Von Buzágh, A. (trans. by Darbishire, O. B.): Colloid Systems, London, Technical Press, 1947.

Hartman, R. J.: Colloid Chemistry, ed. 2, Cambridge, Houghton Mifflin, 1947.

Hauser, E. A.: Colloidal Phenomena, New York, McGraw-Hill, 1939.

International Society of Leather Trades' Chemists: Technical Aspects of Emulsions, New York, Chemical Pub. Co., 1947.

Jirgensons, Bruno: Organic Colloids, Princeton, Elsevier, 1958.

Kraemer, E. O.: Advances in Colloid Science, Vol. 1, New York, Interscience, 1942.

Kruyt, H. R.: Colloid Science, Vols. I and II, New York, Van Nostrand, 1952, 1949.

Mark, H., and Verwey, E. J. W.: Advances in Colloid Science, Vol. 3, New York, Interscience, 1950.

McBain, J. W.: Colloid Science, Boston, Heath, 1950.

Summer, C. G.: Clayton's The Theory of Emulsions and Their Technical Treatment, ed. 5, Philadelphia, Blakiston, 1954.

Verwey, E. J. W.: and Overbeek, J. Th. G.: Theory of the Stability of Lyophobic Colloids, New York, Elsevier, 1948.

Weiser, H. B.: Colloid Chemistry, ed. 2, New York, Wiley, 1949.

NOEL E. FOSS, PH.D.
Dean, School of Pharmacy, University of Maryland

8

Extraction

GENERAL CONSIDERATIONS
HISTORY
PURPOSES OF EXTRACTION
THEORY OF EXTRACTION
    EXTRACTION OF DRIED DRUGS
    EXTRACTION OF SUBSTANCES FROM
        LIQUIDS
SOLVENTS USED IN EXTRACTION

EXTRACTION APPARATUS
METHODS OF EXTRACTION
    MACERATION
    DECOCTION, INFUSION AND DIGESTION
    PERCOLATION
RECOVERY OF MENSTRUA
EXTRACTION BY IMMISCIBLE SOLVENTS

GENERAL CONSIDERATIONS

Extraction, from the Latin *extractio*, derived from *extrahere*, to draw out, is the act of withdrawing something from an organized structure or disorganized mass by traction, suction, expression, distillation, treatment with a solvent or other physical or chemical means. In pharmacy, the term is used almost exclusively to designate the operations involved in the withdrawal of the soluble constituents from crude or partially refined drugs by treatment with suitable solvents and *frequently* to the removal of these constituents from liquids in which they are held in solution by treatment of the solutions with immiscible solvents.

The withdrawal of the iron from a mixture of iron filings and sulfur by means of a magnet, the expression of liquids from vegetable drugs as in the preparation of lemon juice or the separation of a volatile oil, such as caraway, from the fruit by distillation are not extraction processes in the pharmaceutical sense because they do not require the use of a solvent.

The solvent used in the extraction of a drug is called the *menstruum* and the drug residue which remains after extraction is called the *marc*. The liquid drained off from the marc in the maceration process of extraction commonly is referred to as the *macerate liquid* or *solution*, and the liquid which flows from the percolator in extraction by the percolation process is called the *percolate*. The material dissolved by the menstruum, regardless of which of the 2 extraction processes is involved, is called the *extractive*.

HISTORY

The first attempts in the extraction of drugs probably were made soon after primitive man discovered that certain vegetable materials were useful for the alleviation and the cure of bodily ills. Herbs collected for medicinal purposes soon dried out, and it is logical to assume that attempts were made to restore the qualities of the fresh plant by steeping in water. From this, it was a simple step to the discovery that soaking in certain liquids dissolved the active constituents of drugs and permitted their administration in a convenient if not always palatable form.

Subsequently, by employing heat, specialized methods of maceration with water were introduced: i.e., infusion, decoction and digestion. Later still, the superior solvent and preservative properties of vinegar and wine were recognized. References to maceration in these solvents are numerous in ancient writings—e.g., Egyptian papyri and the Bible. However, alcohol was not available to the ancients. It first was obtained by the distillation of wine in the 12th century. The reference to Raimundus Lullus (1235–1315) as an early advocate of the preparation of tinctures by macerating crude drugs in "spirit," found in the older literature, has not been substantiated by recent research. We know now that none of the chemical writings attributed to Lullus was actually his work. It was only in the 16th century, through the influence of Paracelsus, that tinctures and "quintessences" attained widespread use.

Aristotle (384–322 B.C.) described a method of obtaining crude potash by leaching the ashes of plants. Undoubtedly, this process of leaching or lixiviation is the prototype of percolation. Even today, percolation is referred to as lixiviation in the French and the Spanish pharmacopeias. However, its introduction as a pharmaceutical process must have been much more recent, since the *Pharmacopée Universelle* of Nicolas Lémery, published in 1698, fails to mention it.

In 1813, Benjamin Thompson first used the term *percolation* to distinguish a process for preparing coffee. His procedure closely resembled the present method of percolation. Three years later, a Frenchman, Count Réal, developed a pressure percolator in which the solvent, contained in a vertical tube 12 ft. tall, was forced through the drug by its own hydrostatic pressure. In 1831, Boutron and Robiquet published an account of the extraction of the volatile oil of mustard with ether, a case of true displacement. Later, in 1834, Robiquet claimed that he had used this method of extraction in an earlier investigation of bitter almond oil.

In 1833, the Boullays, father and son, read a paper before the Pharmaceutical Society of Paris, in which they established the uselessness of the hydrostatic-pressure method of Réal and stressed the importance of the principle of displacement. Two years later, they published an account of investigations in which they applied the principle of displacement to the extraction of a whole series of drugs. In a thesis published later in the same year, Guillemond, of the School of Pharmacy of Paris, established the superiority of the process of displacement over that of maceration. He gave credit to Robiquet and Boutron for introducing the process to organic chemistry, but the introduction of percolation as a pharmaceutical process was ascribed to the Boullays.

The papers of Guillemond and others, published in the *American Journal of Pharmacy* shortly after their appearance in France, caused Elias Durand of Philadelphia to become interested in the process, and he probably was the first American pharmacist to employ percolation for the extraction of drugs. In 1838, Augustine Duhammel published the first American article on the subject, and, from that time to the present, American pharmacists became the leaders in studying and applying the principle of displacement.

Israel G. Grahame, in a paper presented before the American Pharmaceutical Association in 1858, suggested the use of the funnel as a percolator, advocated the use of drugs of uniform and definite degrees of fineness and emphasized the importance of moistening the drug properly before packing into the percolator.

Squibb, in 1864, introduced the process of repercolation to effect an economy in the quantity of menstruum required and to eliminate the use of heat.

Among the other Americans who conducted experiments in extraction and made noteworthy contributions to the early development of the process of percolation were Procter, Parrish, Diehl, Oldberg and Lloyd.

In 1868, Dr. S. P. Duffield, of Detroit, Mich., published a description of his process of vacuum maceration and expression for the preparation of fluidextracts. In this process, the drug was subjected to vacuum action to remove air from the cells so that there would be better penetration by the menstruum and more rapid and complete extraction of the soluble constituents.

In 1883, W. M. Thompson described a method of extraction in which the menstruum was made to travel upward through the drug by using both vacuum and pressure.

The 2 foregoing extraction processes were forerunners of a method described in 1930 by H. Breddin, a German apothecary, to which he gave the name *diacolation*. The method is the same in principle as Thompson's process for extraction by upward displacement, but there are differences in technical details. *Mulcolation*, described by Kessler in 1934, and *evacolation*, which he developed a year later, are modifications of the diacolation method.

Other methods based on the evacuation of the drug before extraction or on the use of a partial vacuum or pressure to force the menstruum through the drug have been developed by other workers in more recent times. Notable among them is the pressure method developed by William J. Husa, of Florida, which is now official in the *N.F.*

The process of percolation was described in the *French Codex* in 1837 and in the *Edinburgh Pharmacopeia* in 1839. It appeared for the first time in *U.S.P. II*, which was published in 1840.

PURPOSES OF EXTRACTION

Crude vegetable and animal drugs are complex structures composed of a variety of substances. Some of these substances are pharmacologically active and are soluble in one or more of the solvents which have been found to be suitable for use in extraction. Among the more important classes of plant and animal principles comprising this group are alkaloids, glycosides, tannins, resins, oleoresins, fatty oils and essential oils. Other substances—and these constitute by far the larger part of the bulk of crude drugs—are inert pharmacologically. Unfortunately, from a pharmaceutical standpoint, most of them also are soluble to some extent in the solvents usually employed in extraction. The more important classes of materials comprising this latter group of plant and animal drug constituents are sugars, starches, gums, mucilages, albumins, proteins, pectins and cellulose.

The primary purpose of extraction is to separate the pharmacologically active substances from those which are inert in order to obtain the active substance, or substances, in a form more concentrated, more rapidly absorbable, more palatable and more convenient for administration than the crude drug. Where there is only one pharmacologically active constituent present in a drug, and the difficulties involved in extraction and purification are not too great, the object of extraction as a rule is to isolate the active constituent in pure form, as is done in the case of many of the plant alkaloids and some glycosides. In the case of most plant and animal drugs, however, there is more than one pharmacologically active constituent present, and the isolation of any one of the constituents may be difficult and expensive. Therefore, the usual objective is to obtain the active principle, or principles, in some form which is as free as practicable from inert material as exemplified in the galenical preparations, i.e., infusions, decoctions, tinctures, fluidextracts, extracts, resins, oleoresins and others. It is with the extraction processes involved in making these preparations that the pharmacist is concerned primarily.

In certain cases, extraction is employed to remove inert or objectionable constituents, such as fats and waxes, from the drug prior to extraction of the active constituents, as in the preparation of Ergot Fluidextract, N.F., in which case solvent hexane is used to remove the fat prior to extraction of the active alkaloids with an alcoholic menstruum.

THEORY OF EXTRACTION

Some knowledge of the forces operating in the extraction of drugs is necessary for a proper understanding of the different methods employed in extraction, such as maceration, infusion, decoction, digestion and percolation. These methods differ widely with respect to the procedures involved, but the main purposes of each are essentially the same—that is, to accomplish the solution of the soluble constituents of the drug and to separate the solution from the residue or marc. In extraction by maceration, the forces which are active in these 2 steps are mainly osmosis and diffusion. In percolation, the force of gravity, hydrostatic and atmospheric pressures, surface tension, adhesion and capillary attraction also play a part. The relative importance of each of these will vary with the particular process of extraction employed, and, in many cases, one or more of these forces actually may be opposing extraction. It is the algebraic sum of the resultants of all the forces involved in a given procedure that determines the force of extraction.

Extraction of Dried Drugs

When a fresh drug is dried, the moisture present in the tissues evaporates, and the walls of the cells and the ducts shrink; at the same time, the substances held in solution by the water in the tissues precipitate or crystallize out or dry to a solid amorphous mass inside the cells. When a dry drug is immersed in an aqueous or a hydroalcoholic menstruum, the process is reversed. The menstruum is absorbed, causing the tissues to swell and the soluble matter inside the cells to go into solution. In the case of drugs whose tissues are soft and spongy, such as belladonna root, this takes place comparatively rapidly, but when a drug is hard or horny, as in the case of nux vomica, considerable time is required. Before the tissues of such drugs can absorb an appreciable amount of menstruum, they must be broken up in fine pieces so as to expose the softer internal tissues to the action of the menstruum. This also is true of many seeds and leaves, the walls of whose outer layers of cells are impervious to water, but the walls of whose inner cells are permeable and permit the menstruum to diffuse through them and to dissolve the soluble portion of the cell contents.

Regardless of the materials of which the cell walls of a drug are constructed, the diffusion of the soluble constituents through the walls is a slow process. It can be hastened by increasing the surface area of the drug before extraction is begun. This is accomplished by powdering, which not only increases the area of the exposed surface but also causes many of the surface cells to be broken so that the menstruum can come in direct contact with the cell contents.

However, even after a drug is reduced to a powder, some of the cells still are unbroken. The cellulose composing the walls of these cells is of a semipermeable nature—that is, it permits the diffusion of menstruum and its molecular solutions while obstructing the passage of colloidally suspended or emulsified particles. Whenever such a semipermeable membrane separates a dilute and a more concentrated solution, the dilute solution passes through it at a more rapid rate than the concentrated one. Consequently, in the case of extraction of drugs, the solvent will pass into the cell at a more rapid rate than the liquid or the dissolved cell contents pass out. The cell will swell and frequently rupture, allowing direct solution of the contents. If the cell wall remains unbroken, the replacement of concentrated solution by solvent will continue until the concentration on both sides of the membrane is the same. This process is called osmosis. It can be seen that extraction by osmosis, without first grinding the drug, would be a long-drawn-out and wasteful process resulting in weak percolates which would require concentration to an impractical degree to even approximate the strength of weak tinctures.

Because of the relatively enormous area of exposed surface with its broken cells in the powdered drug and because of bursting of the cell walls which occurs during the extraction as described above, it is doubtful whether the osmotic interchange of solvent for solution actually is responsible for any more than a small percentage of the extractive obtained. That the proportion of broken cells is extremely large is indicated by the large amount of colloidally suspended material generally present in percolates.

In percolation, the combination of the pressure of the atmosphere and the hydrostatic pressure of the solvent causes a downward displacement of the menstruum just as long as there is an outlet at the lowest point in the system. As a unit quantity of liquid is drawn out of the percolator by the forces of gravity acting on its mass, there is a tendency toward the formation of a partial vacuum in the area vacated. To overcome this, the atmospheric pressure, supplemented by the force of gravity, presses more liquid down to relieve the vacuum and to restore average pressure conditions, resulting in a continuous, automatic, downward displacement.

The force of gravity also plays a part in other extraction methods. For example, in the processes of infusion, decoction and digestion, the drug frequently is suspended just below the surface of the solvent. As this portion of the solvent becomes saturated with extractive material, its specific gravity increases beyond that of the substratum liquid. As a result, the heavier surface layer drops to the bottom and is replaced by lighter, less saturated solvent. This results in a regular continued circulation of solvent until extraction is complete.

When a small quantity of liquid is poured onto a solid surface, 2 forces at once are manifest. One, the force of surface tension, or the cohesive force, tends to draw the liquid up into a number of spherical droplets so as to reduce the area of surface exposed. The other, the force of adhesion, causing the liquid to cling to or wet the surface, represents the molecular attraction between the liquid and the solid surfaces. It can be seen that these 2 forces, while closely associated and best considered together, are opposite in direction. As there are all degrees of adhesive or wetting qualities as well as wide range of surface tensions, the resultant of forces here is a study of several factors. For example, molecular attraction or adhesion varies from practically zero for interfaces such as exist between mercury and glass or water and paraffin wax, to the very measurable attraction of water to a clean glass surface. The greater this molecular adhesion or wetting power, the better the contact power of the solvent with reference to a given solid. On the other hand, the less the force of surface tension of a liquid, the greater its power to penetrate into the interstices of the material being extracted.

Capillary attraction, or the force causing liquids to rise in capillary tubes against the force of gravity, accounts in part for the ability of solvents to penetrate the interstices of drugs during extraction. This phenomenon is a function of surface tension and varies directly with it; hence, it might be argued that, in order to increase penetration and absorption, a solvent of high surface tension should be chosen. However, surface tension of a high order often is associated with high viscosity, the latter being a drawback outweighing the advantage of greater capillary force. In addition, a closer analysis of capillary rise shows that it is an equilibrium condition and, once established, is difficult to unbalance. In other words, a liquid which has penetrated the capillary spaces of a drug by virtue of the force of capillary rise is held there and cannot be displaced readily. On the other hand, a liquid of lower surface tension can penetrate the tiny interstices much more readily and, not being held by the capillary force, can be displaced with its solute much more readily. From these considerations, it may be concluded that, other things being equal, the ideal solvent is one having a rather low surface tension and a high wetting power.

In extraction by maceration, the drug is allowed to remain in contact with a relatively large volume of menstruum until the extractive matter is distributed uniformly throughout the liquid, and a state of equilibrium is set up. The liquid then is decanted, and the marc is pressed. This procedure may be repeated one or more times, depending on the degree of exhaustion sought.

In the light of the foregoing discussion, percolation may be looked on as an automatically repeated maceration process in which there are no interruptions due to pressing of the marc. The usual procedure in percolation is to pack the drug in a percolator after preliminary moistening. Then the menstruum is added, and the drug is macerated for a period of time before percolation is begun. During this period of maceration, diffusion takes place between the liquid content of the drug tissues and the liquid on the outside. When percolation is begun, the liquid between the particles of drug is displaced by fresh menstruum, and diffusion takes place between the more saturated liquid in the tissues and the fresh menstruum. Therefore, a state of equilibrium will not be reached until the drug is exhausted.

Maceration is the process in general use in European countries for the extraction of drugs, whereas percolation is the process most widely used in America. Because of this situation, the question frequently is raised as to which of the two processes is the better. In reply thereto, it is stated that each has advantages and disadvantages over the other. The process of percolation is better adapted than maceration to the extraction, with hydroalcoholic menstrua, of close-grained drugs which swell but little when moistened. It also has an advantage, where complete extraction of the drug is desired, but its use in these cases is not always practicable. It is not suitable for the extraction, with aqueous menstrua, of drugs containing large amounts of gum or mucilage, such as squill. For the extraction of drugs of this type, the process of maceration usually is resorted to. The latter process also is preferred for the extraction of drugs containing large amounts of resins and gum-resins.

EXTRACTION OF SUBSTANCES FROM LIQUIDS

Up to this point, the discussion of theories has been confined to those applicable to the extraction of soluble substances from solids, but it frequently becomes necessary to extract substances held in solution in liquids. This is a condition encountered in many of the official assays for alkaloids and also in some large-scale manufacturing operations—as for instance, the recovery of alkaloids from waste liquors or the purification of benzoic and salicylic acids. Extraction in these cases usually is effected by the use of a solvent or solvents immiscible with the liquid in which the desired substance is held in solution, and is based on the principle established by Nernst.

According to Nernst's law, if 2 practically immiscible solvents are in contact and a substance which is soluble in both liquids is added to them, the substance will be distributed between the liquids in such a way that the ratio of the concentration of the 2 solutions is a constant irrespective of the quantity of solute. This constant usually is called the *partition coefficient* but also is known as the *distribution ratio* or *constant*.

If C_1 is used to designate the concentration of a substance in chloroform, and C_2 to designate the concentration of the same substance in an equal volume of its aqueous solution, Nernst's law may be formulated as follows: $C_2/C_1 = K$, where K is the distribution constant or coefficient. If there are several substances, such as alkaloids, resins, etc., present in the chloroform solution when it is shaken with acidulated water, the distribution of each substance will take place as if it were present alone.

In actual practice, extraction by the use of immiscible solvents usually is carried out by shaking the liquid to be extracted with several relatively small portions of the immiscible solvent rather than using the whole in one operation. The reason for following this procedure is not the satisfaction of a whim but is based on the principle expressed in Nernst's law, as will become evident from the following explanation:

Assume that 1 Gm. of atropine in 100 ml. of ether solution when shaken with an equal volume of dilute sulfuric acid distributes itself so that 0.1 Gm. remains in the ether layer and 0.9 Gm. in the acid layer of the solvents, $C_{\text{acid}}/C_{\text{ether}} = 9$ (the distribution coefficient). Obviously, only 90 per cent of the atropine present would be extracted from the ethereal solution by extracting it once with 100 ml. of dilute sulfuric acid solution. If the extraction is performed with 200 ml. of the acid solution, the amount of atropine extracted should be

$$\frac{x/200}{\frac{1-x}{100}} = 9$$

and $x = 0.947$ Gm. of atropine.

Where $x =$ the amount of atropine extracted from the ether by the acid solution,

$$C_{\text{acid}} = \frac{x}{200}, \text{ and } C_{\text{ether}} = \frac{1-x}{100}$$

If the original solution is extracted with

several small portions of acid solution, i.e., 50 ml., the amount of alkaloid extracted will be

$$C_{acid} = \frac{x}{50} \text{ and } C_{ether} = \frac{1-x}{100}$$

and since

$$\frac{x/50}{\frac{1-x}{100}} = 9, x = 0.818 \text{ Gm. of atropine}$$

removed by the first extraction with acid, leaving 0.182 Gm. in the ethereal layer. A second extraction with a 50-ml. portion of acid solution will remove

$$\frac{x_1/50}{\frac{0.182 - x_1}{100}} = 9$$

and $x_1 = 0.1489$ Gm. of atropine where x_1 equals the amount of atropine which passes into the acid solution. Thus, in 2 extractions, $0.818 + 0.1489 = 0.9669$ Gm. of atropine is removed from the ethereal solution by 100 ml. of acid solution, whereas a single extraction with 200 ml. of acid solution removed only 0.947 Gm. of the alkaloid.

Since economy in the use of solvents is an important consideration, and large volumes are difficult to handle in shaking out the alkaloids, it is more practical to use several small portions of immiscible solvent than one large portion. In the official assay processes, 15- to 20-ml. portions of the immiscible solvent are used, because it has been found that these quantities serve best to extract the alkaloids quickly and economically. The same principle applies to the extraction of large quantities of materials on a commercial scale.

SOLVENTS USED IN EXTRACTION

Since the objective of practically all extraction procedures used in making the so-called galenical preparations is to dissolve out the pharmacologically active principles of the crude drug with a minimum of inert material, the selection of the solvent, or menstruum, for the extraction of a drug is of fundamental importance.

The total material of all kinds dissolved by a solvent in the process of extraction commonly is known as the *total extractive*. That part of the total which is inert pharmacologically is called the *inert extractive*. It is the latter, because of its composition, which is often a troublesome factor in the preservation of galenicals made by extraction. Some of the constituents comprising this part of the total extractive are prone to absorb oxygen on exposure to air and to undergo change. At first, the change is only one of color, which passes from a greenish or a yellowish brown to a deep brown and finally a black. Ultimately, precipitation takes place. These changes are most noticeable and take place most rapidly in those preparations which require prolonged heating for completion, but they also occur to a lesser degree after long standing in most of the other galenical preparations made by extraction. In addition, some of the substances comprising the inert extractive undergo hydrolysis with the formation of insoluble compounds, and some, which are present as colloidal suspensions, coagulate on standing. Therefore, the less inert extractive dissolved by a solvent in the process of extraction, the more stable the finished product is likely to be.

Numerous solvents have been experimented with in the endeavor to discover one which could be adapted to general use, but it now is conceded that there is no one solvent that is equally satisfactory for all extractions and that the selection of the solvent in each case must be based on the nature of the drug to be extracted and the type of preparation desired. In pharmaceutical manufacturing on the commercial scale, the solvents in actual use are many in number and varied in character, but the following are the more important and are the ones used in the official extraction processes.

Water. This has a wider range as a solvent than any other known liquid. Since it also has the advantage of cheapness, it is used in the extraction of drugs whenever these advantages outweigh the disadvantages of its use.

Cold water is a good solvent for many

plant constituents, such as the alkaloidal salts, glycosides, sugars, mucilaginous substances, pectin, plant acids, coloring matter and mineral salts.

Hot or boiling water causes vegetable tissues to swell and disintegrate, thus permitting the more rapid solution of the soluble matter. It also causes starch grains to burst and a portion of the contents to go into solution. The most frequently encountered disadvantage of its use is that it extracts substances which separate out from the solution on cooling.

Upon the extraction of a drug with water, the sugars, the gums, the plant acids, the mineral salts and the coloring matter, which are the most readily soluble constituents, dissolve first, and thus there is formed a menstruum which has greater solvent action on some substances than does water alone. For instance, such a menstruum will dissolve the resins of cascara bark, which are almost insoluble in pure water. It also may account for the surprisingly large quantities of alkaloids in some aqueous galenicals.

The greatest disadvantage in the use of water as a menstruum in the extraction of drugs is that it extracts large amounts of inert substances and the resulting solutions of plant constituents are usually good media for the growth of yeasts, molds and bacteria. In addition, it causes some drugs to swell to such an extent that extraction by percolation becomes impracticable.

Water weakly acidified with an organic acid, usually acetic or tartaric acid, or a mineral acid such as hydrochloric acid, or water made weakly alkaline with ammonia has been found to possess advantages over water alone in the extraction of certain drugs. For example, water and alcohol acidified with hydrochloric acid is a better menstruum for the extraction of nux vomica and ergot than is water and alcohol alone, and the resins of cascara bark can be extracted more readily with an alkaline menstruum than with pure water.

Alcohol. This does not have as wide a solubility range as water. It is more selective in its action and, therefore, more useful as a solvent for extraction in the making of galenicals. Alcohol is a good general solvent for alkaloids, glycosides, resins and essential oils, but it does not dissolve gums, sugars or albumins. In addition to its selective solvent properties, it acts as a paralyzer toward enzymes and prevents the growth of yeasts, molds, fungi and most bacteria.

Hydroalcoholic Menstrua. Alcohol-water mixtures possess few, if any, of the disadvantages exhibited by water alone in the extraction of drugs. Some of the active constituents of drugs are almost as soluble in alcohol-water mixtures as in strong alcohol. Hence, for economic reasons, many galenical preparations are made by extracting the drug with a hydroalcoholic menstruum. In some cases, the alcoholic content of the menstruum used is as low as 30 per cent.

Glycerin. A good solvent for tannins and their oxidation products is glycerin. Therefore, it frequently is added to alcoholic or hydroalcoholic menstrua in the extraction of tannin-containing drugs. Like water, it dissolves gums and albumins. The fact that it is not volatile bars its use in the preparation of extracts and other preparations from which the solvent must be completely removed.

A menstruum consisting of 1 volume of glycerin and 3 volumes of water was directed by *N.F. VIII* to be used in making the fluidglycerates.

Ether is highly selective in its solvent properties. It does not dissolve any of the objectionable plant constituents. On the other hand, it is an excellent solvent for alkaloidal bases, fats, resins and essential oils. Because of its pharmacologic action and its volatility, it is not suitable for the production of liquid preparations intended for internal use or for storage over a considerable period of time.

Solvent Hexane. A good solvent for fats and oils is solvent hexane. Drugs which contain large quantities of fatty matter frequently are defatted with solvent hexane before subjecting them to extraction with the principal menstruum. This is done, for example, in the preparation of Ergot Fluidextract, N.F.

Acetone dissolves many fats, essential oils and resins, but, like water, it also dissolves a host of inert substances. It also has the disadvantage of having a pronounced odor, which is objectionable to some people and is difficult to remove from preparations made with it. Nevertheless, its use is permitted by the *N.F.* in the preparation of Capsicum and Ginger Oleoresins.

Chloroform is a good solvent for alkaloidal bases, resins and fatty and essential oils. It cannot be used as a menstruum in the production of liquid preparations for internal use because of its pronounced pharmacologic action. So far as the official compendia are concerned, it is used as an immiscible solvent for the extraction of alkaloids in some of the official assay processes.

EXTRACTION APPARATUS

From the standpoint of procedure, the apparatus used in the extraction of crude drugs may be separated conveniently into 2 groups: namely, the type used when extraction is effected by maceration and the type used when extraction is accomplished by percolation.

For the maceration of crude drugs in the quantities usually extracted by the pharmacist, a 1,000-ml. wide-mouth bottle fitted with a ground-glass stopper (Fig. 107) or a quart glass jar with a cover that can be closed tightly, such as an ordinary canning jar, will serve admirably (Fig. 108). These containers also are suitable for extraction by digestion if the operation is carried out at temperatures not exceeding 40°. For digestion at higher temperatures, a wide-mouth Erlenmeyer flask made of Pyrex or Jena glass should be used to avoid breakage which may be caused by heat (Fig. 109).

In cases where digestion at pressures above atmospheric pressure is required, an ordinary small autoclave of the type shown in Figure 110 may be used.

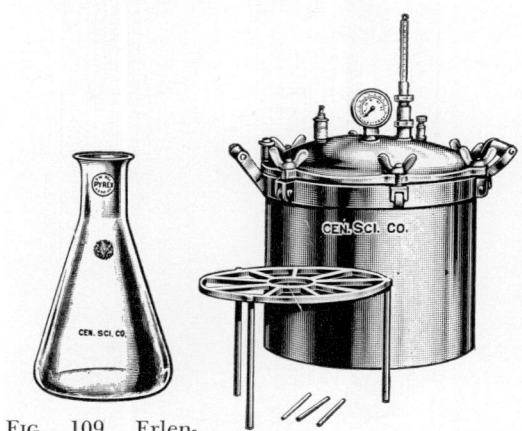

Fig. 109. Erlenmeyer flask.   Fig. 110. Autoclave.

For maceration at temperatures near that of boiling water, as required in the preparation of infusions and decoctions, all that is needed is a teapot or a coffeepot of suitable capacity. However, special earthenware or china pots are available for this purpose. These commonly are called infusion pots (Fig. 111) and usually are fitted with a loose perforated container which rests on a projection near the top of the pot and serves to hold the drug at the top below the surface of the liquid. Under these conditions, displacement of the menstruum in contact with the drug is continuous, and extraction is expedited. If an ordinary teapot is used, the same purpose may be served by placing the drug in

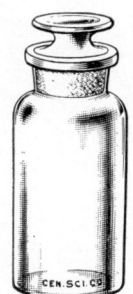 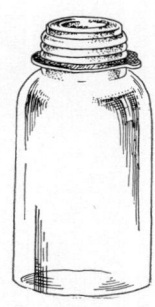 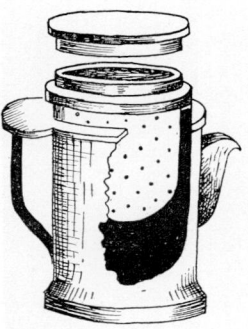

Fig. 107. Wide-mouth bottle.   Fig. 108. Canning jar.   Fig. 111. Infusion pot.

158   Extraction

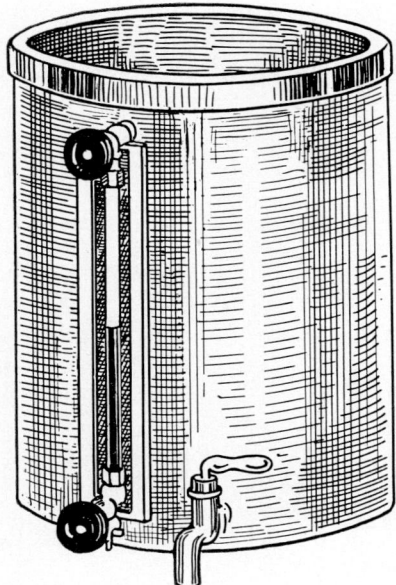

Fig. 112. Maceration tank.

a muslin bag and suspending the latter from the cover.

For the maceration of drugs in the quantities used in manufacturing on a commercial scale, cylindrical tanks of 10, 20, 50 or more gallons capacity are used. These may be made of earthenware, galvanized iron, suitable stainless steel, tinned copper or iron lined with glass or porcelain (Fig. 112). For maceration at temperatures higher than room temperature, these tanks or kettles constructed of the same materials are fitted with jackets so that hot water or steam can be circulated around them (Fig. 113).

For the extraction of drugs by simple percolation, all the apparatus required in addition to a percolator is a container in which to dampen the powdered drug and a container in which to receive the percolate. A shallow porcelain or enameled dish of suitable size will suffice for the former, and a graduated glass bottle of sufficient capacity to contain the amount of percolate required to be retained as finished product will serve for the latter (Fig. 114). In commercial manufacturing, where it is not uncommon to percolate 100 lbs. or more of a drug at a time, the use of a container for the dampening process rarely is resorted to. The drug usually is spread out on a clean tile or concrete floor, where it is sprayed with the dampening menstruum, or it is dampened in a mechanical mixer especially designed for the purpose.

For the preparation of galenicals in the

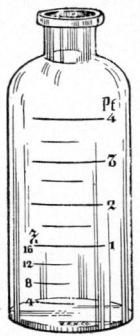

Fig. 114. Graduated percolation bottle.

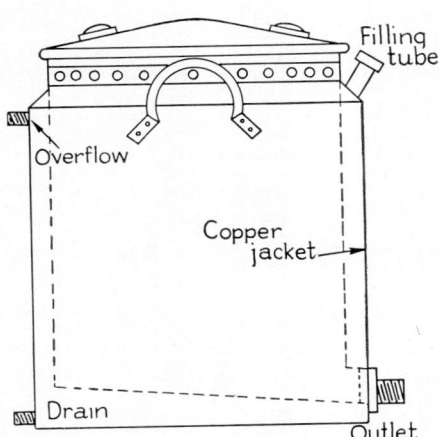

Fig. 113. Kettle with jacket.

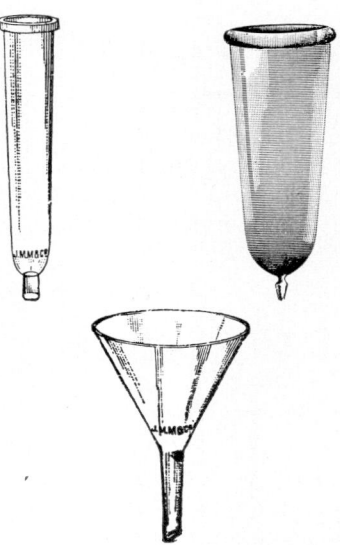

Fig. 115. Percolators. (*Top, left*) Cylindrical. (*Top, right*) Tapering. (*Bottom*) Conical.

quantities for which directions are given in our official compendia, the *U.S.P.* and the *N.F.*, several types of percolators are in general use: namely, the open type, the closed type and the type used in continuous percolation. Each type is represented by several forms, but, because many of these forms are unimportant from a pharmaceutical standpoint, the descriptions given herein are restricted to those forms actually used in pharmaceutical practice.

The open-type percolator may be had in the tapered or cylindrical forms and the comical form, of which the ordinary short-stemmed funnel is a good representative. The narrow cylindrical percolator is reported to have been first recommended by Prof. C. Lewis Diehl but is known more frequently as the Oldberg percolator.

To provide the mechanism necessary for regulating the flow of percolate, percolators of this type are fitted up by inserting a perforated cork or suitable stopper, through which a short glass tube has been passed, into the lower orifice and attaching thereto a piece of rubber tubing. The latter may be slightly longer than the percolator, in which case the flow is regulated by raising or lowering the tube (Fig. 116), or it may be a short piece, in which case the flow is regulated by means of a screw pinchcock (Fig. 117).

The cylindrical form of percolator made of metal, usually copper lined with tin, also is available and should be used when preliminary maceration or percolation with a hot menstruum is required. Metal percolators of this kind usually are supplied with a cover, and the outlet tube at the lower end is fitted with a metal stopcock by which the rate of flow of the percolate can be regulated (Fig. 118).

In selecting a glass percolator, one should be chosen in which the outlet tube does not

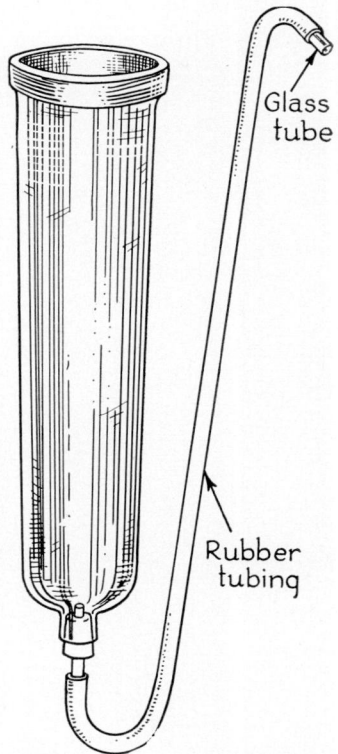

Fig. 116. Percolator with rubber-tube attachment for regulating flow of percolate.

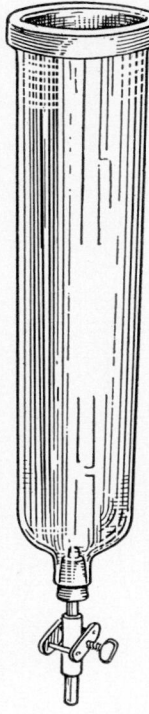

Fig. 117. Percolator with screw pinchcock attachment for regulating flow of percolate.

taper to the end, as shown in Figure 119, but flares slightly outward, as depicted in Figure 120. It is more convenient to equip the percolator with the flaring outlet with the attachments necessary to regulate the flow of the percolate. In the percolator with the tapering outlet these attachments must be put in place from the inside, whereas, in the other, all attachments can be fitted from the outside.

In extraction where more menstruum is required than can be run into the percolator at one time, and where it is desired to collect the percolate in several fractions, the open type of percolator may be fitted up, as shown in Figure 121. The receiver is fitted with a stopper through which pass 2 glass tubes—a short bent tube which is connected with the percolator by a rubber tube and a long straight tube. The latter is adjusted so that, when the desired volume of percolate has flowed into the receiver, the level of the liquid will reach the bottom of the tube. When it reaches this point, percolation ceases because the pressures in the percolator and the receiver are equalized. This apparatus requires attention only when the required volume

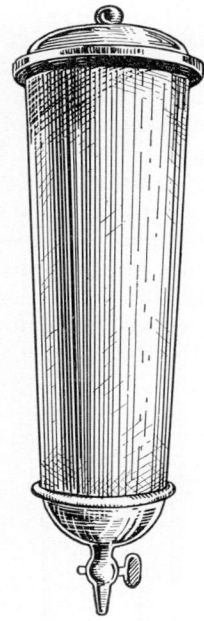

Fig. 118. Small metal percolator.

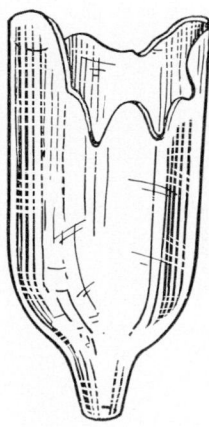

Fig. 119. Percolator with tapering outlet.

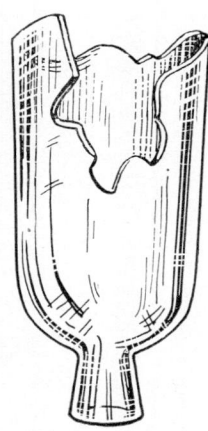

Fig. 120. Percolator with flaring outlet.

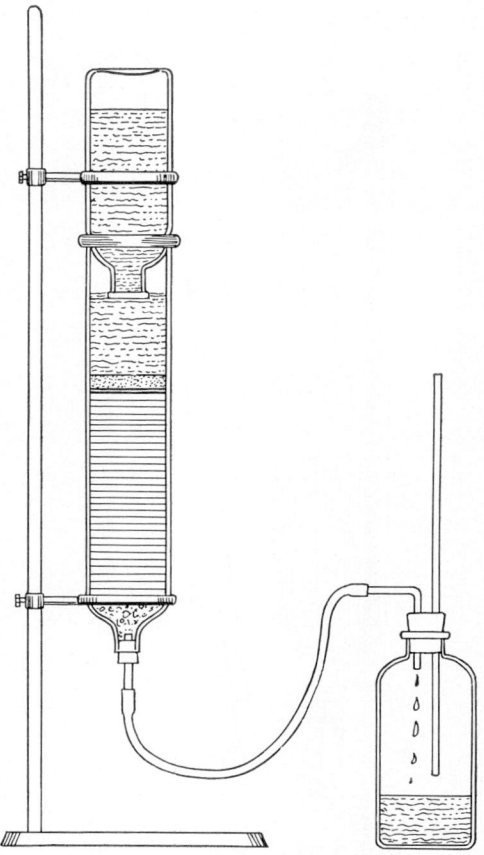

Fig. 121. Fractional percolator.

of percolate has collected. Then the percolate may be transferred to another container and further fractions collected in the same manner.

A modified form of percolator which is more durable than the forms made of glass, which is also said to be economical from the standpoint of the amount of menstruum required, is the so-called well-tube percolator designed by Dr. E. R. Squibb (Fig. 122). This is constructed from an ordinary flat-bottomed crock and operates as follows: after dampening, a thin layer of drug is packed in the percolator. The well-tube, the lower end of which has been covered with a piece of muslin, then is set in position in the crock, and the remainder of the dampened drug packed around it. The menstruum is poured over the drug to a height of several inches. A glass tube which passes through a tightly fitting rubber stopper reaches almost to the bottom of the well-tube and serves as a siphon to withdraw the percolate which passes into it.

Another modification of the open type of percolator is the so-called diacolator. In its original form, this consists of a series of 4 or more glass percolators of small diameter, about 65 cm. long and 3.5 cm. in

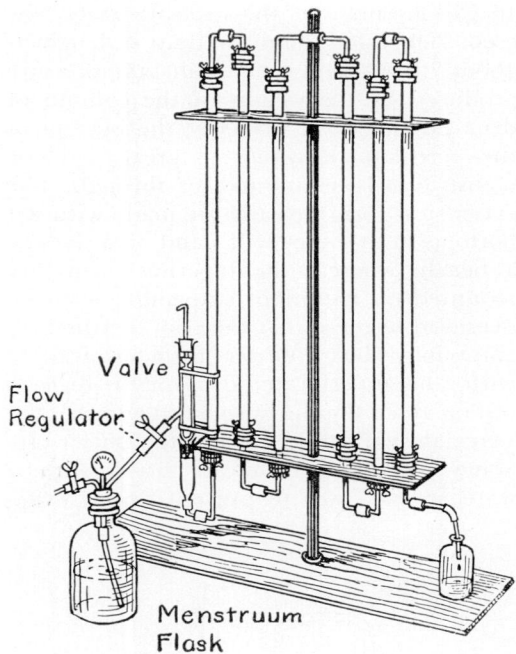

Fig. 123. Breddin diacolator.

diameter, connected alternately at the top and the bottom, as illustrated in Figure 123. To facilitate the passage of the menstruum through the several columns of drug, air pressure is applied at the entrance to the series of percolators or suction is applied at the outlet.

The closed type of percolator is used for the preparation of such galenicals as the ethereal tinctures and the oleoresins, where a highly volatile and flammable solvent is used as the menstruum, to prevent excessive loss of the latter by evaporation and to avoid fire hazards. Figure 124 illustrates an improvised percolator of this type. The side tube connects the percolator with the receiver and serves as a conduit for the necessary air exchange between the two. During the maceration stage, the side tube is closed by means of the stopcock in the glass tube which protrudes from the top of the receiver.

Percolators of the open type for large-scale operations are made of earthenware, suitable stainless steel, galvanized iron or tinned copper and are cylindrical or tapered in shape. They range in fluid capacity from

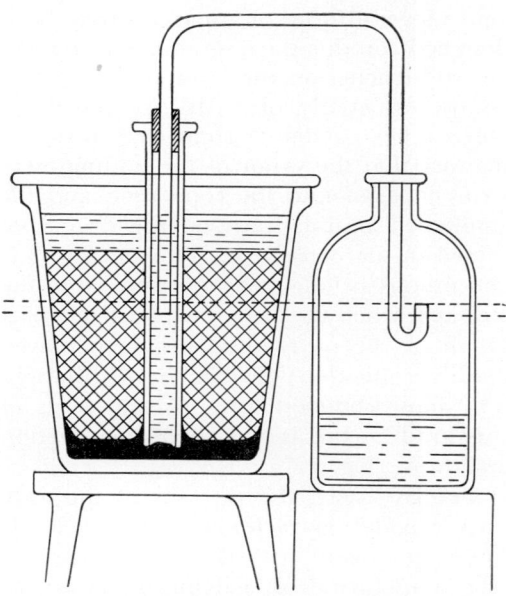

Fig. 122. Squibb well-tube percolator.

10 gallons up, but the capacity rarely exceeds 200 gallons, and the limit in height is about 7 ft. Beyond these limits, the pressure produced by the weight of the column of drug on the lower layers at the bottom of the percolator becomes so great that the menstruum is unable to pass through. The cylindrical forms usually are made with flat bottoms so that they will stand on a shelf or a bench, whereas the tapering forms are mounted on trunnions suspended from an overhead beam so that they can be tilted for emptying. The cylindrical form also is fitted with a loose perforated disk for the drug to rest on and a sloping false bottom so that the percolate will drain toward the outlet tap. Some percolators also are fitted with a water-sealed cover to prevent undue evap-

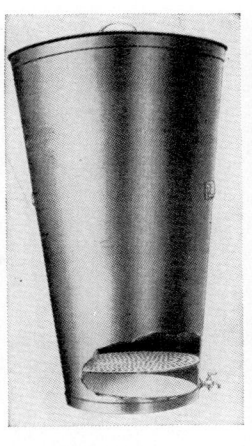

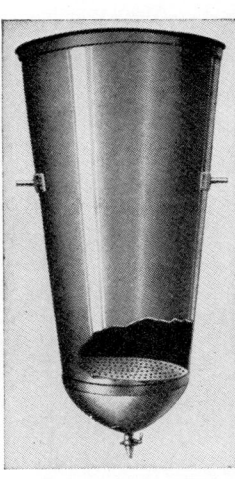

Fig. 125 (*Left*). Large percolator with flat bottom, outlet at side.

Fig. 126 (*Right*). Large percolator with rounded bottom.

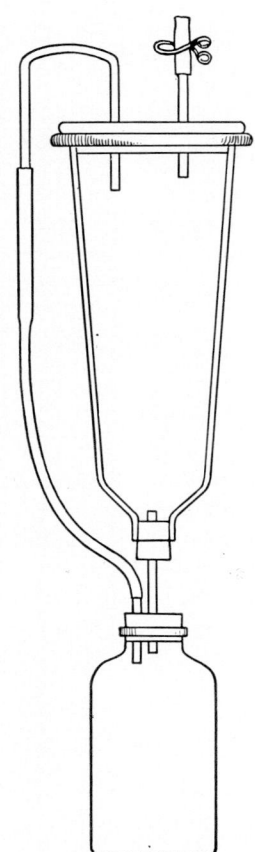

Fig. 124. Closed percolator for extraction with volatile solvents.

oration when a volatile solvent, such as alcohol, is used (Figs. 125, 126).

When a large quantity of a volatile menstruum is required to exhaust a drug by simple percolation, and the greater portion of this must be removed from the percolate by evaporation to make the finished product, continuous extraction may be used to advantage with a saving of time and solvent. Several forms of apparatus have been designed for this purpose, but all of them are constructed on the same principle and consist essentially of a still, a percolator and a reflex condenser connected in such a manner that the vapor of the boiling menstruum passes into the condenser, and the condensed liquid drops on the drug contained in the percolator. This operation is continuous as long as heat is applied to the still and, when the drug is exhausted, a part or all of the menstruum can be removed readily from the percolate by distillation. The most common form of apparatus of this kind in use is the Soxhlet extraction apparatus (Fig. 127).

Unfortunately, the capacity of the ordinary Soxhlet extractor is not sufficiently large to permit its use in making the official quantities of galenicals. However, an apparatus of sufficient capacity to serve this purpose can be constructed easily of a round-bottom flask, an ordinary open glass percolator and a condenser, as illustrated in Figure 128.

For continuous extraction on a commercial manufacturing scale, several forms of apparatus are in use. They are constructed of tinned copper or galvanized iron and are so designed that extraction may be carried out with either a hot or a cold solvent and either continuously by percolation or intermittently by maceration. A common form of apparatus of this type used in this country is the Lloyd extractor (Fig. 129).

METHODS OF EXTRACTION

Like the apparatus used in the extraction of drugs, the methods of extraction employed in the preparation of the galenicals may be divided into 2 general types: namely, the type in which extraction is effected by maceration and the type in which percolation is the process primarily involved. Both types are represented by the methods of extraction which comprise the following processes: maceration, decoction, infusion, percolation, fractional percolation and pressure percolation. For all of these processes, standard methods of procedure are prescribed and should be followed unless specific directions for modification are given or the use of an alternative procedure is permitted.

MACERATION

Maceration, from the Latin *macerare*, to soften, is a process in which a drug is steeped in a liquid, with or without the application of heat, until the tissues become softened and the soluble matter contained in the cells has been dissolved.

As ordinarily conducted, simple maceration requires the use of a bottle or a jar of the types shown in Figures 107 and 108 and is carried out as follows:

Macerate the drug or the mixture of drugs in a moderately warm place with a quantity of menstruum equal to about three quarters of the volume of the finished product, agitating it frequently for several days or until the soluble matter is dissolved. Transfer the mixture to a filter and, when most of the liquid has drained away, wash the residue on the filter with a sufficient quantity of the menstruum, combining the filtrates, to produce the desired volume. Mix the product well.

To avoid the frequent shaking which is necessary during the maceration period, the drug may be placed in a muslin bag and suspended in the menstruum. As the soluble matter dissolves in the menstruum which is in contact with the drug, the liquid increases in specific gravity and sinks to the bottom of the container. Its place is taken by fresh menstruum, and thus there is imparted a circulatory movement to the liquid, and extraction is facilitated.

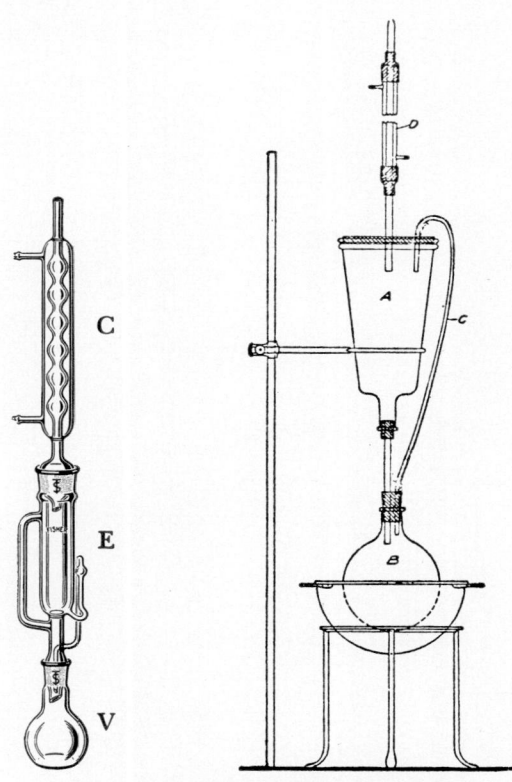

FIG. 127 (*Left*). Soxhlet extraction apparatus. (V, vaporizing chamber; E, extraction chamber; C, condensing chamber).

FIG. 128 (*Right*). Improvised apparatus for continuous extraction. (*A*, percolator; *B*, flask for collecting percolate and vaporizing solvent; *C*, tube for vaporized solvent to pass from *B* to *A*; *D*, condenser.)

164   Extraction

Simple maceration is especially suitable for the extraction, with alcohol, of drugs containing little or no cellular tissue, such as benzoin and myrrh, and for the extraction, with aqueous menstrua, of drugs containing mucilaginous and albuminous matter, such as squill. In this country, the process is not used in the preparation of the galenicals of these and other drugs which require complete extraction of the active principles for their completion.

It is the prescribed process for the preparation of 7 of the official tinctures (3 U.S.P. and 4 N.F. tinctures). However, in the preparation of most of the other galenicals the drugs are subjected to simple maceration as a preliminary step to extraction by percolation.

The process is not used in this country for the preparation of such concentrated galenicals as the extracts and the fluidextracts because it is not possible to extract completely all of the soluble matter from the cellular tissues of a drug in a single maceration. Even if the marc is pressed after the liquid has been drained off, as is done in European countries where maceration is the preferred process of ex-

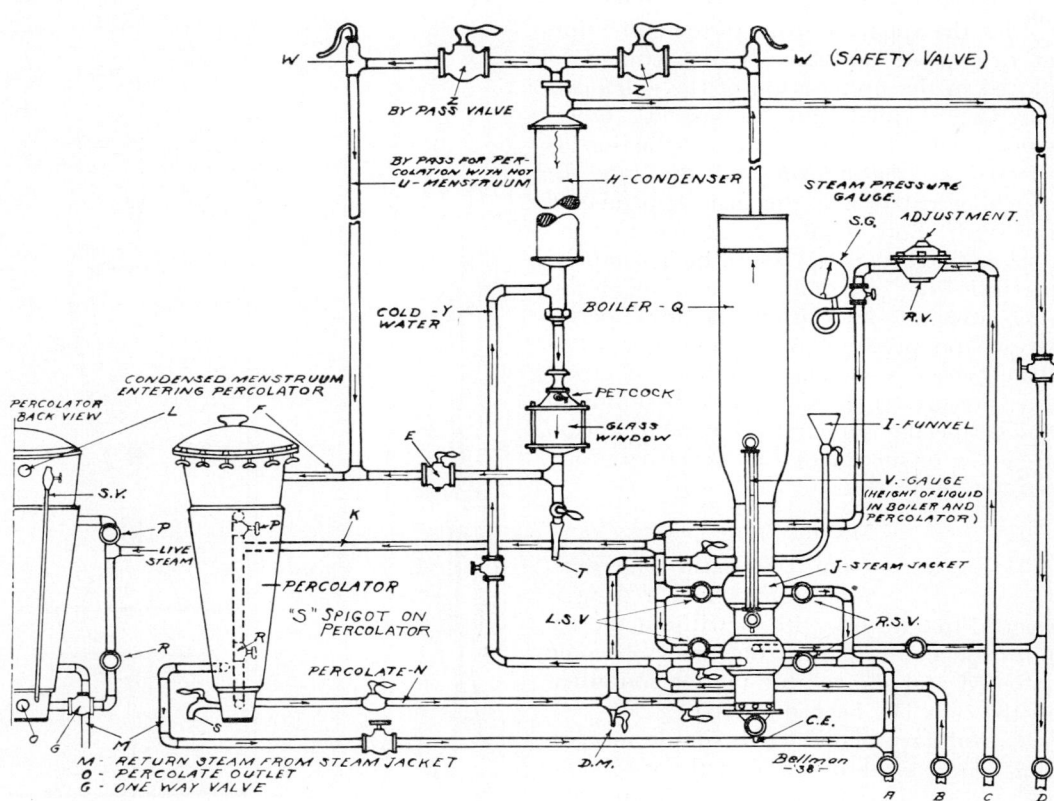

FIG. 129. Lloyd extractor used for continuous extraction.

A.	Return steam	E.	Valve closed when concentrating
B.	Cold water	C.E.	Collection of extract
C.	Live steam	R.	Live steam to percolator to clean system
D.	Waste water	L.S.V.	Live-steam valve
P.	Valve for inlet of steam to percolator jacket	R.S.V.	Return-steam valve
S.V.	Safety valve	D.M.	Collection of menstrua
R.V.	Reducing valve	T.	Collection of distillate on concentration

traction, a certain amount of liquid still will be left in the drug tissues, and this liquid will contain in solution as much of the soluble constituents, in proportion to its volume, as the liquid which was drained off. Obviously, however, the process of simple maceration may be used to effect exhaustion of a drug if it is repeated a sufficient number of times and fresh menstruum is used for each maceration, but this is laborious and time-consuming.

DECOCTION, INFUSION AND DIGESTION

Decoction, from the Latin *decoquere,* meaning to boil down or away, is the process of boiling drugs in water to extract the soluble principles. The process usually is carried out as follows in the preparation of decoctions:

Place the drug in a suitable vessel provided with a cover (see Fig. 111), pour on it an amount of cold purified water equal in volume to that of the finished product, cover it well and boil the mixture for about 15 minutes. Then allow it to cool to about 40°, express, strain the expressed liquid, and pass enough cold purified water through the strainer to make the product measure the desired volume.

The process of decoction, although not prescribed for the preparation of any official galenical, is used in the extraction of drugs of a hard and woody nature, the tissues of which are softened more readily by boiling than by merely steeping in hot water. It is not suitable for the extraction of drugs where these have active constituents which are volatile and would be driven off by boiling.

For the preparation of decoctions, the drug, depending on its nature, should be bruised, cut into small pieces or coarsely powdered, so that penetration of the tissues by the water will be fairly rapid.

Due to the marked swelling of the tissues and the coagulating effect of boiling on the albuminous matter present in plant drugs, the liquid will not drain off from the marc as readily as when extraction is effected by infusion; therefore, the official method required that the liquid be expressed from the marc. This usually is accomplished by folding the straining cloth over the marc deposited thereon and twisting the ends in opposite directions.

Since water extracts sugars and mucilaginous and albuminous matter in addition to the pharmacologically active principles of drugs, decoctions do not keep well and should be prepared freshly when ordered. Unless a preservative is added, they should not be dispensed in quantities that require more than a few days, at most, to consume.

Infusion, from the Latin *infundere,* meaning to pour in, is the process of steeping or drenching a drug in water so as to extract the active principles. Although not prescribed for the preparation of any official galenical, the following is the usual method for making infusions:

Moisten the drug in a suitable vessel, preferably of earthenware and provided with a cover (see Fig. 111), with a quantity of cold purified water about equal in weight to that of the drug and allow it to stand for 15 minutes. Then add boiling purified water in an amount equal to about nine tenths of the desired volume of the finished product, cover the vessel tightly and allow it to stand for 30 minutes. Strain the mixture and pass enough purified water through the strainer to make the infusion measure the desired volume. If the activity of the infusion is affected by the temperature of boiling water, cold purified water should be used.

In contradistinction to extraction by decoction, extraction by infusion is applicable only to drugs with a light structure and comparatively soft tissues. Since the process does not require boiling, it can be used for the extraction of drugs, the constituents of which are volatile.

As is done in the preparation of decoctions, the drug should be prepared for extraction by bruising, cutting or breaking into small pieces, or grinding to a coarse powder.

Since sugars and mucilaginous and albuminous substances are extracted by the process of infusion as well as by the process of decoction, infusions are subject to the same changes as decoctions; therefore, the same precautions should be observed in preparing and dispensing them.

The so-called "concentrated infusions" which have met with some favor in England are not, as might be inferred, preparations made by evaporating down freshly prepared infusions, but rather infusions made by a variety of processes, including percolation. They are intended to be used primarily for the rapid preparation of ordinary infusions and are usually of such a concentration that, when diluted with 7 times their volume of purified water, they will yield preparations which are approximately equivalent in strength to the freshly prepared infusions.

Digestion, from the Latin *digerere,* meaning to separate or dissolve, is another maceration process in which the menstruum is heated. It differs from the processes of decoction and infusion in that the period of maceration is much longer, and the temperature at which the operation is conducted is much lower, usually between 40° and 60°. In the commercial preparation of malt extract, for instance, the malt is infused with water at a temperature not exceeding 60°.

For the apparatus used in the extraction of drugs by digestion, see Figures 109 and 110.

The process, although not prescribed for the preparation of any of the official galenicals, is used widely in chemical and pharmaceutical manufacturing.

Percolation

Percolation, from the Latin *per,* meaning through, and *colare,* meaning to strain, is the process of extracting the soluble constituents from the nonsoluble cellular tissues of a drug by the slow passage of a suitable solvent through a column of the powdered drug packed in a special form of apparatus known as a percolator. In the process as usually conducted, the solvent (mainly as a result of the pull exerted by gravity) passes downward through the drug, but, in some of the more modern modifications of the process (as in diacolation, for instance), the solvent is forced to pass upward through portions of the drug by the application of air pressure at the inlet to the apparatus or suction at the outlet.

As stated above, a percolator is the only special apparatus required for carrying out the process of percolation. (For descriptions of the forms in general use, and their fittings, see Figs. 115-118.)

As usually conducted, the process of percolation comprises the following stages:
1. Preparation of the drug.
2. Dampening of the powder with the menstruum to soften and swell the tissues.
3. Packing the dampened powder into a percolator and adding sufficient menstruum to saturate the drug.
4. Period of maceration.
5. Percolation regulated to produce a specified volume of percolate in a specified period of time.

Preparing the Drug. To obtain the best results in percolation, the drug must be finely subdivided (powdered) in order that as much of the cell contents as possible will come in intimate contact with the solvent and so that there will be as little unbroken tissue as possible to obstruct the passage of the dissolved extractive through the cell walls. The particles should be uniform in size so that the spaces between them will be approximately the same, allowing the menstruum to flow evenly throughout the entire mass contained in the percolator.

The degree of fineness to which a drug should be subdivided for efficient extraction by percolation depends mainly on the nature of the drug, the solvent and the degree of exhaustion to be attained. In general, it may be said that the more compact the drug, the harder are its tissues and the finer should be the state of subdivision; and that a drug having active principles sparingly or difficultly soluble should be in a finer state of subdivision than one having active constituents which are readily soluble. Likewise, a drug which is to be extracted with alcohol should be in a finer powder than one which is to be extracted with water, because the former hardens the tissues and makes penetration by the solvent more difficult, whereas the latter softens and expands the tissues, thus making penetration by the solvent less difficult. As a rule, the finer the state of subdivision, the easier it is to effect complete extraction of the soluble principles of a drug. However, there are practical limitations to be considered; e.g., if the powder is too fine, it will clog the percolator.

Because of these conditions, the official compendia specify the degree of fineness of the powder to be used in the preparation of each galenical made by the percolation process. However, in most cases a moderately coarse powder is directed to be used.

Dampening the Drug. The powdered drug is dampened with menstruum and set aside for about 15 minutes before packing it into the percolator to prevent blocking of the percolator. If the powder were packed into the percolator in the dry state, in many instances upon addition of the menstruum the drug would swell to such an extent that the pressure developed within the percolator would cause an upheaval of the drug at the surface level or a block at lower levels, thus making it impossible for the menstruum to penetrate through to the lower layers.

The quantity of menstruum required to dampen a drug to the proper degree prior to packing it into the percolator is dependent on a number of factors, the most important of which are the nature of the

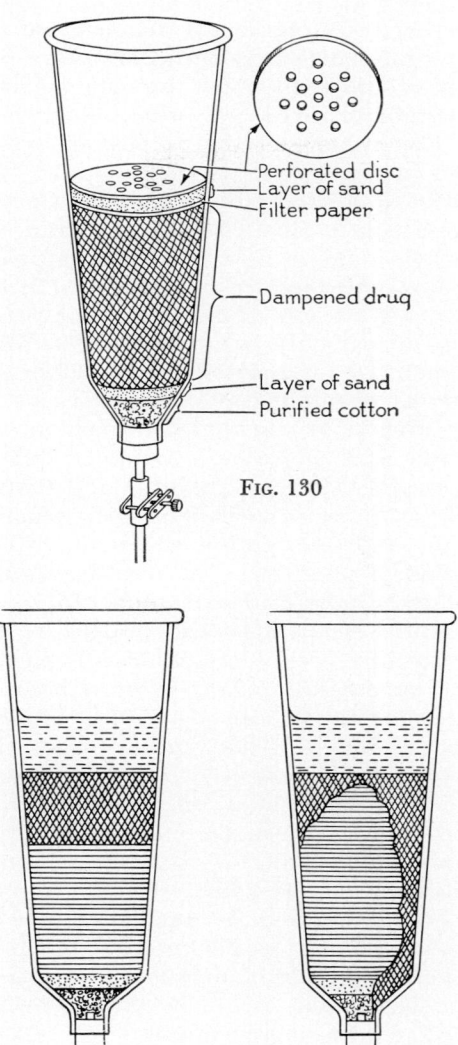

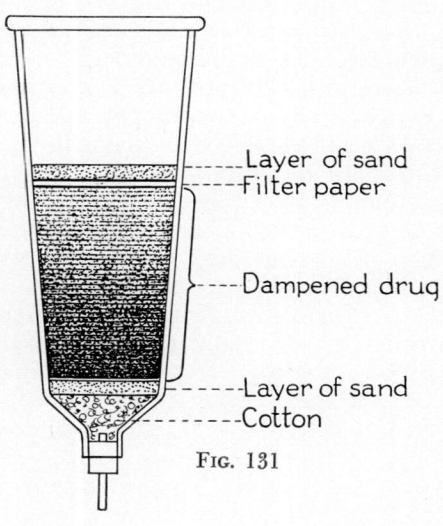

Fig. 130 (*Top, left*). Percolator fully equipped and packed with drug.

Fig. 131 (*Top, right*). Percolator showing proper packing with respect to density.

Fig. 132 (*Bottom, left*). Even flow in percolator with proper packing.

Fig. 133 (*Bottom, right*). Uneven flow in percolator due to uneven packing.

drug, the nature of the menstruum and the scale on which the operation is conducted. For the preparation of extracts and fluidextracts, the official compendia require that 600 to 800 ml. of menstruum be used for 1,000 Gm. of drug, but the quantity to be used in the preparation of tinctures is left to the discretion of the pharmacist. A larger proportion of menstruum may be used in dampening a drug in large-scale operations than is used in small-scale operations, because the percolators used in the former operations are packed less firmly than those used in the latter.

Packing the Percolator. The following is the procedure usually followed in packing a percolator for small-scale operations: A pledget of cotton, large enough to plug the orifice and to form a thin layer above it, is placed in the bottom of the percolator. This is leveled off by the addition of a thin layer of clean sand, after which a small quantity of the dampened drug is run in and pressed down lightly but uniformly. The remainder of the dampened drug then is added in small portions at a time, each successive portion being pressed down in the same manner, but more firmly than the preceding portion. A serviceable tamper for the pressing operation may be made of a cylindrical piece of hard wood, such as a broom handle, by sawing it off squarely at the end. To prevent disturbance of the top stratum of drug when the menstruum is poured in, it should be covered with a filter paper and this in turn with a thin layer of sand or with a perforated plate or a circular piece of wire gauze to weight it down (see Figs. 130-133).

Packing a percolator so that the best results will be obtained in percolation is an art which can be acquired only by experience. When properly performed, the menstruum will descend slowly and evenly throughout the moistened drug, carrying with it the extractive. If the percolator is packed badly, the menstruum will take the path of least resistance, forming channels through the more loosely packed portions, and will descend through these portions more rapidly than through the tightly packed portions. If the drug is packed too tightly, the menstruum will not pass through it; conversely, if it is packed too loosely, the menstruum will pass through so rapidly that extraction will be incomplete. As a rule, spongy drugs should be packed more loosely than those whose tissues are hard and compact, and drugs which are to be extracted with water should be packed more loosely than those to be percolated with an alcoholic menstruum.

After the drug has been packed into the percolator, sufficient menstruum is added to saturate it and to leave a layer on the surface; this condition should be maintained until the last portion of menstruum has been added. The latter is essential to prevent the formation of channels and the subsequent deflection of the downward passage of the menstruum through the drug into these channels of least resistance where its effectiveness for the purpose of extraction would be lost.

Period of Maceration. As soon as percolate begins to drop from the percolator, the outlet should be closed and sufficient menstruum added to form a layer several inches in depth on top of the drug. The percolator then should be covered and set aside to macerate for a period of time sufficiently long to permit the soluble constituents of the drug to be distributed throughout the liquid with which it is saturated. Here, again, the nature of the drug and that of the menstruum used must be reckoned with, and the optimum length of the period of maceration must be determined for each individual extraction. In actual practice, the period varies widely. In the percolation process of the official compendia, for instance, it ranges from 2 hours in the preparation of Glycyrrhiza Fluidextract, U.S.P., to 72 hours in the preparation of Ipecac Fluidextract, U.S.P. However, in the case of most of the official tinctures, the length of the maceration period is 24 hours, and for most of the other galenicals it is 48 hours.

Percolation and Its Regulation. At the end of the period of maceration, the lower orifice of the percolator should be opened, and percolation should be allowed to proceed at a definite rate of speed. The rate of flow of the percolate must be regulated if satisfactory results are to be obtained. If it is too rapid, there will not be sufficient time for the menstruum to penetrate the cells of the drug and dissolve out the soluble principles. On the other hand, if it is too slow, the liquid may become so thick, due to the large amount of extractive dissolved, that it will not pass through the lower strata of the drug, and a block will result.

In the official compendia, the percolation process is directed to be used in the preparation of certain tinctures, fluidextracts, extracts, oleoresins and resins and, in most instances, the rate of flow of the percolate is specified. The following are the terms used in stating these specifications, and their meanings: "Percolate slowly" means at a rate of speed not exceeding 1 ml. per minute; "percolate rapidly," a rate of 3 to 5 ml. per minute; "percolate at a moderate rate," a rate of 1 to 3 ml. per minute.

In the preparation of most of the official galenicals, the directions specify percolation at a moderate rate, but in the preparation of Ipecac Fluidextract, U.S.P., for instance, the directions specify percolation at a slow rate of speed, and, in the case of Rhubarb Fluidextract, N.F., percolation is directed to be conducted rapidly. Obviously, the rate of flow of percolate, other essential requirements having been met, will depend on the quantities of drug and menstruum involved. The larger these quantities, the more rapid the flow of percolate should be. This condition is recognized by the official compendia, in which it is stated that the rate of flow of the percolate may be increased when the quantities of drug and menstruum are greater than those directed to be used in the official monographs.

In the preparation of the weaker galenicals, such as the tinctures, the official compendia direct that percolation be continued until the specified volume (usually 1,000 ml.) of percolate has been obtained, unless the tincture is to be adjusted to a prescribed standard. In the latter case, percolation is stopped when a volume of percolate equal to 95 per cent of the specified volume of the finished product is obtained. When the strength of the percolate has been determined, all that is then required to adjust it to the specified standard is the addition of the proper amount of menstruum. For the preparation of the more concentrated galenicals, such as the fluidextracts and the extracts, percolation is directed to be continued to exhaustion of the drug, which is determined by removing a small quantity of the percolate and testing it for active constituents. To avoid the possibility of causing injury to the active principles in cases where such principles might be harmed by prolonged heating, the official compendia direct that the first 850 ml. of the percolate be reserved, that the remainder be concentrated to a soft extract by evaporation at a temperature not exceeding 60° and dissolved in the reserved portion and that, if no assay is directed, sufficient menstruum be added to the whole to make the finished product measure 1,000 ml.

In most extractions by percolation, one menstruum is used throughout—i.e., for dampening, macerating and percolating the drug—but sometimes better results can be obtained by using two menstrua instead of one: one for maceration and the beginning of percolation and another for completing the process. This applies particularly to drugs containing large amounts of tannin, such as krameria, chestnut leaves, witch-hazel leaves, wild cherry bark, etc., and to certain drugs, the alkaloidal constituents of which can be extracted best with an acid menstruum, but where an excess of acid in the finished product is objectionable, such as nux vomica. In the extraction of drugs of the first type, glycerin is directed by the official compendia to be a component of the menstrua used in the beginning and an acid, such as acetic or hydrochloric, is directed to be a component of the initial menstrua used in the extraction of drugs of the second type.

Fractional Percolation. Fractional or divided percolation, also called repercolation, is a modification of the ordinary process of percolation, in which the drug is divided into several portions and each portion extracted separately as follows: Portion number one is dampened, macerated and percolated in the usual way, except that the percolate is collected in a number of fractions each of definite volume. Portion number two then is dampened with fraction number two of the percolate obtained from the first portion of drug, fraction number one of this percolate being reserved as finished product. Percolation then is continued in the usual manner, but again the percolate is collected in fractions, the first of which is reserved as finished product and is larger in volume than that collected from the first portion of drug extracted, and the remainder of which are the same in number as those collected in the first percolation but smaller in volume. The remaining portions of drug are treated in the same manner, the size of the reserve fraction of percolate being increased in each case.

In the official compendia, the drug is directed to be divided into 3 portions, the percolate from each portion being collected in fractions of definite volume; these fractions are directed to be used in the percolation of the succeeding portions of drug as indicated in the diagrammatic representation in Figure 134.

The principal advantages of this process over that of ordinary percolation are that a concentrated preparation can be produced without subjecting any part of the percolate to heat and that it is more economical in the use of menstruum. However, as a rule it cannot be used for the extraction of drugs where percolation to exhaustion is the objective, because this requires a drug-percolate ratio of at least 1:3 on the average and, in the process of fractional percolation, the ratio is 1:1.

In the official compendia, the process is made use of in the preparation of the fluidextract of a drug whose active principles might be injured by heat, i.e., ergot. It is also used in the preparation of fluidextracts of unofficial drugs containing essential oils such as buchu, thyme, etc.

Pressure Percolation. Another modification of the ordinary percolation process, pressure percolation is in reality a modified diacolation process and is carried out in a specially designed apparatus called a diacolator. It differs from simple percolation in that it is conducted on a column of drug much greater in length and much smaller in diameter than usually is worked with, and in that the menstruum is forced through the drug under pressure. In addition, the rate of percolation is slower—about one half the rate at which the other types of percolation usually are conducted. For convenience, a series of comparatively short percolators is used instead of one long percolator, because the latter, which should be sufficient in length to ensure complete extraction of the drug when 1,000 ml. of percolate have been collected, would be unwieldy. (See Fig. 123.)

A drug to be extracted by this process should be ground to a coarse powder, approximately 70 per cent of which is a No. 4 powder and the remainder of which is a No. 6 powder. About 200 Gm. of the powder is dampened, packed in each percolator, macerated for the required period of time and percolated at the rate of about 6 drops per minute. Instead of operating each percolator separately, 4 or more are joined together by means of connecting tubes, so that percolate flowing from the bottom of the first will pass into the bottom of the second, up through the drug, out of the

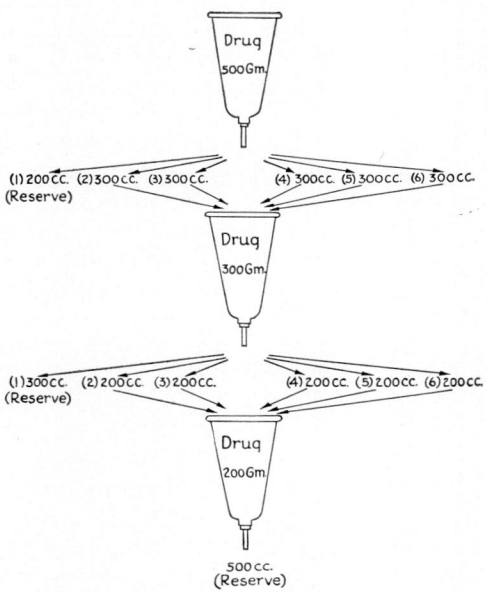

FIG. 134. Diagram of fractional percolation.

top into the top of the third, and so on to the end of the series.

Although described in the N.F., the process is not prescribed for the preparation of any of the official galenicals. It is merely stated that it may be used as an alternative for simple or fractional percolation where these are the prescribed processes.

Although the N.F., in which the process is described, states that it can be used as an alternative for simple or fractional preparations, the process is prescribed as an alternative method only in preparation of Belladonna Leaf Fluidextract, N.F.

Continuous Extraction. Another modification of the percolation process is continuous extraction. Although not prescribed for making any of the official galenicals, it is used widely. It is effected by the use of an extractor of the Soxhlet type (see Figs. 127, 128), whereby a relatively small quantity of menstruum through repeated vaporization and condensation is made to percolate again and again through the drug.

The process can be used to advantage for the extraction of drugs the active principles of which are not injured by heat and in which a highly volatile solvent, such as ether, acetone or solvent hexane is used. It is the process generally used in the preparation of the galenical oleoresins, and is well suited for defatting drugs, such as nux vomica, with solvent hexane or ether prior to extraction of the active principles by one of the other percolation processes.

RECOVERY OF MENSTRUA

In most extraction processes, alcohol or a mixture of alcohol and water are the menstrua used and, therefore, conservation of the menstrua is essential to economic manufacture. In addition to loss through evaporation, a considerable amount of menstruum is retained by the marc. The greater portion of this can be recovered by displacing it with water after percolation has been completed or by pressing the marc in an ordinary tincture press when the quantity is small or in a hydraulic press when the quantity is large, as in commercial manufacturing. Then the alcohol can be separated from the other components of the menstruum by fractional distillation. In some manufacturing plants, the percolator and its contents are placed directly in a large vacuum still, thus eliminating the time and the labor required to press the marc. Menstrua composed of other volatile solvents may be recovered in the same manner.

EXTRACTION BY IMMISCIBLE SOLVENTS

Extraction by immiscible solvents is the process of separating a constituent from the other constituents of a solution by shaking the latter with an immiscible solvent in which the constituent is soluble. It is the means commonly used in alkaloidal assaying for extracting alkaloids from liquids. The liquid to be extracted is shaken vigorously with the immiscible solvent, the mixture allowed to stand until separation of the liquids has taken place and the lower layer drawn off. The process is repeated with fresh portions of immiscible solvent until extraction is complete. The process also is employed on a manufacturing scale for the extraction of alkaloids from aqueous wash liquors and for the extraction of some organic acids which are sparingly soluble in water, such as benzoic and salicylic acid.

For extractions by this process on a small scale, as in alkaloidal assaying, a separatory funnel usually is employed.

BIBLIOGRAPHY

MACERATION

Webb: Drug. Circ. **42:**216, 1898.

PERCOLATION

Boullays: J. Pharm. Chim. **19:**281, 393, 1833; **21:**1, 1835.
Buchner: Repert. f. d. Pharm. **2:**356, 1816.
Cadet-Gassicourt: J. Pharm. Chim. **2:**165, 468, 1816.
Couch: Am. J. Pharm. **91:**16, 92, 1919; **92:**770, 853, 1920.
Diehl: Proc. Am. Pharm. A. **27:**727, 1879.
Dobereiner: Trommsdorffs' J. d. Pharm. New Ser. **1, 2:**458, 1817.

Duffield: Am. J. Pharm. **41**:2, 1869.
Duhamel: Am. J. Pharm. **10**:1, 1838.
Grahame: Am. J. Pharm. **30**:354, 1858.
Greco and Dumez: J. Am. Pharm. A. **39**: 560, 1950.
Guillermond: J. Pharm. Chim. **21**:349, 1835.
Hatcher and Lichtman: Am. J. Pharm. **93**: 534, 1921.
Husa, *et al.*: J. Am. Pharm. A. **23**:1, 891, 980, 1097, 1187, 1934; **24**:446, 538, 615, 839, 1935; **25**:10, 110, 311, 391, 1936; **26**: 20, 121, 220, 319, 1246, 1937; **27**:105, 205, 211, 290, 852, 859, 862, 1938; **28**:5, 593, 1939; (Sci. Ed.) **29**:455, 1940; (Sci. Ed.) **30**:635, 1941.
Huyck, J. Am. Pharm. A. (Sci. Ed.) **37**: 191, 1948.
Kremers and Brandel: Pharm. Rev. **24**:200, 311, 340, 1906; **25**:57, 242, 273, 317, 348, 1907.
Lloyd: Proc. Am. Pharm. A. **27**:682, 1879.
Oldberg: Proc. Am. Pharm. A. **32**:388, 1884.
Procter: Am. J. Pharm. **11**:189, 1839; **31**: 317, 1859.
Robiquet: J. Pharm. Chim. **20**:79, 1834.
Romershausen: Abstract. Repert. d. Pharm. **6**:316, 1819.
Scoville: J. Am. Pharm. A. **9**:864, 1920; **10**:844, 1921; **12**:104, 1923; **21**:877, 1932.
Self and Corfield: Pharm. J. **125**:98, 1930.
Soubeiran: Am. J. Pharm. **8**:221, 1836.
Squibb: Am. J. Pharm. **30**:97, 1858; **38**:109, 1866; **40**:1, 1868.
Thompson: Rep. Arts, Mfg. and Agric., Ser. 2, **22**:274, 339, 1813.
Thomson: Am. J. Pharm. **55**:537, 1883.
Wruble: J. Am. Pharm. A. **22**:641, 1933; **23**:208, 1934.

PART TWO

Pharmaceutical Preparations

ROY A. BOWERS, PH.D.
Dean, College of Pharmacy, Rutgers University

9

Waters

INTRODUCTION
STANDARDS FOR WATER
AROMATIC WATERS

OFFICIAL AROMATIC WATERS
STORAGE AND PRESERVATION OF AROMATIC WATERS

INTRODUCTION

Waters for pharmaceutical use, the standards for which are contained in the *U.S.P.* and the *N.F.*, embody a group of flavored and medicated waters known as aromatic waters as well as water, H_2O, in several grades of purity.

Aromatic waters are defined as saturated solutions (unless otherwise specified) of volatile oils or other aromatic or volatile substances in water. They are colorless, clear and free from empyreumatic and other foreign odors. In former revisions of the official compendia and in some modern foreign pharmacopeias, waters embodied many chemicals in aqueous solution. One such water is retained, Chloroform Water, N.F. Unlike most waters, Rose Water, U.S.P., is not saturated, and Hamamelis Water, N.F., is hydroalcoholic. Orange Flower Water, N.F., is the only water not perfectly clear. It is faintly opalescent.

Water is official in 4 degrees of purity, ranging from ordinary drinking water (tap water) to that which is used as a vehicle or diluent for medication administered by injection. These are as follows:

Water, U.S.P.
Purified Water, U.S.P.
Water for Injection, U.S.P.
Sterile Water for Injection, U.S.P.

STANDARDS FOR WATER

Water, U.S.P. Pharmaceutical manufacturers are permitted to use drinking water that conforms to the standards listed under Water, U.S.P., in the washing and the extraction of crude drugs and in the preparation of products for external use and other preparations in which the difference between water and purified water is of no consequence. This choice is necessitated because of the difficulties entailed in maintaining proper production and storage facilities required for the huge amount of water employed in this phase of drug manufacturing.

Purified Water, U.S.P., is used in the preparation of all medication containing water except ampuls, injections, some official external preparations such as liniments, and other specialized products. Water for Injection, U.S.P., must be used for aqueous solutions intended for injection.

Water, U.S.P., is not suitable for general pharmaceutical use because of the considerable amount of dissolved solids present. A 100-ml. portion of official water contains not more than 100 mg. of residue (0.1%) after evaporation to dryness on a steam bath and subsequent drying to constant weight in an oven at 105°, while an equal amount of purified water yields not more than 1 mg.

of residue under the same conditions. These dissolved solids consist chiefly of the chlorides, sulfates and bicarbonates of sodium, potassium, calcium and magnesium. Practically the only difference between water and purified water lies in the amount of total dissolved solids. The development of precipitates and effervescence which occurs when preparing medicinals with water in place of purified water is the major objection to its use. Water is clear, colorless and practically tasteless and odorless even near the boiling point. It meets the U.S. Public Health Service regulations for potable water with respect to bacteriologic purity. A pH range is given, but most tap water is neutral or just slightly alkaline. The deviation from neutrality to slight acidity or alkalinity is due not only to the composition of the dissolved solids but also to dissolved carbon dioxide or ammonia.

Purified Water, U.S.P. With the exception of the amount of dissolved solids present, and a limitation of oxidizable substances, the standards for Purified Water, U.S.P., are similar to those for water. Purified Water, U.S.P., formerly official as Distilled Water, may be prepared by distillation or deionization. No red color is produced when 2 drops of methyl red pH indicator are added to 10 ml. of purified water in a test tube. A 10-ml. portion shows no blue color on the addition of 5 drops of bromothymol blue pH indicator. This indicates a pH range of approximately 5 to 7. Freshly distilled water has a pH of about 5.6 and usually changes to about pH 6 on storage. Distilled water may be rendered carbon-dioxide-free by boiling after it is freshly prepared. Since purified water is obtained by distillation or deionization, it must be labeled to indicate the method of preparation.

Although deionization or demineralization procedures for the removal of dissolved salts from water have been used for more than 20 years, water purified in this manner was not given official recognition until the fourth and final supplement to U.S.P. XIV.

The deionization methods for the production of water of distilled-water quality possess a number of advantages over distillation for the manufacturer, the laboratory worker and the prescriptionist. These include: (1) the elimination of the use of heat, (2) simpler equipment with less maintenance, (3) lower long-term costs and (4) ease of production and storage.

The deionization methods in use today no doubt resulted from the well-known zeolite process for "softening" water of high mineral content. The "exchangers" used are synthetic, polymeric, high-molecular-weight resins which are insoluble in water and characterized by an unusually high content of free amino, sulfonic acid or phenolic functions. These resins are of 2 main types: the cation or acid exchangers which permit the replacement of the cations in solution with hydrogen ion, and the anion or base exchange resins which permit the removal of anions.

The manner in which these resins function may be summed up, in simplified form, as follows:

1. Acid or Cation Exchange Step: In this step, the cation(s) of the salt(s) are replaced with hydrogen ions. The cations so replaced remain behind "fixed" to the resin.

$$\text{H Resin} + M^+ + X^- \rightarrow M \text{ Resin} + H^+ + X^-$$

where M^+ and X^- are the cation and the anion of a salt present in solution.

2. Base or Anion Exchange Step: The water is then passed through a basic resin (usually a polyamine) and the anion remaining, after step (1), is removed according to:

$$\text{Resin}-NH_2 + H^+ + X^- \rightarrow \text{Resin}-NH_2 \cdot HX$$

This anion exchange step also may be represented as:

$$\text{Resin}-NH_3OH + H^+ + X^- \rightarrow \text{Resin}-NH_3X + H_2O$$

Ion exchange as shown above thus effects the removal of dissolved salts and only water remains behind. In those instances where the anion is a carbonate or a bicarbonate, the carbon dioxide formed usually remains dissolved and most often is present in amounts too small to alter the purity of the water. However, if large quantities of carbonates or bicarbonates give rise to substantial amounts of carbon dioxide, the gas may be removed by aeration.

Many types of ion-exchange resins are available. Simple units of the "mixed-bed" type easily are installed in any prescription department or laboratory, thus making available a ready supply of purified water. Regeneration of the units is a simple procedure and does not involve substantial quantities of time or material.

In addition to the permanent units, "cartridges" of mixed resins which fit into the top of a polyethylene bottle can be obtained from any chemical supply house. Such units provide a simple means for readily converting tap water into purified water.

With the exception of preparations intended for parenteral administration for which Water for Injection is specifically intended, purified water prepared by deionization may be used in any formulation, preparation or prescription calling for distilled water.

Water for Injection, U.S.P. This is sterile, pyrogen-free water purified by distillation for the preparation of products for parenteral use. It contains no added substance and meets the requirements of the tests under purified water. When previously rendered isotonic by the addition of 900 mg. of pyrogen-free sodium chloride for each 100 ml., it must meet the requirements of the Pyrogen Test. The preparation is to be packaged in tight containers and may be stored at a temperature below or above the range in which microbial growth occurs.

"Sterilization" refers to the destruction of all living organisms and their spores in, or their removal from, materials. This may be accomplished in various ways, but the preferable method in this case is *U.S.P. XIII* Process C, i.e., steam under pressure (heating in an autoclave). If an autoclave is not available, freshly distilled water may be sterilized by boiling the water for at least 60 minutes in a flask stoppered with a plug of purified nonabsorbent cotton covered with gauze, tinfoil or stout nonabsorbent paper; or the neck of the flask may be covered with cellophane and tightly fastened with cord. The water is allowed to cool without removing the stopper. If the cotton plug is used as a stopper, the top of the flask may be wrapped with paper in order to protect the mouth of the flask.

Pyrogens are nitrogenous, fever-producing substances of probable bacterial origin. They usually are considered to consist of disintegrated or intact dead bacteria as well as liberated endotoxins and exotoxins. Pyrogens are nonvolatile, and are produced by specific bacteria which grow in water. Ordinary distillation will not cause the removal of these pyrogenic substances. The manufacturer of pyrogen-free sterile water may employ any suitable method of preparation that will produce a product that conforms to the *U.S.P.* Sterility Test for Liquids, the Pyrogen Test, and the requirements of the tests prescribed in the official monograph of Water for Injection.

One procedure in common use consists of at least 3 or 4 distillations. The first distillation may be carried out in a block tin still operated so that about 10 per cent of the distillate escapes as vapor, thus eliminating most of the volatile impurities. The next 2 or 3 distillations are carried out in an all-Pyrex resistant-glass apparatus under aseptic conditions. The final distillation is carried out according to the procedure suggested in the *N.F. VII* monograph on redistilled water. The method consists of a fractional distillation in which potassium permanganate and either sodium or barium hydroxide has been added to the multidistilled water. When 50-ml. samples of the distillate contained in a Nessler tube no longer give a yellow coloration upon the addition of alkaline mercuric potassium iodide solution, water free from pyrogens and other organic matter is collected under aseptic conditions. These oxidizable substances present in distilled water are oxidized and rendered nonvolatile in the alkaline potassium permanganate medium. The nitrogen escapes with the water vapor as ammonia. The ammonia in the distillate gives the color reaction by reacting with the alkaline mercuric potassium iodide to form the yellowish-orange-colored compound of the composition

HgO·Hg(NH$_2$)I. The absence of the ammonia in the distillate indicates that all of the nitrogenous substances in the water have been destroyed and rendered nonvolatile.

Recently, pyrogen and bacterial retentive filters have been developed and are used widely. Models can be obtained with a steam-generating unit from which steam may pass through the filter to ensure complete sterilization of the circulatory passages as well as the filter disks themselves.

Water for injection prepared for immediate use must be distilled and sterilized within 24 hours and may be stored for not more than 24 hours in well-cleansed, tight containers at a temperature below or above that at which bacterial growth may take place. Unused portions are to be discarded or resterilized, unless following sterilization the container is kept closed at all times and nothing enters except the filtered air needed for replacement as the water for injection is drawn off. When this freshly prepared water is stored and sterilized in hermetically sealed containers, it will remain in good condition indefinitely.

Sterile Water for Injection U.S.P. Specifications are provided in this monograph for water for injection, sterilized and packaged in suitable containers, preferably of Type I glass, of not larger than 1,000-ml. size. When in containers of not larger than 30-ml. size, it may contain a bacteriostatic agent, the label of which indicates the name and the proportion of the added agent.

The preparation must meet the requirements of the Sterility Tests and the Pyrogen Test and the other tests under Purified Water. The following limits for total solids apply for Sterile Water for Injection in glass containers: up to and including 30-ml. size, 40 parts per million; from 30-ml. up to and including 100-ml. size, 30 parts per million; and for larger sizes 20 parts per million.

AROMATIC WATERS

History. Aromatic waters were known in antiquity, and distilled waters were prepared in Egypt as early as the 4th century. Distilled rose water was an important article of export in Persia in the 8th and the 9th centuries. The introduction of distillation and of distilled waters into Europe generally has been attributed to the renowned Catalanian physician, Arnaldus de Villanova (1235–1312), who for some time taught at the University of Montpellier (France). Around 1500, the distilled aromatic waters were accorded much recognition in therapy. There developed a special trade of so-called "water-brenners," and a number of books on the art of distilling appeared, of which those written by Hieronymus Brunschwygk—spelled also Brunschwig, Brunschwyk, etc.—(1430–1512) are known best. Until the end of the 18th century, the official pharmacopeias of all countries vied with each other in the number and the variety of their formulas for distilled waters.

Application. Aromatic waters provide a pleasingly flavored medium for the liquid administration of water-soluble remedial agents and for the liquid phase of suspensions and emulsions. Hospital pharmacists have recommended aromatic waters as vehicles for stock solutions of sodium citrate, potassium citrate and methenamine to prevent development of fungi and molds. The medical practitioner possesses in aromatic waters not only the solvent powers of water but also the enhancing aroma and the flavor of natural well-known plant essences or other volatile matter which mask the undesirable tastes and physical characteristics of many medicinal substances.

Preparation. Most aromatic waters are prepared extemporaneously according to the simple methods of the *U.S.P.* and the *N.F.* The aromatic or volatile principles are very slightly soluble in water, thus only small amounts of the aromatic principles are necessary to produce a saturated solution. The *U.S.P.* prescribes 3 general methods: distillation, solution and alternate solution.

DISTILLATION. The distillation method can be considered as an over-all method. That is, from a theoretical point of view, most of the waters can be prepared by distillation. But it is not practical or economically feasible to use this method when in most cases, just as satisfactory a product can be prepared when needed in the prescription laboratory at small cost and with little

Aromatic Waters

apparatus. Stronger Rose Water, U.S.P., Orange Flower Water, N.F. and Hamamelis Water, N.F., are prepared directly from fresh plant material and thus cannot be prepared by any method other than distillation. The distillation method consists of placing the odoriferous portion of the plant or the drug from which the aromatic water is to be prepared in a suitable still with sufficient purified water, and distilling most of the water, carefully avoiding the development of empyreumatic odors through charring or scorching of the substances. The excess oil is separated from the distillate, and the clear aqueous portion is preserved or used, thus representing the product. If necessary, the aromatic water is filtered. (For a discussion on distillation, see p. 59.)

The aromatic principles of most plants can be separated from the crude material by steam distillation and thus be available for use in the extemporaneous preparation of waters. Such being the case, for most waters the *U.S.P.* prescribes the following method:

SOLUTION:
    The Volatile Oil, or Other Specified Volatile Substance, 2 ml. or 2 Gm.
    Purified Water, a sufficient, quantity,
        To make .... 1,000 ml.

Shake the volatile substance (suitably comminuted if a solid) with 1,000 ml. of purified water in a capacious bottle, and repeat the shaking several times during a period of about 15 minutes. Set the mixture aside for 12 hours or longer, filter through wetted filter paper and pass enough purified water through the filter to make the product measure 1,000 ml.

Upon preparing a water by this method, it will be observed that 2 ml. or 2 Gm., liquid or solid as the case may be, is a considerable excess. The excess creates a greater exposure between the solute and the solvent phases. The time element involved takes advantage of the high vaporization rates of the volatile substance, thus developing increased exposure. In filtering, the filter paper must be wet to prevent the passage of excess oil into the filtrate and to eliminate absorption of the dissolved aromatics.

The disadvantage of this method is that it is difficult to obtain a brilliantly clear preparation, due to the formation of extremely fine particles, in spite of repeated filtration. This may be obviated by using boiling purified water. Also, it is hardly suitable, when a saturated solution is sought, to make up to volume with purified water as the official method directs. Making up to volume may not be necessary since the loss in volume is slight.

ALTERNATE SOLUTION. The *U.S.P.* has recognized the clarification and time-consuming factors by offering as an alternative the following method:

"Thoroughly incorporate the volatile oil (or the suitably comminuted volatile solid) with 15 Gm. of purified talc or with a sufficient quantity of purified siliceous earth or pulped filter paper. Add 1,000 ml. of purified water, and thoroughly agitate the mixture several times during 10 minutes. Then filter the mixture, returning the first portions, if necessary, to obtain a clear filtrate, and add enough purified water through the filter to make the product measure 1,000 ml."

The principle of adsorption and distribution of the volatile substance with an inert, insoluble solid such as prescribed is displayed here. There will be an increased exposure of the aromatic substance since it will be in a finer state of subdivision, and repeated shakings produce a milklike suspension of the aromatic-adsorbed solid. In addition, the adsorptive agent acts as a clarifier in filtration in that the undissolved volatile material will remain adsorbed in the insoluble solid and be prevented from passing through the filter. The time-saving factor is an important advantage.

Unfortunately, the alternative method has not proved to be entirely satisfactory due to the problem of the purified talc or purified siliceous earth passing through even dense-textured filter paper. Purified talc on the market is subdivided too finely, and it is difficult to obtain good purified siliceous earth free from soluble and finely divided extraneous matter. The use of pulped filter paper does not solve the clarification problem. Several other substances have been recommended as intermediate agents. Calcium phosphate showed great promise at first, since not only did it produce a clear water but also the preparations possessed a more sparkling clarity. However, these waters developed a yellow tinge in aging due to the slightly alkaline reaction of dissolved calcium phosphate with the dissolved volatile principles. This alkaline reaction presented incompatibility problems. Magnesium and calcium carbonates were ruled out for the same reason as calcium phosphate.

The ultimate goal in preparing any pharmaceutical is that of obtaining a product that adheres to official standards. The *U.S.P.* and the *N.F.* permit deviation of detail from the official methods, provided that the final product meets official requirements. As for preparing waters, not only may a superior product be obtained by using boiling purified water in the official method of solution, but also this method obviates the difficulty of clarification.

Use of Aromatic Waters. Aromatic waters are not therapeutically potent because of the very small proportion of active substance present in them. Their chief function is that of aqueous, flavored, aromatized vehicles. Since aromatic waters are saturated solutions, some of the aromatic becomes "salted out" when a considerable quantity of solute is added. The insoluble material detracts from the elegance of the preparation. It collects on the top of the liquid to impart a burning nauseous taste to the first doses taken. This incompatibility may be avoided by diluting the aromatic water with an equal quantity of purified water before dissolving the solute or by removing the insoluble portion by filtration.

Official usual doses are given for Chloroform Water (15 ml.) and Peppermint Water (15 ml. 3 times a day). For other aromatic waters practitioners usually prescribe 5 to 15 ml. per dose.

OFFICIAL AROMATIC WATERS

The official aromatic waters are as follows:

United States Pharmacopeia XVI
Peppermint Water
Rose Water
Stronger Rose Water

National Formulary XI
Camphor Water
Chloroform Water
Cinnamon Water
Hamamelis Water — *Preserved c̄ 15% alcohol*
Orange Flower Water

Chloroform Water. This is not prepared according to the general methods. There is no clarification problem involved, and a slight excess of chloroform must remain in the bottle. A saturated solution is prepared and maintained by adding an excess of chloroform in a dark amber-colored bottle to a given quantity of purified water, shaking vigorously and taking care that a slight excess of chloroform is always present. Since chloroform is heavier than water, the excess will remain on the bottom of the container. The high volatility of chloroform creates an equilibrium of loss and restoration of strength by evaporation. Naturally, when dispensing, the bottle should not be shaken, and only the supernatant liquid used. The bottle may be refilled with purified water and shaken after each decantation. Chloroform water is stored in a light-resistant bottle since light causes chloroform to be oxidized to the obnoxious, poisonous gas, phosgene, according to the following formula:

$$CHCl_3 + O \xrightarrow{light} \underset{phosgene}{COCl_2} + HCl$$

In addition to its use as a vehicle, chloroform water is used as an expectorant, a stomachic and an antiemetic in an average dose of 15 ml.

Distilled Aromatic Waters. The official Orange Flower Water, Stronger Rose Water and Hamamelis Water cannot be prepared extemporaneously by the pharmacist. These represent saturated aqueous solutions of the water-soluble odoriferous principles of the fresh material and are prepared by distillation. Rose Water is prepared by dilution of stronger rose water with an equal volume of purified water. While orange flower water and stronger rose water are prone to mold formation and general loss of fine aroma, hamamelis water is preserved by the addition of 15 per cent alcohol. For this reason many pharmacists prefer to use an orange flower water prepared from the orange flower oil as an unofficial replacement. Also, a large proportion of the rose water in general use is not prepared from the official stronger rose water as the *U.S.P.* directs but is made by diluting a specially prepared solution of 50 per cent alcohol and rose oil or rose synthetic. Neither of these artificial substitutes compares in quality with the official products.

Hamamelis Water. This also is known as Witch-hazel Water, Distilled Witch-hazel Extract and Witch Hazel. Frequently, the label on the commercial product will contain one or more X's. Each X represents one distillation. For example, XXXX means that the water is a quadruple-distilled product. That is, the distillate of the first distillation is returned to a fresh quantity of the drug and redistilled. The procedure, in this instance, is carried out 4 times. It is believed that the first distillation does not yield a saturated water, and subsequent distillations are necessary. The other waters prepared by distillation are treated in like manner. Hamamelis water is used as an astringent and perfume in aftershave lotions and other cosmetic products.

Camphor Water. This is the only aromatic water prepared from a solid. Camphor presents a comminution problem. It is available in granular or crystalline tough masses or in the form of compressed cakes. A fine powder can be obtained by allowing a small quantity of alcohol, ether or chloroform to drop on the broken masses of camphor in a dry mortar followed by rapid and light trituration. Prolonged or heavy trituration causes the camphor to become gummy. The fine powder is spread on a paper to permit the solvent to evaporate spontaneously. Synthetic camphor will produce a fine powder with much less difficulty than will natural camphor.

An older method preferred by some pharmacists involves actual liquefaction of the camphor with a minimum amount of alcohol followed by adsorption with purified talc. The disadvantage is the retention of some alcohol in the finished product.

Freshly prepared camphor water contains a higher percentage of dissolved camphor, for not only does camphor volatilize with prolonged storage, it also tends to precipitate with depressions in storage temperatures. In addition to its general vehicular use, camphor water frequently is prescribed in eyedrops and eyewashes for its slight refreshing, stimulating effect.

Bitter Almond Water, N.F. VIII. This is prepared by saturating a liter of purified water with 1 ml. of bitter almond oil.

Wintergreen Water, N.F. IX. Involves the use of 5 ml. of gaultheria oil (methyl salicylate) per liter. Unlike other volatile oils, these oils are not complex mixtures but are composed almost entirely of a single constituent. Gaultheria oil has a greater solubility in water and thus requires more to produce a saturated solution.

Phenolated Water, N.F. VIII. This is a 2 per cent aqueous solution of phenol. It will be noted that 22 ml. of liquefied phenol is mixed with 978 ml. of purified water to prepare this product. The apparent excess accounts for 12 per cent water already present in the liquefied phenol. Phenolated water is valued for its topical antiseptic properties and its ability to relieve itching of the skin.

STORAGE AND PRESERVATION OF AROMATIC WATERS

Intense sunlight and changes in temperature cause aromatic waters to lose some of their delightfulness. Freezing effects separation of the aromatics to produce cloudiness. Stoppering with purified cotton allows access of some air but excludes dust. Thus the water will not acquire the characteristic odor of stale air. In general, aromatic waters are not permanently stable preparations since they support the growth of molds and other organisms. Waters prepared aseptically from recently boiled purified water and filtered through a Chamberland L3 filter into a sterilized resistant-glass container have remained in perfect condition for a year.

EDWARD ARMOND BRECHT, Jr., Ph.D.
*Dean and Professor of Pharmacy,
University of North Carolina*

10

Syrups and Juices

SYRUPS
SYRUPS OF U.S.P. XVI

SYRUPS OF N.F. XI
JUICES OF U.S.P. XVI

SYRUPS

A syrup is a nearly saturated aqueous solution of a sugar, with or without medicinal or flavoring ingredients. The syrups constitute a class of liquid preparations of pleasing appearance and palatability well suited as vehicles for systemic medication to be taken internally. They are characterized by a sweet taste and a relatively high specific gravity (1.18 to 1.37).

Medicinally, the syrups are divided into 2 groups: the *flavoring* syrups, which are used as vehicles, and the *medicated* syrups, which contain ingredients giving them therapeutic value. Pharmaceutically, the syrups may be grouped according to the method of preparation: those made by the addition of ingredients to syrup and those made by the solution of sugar in an aqueous solution of the ingredients. A third class of official syrups is composed of those legally protected by patents, copyrights and trademarks. These products are included in the official compendia on the basis of important usage in medical practice to provide legal standards for their content of the active ingredients. For these syrups there are no official formulas for their preparation and no descriptions of the products.

Although there is a large group of organic compounds known as sugars, the sugar of importance in the preparation of syrups is sucrose, the official name of common sugar. Sucrose usually is produced from either the sugar cane or the sugar beet, although the *U.S.P.* recognizes that it may be produced from other sources, such as the sugar maple. Before the Food and Drug Act of 1906, the sucrose ordinarily obtainable was often unsuitable for pharmaceutical use due to the addition of harmful whitening agents, such as ultramarine, or the use of bleaching chemicals. At that time, crystal sugar was preferred for pharmaceutical use. At the present time, the quality of sugar is not subject to this difficulty.

Sucrose is a disaccharide. It undergoes hydrolysis to give a molecule each of the monosaccharides dextrose (glucose) and levulose (fructose, fruit sugar).

$$C_{12}H_{22}O_{11} + H_2O \rightarrow$$
sucrose
$$C_6H_{12}O_6 + C_6H_{12}O_6$$
dextrose levulose

This reaction also is called inversion because a solution of sucrose rotates polarized light to the right, while the same solution after hydrolysis rotates the light to the left because the levulose has a greater rotating power than the dextrose. This reaction is interesting for 3 reasons: (1) Solutions of invert sugar are more subject to fermentation than solutions of sucrose. (2) After inversion, the solution is sweeter; if sucrose is rated with a sweetness of 100, dextrose is rated 74 and levulose 173. (3) Finally, the levulose formed by inversion seems to be responsible for the brown discoloration which develops in some of the colorless syrups. This change is called *caramelization*, and it takes place in the syrups containing strong acids because the hydrogen ion catalyzes the inversion of sucrose.

To eliminate the discoloration of certain colorless syrups containing acids, formulas were adopted for *N.F. VII* of 1942 in which dextrose was used in place of sucrose in Syrup of Hypophosphites and Compound Syrup of Hypophosphites. These syrups do not become brown, but other difficulties are introduced. Dextrose forms a saturated solution at 50 per cent, while sucrose dissolves to the extent of 65 per cent. Dextrose dissolves more slowly. The saturated solution of dextrose readily supports the growth of micro-organisms. To improve the keeping qualities of these syrups, fairly large amounts of glycerin are added. The glycerin also serves to increase the viscosity of dextrose syrups to compare favorably with sucrose syrups. Compound Hypophosphites Syrup *N.F. X* was the last of these syrups to be official.

The concentration of sucrose in a syrup is an important factor controlling its keeping quality. As a carbohydrate, sucrose in dilute aqueous solutions provides a nutrient pablum which well supports the growth of many micro-organisms, especially yeasts and molds. The ability of these organisms to grow is decreased as the concentration of sucrose is increased. Therefore, syrups should contain enough sucrose to approach saturation. It is undesirable to attain true saturation because slight cooling might start crystallization, which results in the formation of large crystals which are difficult to redissolve, and this proceeds sufficiently to yield a sucrose concentration greatly below saturation.

Many of the official syrups do not contain any preservative other than an adequate sucrose concentration to prevent fermentation or the growth of other organisms. A few syrups contain 0.1 to 0.2 per cent of sodium benzoate or benzoic acid, which is efficient for this purpose.

Glycerin is used in some of the syrups, especially those made with dextrose, as a preservative against the growth of micro-organisms, and is effective if the concentration is sufficient (30% by volume, with dextrose). Glycerine is efficient as a solvent for tannins and as a preservative against the precipitation of vegetable extractive. Although glycerin has a sweet taste, its sweetness is not so pleasing as that of sucrose.

Alcohol is present in dilute concentrations in some of the syrups. It serves as a solvent for the addition of alcohol-soluble ingredients. The concentration of alcohol is not sufficient to prevent the growth of organisms, although some pharmacists believe that the alcohol concentrates in the vapors above the syrup and thus prevents the growth of surface molds.

TABLE 8. PRESERVATIVES FOR PHARMACEUTICAL PREPARATIONS

PRESERVATIVE	PREPARATIONS		
	Acid	*Neutral*	*Alkaline*
Benzoic acid....	0.1%	0.2%	
Alcohol........	15.0	17.5	17.5%
Glycerin.......		45.0	45.0

The concentrations of preservatives suitable for pharmaceutical preparations are summarized in Table 8.[1] Knowing that 65 per cent of sucrose is self-preserving, it is possible to predict the amounts of accessory preservatives needed in those syrups containing reduced sugar concentrations on the basis of calculated "free water."[2] These calculations show that all of the official syrups are preserved adequately. The fact that some syrups are subject to deterioration by the growth of micro-organisms is explainable on the basis of the differences in the nutritive value of the ingredients.

In a screening of more than 200 chemicals, volatile oils and synthetic flavoring agents as preservatives for syrups, especially as antimolding agents, many compounds were found to be effective at concentrations less than those required with sodium benzoate and benzoic acid.[3] Examples of effective minimum concentrations are the following:

Sodium Benzoate, U.S.P.	1:500
Benzoic Acid, U.S.P.	1:1,000
Methylparaben, U.S.P.	1:1,000
Propylparaben, U.S.P.	1:2,000
Butyl *p*-hydroxybenzoate	1:5,000
Cinnamaldehyde, N.F. IX	1:10,000
8-Hydroxyquinoline Sulfate	1:100,000

Further studies showed a definite potentiating effect with mixtures of *p*-hydroxybenzoic esters, and a concentration of 1:4,500 of a mixture of equal parts of methylparaben and butylparaben was recommended for syrups.[4] For a single substance as the preservative 1:7,500 of *o*-phenylphenol was recommended.[5] These agents can be used only after careful evaluation of their effects on taste and the incompatibilities of the final products.

Syrups usually are stored at room temperature, but some of them do not keep well. At a risk of causing crystallization of sugar, their original quality is maintained for a longer time if they are kept in a refrigerator.

SYRUPS OF *U.S.P. XVI*

Syrup

Simple Syrup; Sirup

Syrup contains 85 per cent w/v of sucrose, corresponding to 64.74 per cent. The specific gravity is 1.313.

Syrup is made by dissolving sucrose in boiling water or, preferably, without heat by percolation with purified water (about 465 ml. total). Cotton is packed loosely in the neck of the percolator to remove mechanical impurities such as lint. The cotton is moistened after packing and before the sucrose is placed in the percolator so that the first, concentrated syrup will pass through satisfactorily. In making small quantities it is always necessary to pass the percolate through the percolator several times before all of the sucrose is dissolved. This process has the advantage of requiring little attention and is well suited to the manufacture of large quantities of syrup. Also, syrup made by this process, without heat, is practically colorless.

A quicker method for making syrup consists of placing the properly weighed sucrose in a graduated bottle, adding purified water and hastening solution by frequent shaking. Finally, the product should be strained through a flat pledget of cotton over the orifice of a large funnel.

A formerly official, so-called *hot process* for making syrup was omitted from U.S.P. XVI. It required heating the syrup to 100° to hasten the solution of the sucrose. There was also the advantage of some degree of sterilization by the heat. Although the use of boiling water is permitted, there are two disadvantages in the use of heat. There is more inversion of the sucrose, reducing the keeping quality of the product by the increased content of monosaccharides which better support the growth of micro-organisms, and the product has a pale amber color due to carmelization.

Syrup is a very simple preparation, but it should be made with care. The official concentration is very important in gaining a self-preserving product with minimum possibilities of crystallization (if too concentrated) and of support for the growth of yeasts, molds and bacteria (if too weak).

Syrup has a nutrient value as a carbohydrate. It is used as a vehicle, a base for other syrups, a sweetening agent and a pill excipient. No usual dose is given; it may be used *ad libitum*.

Cacao Syrup

Cocoa Syrup

The liquid glucose is used to prevent the undissolved cacao powder from settling. The vanillin accentuates and augments the chocolate flavor. Official cacao may contain from 10 to 22 per cent of nonvolatile, ether-soluble extractive which is chiefly cocoa butter, a fat. Breakfast cocoa contains near the upper limit of fat and gives a less satisfactory syrup (which tends to increase in viscosity due to coalescence of the fat) than commercial cocoa, which contains near the lower limit of fat.[6]

Because of the universal popularity of chocolate and because this preparation is efficient in masking tastes, Cacao Syrup is an excellent vehicle. It sometimes has the disadvantage, psychologically, of failing to "taste like medicine." No usual dose is given.

Cherry Syrup

Syrupus Cerasi

Cherry Syrup is made by dissolving sucrose in cherry juice with the aid of the heat of a water bath. The small quantity of alcohol is used as a preservative against fermentation and the growth of surface molds.

Cherry Syrup is a brilliant red syrup with a pleasant taste well suited for use as a vehicle. It has the advantage over wild cherry syrup in being free from tannin, the source of some incompatibilities. It has been recommended especially as a vehicle for iron preparations and bitter and salty drugs. This syrup is acidic, due to the malic acid content of cherries. No usual dose is given.

Chlorpheniramine Maleate Syrup

Chlor-Trimetron Maleate Syrup is the proprietary name for this product. This syrup contains from 6 to 8 per cent of alcohol. The syrup contains 0.5 mg. of the antihistaminic drug per ml. The usual oral dose of chlorpheniramine maleate is 4 mg. up to 4 times a day. A prescription is required for the dispensing of this product.

Chlorpromazine Hydrochloride Syrup

Thorazine Hydrochloride Syrup is the proprietary name for this product. The syrup contains 2 mg. of the tranquilizer per ml. The usual oral dose is 100 mg. daily in divided doses.

Thorazine Syrup is light-sensitive and must be kept and dispensed in amber bottles. It may be sold only on prescription.

Citric Acid Syrup

Citric Acid Syrup also is called Lemon Syrup. However, it should not be confused with the lemon syrup used at the soda fountain, which has a more pronounced flavor. A small quantity of water is used to hasten the solution of the citric acid. This solution is mixed with syrup, the lemon tincture is added, and finally enough syrup is added to make the required volume. This preparation has a faint opalescence caused by the precipitation of the inert terpenes contained in the lemon tincture.

The *U.S.P.* cautions that this syrup should not be used if it has a terebinthinate odor or taste (caused by the oxidation of the terpenes) or shows other signs of deterioration (fermentation).

The official syrup has been criticized for lacking a pronounced flavor, for being cloudy and for susceptibility to fermentation and the growth of molds. Stoklosa[7] recommended a formula using 5 per cent of lemon tincture to be diluted with purified water and filtered clear with the aid of talc before adding citric acid and sucrose. It was recommended that this syrup be stored in a refrigerator.

Citric Acid Syrup is used as a pleasantly flavored vehicle. It has an acidity of pH 3 and has been recommended as a vehicle for ascorbic acid. The oxidation of the vitamin is limited adequately by the acidity to guarantee a shelf-life of 12 months when a 20 per cent excess of ascorbic acid is added at the time of compounding.[8] The weak acidity of Citric Acid Syrup may be sufficient to cause incompatibilities with some medicinal agents such as phenobarbital sodium and sodium salicylate. No usual dose is given.

Diethylcarbamazine Citrate Syrup

Hetrazan Syrup contains 24 mg. of the antifilarial drug per ml. It is effective against Bancroftian filariasis, Malayan filariasis, and loiasis; and useful in infestations by roundworms (ascariasis) but not adult hookworms, whipworms, tapeworms or pinworms. Toxic reaction may be due to worm absorption; inherent toxicity is very low. An antihistamine is helpful when toxicity occurs. The usual dose is 2 mg. per Kg. of body weight 3 times a day for 7 to 21 days. A prescription is required.

Dimenhydrinate Syrup

Dramamine Liquid is the proprietary name for this product. It is more like an elixir in terms of specific gravity and viscosity but not in alcohol content, which is only 5 per cent. The syrup contains about

3.1 mg. per ml. Dramamine is used to prevent motion sickness and nausea and vomiting from other causes, such as pregnancy and anesthesia. The usual oral dose is 50 mg. 4 times a day. A prescription is not required.

GLYCYRRHIZA SYRUP

Licorice Syrup

Glycyrrhiza Syrup is made by simple mixture. A "bouquet" of fennel oil and anise oil is dissolved in the glycyrrhiza fluidextract, to which is added enough syrup to make the required volume. The volatile oils complement the flavor of glycyrrhiza. This syrup is dark brown and not necessarily clear.

Glycyrrhiza Syrup is used as a vehicle. It has been rated as very efficient for masking both salty and bitter tastes. However, this syrup is not pleasing to the tastes of all people. No usual dose is given.

IPECAC SYRUP

Ipecac Syrup is made by mixing ipecac fluidextract and glycerin, then adding enough syrup to make the required volume. The active constituents of this preparation are the alkaloids emetine and cephaëline in the form of their hydrochlorides.

Ipecac Syrup is used as an emetic, especially in pediatric practice, for the relief of spasmodic croup by causing the removal of thickened mucus from the larynx. In smaller doses, it is used as a nauseant expectorant and diaphoretic in the treatment of coughs and colds. In still smaller doses, it is used as a stomachic to stimulate the appetite and digestion. Although emetine and, to a lesser extent, cephaëline have a specific amebicidal action, this preparation does not contain enough of them to be used against infections by ameba. The usual emetic dose is 8 ml., and the expectorant dose is 1 ml.

ORANGE SYRUP

Syrupus Aurantii

Orange Syrup is made by a process resembling the manufacture of an aromatic water with subsequent solution of the sucrose. A clear aqueous solution is made from the sweet orange peel tincture and citric acid, using talc as a distributing agent and filtering aid. The solution must be filtered until clear as it is very difficult to remove any cloudiness after the sucrose has been added. The sucrose is then dissolved in the filtrate by agitation. Heat must be avoided because the flavor of the finished product would be reduced by volatilization of the orange oil. Purified water should be added to maintain the required volume to obtain solution of the sucrose with minimum effort. The sucrose concentration, 82 per cent w/v, is slightly low due to the content of alcohol, 2 to 5 per cent by volume, in which sucrose is not soluble. The citric acid is present to impart a pleasant tart taste.

Sweet orange peel tincture is preferred as the source of the volatile oil of orange rather than the pure orange oil, which is also official, because the latter tends to oxidize, thereby developing a turpentine-like odor which is unpleasant and objectionable.

Orange Syrup should be perfectly clear, having this advantage in appearance over the similar product, citric acid syrup. This syrup should not be used if it has developed a terebinthinate odor or taste, or shows signs of fermentation by cloudiness.

Orange Syrup is used as a pleasantly flavored vehicle. It is slightly acidic. No usual dose is given.

PHENINDAMINE TARTRATE SYRUP

Thephorin Tartrate Syrup contains 2 mg. of the antihistaminic drug per ml. The usual dose is 25 mg. up to 4 times daily. A prescription is required.

PIPERAZINE CITRATE SYRUP

Although there is no patent on piperazine citrate, this syrup is available under trade names as follows: Antepar Syrup, Multifuge, Parazine Liquid, Pipizan Citrate Syrup, Ta-Verm and Vermago. The syrup contains 100 mg. of anhydrous piperazine citrate per ml. This is the lower limit permitted by the official monograph, but a concentration as high as 120 mg. per ml. is allowed. Piperazine citrate is a useful anthelmintic against pinworms and roundworms. It is relatively nontoxic to humans. The usual dose is 50 mg. per Kg. of body weight but not more than 2 Gm. daily. The daily dose is divided into 2 equal portions given morning and night for 14 days or for 7 days followed by a week's rest and a second course for 7 days. A prescription is required for this syrup.

Prochlorperazine Ethanedisulfonate Syrup

Compazine Syrup contains the equivalent of 1 mg. of Compazine base per ml. This drug is a tranquilizer and antiemetic. The usual oral dose is the ethanedisulfonate equivalent to 5 mg. A prescription is required.

Promethazine Hydrochloride Syrup

Phenergan Hydrochloride Syrup contains 1.25 mg. of this antihistaminic per ml. Phenergan is one of the most potent antihistamines. It is used for the control of allergies and for preoperative, operative and postoperative care. In ambulatory use, if drowsiness occurs, the patient should not drive an automobile. There is also a Phenergan Syrup Fortis which contains 5 mg. per ml. The usual oral dose is 25 mg. up to 3 times a day. A prescription is required.

Raspberry Syrup

Syrupus Rubi Idæi

Raspberry Syrup is made by dissolving sucrose in raspberry juice (see p. 193). The heat of a water bath is used to hasten solution. A small amount of alcohol is added as an aid in preventing fermentation and the growth of surface molds.

Raspberry Syrup provides a clear red vehicle with a very pleasant taste. This syrup has an acid reaction due to the citric acid contained in raspberries. No usual dose is given.

Wild Cherry Syrup

Syrupus Pruni Virginianæ

Wild Cherry Syrup is prepared from the dried stem bark of *Prunus serotina* Ehrhart (*Rosaceæ*) by the process of percolation. The extractive from 15 per cent w/v is represented in this syrup.

The percolator is prepared by equipping the lower orifice with a rubber tube and a screw clamp to regulate the flow of percolate. A thin layer of cotton is placed across the shoulder of the percolator, a thin layer of washed sand is placed on the cotton to produce a level surface, and a close-fitting piece of filter paper is placed on the sand to separate the drug and the sand if the drug must be repacked later. The wild cherry, in coarse powder, is moistened with water before introduction into the percolator to allow for the swelling of the drug which might prevent the flow of menstruum if the swelling took place after the drug was packed in the percolator. The moistened wild cherry is packed in the percolator with steady, even strokes. Since the menstruum is aqueous, causing the cells to swell, this drug should not be packed tightly. The drug is covered with a close-fitting filter paper and a layer of sand to prevent unpacking of the drug when the menstruum is added. Water is added as the menstruum. The lower orifice must be open to allow the displaced air to escape, otherwise the air would rise through the drug, causing it to become channeled, thus interfering with the even flow of the menstruum. Once the menstruum has been added, a layer of it must be maintained above the drug to prevent the trapping of air which would cause channeling when more menstruum is added. (See Chap. 8 for detailed treatment and illustrations of percolation.)

When the percolate begins to flow from the lower orifice, it is closed, and the drug is macerated for 1 hour to allow for chemical reaction to take place and for equilibrium to be established in the solution of the active constituents. The percolation is then allowed to proceed rapidly by opening the lower orifice. A rapid rate of flow in this case means the completion of percolation in about 4 hours. Thus, in making a liter of this syrup, the rate of flow should be 1.6 ml., about 25 drops, per minute. The percolate should be collected in a narrow-mouth container large enough to hold the final volume of syrup and graduated to show the required volume of percolate and the final volume of syrup. It should not be necessary to filter the percolate because it is filtered by the cotton. The sucrose is added to the percolate, and dissolved by agitation without the aid of heat because this syrup contains volatile constituents. Finally, the glycerin, the alcohol and sufficient water to make the required volume are added. The glycerin is added to prevent the formation of a sediment from the tannins dissolved by the water. Formerly, glycerin was used in the menstruum, but the increased extraction of tannins produces an undesirable degree of bitterness. The present method for preparing this syrup is also better because the reduced content of tannin causes less precipitation of the alkaloids, such as codeine, which frequently are prescribed in this vehicle.[9,10] The small amount of alcohol is used to aid in preservation against fermentation and the growth of surface molds.

It formerly was stated that wild cherry contains the glycoside amygdalin, but it now appears that wild cherry actually contains the glucoside of *d*-mandelonitrile. The only difference is that amygdalin hydrolyzes to yield 2 molecules of glucose while a molecule of *d*-mandelonitrile glucoside gives 1 molecule of glucose. Wild cherry also contains a thermolabile enzyme, emulsin, which catalyzes the hydrolysis.

$$\underset{\substack{d\text{-mandelo-}\\ \text{nitrile}\\ \text{glucoside}}}{C_{14}H_{17}O_6N} + \underset{\text{water}}{H_2O} \xrightarrow{\text{emulsin}}$$

$$\underset{\text{benzaldehyde}}{C_6H_5CHO} + \underset{\substack{\text{hydro-}\\\text{cyanic}\\\text{acid}}}{HCN} + \underset{\text{glucose}}{C_6H_{12}O_6}$$

Benzaldehyde (synthetic bitter almond oil) contributes to the odor and the flavor of this syrup. The amount of hydrocyanic acid is very small, but it may be sufficient to stimulate respiration slightly.

Wild Cherry Syrup is a pleasantly flavored vehicle with a slight therapeutic value and is popular in remedies for coughs and colds. No usual dose is given.

The formula for a wild cherry syrup free of carbohydrates and glycerin has been developed for diabetics. Sodium alginate, 5 per cent w/v, was used for obtaining a syrupy viscosity, 0.2 per cent w/v of saccharin sodium as a sweetening agent and 0.1 per cent w/v of methylparaben as the preservative.[11]

SYRUPS OF *N.F. XI*

Acacia Syrup

The dry, solid ingredients, powdered or granulated acacia (10% w/v), sodium benzoate and sucrose first are mixed to avoid the lumping that would occur if the acacia were moistened separately. Purified water is added to the mixture, and solution is hastened by heating on a water bath. Gentle stirring also will increase the speed of solution. Vanilla tincture is added to the solution after cooling to impart a pleasant flavor. Sodium benzoate, 0.1 per cent w/v, is used as a preservative against fermentation, but this syrup does not keep well at room temperature.

Acacia Syrup is used as a vehicle when a demulcent action is desired in the throat. It also is used as a vehicle for insoluble powders when the suspending action of acacia is advantageous. No usual dose is given.

Bromides Syrup

Bromides Syrup represents a solution of 5 bromides: sodium, potassium, ammonium, calcium and lithium. These are dissolved in purified water with the aid of heat. The sucrose is then dissolved in the hot solution. After the primary solution is cool, vanilla tincture is added for flavor in addition to that imparted by the compound sarsaparilla syrup. Compound amaranth solution is used to darken the brown color of the preparation.

Bromides Syrup is a popular, agreeable form for administering the bromide ion for its sedative action. A full therapeutic amount (about 1.25 Gm.) of bromides is represented in the usual dose, 5 ml.

The Federal Food and Drug Administration requires the following statement on the label of preparations containing bromides when sold at retail without a prescription: "*Caution:* Not to be given to children. Do not take more than the dose recommended. If rash or daytime drowsiness or any unusual symptoms occur, discontinue use at once. Not to be taken by those suffering from kidney disease. Frequent or continuous use may be dangerous."

DEXTROMETHORPHAN HYDROBROMIDE SYRUP

Romilar Hydrobromide Syrup is a proprietary form of this syrup. There are many other syrups, tablets, capsules, and a lozenge with this ingredient along with other active ingredients.

Dextromethorphan Hydrobromide Syrup contains 15 mg. in 5 ml. Dextromethorphan is a synthetic morphine derivative which has the same relationship to racemorphan that codeine has to morphine. Both levomethorphan, an optically active isomer, and racemethorphan, the racemic mixture, are Class A narcotics as based upon the 1954 amendment to the Harrison Narcotics Act. Dextromethorphan is not a narcotic drug.

Dextromethorphan is used exclusively as an antitussive drug to control the cough reflex. Its action is equal on a weight-to-weight basis to that of codeine. Dextromethorphan produces a little or no central depression and no analgesia. It appears to have no addicting effect even after prolonged use of large doses.

The usual dose is 10 to 20 mg., given 1 to 4 times a day. This preparation can be sold without a prescription.

DIHYDROCODEINONE BITARTRATE SYRUP

Dicodid Bitartrate and Hycodan are proprietary names for dihydrocodeinone bitartrate.

This syrup is made very simply by first dissolving the bitartrate in a small amount of purified water with the aid of gentle heat and adding a sufficient amount of cherry syrup to make the required volume.

It should be noted that the official syrup contains 10 mg. of the narcotic in each 4 ml. while a proprietary syrup contains only 4 mg. in 4 ml.

This syrup is a taxable narcotic and can be dispensed only on properly written original prescriptions because it contains no other active ingredient.

Hycodan Syrup contains 5 mg. of dihydrocodeinone bitartrate and 1.5 mg. of homatropine methylbromide (Mesopin) in 5 ml. It is a Class B narcotic for which prescriptions may be accepted by telephone because it does not contain more than $1\frac{1}{3}$ grains of the narcotic per fluid ounce and does contain a non-narcotic drug in full therapeutic dose. There are many additional proprietary antitussive syrups containing lesser amounts of dihydrocodeinone bitartrate and other therapeutic ingredients. These are Class X narcotics, exempt preparations, if the amount of dihydrocodeinone bitartrate does not exceed $\frac{1}{6}$ grain per fluid ounce.

Dihydrocodeinone is a narcotic having analgesic and sedative actions similar to codeine but, weight for weight, is more active and more addicting. In doses smaller than the official usual dose of 10 mg., it is used for its antitussive action by depressing the cough reflex. Dihydrocodeinone Bitartrate Syrup contains 2.5 mg. per ml. The usual dose of the drug is 10 mg.

EPHEDRINE SULFATE SYRUP

Ephedrine Sulfate Syrup contains 0.4 per cent w/v of ephedrine sulfate dissolved in a synthetic vehicle flavored with lemon oil, orange oil, benzaldehyde and vanillin. It is given a tart taste with citric acid and is colored with amaranth solution and caramel. A small amount of alcohol is included as a preservative against fermentation and the growth of surface molds.

This syrup formerly was prepared with cherry syrup as the vehicle, but the limited seasonal supply of the fresh fruit caused the adoption of this suitable substitute.

The usual dose of Ephedrine Sulfate Syrup contains 20 mg. of ephedrine sulfate. It is used to prevent or relieve the symptoms of asthma or to prevent narcolepsy. The usual dose is 5 ml.

AROMATIC ERIODICTYON SYRUP

Aromatic Yerba Santa Syrup, Syrupus Corrigens

Eriodictyon fluidextract contains a resin which is made water-soluble by the alkalis, potassium hydroxide solution and magnesium carbonate. The magnesium carbonate also serves as a distributing agent and filtering aid. The compound cardamom tincture, sassafras oil, lemon oil and clove oil are used for their flavor.

Aromatic Eriodictyon Syrup is used as a vehicle, especially for masking bitter tastes, such as those of quinine and strychnine. The eriodictyon resin is supposed to paralyze the taste buds and to adsorb the alkaloids. The alkalinity of the syrup is helpful in reducing the tastes of alkaloid salts. This syrup has a mild expectorant action. The usual dose is 8 ml.

Ferrous Iodide Syrup

Ferrous Iodide Syrup contains 6.5 to 7.5 per cent w/v of FeI_2, corresponding to approximately 5 per cent. The ferrous iodide is prepared by the direct combination of iron, in the form of bright wire, and iodine. Official iron is often obtained in the form of "card teeth." To prevent rusting, the iron usually is covered with a thin layer of oil, which must be removed by rinsing with petroleum benzin to obtain a rapid reaction. If official iron is not available, reduced iron can be used satisfactorily and has the advantage of giving a more rapid reaction. The rate of reaction may be controlled by warming to speed it and cooling to retard it. Completion of the reaction is shown by the absence of the odor or the brown color of iodine.

$$Fe + I_2 \rightarrow FeI_2$$

The solution is heated to boiling to complete the reaction and to drive off dissolved oxygen. Part of the sucrose is added before filtering to aid in preventing the oxidation of the ferrous iodide. Either hypophosphorous acid or citric acid may be added as a preservative against oxidation. Either one is effective for this purpose, but citric acid is preferable because it does not cause caramelization. This syrup becomes brown in a few months when preserved with hypophosphorous acid. Ferrous Iodide Syrup should be kept in well-filled, colorless glass containers exposed to light. Light has a reducing action. This syrup is one of the heaviest syrups, having a specific gravity of 1.37.

A ferrous iodide syrup which will retain its original color for a longer time can be made by replacing the sucrose in the official formula with 600 Gm. of dextrose, 0.8 Gm. of sodium benzoate and 0.8 Gm. of saccharin sodium.[12]

Ferrous Iodide Syrup has a pronounced ferruginous taste. It is used for both ions, the ferrous ion being hematinic and the iodide ion tonic, but chiefly for the latter. It should be taken in water through a drinking tube to avoid staining of the teeth. The usual dose is 1 ml.

Ferrous Sulfate Syrup

Ferrous Sulfate Syrup contains 4 per cent w/v of $FeSO_4 \cdot 7H_2O$. This preparation is made by a method which roughly parallels that for ferrous iodide syrup. The method is simpler because ferrous sulfate is sufficiently stable to be an article of commerce. The first portion of sucrose is included in the preliminary solution of ferrous sulfate (green vitriol) to protect the ferrous ion from atmospheric oxidation. If all of the sucrose were added, the solution would be too viscous to allow perfect filtration. The citric acid prevents discoloration by the ferric ion which might be produced by atmospheric oxidation. The peppermint spirit gives a persisting flavor which greatly masks the somewhat unpleasant ferruginous taste of the ferrous ion.

Ferrous Sulfate Syrup simulates proprietary products which have found extensive use in pediatric practice for the treatment of anemia caused by the dietary deficiency of iron. The usual dose of 10 ml. contains about 400 mg. of Fe. (Ferrous iodide syrup, used primarily for its iodide content, contains in a usual dose 12.6 mg. of Fe.) The usual dose is 10 ml.

Hydriodic Acid Syrup

Hydriodic Acid Syrup contains 1.3 to 1.5 per cent w/v of HI. It is made by dissolving the sucrose in a mixture of diluted hydriodic acid, containing 10 per cent w/v of HI, and purified water.

This syrup is subject to 2 kinds of deterioration, both producing a color change from colorless to brown. One change is due to atmospheric oxidation of iodide ion to free iodine. This deterioration is prevented by the hypophosphorous acid contained in the diluted hydriodic acid, because hypophosphorous acid is oxidized more easily than iodide ion. The second is due to caramelization, which takes place after the sucrose has been inverted. The latter source of discoloration is greatly minimized by reducing the sucrose concentration, accounting for the unusually low concentration, 45 per cent w/v, in this syrup. The acidity of the syrup prevents the growth of organisms. An unofficial hydriodic acid syrup which will remain colorless for a longer period of time can be made by substituting 600 Gm. of dextrose for the sucrose called for in the official formula.[13]

Hydriodic Acid Syrup is used for the tonic effect of iodide ion. It should be taken well diluted with water through a drinking tube to protect the teeth. The acidity is sufficient to cause softening of the dentin. This preparation is categorized as an expectorant. The usual dose is 5 ml.

Compound Sarsaparilla Syrup

Compound Sarsaparilla Syrup is made by simple admixture. The aromatic flavoring substances, sassafras oil, anise oil and methyl salicylate (synthetic wintergreen oil) are dissolved in a small quantity of alcohol. This solution is added to the mixture of the sarsaparilla fluidextract and the glycyrrhiza fluidextract. Finally, this mixture is added to the syrup.

Compound Sarsaparilla Syrup is a dark-brown, slightly cloudy liquid with a taste closely resembling that of root beer. On the basis of the theory of precipitation when mixing liquids, it would be more logical to add the syrup to the alcoholic mixture of the fluidextracts and the volatile oils. The alcohol seems to be unnecessary in this preparation, as the fluidextracts might be used to dissolve the volatile oils.

Sarsaparilla contains saponins which aid in the absorption of medicinal substances from the digestive tract. Compound Sarsaparilla Syrup is used as a vehicle. No usual dose is given.

Senna Syrup

Senna Syrup is prepared by dissolving the coriander oil in the senna fluidextract. Purified water is added, and the mixture is allowed to stand for 24 hours with occasional agitation to allow for the solution of the active constituents and precipitation of inert extractive from the fluidextract. The solution is then filtered clear, and the sucrose is dissolved by agitation. Enough distilled water is added to make the required volume. The coriander oil imparts a pleasant flavor, masking the taste of senna. The stimulating action of the coriander oil in the intestine reduces the griping action of the senna. The sucrose concentration is low, due to the presence of 5 to 7 per cent by volume of alcohol. The active constituent is emodin, including emodin glycosides.

Senna Syrup is used as a laxative, especially for children. The usual dose is 8 ml.

Tolu Balsam Syrup

Syrup of Tolu

Tolu Balsam Syrup is prepared by a method in which an aromatic water is made with the aid of a distributing agent, and the sucrose is dissolved in the clear filtrate. Magnesium carbonate is used as the distributing agent for the tolu balsam tincture because its alkalinity aids in dissolving the resinous constituents of tolu balsam. A small part of the sucrose is added, also to aid in the solution of the resins. The aqueous solution must be filtered until perfectly clear because it is very difficult to remove a slight cloudiness after all of the sucrose has been added. The remainder of the sucrose may be dissolved in the filtrate either by agitation with the aid of gentle heat, not over 50°, or by percolation. The sucrose concentration, 82 per cent w/v, is slightly lower than usual due to the 2 to 4 per cent by volume of alcohol introduced in the tincture.

On aging, Tolu Balsam Syrup may develop an unpleasant odor resembling that of coal gas or benzene. This is caused by the growth of molds which reduce cinnamic acid to cinnamene.

Tolu Balsam Syrup is used as a vehicle and is especially popular in remedies for coughs and colds. Its slightly alkaline reaction may cause incompatibilities. No usual dose is given.

The British Pharmaceutical Codex, 1959, gives a formula for Solution of Tolu (*Liquor Tolutanus*): 50 Gm. of tolu balsam is dissolved in 300 ml. of 90 per cent alcohol. To this is added purified talc and 350 ml. of water heated to 70°. The mixture is agitated vigorously, set aside for 24 hours, and then filtered. With the aid of gentle heat, 500 Gm. of sucrose is dissolved in the filtrate, and sufficient purified water is added to make 1,000 ml. One volume of this solution, when mixed with 7 volumes of syrup, yields a tolu syrup with good aromatic qualities. The tolu solution keeps better than the tolu syrup and thus provides a convenient method for the extemporaneous preparation of the syrup. This formula is interesting as revealing the nature of the soluble tolu extracts which are available commercially for making unofficial tolu syrups.

Compound White Pine Syrup

Compound White Pine Syrup is prepared by the percolation of a mixture of 6 botanic drugs: white pine, wild cherry, aralia, poplar bud, sanguinaria and sassafras. (For details of the percolation process, see wild cherry syrup, pp. 187-188.)

Amaranth solution is added to darken the color of the preparation. A small amount of chloroform is included both to act as a preservative against the growth of organisms and to give its sedative effect locally in the throat. This syrup contains from 10 to 12 per cent of alcohol to aid in the extraction of the active constituents which are resinous for the most part.

Compound White Pine Syrup is a very popular, pleasant-tasting preparation used in the treatment of coughs and is classified as antitussive. It also is used as a vehicle for the same purpose. The usual dose is 5 ml.

Compound White Pine Syrup with Codeine

Compound White Pine Syrup with Codeine is an exempt narcotic preparation because it contains a little less than 1 gr. of codeine phosphate to the fluidounce. Codeine phosphate is a good selection of the salt to be used in this preparation because it is more soluble than the sulfate. The small amount of purified water is used to hasten the solution.

Compound White Pine Syrup with Codeine is an efficient antitussive preparation to control the cough reflex and to relieve the unpleasant symptoms of coughs and colds. The usual dose is 5 ml.

Diabetic Syrups

Persons suffering from the disease diabetes mellitus must regulate their caloric intake accurately, and syrups are troublesome to them either as something to be avoided (even though medicinal) or another item to be included in their calculations. For this reason, pharmaceutical preparations have been developed which contain no (or very little) carbohydrates.

In the case of syrups, the sweetness is obtained by the use of saccharin sodium which is rated 300 to 550 times as sweet as sucrose, or cyclamate sodium (Sucaryl Sodium) which is 30 to 40 times as sweet as sucrose, and the characteristic viscosity is obtained by the use of such thickening agents as acacia, tragacanth, sterculia gum, sodium alginate and methylcellulose. Such preparations must contain preservatives against the growth of micro-organisms.

Woo and Huyck[14] developed and tested formulas for nonnutritive "syrups" of which the following was recommended:

Tragacanth, powdered	1.5
Glycerin	6.0
Saccharin sodium	0.1
Methylparaben	0.1
Distilled water, to make	100.0

General

Syrups as vehicles for proprietary drugs such as antibiotics, antihistaminics, antitussives and vitamins have received increased use. There is a tendency to depart from the standard flavors of orange, lemon and peppermint to adopt more interesting flavors such as lime, pineapple, root beer and distinctive mixtures. Research has shown the feasibility for preparing syrups of pleasing taste from fresh fruits[15] such as grapes, peaches, etc., and from compounded imitation flavor concentrates[16] such as cream soda, grape, maple, raspberry and wild cherry.

Sorbitol, $C_6H_{14}O_6$, is a polyhydric alcohol made by the hydrogenation of glucose. Although this compound is not chemically a sugar or carbohydrate it has similar physical and physiologic characteristics, such as being a colorless crystal, very soluble in water, sweet to the taste, and metabolized (50% in dogs). Its use is most economical in the form of the 70 per cent solution which is official in *U.S.P. XVI* as a pharmaceutic necessity: vehicle; humectant; sweetener. A trade name for the solution is Sorbo. Sorbitol solution is used in a number of commercial preparations which are like syrups in taste, viscosity, and appearance. The advantages include taste improvement, reduced sweetness, less crystallization and locking of screwcaps, and improved stability for some active ingredients.

JUICES

A juice is the liquid obtained by expression from the fresh part of a plant. The *U.S.P.* contains 2 monographs for juices, both made from fresh fruits, and the *N.F.* contains none. Some of the foreign official compendiums contain juices made from fresh leaves, succulent bulbs, etc. The *British Pharmaceutical Codex, 1949*, contained monographs for the juices of garlic, lemon and taraxacum.

JUICES OF *U.S.P. XVI*

Cherry Juice

Succus Cerasi

Cherry Juice is the liquid expressed from the fresh ripe fruit of the sour red cherry, *Prunus Cerasus* Linné *(Rosaceæ)*. It contains not less than 1.0 per cent of malic acid.

The cherries are stemmed but not pitted, washed with water, passed through a grinder to crush the kernels, and 0.1 per cent of benzoic acid added to prevent fermentation. The kernels are crushed to add to the flavor of the juice. The mixture is allowed to stand at room temperature for several days to allow for the removal of pectin, a water-soluble product naturally present in fresh cherry juice. Upon standing, the pectin is hydrolyzed to pectic acid, which is insoluble in water. The hydrolysis is catalyzed by the enzyme, pectase. (A small amount of methyl alcohol also results from the hydrolysis of pectin.) The absence of pectin is shown when a filtered portion of the juice gives a clear solution when mixed with one half its volume of alcohol. This solution should not become cloudy within 30 minutes if pectins are absent. The juice is then expressed and filtered. If the pectin is not removed from cherry juice, a syrup made from it is likely to gel.

Since fresh cherries are available during only a short season of the year, Cherry Juice has been made official as the ingredient for making cherry syrup.

Raspberry Juice

Succus Rubi Idæi

Raspberry Juice is the liquid expressed from the fresh ripe red raspberry, varieties of *Rubus idæus* Linné or of *R. strigosus* Michaux *(Rosaceæ)*. It contains not less than 1.5 per cent of citric acid.

The process of preparation is similar to that used for cherry juice (see above).

Since raspberries are available during only a short season each year, Raspberry Juice has been made official as the source for raspberry syrup.

BIBLIOGRAPHY

Boothe, E., and Kaufman, K. L.: Masking bitter drugs, J. Am. Pharm. A. (Pract. Ed.) **8**:68, 1947.

Fantus, Bernard: Advances in therapeutic technique, J.A.M.A. **105**:879, 1935.

Moncrieff, R. W.: Chemical Senses, ed. 2. London, Hill, 1951.

Purdum, W. A.: Method of evaluating relative efficacy of disguising agents for distasteful drugs, J. Am. Pharm. A. (Sci. Ed.) **31**:298, 1942.

———: A comparison of two methods for evaluating the relative efficacy of disguising agents for distasteful drugs, J. Am. Pharm. A. (Sci. Ed.) **32**:103, 1943.

Wright, H. N.: The comparative efficiency of the commonly used flavoring agents, J.A.M.A. **108**:959, 1937.

REFERENCES

1. **Gabel, L. F.:** The relative action of preservatives in pharmaceutical preparations, J. Am. Pharm. A. **10:**767, 1921.
2. **Grote, I. W., and Walker, Peggy:** Studies in the preservation of liquid pharmaceutical preparations: I. The relationship between the preservative action of alcohol and the solid content of the preparation, J. Am. Pharm. A. (Sci. Ed.) **35:**182, 1946.
3. **Lord, C. F., Jr., and Husa, W. J.:** Antimolding agents for syrups, J. Am. Pharm. A. (Sci. Ed.) **43:**438, 1954.
4. **Littlejohn, O. M., and Husa, W. J.:** The potentizing effect of antimolding agents in syrups, J. Am. Pharm. A. (Sci. Ed.) **44:**305, 1955.
5. **Schimmel, J., and Husa, W. J.:** The effect of various preservatives on microorganisms isolated from deteriorated syrups, J. Am. Pharm. A. (Sci. Ed.) **45:**204, 1956.
6. **Nariar, G., Ohmart, L. M., and Stoklosa, M. J.:** An improved cacao syrup, J. Am. Pharm. A. (Pract. Ed.) **15:**97, 1954.
7. **Stoklosa, J. M.:** Lemon syrup: an improved vehicle, J. Am. Pharm. A. (Pract. Ed.) **9:**556, 1948.
8. **Bandelin, F. J., and Tuschhoff, J. V.:** Ascorbic acid syrup, J. Am. Pharm. A. (Pract. Ed.) **15:**761, 1954.
9. **Reed, C. C., Burrin, P. L., and Bibbins, F. E.:** Syrup of wild cherry in prescriptions, J. Am. Pharm. A. (Pract. Ed.) **1:**73, 1940.
10. **Rasanen, P. R., and Burt, J. B.:** Syrup of wild cherry, Am. J. Pharm. **115:**292, 1943.
11. **Swafford, W. B., and Nobles, W. L.:** Modifications in the formula of wild cherry syrup, J. Am. Pharm. A. (Pract. Ed.) **15:**99, 1954.
12. **Husa, W. J., and Pedrero, E., Jr.:** The stabilization of ferrous iodide syrup, N.F. VIII, J. Am. Pharm. A. (Sci. Ed.) **39:**67, 1950.
13. **Ewing, C. O., and Graves, D. B.:** Stabilizing hydriodic acid syrup, U.S.P., Drug Standards **19:**102, 1951.
14. **Woo, M., and Huyck, C. L.:** Diabetic syrups, Bull. National Formulary Committee **16:**140, 1948.
15. **Drommond, F. G., and DeKay, H. G.:** Fresh fruit syrups and elixers as vehicles. J. Am. Pharm. A. (Pract. Ed.) **15:**232, 1954.
16. **Lankford, B. L., and Becker, C. H.:** The use of some imitation flavors for masking distasteful drugs: I. Ammonium chloride, II. Quinine hydrochloride, J. Am. Pharm. A. (Sci. Ed.) **40:**77, 1951.

MITCHELL JOHN STOKLOSA, A.M.

Professor of Pharmacy, Massachusetts College of Pharmacy

11
Solutions

HISTORY
GENERAL CONSIDERATIONS
SOLUTIONS PREPARED BY SIMPLE SOLUTION
SOLUTIONS PREPARED BY CHEMICAL REACTION
SOLUTIONS PREPARED BY SIMPLE SOLUTION WITH STERILIZATION
ANTICOAGULANT AND PHYSIOLOGIC SOLUTIONS
OPHTHALMIC SOLUTIONS
OPHTHALMIC SOLUTIONS PREPARED FROM STERILE OPHTHALMIC POWDERS
SOLUTIONS PREPARED BY EXTRACTION
UNOFFICIAL SOLUTIONS

SOLUTIONS (LIQUORES)

HISTORY

The word "liquor" was introduced into the language of the chemist in the 17th century and originally meant anything liquid. Thus, Glauber in 1648 gave the name *liquor silicum* to a compound of silica and tartar manufactured by Van Helmont in 1640. In like manner, the iron "liquor," the red and yellow "liquor" of the calico printers, the ammoniacal "liquor" of the gas works and the "liquor" of the tanneries—all are reminiscent of special uses in those arts in which chemical processes play an important part. There is no doubt that the pharmaceutical terms *liquor ammoniæ*, *liquor potassæ*, etc., originated from such usages as those mentioned above.

One of the earliest, if not the earliest, explanations of "liquor" as a generic pharmaceutical term was given by J. A. Buchner in 1822 in his *Einleitung in die Pharmacie* (p. 277) as follows: "Under this name are comprehended a variety of liquids, some of which are obtained by solution, others by mixture, still others by distillation. In common they have their transparency and relative stability, hence they can be kept in stock." Eight years later, in 1830, P. L. Geiger, in the second edition of his *Handbuch der Pharmacie* (p. 149) stated that "at present one comprises within this term [liquor] mostly aqueous solutions of salts and other mostly colorless aqueous compounds." The first edition of the *U.S.P.* included 7 preparations titled liquors. The *U.S.P.* of 1860 created the class "liquores" in which 21 preparations were classified under such a heading. This arrangement was maintained so long as Latin titles were retained by the *U.S.P.*

GENERAL CONSIDERATIONS

DEFINITION

A solution may be defined as a 1-phase system of 2 or more chemical components. For example, the addition of alcohol to water produces a single-phase system that is composed of 2 different chemical substances which are so intimately mixed with each other that a physically homogeneous system results. Although such a system may be solid, liquid or gaseous in nature, the pharmacist deals most frequently with solutions in which the solvent is a liquid.

The term "liquor," or "solution," as used by recent revisions of the *U.S.P.* and the *N.F.* has a more limited meaning than the general definition stated above. All official solutions are liquid preparations involving liquid solvents. Although many of the liquid galenicals could be classified as solutions if the broad definition were to be used, the official compendia do not recognize them in this category. Certain groups of galenicals form distinctive or traditional classes of their own, such as syrups, elixirs, tinctures and others.

The solvent most commonly used in preparing the official solutions is water. Other liquids, such as alcohol and glycerin, are specified in some of the monographs. The solutes vary widely as to their nature and include solids, liquids and gases. Consequently, the nature of this group of preparations is too diverse to permit an accurate definition of the class. However, the following one embraces all of the solutions of the official compendia: Solutions are liquid preparations which contain one or more solutes dissolved in a liquid solvent and do not by reason of their components or their method of manufacture fall into some other group of official products. This is a much broader definition than the older one, allowed by revisions of the *U.S.P.* of the early 20th century, in which the term "liquor" was limited, with few exceptions, to aqueous solutions of nonvolatile substances.

Uses

The official solutions are used for many and varied purposes. Some are intended to be administered per se for the medicinal action, internally or externally, of the ingredients which they contain; others are used as ingredients in the compounding of prescriptions or in the formulation of other official preparations; and still others serve as reagents in various processes, as solvents for certain substances, and as coloring agents for pharmaceutical products.

Preparation and Classification

The methods by which the official solutions are prepared are no less varied than the uses for which they are intended. Because the concentration of solutions varies widely, from one tenth of 1 per cent to 100 per cent on a weight-to-volume basis, and because nearly every solution is prepared by a special method, there is no general formula for the class, and no type processes can be given for the manufacture of the group as a whole. However, for the purpose of study, the following classification based on the type of procedure involved in the preparation of solutions seems to be practicable:

1. Solutions prepared by simple solution
2. Solutions prepared by chemical reaction
3. Solutions prepared by simple solution with sterilization
   A. Anticoagulant and physiologic solutions
   B. Ophthalmic solutions
   C. Ophthalmic solutions prepared from sterile ophthalmic powders
4. Solutions prepared by extraction

It is not intended to imply in the division given above that there is any fundamental difference in character between a simple solution and a chemical solution. Identical solutions of calcium hydroxide can be prepared by dissolving calcium hydroxide [$Ca(OH)_2$] in water or by slaking lime (CaO) with an excess of water in which it dissolves after first reacting to form calcium hydroxide. On the other hand, a solution made by chemical reaction is often more complex than a corresponding simple solution because it contains all the products of the reactions that have taken place during the method of preparation. For example, a solution of ammonium acetate could be prepared by simply dissolving the salt in water, but it would not be a satisfactory substitute for the carbonated solution which was formerly official and was prepared by the reaction of acetic acid with ammonium carbonate.

The official compendia direct the preparation of certain solutions by methods involving chemical reactions for 4 principal reasons:

1. The desired therapeutic substance may not be obtainable or readily usable in a form other than that of a solution (formaldehyde solution, hydrogen peroxide solution and others).

2. The pure substance may be susceptible to chemical changes or decomposition when in the solid state (ferric chloride solution, lead subacetate solution and others).

3. The pure solute may not dissolve readily from the solid state (ferric subsulfate solution, lead subacetate solution, aluminum subacetate solution and others).

4. The several products resulting from the chemical reaction may be desirable constituents of the preparation (magnesium citrate solution).

Some of the official solutions are prepared in sterile form for special uses. These include ophthalmic solutions, anticoagulant solutions for mixing with blood, and physiologic solutions that are intended to be used per se or as vehicles for other medicaments for application to delicate mucous membranes. Sterile solutions intended for parenteral administration are now classified as Injections regardless of the dosage used; previously, solutions used in large volume for the replacement of blood or fluid were classified as Sterile Solutions.

Ophthalmic solutions are required by the U.S.P. and the N.F. to be sterile and, if packaged in multiple-dose containers, to contain a suitable substance or mixture of substances to prevent the growth of, or to destroy, micro-organisms accidentally introduced when the containers are opened in use. These requirements are consistent with a ruling from the Food and Drug Administration concerning liquid preparations for ophthalmic use.

Autoclaving in the final container is the preferred method of sterilizing ophthalmic solutions. However, since no specific procedure is directed in any instance (see monograph on Ophthalmic Solutions in both the U.S.P. and the N.F.), the methods of attaining sterility are determined by the character of a particular product. Sterilization methods and procedures are discussed in detail under Preparation of Injections, Chapter 12, pages 234-241.

Several preservatives have been suggested for use in ophthalmic solutions. These include: (1) phenylethyl alcohol in a concentration of 0.5 per cent; (2) chlorobutanol in a concentration of 0.5 per cent; (3) benzalkonium chloride in a concentration of 0.01 per cent (1 in 10,000); and (4) phenylmercuric nitrate in 0.001 per cent concentration (1 in 100,000). However, any preservative which is harmless yet effective in the concentration employed is acceptable. Ophthalmic solutions that are intended for surgical use must be sterile and must not contain any preservative. Such solutions should be packaged in single-use disposable containers.

In the extemporaneous compounding of ophthalmic solutions, it is recommended that aseptic conditions be maintained throughout if contamination is to be avoided. All intermediate containers used in their preparation and the final container should be sterilized. If the dispensing container is a dropper-bottle unit, the accompanying dropper top may be stapled into a stiff paper envelope and autoclaved separately. The solvents used should be sterile distilled water or water for injection. Careful consideration should be given to the use of buffering agents which are used to produce definite pH levels, and tonicic agents which are often added to make solutions isotonic.

The U.S.P. recognizes 2 ophthalmic powders, Chloramphenicol and Tetracycline Hydrochloride, and the N.F. includes Ophthalmic Chlortetracycline Hydrochloride and Ophthalmic Oxytetracycline Hydrochloride, which are intended for preparing solutions for use in the eye. Each of these preparations is official as a sterile, dry mixture with suitable buffers, preservatives and diluents. Prior to dispensing, sterile distilled water is added to the dry powder to make a solution of the desired concentration.

Two official solutions, Epinephrine Solution and Liver Solution, are prepared by extraction of the active principles from suitable animal tissues.

In the discussion to follow, no attempt will be made to repeat in detail the U.S.P. and the N.F. directions for the preparation of the official solutions. Rather, the discussion will be limited to: (1) brief comments concerning special technics and the reasons therefor; (2) a consideration of chemical reactions; (3) a presentation of significant information concerning packaging, storage and dispensing of certain solutions; (4) commercial counterparts, if available; and (5) comments on the uses of individual members of the class.

SOLUTIONS PREPARED BY SIMPLE SOLUTION

Amaranth Solution, U.S.P.
Liquor Amaranthi

Amaranth Solution is a solution of amaranth in purified water. It contains, in each 100 ml., not less than 0.9 Gm. and not more than 1.1 Gm. of the dye. Amaranth, also known as FD&C Red No. 2, is a comparatively nontoxic dye which is certified for coloring foods, drugs and cosmetics.

Uses. The official solution, described as a clear, vivid red liquid, is categorized as a coloring agent and was recommended by the Committee of the National Formulary as a substitute for cudbear tincture. In concentrations of approximately 1:1,000, amaranth imparts a pleasing red color to clear liquid preparations. Its color stability is fairly good in either acid or alkaline solutions.

Compound Amaranth Solution, N.F.

Compound Amaranth Solution is a hydroalcoholic solution of amaranth and caramel. It is prepared by adding amaranth solution to a dilution of caramel and water, and diluting with alcohol and purified water to the designated volume.

Uses. It is used as a coloring agent in certain official preparations to replace compound cudbear tincture. It imparts a reddish-brown color to liquid galenicals.

Diluted Ammonia Solution, U.S.P.
Ammonia Water; Diluted Ammonium Hydroxide Solution; Liquor Ammoniæ Dilutus

Diluted Ammonia Solution is a solution of ammonia containing, in each 100 ml., not less than 9 Gm. and not more than 10 Gm. of NH_3. It is prepared by diluting 398 ml. of strong ammonia solution to 1,000 ml. with purified water.

Upon exposure to air it loses ammonia rapidly; hence, it should be stored in tight containers, preferably at a temperature not above 30°. Cork stoppers should not be used, because the ammonia water invariably dissolves coloring matter from the cork and becomes discolored.

Uses. Because of the ammonium ion which it contains, this solution possesses stimulant properties. Actually, it is too irritating for either internal or external use without dilution. Its rubefacient properties make it useful as an ingredient in the formulation of stimulating liniments, especially when it is combined with certain vegetable oils. It is used as an ingredient in Aromatic Ammonia Spirit in which it serves as a reagent and stimulant. It is a good solvent for carmine, the resulting solution having a deep-red color. The vapors of the solution may be inhaled cautiously for their stimulating effect in sudden syncope of nervous origin.

Strong Ammonia Solution, U.S.P.
Stronger Ammonia Water; Stronger Ammonium Hydroxide Solution; Liquor Ammoniæ Fortis

Strong Ammonia Solution is an aqueous solution of ammonia containing not less than 27 per cent and not more than 30 per cent, by weight, of NH_3.

It is prepared by dissolving ammonia gas in water until the desired concentration has been reached. No official method is given for its manufacture, since it is not adapted to small-scale production and is available in unlimited quantities from the chemical industry. The ammonia gas is obtained from coke-oven gas, coal gas and oil gas, and from the fixation of nitrogen from the air.

The solution is a complex preparation containing not only dissolved ammonia but also hydrates of ammonia, ammonium hydroxide and ammonium (NH_4+) and hydroxyl ($OH-$) ions. It deteriorates rapidly when exposed to the air. Therefore, it should be stored in tight containers, preferably at a temperature not exceeding 25°.

The following caution is given by the *U.S.P.* for this solution: *"Use care in handling Strong Ammonia Solution because of the caustic nature of the solution and the irritating properties of its vapor. Cool the container well before opening, and cover* the closure with a cloth or similar material while opening. Do not taste Strong Ammonia Solution, and avoid inhalation of its vapor."

Uses. Strong Ammonia Solution is too potent for medicinal use in the undiluted state. It is a powerful reagent and solvent and is used in many technical processes. Vapors from the solution are capable of producing severe irritation of the respiratory tract. Perhaps the most important pharmaceutical use of the solution is in the preparation of the diluted solution.

N.F. Antiseptic Solution

N.F. Antiseptic Solution is a hydro-alcoholic solution containing boric acid, thymol, chlorothymol, menthol, eucalyptol, methyl salicylate and thyme oil.

Since this solution contains both water-soluble and alcohol-soluble ingredients, the *N.F.* directs that the boric acid be dissolved in purified water and the other ingredients in the alcohol. The two solutions are mixed, allowed to stand for 2 hours or more to ensure complete saturation and then are filtered to remove the excess of volatile principles. Purified talc may be used, if necessary, to clarify the product. The *N.F.* directs that the solution be cooled to 10° and maintained at this temperature during filtration. This is done so that the solution will not become cloudy when it is stored in a cool place.

NOTE: Specially denatured alcohol Formula No. 38-B, containing 6 lbs. of boric acid and 1⅓ lbs. each of thymol, chlorothymol and menthol added to 100 gallons of ethyl alcohol, has been approved for use in this preparation, provided that adjustment is made for the quantities of the formula ingredients present in the denatured alcohol.

Attention is called to the antibacterial test which requires that the solution (undiluted) kill *Staphylococcus aureus* in 5 minutes under the conditions of the test.

This solution is popularly used as a mouthwash. When employed for this purpose, the wash should be used undiluted. It is interesting to note that, according to authoritative medical and dental opinions, the solution does not function as a germicide when used as a mouthwash. However, it is a pleasant and refreshing deodorant wash.

Alkaline Aromatic Solution, N.F.
Liquor Aromaticus Alkalinus

Alkaline Aromatic Solution is a hydro-alcoholic solution containing thymol, eucalyptol, glycerin and methyl salicylate, alkalinized by sodium borate and potassium bicarbonate, and colored by amaranth solution. The procedure for its manufacture is essentially the same as that used in preparing N.F. Antiseptic Solution, except that the mixed ingredients are allowed to stand for 24 hours at room temperature and then filtered without chilling.

It should be noted that a chemical reaction occurs in the manufacture of this solution; however, the preparation is discussed here because it is so closely related to N.F. Antiseptic Solution. The chemical reaction which occurs between glycerin, sodium borate and potassium bicarbonate is essentially the same as the one that takes place in the manufacture of Compound Sodium Borate Solution, which is discussed on pages 214-215.

Uses. The uses of Alkaline Aromatic Solution are the same as those for N.F. Antiseptic Solution. It possesses a mild alkalinity and, when diluted with an equal volume of water, it is claimed to be almost isotonic with body fluids.

For oral use, the solution should not be diluted; for use in the dental spray bottle, it should be diluted with 5 volumes of water.

Benzalkonium Chloride Solution, U.S.P.
Liquor Benzalkonii Chloridi

Benzalkonium Chloride Solution contains not less than 93 per cent and not more than 107 per cent of the labeled amount of benzalkonium chloride. It may be buffered by the addition of ammonium acetate in a quantity not exceeding 40 per cent of the weight of the benzalkonium chloride. It may contain a suitable coloring agent.

Benzalkonium chloride is a quaternary ammonium compound and is a highly active cationic detergent and germicide. Its aqueous solutions are alkaline to litmus and foam strongly when shaken. The official preparation is a clear liquid. It is colorless unless a color has been added, and it has an aromatic odor and a bitter taste.

Benzalkonium Chloride Solution is available commercially under the name Zephiran Chloride Solution in a concentration of 1:1,000. A 12.8 per cent aqueous solution of Zephiran Chloride is marketed as a convenient concentrate for the extemporaneous preparation of dilute solutions.

Uses. Benzalkonium Chloride Solution is an effective surface disinfectant for general use in the prophylactic disinfection of the intact skin and the mucous membranes. It is used in a concentration of 1:1,000 for the preoperative disinfection of the unbroken skin and in concentrations of 1:2,000 to 1:10,000 for application to mucous membranes and abraded skin. Dilutions of 1:2,000 to 1:5,000 are used for instillation into and irrigation of the eye or the vagina. For urinary bladder and urethral irrigation, a concentration not stronger than 1:20,000 is recommended, and for retention lavage of the bladder, the concentration should not exceed 1:40,000. Benzalkonium chloride in dilutions of 1:1,000 to 1:5,000 is used for the sterile storage of metallic instruments. When used for this purpose, 0.5 per cent of sodium nitrite may be added to prevent the corrosion of the metallic instruments.

Since benzalkonium chloride is a cationic detergent, ordinary soaps which are anionic detergents may interfere with its germicidal action. For this reason, it is suggested that areas which may have been scrubbed with a soap solution be carefully rinsed free of soap before the disinfectant solution is applied. Since alcohol diminishes the ionization of ordinary soap solution and thus protects the benzalkonium chloride to some extent, it is suggested that the scrubbing with soap solution may be followed by the application of 70 per cent alcohol before the disinfectant is applied.

BENZETHONIUM CHLORIDE SOLUTION, U.S.P.

Benzethonium Chloride Solution contains not less than 93 per cent and not more than 107 per cent of the labeled amount of benzethonium chloride.

This solution resembles Benzalkonium Chloride Solution, its active ingredient being a quaternary ammonium germicide of the type known as hyamines. The official product is a clear, colorless and odorless liquid and has a bitter taste. It is slightly alkaline to litmus. The activity of benzethonium chloride, like that of other quaternary ammonium compounds, is decreased by soap and other detergents. The commercial counterpart of the official solution is available as Phemerol Chloride Solution in a concentration of 1:1,000.

Uses. Benzethonium Chloride Solution is used as a general surface-active germicide and antiseptic. A 1:1,000 solution is recommended for topical use to the skin, and a 1:5,000 solution is suggested for use in the eyes or the nose. Like other compounds of this type, it is not highly effective when used for surgical disinfection because it tends to form a film under which viable bacteria can survive.

BORIC ACID SOLUTION, N.F.

"Saturated" Boric Acid Solution;
Liquor Acidi Borici

Boric Acid Solution contains, in each 100 ml., not less than 4.25 Gm. of H_3BO_3.

Although the synonym, "Saturated" Boric Acid Solution, implies that the official solution is saturated at room temperature, it is actually undersaturated, since the solubility of boric acid is given as 1 Gm. in 18 ml. of water at 25°. A degree of unsaturation is allowed to prevent crystallization if the solution is kept in a cool place or if part of the solvent evaporates. The *N.F.* warns against the dispensing of this solution if it contains any crystals of boric acid and states that it must be dispensed perfectly clear. This precaution is given because the solution is used widely as a wash for the eyes, and any crystals of boric acid that might be present could irritate the conjunctiva.

Although Boric Acid Solution often is used in the eyes, it is employed also for other purposes and, apparently for this reason, has not been classified as an Ophthalmic Solution.

Uses. Boric Acid Solution is used as a wash or a wet dressing for wounds, skin inflammations and similar conditions. It is also used as a soothing and cleansing wash for the eyes and as a vehicle in the preparation of collyria and eyedrops.

For external use, it may be used undiluted. For ophthalmic use, it may be diluted with an equal volume of water so as to produce a solution that is very nearly isotonic with tear fluid.

The official solution, or a dilution of it, is frequently prescribed as an ingredient in dermatologic ointments and lotions.

CALCIFEROL SOLUTION, U.S.P.

Calciferol Solution is a solution of calciferol in an edible vegetable oil or in polysorbate 80 or in propylene glycol. It contains, in each Gm., not less than 0.25 mg. (10,000 U.S.P. Vitamin D Units) of calciferol.

Calciferol or crystalline Vitamin D_2 is an activated sterol derived from ergosterol. The official solution is a clear liquid, having the characteristics of the solvent used in preparing it. A brand of crystalline vitamin D_2 is marketed under the name Drisdol. A Solution of Drisdol in propylene glycol is available commercially and is described as a clear liquid, odorless and tasteless, easily miscible with milk, water and other liquids.

Uses. Calciferol Solution exhibits antirachitic properties and is used in the prevention and the treatment of conditions that usually respond to vitamin D therapy.

COMPOUND CALCIUM CYCLAMATE SOLUTION, U.S.P.

Compound Calcium Cyclamate Solution contains, in each 100 ml., not less than 5.4 Gm. and not more than 6.6 Gm. of calcium cyclamate, and not less than 0.54 Gm. and not more than 0.66 Gm. of saccharin calcium. It may contain suitable preservatives.

Commercially, this is marketed as Sucaryl Calcium Sweetening Solution.

Uses. Like Compound Sodium Cyclamate Solution, N.F., this preparation is a non-caloric sweetener. However, it possesses the added advantage in that, because of the absence of sodium ion, it may be used by persons on low-sodium diets.

CALCIUM HYDROXIDE SOLUTION, U.S.P.

Lime Water; Liquor Calcis; Liquor Calcii Hydroxidi

Calcium Hydroxide Solution is a solution containing, in each 100 ml., not less than 140 mg. of $Ca(OH)_2$ at 25°. It is prepared by vigorously and repeatedly agitating 3 Gm. of calcium hydroxide with 1,000 ml. of cool purified water during 1 hour, allowing the excess of calcium hydroxide to settle and decanting the clear, supernatant liquid which is to be dispensed. Cold water is specified in preparing the solution because calcium hydroxide is more soluble at lower than at higher temperatures. Thus, the calcium hydroxide content of lime water which is stored at 15° is about 170 mg. per 100 ml. The *U.S.P.* does not allow the excess of calcium hydroxide to be used in preparing additional quantities of the solution, hence the practice by some pharmacists of repeatedly adding water to a bottle containing the residue from a previous portion of the solution is condemned. Since the excess of calcium hydroxide is quickly converted to the carbonate, the resulting solution would be substandard in strength.

The solution should be stored in well-filled, tight containers so as to prevent entry of air which, because of its carbon dioxide content, will cause precipitation of the lime as calcium carbonate.

Uses. Lime water is sometimes used as an antacid, although its calcium hydroxide content is so low that large quantities of it are required. Occasionally, it is added to infants' feeding formulas for this purpose. For internal use, it has been given in doses ranging from 15 ml. to 120 ml. More frequently, it is employed as an ingredient in dermatologic preparations in which it serves as a reagent or supplies alkalinity. In order that lime water may serve its function as a reagent in lotions and liniments, it must be of proper strength. The *U.S.P.* categorizes the solution as an astringent.

CARBOL-FUCHSIN SOLUTION, N.F.

Castellani's Paint

Carbol-Fuchsin Solution is a solution of basic fuchsin, boric acid, phenol and resorcinol in a solvent consisting of acetone, alcohol and purified water. It is prepared by dissolving the basic fuchsin in a mixture of acetone and alcohol, adding to it the aqueous solution of boric acid, phenol and resorcinol, and diluting the liquid to volume with purified water.

The solution is a dark purple liquid which appears purplish red when spread in a thin film. It is a stabilized preparation of the original *Castellani's Paint*. A brand of carbol-fuchsin paint is available under the commercial name Carfusin.

Uses. The solution is an antimycotic and is employed for topical application to superficial fungal infections of the skin, particularly dermatophytosis of the feet. Test applications of the preparation diluted with one or two volumes of water may be advisable. Unfortunately, the solution stains clothing.

Cetylpyridinium Chloride Solution, U.S.P.

Cetylpyridinium Chloride Solution contains not less than 95 per cent and not more than 105 per cent of the labeled amount of cetylpyridinium chloride.

Cetylpyridinium chloride is a quaternary ammonium salt. It is a cationic detergent that possesses surface-active and antiseptic properties against sensitive nonsporulating bacteria. As with other cationic detergents, its effectiveness as a germicide is reduced by ordinary soap and other anionic surfactants. The official solution is a clear liquid having an aromatic odor and a bitter taste. It is colorless unless a color has been added. Its commercial counterpart, Ceepryn Chloride Aqueous Solution, is available as a 1:1,000 solution made isotonic with alkaline phosphates. A 10 per cent aqueous solution of Ceepryn Chloride with monobasic sodium phosphate is marketed as a concentrate from which weaker solutions may be conveniently prepared.

Uses. The solution possesses marked local anti-infective properties. It is used topically in concentrations ranging from 1:100 to 1:1,000 for application to intact skin. In more dilute concentrations, 1:5,000 to 1:10,000, it is employed on mucous membranes by topical application or irrigation.

Coal Tar Solution, U.S.P.

Liquor Carbonis Detergens;
Liquor Picis Carbonis

Coal Tar Solution is an alcoholic solution of coal tar and polysorbate 80. It is prepared by mixing 200 Gm. of coal tar with 500 Gm. of washed sand and adding 50 Gm. of polysorbate 80 and 700 ml. of alcohol. This mixture is macerated for 7 days in a closed vessel, with frequent agitation. At the end of the maceration period, the mixture is filtered to remove the sand and other undissolved materials, and the vessel and the filter are washed with sufficient alcohol to make the product measure 1,000 ml.

In extemporaneous compounding, the solution is frequently diluted with water or with essentially aqueous liquids. When so diluted, the satisfactory dispersion of the alcohol-soluble constituents of the coal tar may be ensured to a greater degree by the presence of a suitable dispersing agent in the solution. In the official product, this function is served by the polysorbate 80, a nonionic surfactant, which is commercially available as Tween 80. In earlier official texts quillaja, from which the saponins were extracted during the maceration process, was used for the same reason. Washed sand is employed in the official procedure for the purpose of mechanically dispersing the coal tar so that a greater surface area is exposed to the solvent.

Uses. Coal Tar Solution is very commonly prescribed as an ingredient in extemporaneous lotions, liniments, ointments, creams and pastes that are intended for use in the treatment of many skin conditions, notably psoriasis and eczema.

Cyclopentamine Hydrochloride Solution, N.F.

Cyclopentamine Hydrochloride Solution contains not less than 95 per cent and not more than 105 per cent of the labeled amount of cyclopentamine hydrochloride.

The commercial counterpart of the official product is marketed as Clopane Hydrochloride Solution. It is available as an isotonic aqueous solution in 2 concentrations: 0.5 and 1.0 per cent.

Uses. The solution possesses vasoconstrictor properties and is used intranasally for the relief of congestion due to allergic or vasomotor rhinitis or sinusitis. For this purpose the solution may be applied to the nose by spray, by dropper, or by tampon.

EPHEDRINE SULFATE SOLUTION, N.F.

Ephedrine Sulfate Solution yields, from each 100 ml., not less than 2.7 Gm. and not more than 3.2 Gm. of ephedrine sulfate. It contains 0.5 per cent of chlorobutanol as a preservative and sufficient sodium chloride to render it nearly isotonic with body fluids.

The solution is a clear, colorless liquid having a slightly camphoraceous odor and taste.

Uses. Ephedrine Sulfate Solution is used as a source of the ephedrine salt in the preparation of aqueous sprays and nose drops. It is usually too strong for application to nasal membranes in the undiluted form. For use on mucous membranes of the nose, it should be diluted with an equal volume of isotonic sodium chloride solution. In this concentration, it is used to relieve nasal congestion and swelling due to hay fever and upper respiratory infections.

ETHYLENEDIAMINE SOLUTION, U.S.P.

Liquor Æthylenediaminæ

Ethylenediamine Solution contains not less than 67 per cent of ethylenediamine.

Ethylenediamine may be prepared by reacting ethylene chloride with ammonia at elevated temperature and pressure. The official solution is a clear, colorless or slightly yellow liquid, having an ammonia-like odor and a strong alkaline reaction. The following note concerning its storage is given in the pharmacopeial monograph: *"Ethylenediamine Solution is strongly alkaline and may readily absorb carbon dioxide from the air to form a nonvolatile carbonate. Protect Ethylenediamine Solution against undue exposure to the atmosphere."*

Uses. It is used as a solvent for theophylline in the preparation of aminophylline, which is officially described as a mixture of the two substances. The *U.S.P.* categorizes this preparation as a pharmaceutic necessity for Aminophylline Injection, in which it is used for the purpose of stabilization.

HEXYLCAINE HYDROCHLORIDE SOLUTION, N.F.

Hexylcaine Hydrochloride Solution contains not less than 93 per cent and not more than 107 per cent of the labeled amount of hexylcaine hydrochloride.

A 5 per cent isotonic solution of hexylcaine hydrochloride is available commercially under the name Cyclaine Hydrochloride Solution. It is a clear, colorless solution having a slightly acidic reaction.

Uses. The solution, in 1 to 5 per cent concentrations, is used as a local anesthetic for topical application by spray, cotton applicator, or tampon to mucous membranes. When used in this manner, the solution is as potent as equal concentrations of cocaine.

IODINE SOLUTION, N.F.

Iodine Solution contains, in each 100 ml., not less than 1.8 Gm. and not more than 2.2 Gm. of iodine, and not less than 2.1 Gm. and not more than 2.6 Gm. of sodium iodide.

It is prepared by dissolving 2 per cent of iodine in a concentrated aqueous solution of sodium iodide and diluting with purified water to the required volume.

Iodine is very slightly soluble in water but dissolves freely in solutions of iodides. Sodium iodide is used in the manufacture of the official preparation to effect the solution of the iodine.

Iodine Solution is a transparent, reddish-brown liquid having the odor of iodine. The *N.F.* directs that it be stored in tight, light-resistant containers, preferably at a temperature not above 35°.

Uses. The solution contains the same concentrations of iodine and sodium iodide as Iodine Tincture in which diluted alcohol is the solvent. Like the tincture, it is an antibacterial and is used as a skin and surgical disinfectant.

STRONG IODINE SOLUTION, U.S.P.

Compound Iodine Solution;
Lugol's Solution; Liquor Iodi Fortis;
Solutio Iodi Aquosæ

Strong Iodine Solution contains, in each 100 ml., not less than 4.5 Gm. and not more than 5.5 Gm. of iodine and not less than 9.5 Gm. and not more than 10.5 Gm. of potassium iodide. The solution is made by dissolving 5 per cent of iodine in a concentrated aqueous solution of potassium iodide and diluting with purified water to the required volume. The potassium iodide serves the same purpose in this preparation as does sodium iodide in Iodine Solution.

Uses. Lugol's solution is administered internally for the systemic effect of iodine. The usual dose is 0.3 ml. (5 minims), diluted with water or milk, 3 times a day.

MERBROMIN SOLUTION, N.F.

Merbromin Solution contains, in each 100 ml., not less than 1.8 Gm. and not more than 2.2 Gm. of merbromin.

Merbromin is the official name for the compound that is commercially available as Mercurochrome. The solution is prepared by dissolving 2 per cent of merbromin in sufficient water to make the required volume. The resulting product is a clear, red liquid having a yellow-green fluorescence. The solution has a pronounced staining property; however, such stains may be removed by the use of a solution of chlorinated soda. When Merbromin Solution is combined with acids or acid salts, an incompatibility, evidenced by precipitation, results.

Uses. It is used as a nonirritating antiseptic for local application to minor wounds. When used for this purpose, its reliability is open to question, since merbromin, in aqueous solutions, has been shown to have a low phenol coefficient. (See Surgical Merbromin Solution, below.)

SURGICAL MERBROMIN SOLUTION, N.F.

Surgical Merbromin Solution contains, in each 100 ml., not less than 1.8 Gm. and not more than 2.2 Gm. of merbromin in a vehicle of acetone, neutralized alcohol and water.

The solution is prepared by dissolving 2 per cent of merbromin in 35 per cent of water and adding 10 per cent of acetone and sufficient neutralized alcohol to make the required volume. Neutralized alcohol is used so that the alkalinity of the solution may be maintained, thus preventing precipitation of the merbromin. A mixture of acetone, alcohol and water is used as the solvent because merbromin has been shown to be more effective as a germicide in this vehicle than it is in aqueous solutions. *Scott's Solution* is a synonym that is commonly used for the official preparation.

Uses. It is used as a skin disinfectant, particularly in preparing the skin for surgical operations.

METHYLROSANILINE CHLORIDE SOLUTION, U.S.P.

Methylrosaniline Chloride Solution contains, in each 100 ml., not less than 0.95 Gm. and not more than 1.05 Gm. of methylrosaniline chloride, calculated as hexamethylpararosaniline chloride.

Methylrosaniline Chloride, variously known as Gentian Violet, Crystal Violet and Methyl Violet, is a medicinal dye consisting of a mixture of rosanilines. A brand of gentian violet is available commercially under the name Pyoktanin. The official preparation is made by dissolving 1 per cent of the dye in a hydro-alcoholic solvent containing 10 per cent of alcohol. The resulting solution is a purple liquid having a slight odor of alcohol.

Uses. The solution is a local anti-infective. It is used topically, in undiluted form, in conditions of the skin and the mucous membranes where the infection is caused by gram-positive bacteria or by certain parasitic fungi.

NAPHAZOLINE HYDROCHLORIDE SOLUTION, N.F.

Naphazoline Hydrochloride Solution is a solution of naphazoline hydrochloride in water adjusted with suitable buffers and with sodium chloride and/or potassium chloride to a suitable pH and tonicity. It may contain a preservative. It contains, in each 100 ml., not less than 45 mg. and not more than 55 mg. of naphazoline hydrochloride.

This preparation corresponds, in strength, to the one formerly official as Mild Naphazoline Hydrochloride Solution and is marketed under the name Privine Hydrochloride Nasal Solution. It is an isotonic, buffered, aqueous solution having a pH of

6.2 to 6.3. The solution should be preserved in tight, light-resistant containers. A 0.1 per cent solution of naphazoline hydrochloride is also available commercially as Privine Hydrochloride Ophthalmic Solution.

Uses. Naphazoline Hydrochloride Solution is a powerful vasoconstrictor, possessing the chief pharmacologic properties of ephedrine. It is used to relieve the congestion and the swelling of the nasal mucosa due to colds, hay fever, rhinitis and other allergic conditions.

Nitrofurazone Solution, N.F.

Nitrofurazone Solution contains, in each 100 Gm., not less than 190 mg. and not more than 210 mg. of nitrofurazone.

Nitrafurazone is a substituted furan compound which is soluble in polyethylene glycol mixtures up to about 1 per cent. The solution is prepared by dissolving 0.2 per cent of nitrafurazone in a mixture of equal parts of polyethylene glycol 1540 and polyethylene glycol 300, which has been previously heated to a temperature of between 60° and 70°. When solution is effected (about 30 minutes), the liquid is allowed to cool to 45°, and a solution of octylphenoxy polyethoxyethanol in water is added to it at this temperature with continuous stirring.

The resulting solution is a light-yellow, clear, somewhat viscous, water-miscible liquid having a faint characteristic odor. It should be preserved in tight, light-resistant containers, and contact at all times with direct sunlight, excessive heat, and alkaline materials should be avoided.

The commercial counterpart of the official solution is available as Furacin Solution.

Uses. Nitrofurazone Solution possesses antibacterial properties and is used topically in the prophylaxis and the treatment of mixed infections. It is applied directly to the infected area or to bandages with which the area is to be covered. Some of the conditions in which it is recommended are burns, ulcerations, contaminated wounds and pyodermas, especially impetigo and ecthyma.

Nitromersol Solution, N.F.

Nitromersol Solution yields, from each 100 ml., not less than 180 mg. and not more than 220 mg. of nitromersol.

The solution is prepared by dissolving nitromersol in purified water which has been made alkaline with sodium hydroxide and monohydrated sodium carbonate. The resulting solution is a clear reddish-orange liquid which is affected by light. It should be preserved in tight, light-resistant containers.

The following caution concerning the preparation of dilutions of the solution is given in the official monograph: *"Dilutions of Nitromersol Solution should be prepared as needed since they tend to precipitate on standing."*

The commercial counterpart of nitromersol is known as Metaphen, and a 1:500 solution of nitromersol with 3 per cent of benzyl alcohol is available under the name Metaphen First Aid Solution.

Uses. Nitromersol Solution is used as an antiseptic for the skin and the mucous membranes. It is relatively free from irritation and it is reported to be more effective than inorganic mercurials.

Paramethadione Solution, N.F.

Paramethadione Solution is a solution of paramethadione is diluted alcohol. It contains not less than 94 per cent and not more than 106 per cent of the labeled amount of paramethadione.

Paramethadione, a homologue of trimethadione, is a colorless, oily liquid having an esterlike odor. It is slightly soluble in water and freely soluble in alcohol. The official preparation is available commercially as a 30 per cent solution under the name Paradione Solution.

Uses. Paramethadione Solution is an anticonvulsant which is indicated in the treatment of petit mal, myoclonic and akinetic epilepsy. The solution should be diluted before being administered.

Phenylephrine Hydrochloride Solution, U.S.P.

Phenylephrine Hydrochloride Solution contains not less than 95 per cent and not more than 105 per cent of the labeled amount of phenylephrine hydrochloride.

The official preparation is available under the trade name Neo-Synephrine Hydrochloride Solution. It is marketed as an isotonic solution in concentrations ranging from 0.25 to 1 per cent for topical and intranasal use, and as a low surface tension solution in concentrations ranging from 0.125 to 10 per cent for ophthalmic use.

Uses. Phenylephrine Hydrochloride Solution is a vasoconstrictor for topical application to the mucous membranes and is used to relieve congestion due to colds, hay fever and certain upper respiratory infections. It is also an effective decongestant and mydriatic in the eye.

POTASSIUM IODIDE SOLUTION, N.F.

Saturated Potassium Iodide Solution

Potassium Iodide Solution contains, in each 100 ml., not less than 97 Gm. and not more than 103 Gm. of potassium iodide.

The solution is prepared by dissolving 1,000 Gm. of potassium iodide in 680 ml. of hot purified water, cooling to about 25°, and adding sufficient purified water to make the product measure 1,000 ml. If the solution is not to be used within a short time, 500 mg. of sodium thiosulfate should be added to each liter.

The official preparation is recognized as a saturated solution and offers a convenient dosage form for the administration of potassium iodide, since each ml. of the solution contains 1 Gm. of the salt.

When the solution is exposed to light and air, free iodine is liberated very slowly as a result of oxidation. The objective evidence of this deterioration is a yellow color. If a small amount of sodium thiosulfate is added to the solution, the free iodine is converted to sodium iodide as it is formed, and the solution remains colorless. The *N.F.* directs that the solution be preserved in tight, light-resistant containers.

Uses. This preparation is prescribed rather commonly as an alterative in a variety of conditions, including some forms of goiter, tuberculosis, syphilis, bronchitic asthma and rheumatism. The usual dose is 0.3 ml. (approximately 5 minims).

PRAMOXINE HYDROCHLORIDE SOLUTION, N.F.

Pramoxine Hydrochloride Solution is a solution of pramoxine hydrochloride in purified water made isotonic by the addition of sodium chloride. It contains not less than 95 per cent and not more than 105 per cent of the labeled amount of pramoxine hydrochloride.

Pramoxine Hydrochloride is the official name for Tronothane Hydrochloride, a topical anesthetic. A 1 per cent isotonic aqueous solution of pramoxine hydrochloride is marketed as Tronothane Hydrochloride Topical Solution and is packaged in low-pressure aerosol containers for convenient use.

Uses. The solution is a surface anesthetic intended for topical application as a spray. It is used for the temporary relief of surface pain and itching of minor burns and skin irritations.

RACEPHEDRINE HYDROCHLORIDE SOLUTION, N.F.

dl-Ephedrine Hydrochloride Solution

Racephedrine Hydrochloride Solution contains, in each 100 ml., not less than 930 mg. and not more than 1.07 Gm. of racephedrine hydrochloride.

The solution is prepared by dissolving 1 per cent of racephedrine hydrochloride and 0.5 per cent of chlorobutanol in Ringer's Solution. The solution should be filtered, if necessary, until it is clear. Chlorobutanol is included in the formula as a preservative.

Uses. It is used for topical application by dropper or spray to the nasal mucosa as a decongestant.

RADIOCYANOCOBALAMIN SOLUTION, U.S.P.

Radiocyanocobalamin (Co^{60}) Solution

For discussion, see Chapter 26.

RADIOGOLD SOLUTION, U.S.P.

Sterile Radioactive Gold Colloid; Sterile Radiogold (Au^{198}) Colloid

For discussion, see Chapter 26.

COMPOUND SODIUM CYCLAMATE
SOLUTION, N.F.

Compound Sodium Cyclamate Solution contains, in each 100 ml., not less than 5.4 Gm. and not more than 6.6 Gm. of sodium cyclamate, and not less than 0.54 and not more than 0.66 Gm. of saccharin sodium. It may contain suitable preservatives.

Sodium cyclamate is a synthetic, nonnutritional sweetener. It is about 30 times as sweet as sugar. The official preparation is available as Sucaryl Sodium Sweetening Solution.

Uses. The solution is a noncaloric sweetening agent and is used as a substitute for sugar by diabetics and others who are on a restricted carbohydrate diet. It contains sodium ion, and this factor must be considered when the solution is to be used by persons on low salt diets. In sweetening power, each 0.9 ml. (approximately one quarter teaspoonful) is equivalent to about 2 teaspoonfuls of sugar.

SODIUM PHOSPHATE SOLUTION, N.F.

Sodium Phosphate Solution contains, in each 100 ml., not less than 71 Gm. and not more than 79 Gm. of sodium phosphate.

The solution is made by adding 755 Gm. of sodium phosphate, 130 Gm. of citric acid and 150 ml. of glycerin to 150 ml. of purified water, digesting the mixture on a water bath until solution is effected, filtering and adding sufficient purified water through the filter to make the product measure 1,000 ml.

The *N.F.* permits the use of a chemically equivalent quantity of exsiccated sodium phosphate in place of the crystalline salt. If the exsiccated form is used, the quantity should be reduced to 400 Gm., and the amount of water should be increased to 500 ml.

The citric acid imparts a more pleasant taste to the solution and probably reacts at least to some extent with the sodium phosphate to form a mixture of sodium acid citrate and sodium acid phosphate. Glycerin adds to the palatability of the solution and serves as a preservative.

The solution should be kept in tight containers and in a moderately warm place (not under 22°).

Uses. It is a palatable dosage form of sodium phosphate and is used as a mild saline cathartic. The usual dose is 8 ml. (approximately 2 fluidrams).

SODIUM RADIO-IODIDE SOLUTION, U.S.P.

Sodium Radio-iodide (I^{131}) Solution (U.S.P. XV)

For discussion, see Chapter 26.

SODIUM RADIOPHOSPHATE SOLUTION, U.S.P.

Radioactive Phosphorus Solution; Sodium Radio-phosphate (P^{32}) Solution (U.S.P. XV)

For discussion, see Chapter 26.

SORBITOL SOLUTION, U.S.P.

Sorbitol Solution is a water solution containing, in each 100 Gm., not less than 69 Gm. and not more than 71 Gm. of total solids consisting essentially of D-sorbitol, a hexahydric alcohol and a small amount of mannitol and other isomeric polyhydric alcohols. The content of D-sorbitol, in each 100 Gm., is not less than 64 Gm.

The official product is a clear, colorless, syrupy liquid, having a sweet taste and no characteristic odor.

Uses. Sorbitol Solution is a humectant and a sweetener and may be classified as a vehicle. It has many of the properties of glycerin and has been suggested as a replacement for it. It is used as an emollient and moisture-conditioning agent in various cosmetic and pharmaceutical formulations.

TETRAHYDROZOLINE HYDROCHLORIDE
SOLUTION, N.F.

Tetrahydrozoline Hydrochloride Solution is a solution of tetrahydrozoline hydrochloride in water adjusted to a suitable tonicity. It may contain a preservative. It contains not less than 90 per cent and not more than 110 per cent of the labeled amount of tetrahydrozoline hydrochloride.

Commercially, the solution is available in 0.1 per cent concentration as Tyzine Solution or Spray, and in 0.05 per cent concentration as Tyzine Pediatric Nasal Drops.

Uses. The solution is used as a nasal decongestant and is applied topically by dropper or spray.

Thimerosal Solution, N.F.

Thimerosal Solution contains, in each 100 ml., not less than 95 mg. and not more than 105 mg. of thimerosal. The preparation may be colored with one or more coal-tar colors, certified by the Federal Food and Drug Administration for use in drugs.

Ethylenediamine and sodium borate are used in the solution as buffering agents to maintain the alkalinity that is required, and monoethanolamine is added as a stabilizing agent. The *N.F.* cautions that it must be prepared and stored in glass or suitable resistant metal containers.

The official product is similar to the preparation that is marketed as Merthiolate Solution.

Uses. Thimerosal Solution is used as an antiseptic or disinfectant for topical application to wounds or abrasions. It is often applied as a wet dressing.

Tribromoethanol Solution, U.S.P.

Bromethol; Liquor Tribromoæthanolis

Tribromoethanol Solution is a solution of tribromoethanol in amylene hydrate. It contains, in each 100 ml., not less than 99 Gm. and not more than 101 Gm. of tribromoethanol.

The product is a clear, colorless liquid, having a camphoraceous odor and a burning taste. Because it is unstable in the presence of light and air, it should be stored in tight, light-resistant containers dried carefully prior to filling.

Unlike most solvents used in the preparation of official solutions, the amylene hydrate has a definite influence on the physiologic action of the solution. It is a hypnotic and adds its effect to the anesthetic action of the tribromoethanol. Because of this combined action, a greater degree of depression is produced by the solution than by the tribromoethanol alone.

The solution is known commercially as Avertin with Amylene Hydrate and Avertin Fluid.

Uses. It is used as a basal anesthetic, either by itself or as a preliminary to the administration of gaseous anesthetics. The *U.S.P.* directs that the solution be diluted before use with 40 times its volume of warm purified water. It also requires that, when 5 ml. of this dilution is mixed with 1 drop of Congo Red T.S., it must have the same color as a mixture of 5 ml. of purified water and 1 drop of the same test solution. This test detects the presence of free hydrobromic acid, which is present if the solution has decomposed. The test is emphasized here because the solution should *never be used* unless it can meet this requirement. The usual dose for each Kg. of body weight is rectally 0.06 to 0.08 ml., not to exceed 8 ml. for woman and 10 ml. for man.

Trimethadione Solution, N.F.

Trimethadione Solution contains not less than 94 per cent and not more than 106 per cent of the labeled amount of trimethadione.

A flavored aqueous solution containing approximately 4 per cent of trimethadione is available commercially as Tridione Solution. The solution should be preserved at temperatures not exceeding 30° C.

Uses. Trimethadione Solution is used as an anticonvulsant, particularly in the petit mal type of epilepsy. It is particularly useful in administering the drug to children.

Tyrothricin Solution, N.F.

Tyrothricin Solution is a solution of tyrothricin in alcohol. A wetting agent may be added. It has a potency of not less than 90 per cent and not more than 120 per cent of the labeled potency.

The preparation is available commercially under its official name as a 2 per cent solution, and under the trade name Soluthricin Concentrate as a 2.5 per cent solution. These products must be diluted with sterile distilled water before use, usually to a concentration of 30 to 50 mg. per 100 ml. Soluthricin is also marketed as a ready-for-use solution of tyrothricin in a concentration of 0.05 per cent.

Uses. The solution is a topical antibiotic intended for application by irrigation and as a spray or wet dressing. It is effective against a variety of gram-positive organisms and is indicated in the treatment of infected wounds, indolent ulcers, abscesses of the

WATER-MISCIBLE VITAMIN A SOLUTION, U.S.P.

Water-Miscible Vitamin A (U.S.P. XV)

Water-miscible Vitamin A Solution is Vitamin A, in the form of oleovitamin A, rendered water-miscible with the aid of suitable dispersing agents. Its vitamin A content is not less than 95 per cent of that stated on the label. It may contain a suitable flavor.

This solution represents the official counterpart of a number of commercial products in which vitamin A has been solubilized or dispersed and rendered water-miscible. While there are several patented methods for achieving water-miscibility of this oil-soluble vitamin, it would appear that, in at least one of the procedures, compounds of the polysorbate-type are used. The U.S.P. requires that a mixture of the solution and 10 volumes of water be clear or opalescent, and that no oily drops be visible in it after standing 1 hour.

It is claimed that aqueous dispersions of vitamin A are absorbed more rapidly and more completely from the gastrointestinal tract than are the oily preparations.

Commercially, Water-Miscible Vitamin A Solution is available in concentrations of 25,000 to 50,000 U.S.P. Units per ml. under such trade names as Acon Drops, Aquasol A and Vitamin A, Water Soluble.

Uses. Vitamin A is the antixerophthalmic vitamin. The water-miscible solution is administered orally, in prophylactic and therapeutic doses, in vitamin A deficiencies.

SOLUTIONS PREPARED BY CHEMICAL REACTION

Aluminum Acetate Solution, U.S.P.

Burow's Solution; Liquor Alumini Acetatis

Aluminum Acetate Solution yields, from each 100 ml., not less than 1.2 Gm. and not more than 1.45 Gm. of aluminum oxide (Al_2O_3), and not less than 4.24 Gm. and not more than 5.11 Gm. of acetic acid ($C_2H_4O_2$), corresponding to not less than 4.8 Gm. and not more than 5.8 Gm. of aluminum acetate ($C_6H_9AlO_6$).

Officially, the solution is prepared by adding glacial acetic acid to aluminum subacetate solution and diluting with water. The glacial acetic acid reacts with the basic aluminum acetate, converting it to the normal acetate. $(CH_3COO)_2 AlOH + CH_3COOH \rightarrow Al(CH_3COO)_3 + H_2O$.

Other methods for preparing the solution, as by reaction between lead acetate and aluminum sulfate, may be used, but the resulting product must meet the official requirements.

The solution has a distinct tendency to deposit a precipitate of a basic form of aluminum acetate, especially if it is exposed to the air. The U.S.P. allows the use of not more than 0.6 per cent of boric acid for the purpose of retarding or preventing the precipitation of the basic acetate. The solution may be dispensed only when clear.

Burow's Solution is a clear, colorless liquid having a faint acetous odor and a sweetish, astringent taste. It is distinctly acid, having a pH of about 4.0. It should be stored in tight containers.

Uses. Aluminum Acetate Solution, properly diluted, is used as an astringent wash or wet dressing for a variety of dermatologic conditions. For topical application, it is usually diluted with 10 to 40 parts of water. It is commonly employed as an ingredient in dermatologic lotions, ointments and pastes.

Aluminum Subacetate Solution, U.S.P.

Liquor Alumini Subacetatis

Aluminum Subacetate Solution yields, from each 100 ml., not less than 2.30 Gm. and not more than 2.60 Gm. of aluminum oxide (Al_2O_3), and not less than 5.43 Gm. and not more than 6.13 Gm. of acetic acid ($C_2H_4O_2$).

The official solution may be prepared by reacting aluminum sulfate with acetic acid and precipitated calcium carbonate, 24 hours being allowed for the reaction to take place. The equation for the reaction which occurs is as follows:

$Al_2(SO_4)_3 \cdot 18H_2O + 3CaCO_3 + 4CH_3COOH \rightarrow 2(CH_3COO)_2AlOH + 3CaSO_4 + 3CO_2 + 19H_2O$

In order to produce the basic salt, a quantity of acetic acid insufficient to form the normal acetate is used. The calcium carbonate is used to remove the sulfate radical from the solution by precipitating it as insoluble calcium sulfate.

The solution may be prepared by other methods provided that the finished product conforms to pharmacopeial standards.

Aluminum Subacetate Solution is a clear and colorless or faintly yellow liquid having an acetous odor and an acid reaction to litmus. It gradually becomes turbid on standing due to the formation of a more basic salt.

For the purpose of stabilizing the solution the addition of boric acid, in a concentration of not over 0.9 per cent, is allowed.

Uses. The solution, usually diluted with 20 to 40 parts of water, is used as an astringent wash or wet dressing for topical application in the treatment of certain eczematous conditions of the skin.

SAPONATED CRESOL SOLUTION, N.F.

Compound Cresol Solution

Saponated Cresol Solution is an aqueous saponated solution containing, in each 100 ml., not less than 46 ml. and not more than 52 ml. of cresol.

The solution is prepared by the saponification of a mixture of cresol with certain vegetable oils or of the mixed fatty acids derived therefrom, excluding coconut and palm kernel oils. The vegetable oils may be corn, cottonseed, linseed, soya bean or similar oils which have a saponification value not greater than 205 and an iodine value not less than 100.

The vegetable oil is completely saponified with a solution of potassium hydroxide, cresol is mixed with the prepared soap, and sufficient purified water is added to make the required volume. The cresol is probably not truly dissolved in this solution, but merely suspended in an extremely fine state of subdivision. The soap formed aids in the suspension of the cresol which, under ordinary circumstances, is soluble in water only to the extent of about 2 per cent.

Alcohol is used in this formula because it has been shown to have a catalytic effect on the saponification reaction. It may be replaced by a smaller portion of oleic acid, but, if this is done, the oil should be heated to 85° before the addition of the solution of the alkali hydroxide, and the mixture is heated, if necessary, to complete saponification.

The hardness of the soap formed depends on the nature of the fatty acids contained in the oil and on the alkali used in the saponification of the oil. Oils containing rather large percentages of stearin and palmitin usually yield harder soaps, while those containing a large amount of olein yield softer soaps. Potassium hydroxide forms a soft soap with oils; sodium hydroxide forms a hard soap. Although the *N.F.* specifies potassium hydroxide in the formula, it permits the use of a mixture of potassium and sodium hydroxides. The *N.F.* also states that the quantities of potassium and sodium hydroxides have been determined on the basis of official minimum percentages of strength; namely, 85 per cent for potassium hydroxide and 95 per cent for sodium hydroxide. If either or both of the hydroxides used should have a different percentage strength, corresponding changes in the quantities should be made.

Uses. Saponated Cresol Solution is employed for its antiseptic or germicidal effect, usually diluted with 50 to 100 parts of water. It is used commonly as a disinfectant and deodorant for washable fixtures in sickrooms, toilets and shower rooms. It is used to some extent as a personal antiseptic and as a surgical disinfectant.

FERRIC CHLORIDE SOLUTION, N.F.

Iron Perchloride Solution

Ferric Chloride Solution is a water solution containing, in each 100 ml., not less than 37.2 Gm. and not more than 42.7 Gm. of $FeCl_3$, and not less than 3.85 Gm. and not more than 6.6 Gm. of HCl.

No official method is given for the preparation of this solution. Usually it is prepared by the oxidation of ferrous chloride, using either nitric acid, chlorine or hydrogen peroxide. Chlorine and hydrogen peroxide generally are favored as the oxidizing agents, since they are removed more easily from the finished solution than is nitric acid. Ferric Chloride Solution is a yellowish-orange liquid, having a faint odor of hydrochloric acid and an acid reaction. It is affected by light and should be stored in tight, light-resistant containers.

Uses. The solution is used chiefly for the preparation of ferric chloride tincture, which is used as a hematinic. It is a powerful astringent and is sometimes employed as a styptic. Because of its hydrochloric acid content, the official product should not be used as the source of ferric chloride for the preparation of extemporaneous solutions that are intended for topical application in ivy poisoning. Such solutions should be prepared from ferric chloride crystals.

FERRIC SUBSULFATE SOLUTION, N.F.

Monsel's Solution, Basic Ferric Sulfate Solution

Ferric Subsulfate Solution is a water solution containing, in each 100 ml., basic ferric sulfate equivalent to not less than 20 Gm. and not more than 22 Gm. of Fe.

No official instructions are given regarding the procedure for manufacture of this solution; however, it may be prepared by adding ferrous sulfate to a hot diluted mixture of sulfuric and nitric acids, and boiling the combined reactants until the chemical reaction is complete and the solution is free from nitrate ion. In the chemical reaction which occurs, the nitric acid serves as an oxidizing agent to convert the iron from the ferrous to the ferric state. However, insufficient sulfuric acid is present to allow the formation of normal ferric sulfate, and a basic salt is formed. The basic sulfate has a variable composition, but the following equation has been suggested as being representative of the reaction which occurs.

$$12FeSO_4 + 3H_2SO_4 + 4HNO_3 \rightarrow 3Fe_4O(SO_4)_5 + 4NO + 5H_2O$$

The presence of a black color indicates that sufficient nitric acid has not been added to complete the oxidation of the iron. After the reaction has been completed, the excess nitric acid is removed by boiling the solution until it no longer gives a positive test for the nitrate ion.

Ferric subsulfate solution is a dark, reddish-brown liquid, odorless or nearly so, with an acid, strongly astringent taste. It must be preserved in tight, light-resistant containers and in a moderately warm place (not under 22°). When exposed to low temperatures, crystallization may take place in the solution. The crystals will redissolve upon warming the solution.

Uses. Monsel's Solution is an astringent. In undiluted form, it is used primarily as a styptic for external application by means of cotton swabs.

FORMALDEHYDE SOLUTION, U.S.P.

Formaldehyde Solution contains not less than 37 per cent of formaldehyde (CH_2O), with methanol added to prevent polymerization.

Formaldehyde is a gas that may be prepared by oxidation of methyl alcohol in the presence of catalysts, as indicated by the following equation:

$$2CH_3OH + O_2 \xrightarrow{catalyst} 2HCHO + 2H_2O$$

Aqueous solutions containing up to 40 per cent of formaldehyde are prepared in this way, a variable amount of methanol being left unconverted. Formaldehyde has a pronounced tendency to polymerize into paraformaldehyde, a solid polymer of indefinite molecular weight. The presence of a small amount of methanol in the solution retards this polymerization.

Formaldehyde Solution is a clear, colorless or nearly colorless liquid, having a pungent odor. Its vapors are very irritating to the mucous membranes of the nose and the throat. On long standing, especially in the cold, the solution may become cloudy due to the formation of paraformaldehyde. This cloudiness disappears when the solution is warmed. It should be stored in tight containers, preferably at temperatures not below 15°. The official preparation is commonly known as Formalin and Formol.

Uses. Formaldehyde Solution is used chiefly as a disinfectant deodorant and fumigant. It may be vaporized for fumigation purposes by spontaneous evaporation of the solution, by volatilization using heat, or by the addition of oxidizing agents, such as potassium permanganate. When an oxidizing agent is added, a portion of the formaldehyde is oxidized, and the heat generated is sufficient to volatilize most of the remainder of the formaldehyde. The solution is used also for cold disinfection of surgical instruments. Highly diluted, it is employed sometimes in the treatment of skin diseases. It is an important tissue fixative and an ingredient of embalming fluids.

Hydrogen Peroxide Solution, U.S.P.

Hydrogen Dioxide Solution; Liquor Hydrogenii Peroxidi

Hydrogen Peroxide Solution contains, in each 100 ml., not less than 2.5 Gm. and not more than 3.5 Gm. of H_2O_2. Suitable preservatives, totaling not more than 0.05 per cent, may be added.

No official procedure is given for the preparation of this solution, since it can be prepared by several methods. The hydrogen peroxide may be generated by decompositions of barium peroxide with phosphoric acid or dilute sulfuric acid.

$$BaO_2 + H_3PO_4 \longrightarrow BaHPO_4 + H_2O_2$$
or
$$BaO_2 + H_2SO_4 \longrightarrow BaSO_4 + H_2O_2$$

It is produced also by the hydrolysis of persulfuric acid, which is prepared by the electrolytic oxidation of sulfuric acid. The solution prepared by this method usually contains 30 per cent of H_2O_2 and is capable of liberating 100 times its volume of oxygen. For this reason, it is called "100 volume peroxide." This concentrated solution is diluted with water to the strength of the official product, which contains 3 per cent of H_2O_2 and is capable of liberating 10 times its volume of oxygen.

The solution has a great tendency to decompose, with the formation of oxygen and water. This deterioration causes a reduction in the content of H_2O_2. Since acetanilid and some other organic compounds have a retarding effect on this decomposition, one of them, in a concentration of about 0.05 per cent, usually is added to the solution. The preparation should be preserved in tight, light-resistant containers, preferably at a temperature not above 35°.

Uses. Because of its ability to liberate nascent oxygen, Hydrogen Peroxide Solution is used widely for the cleansing of wounds and suppurating areas. In such conditions, its value is probably more the result of its ability to remove organic detritus than of its antibacterial powers.

Phenolated Iodine Solution, N.F.

Boulton's Solution; Carbolized Iodine Solution

Phenolated Iodine Solution is prepared by mixing strong iodine solution, liquefied phenol, glycerin and water, and exposing the resulting liquid in a tightly stoppered, glass container to sunlight until it has become colorless or faintly yellow. This reaction may also be accomplished by heating the liquid at a temperature not exceeding 70°.

The exact mechanism of the reaction is not definitely known. However, it has been suggested that either the iodine enters the phenol molecule to produce a colorless compound or that it is converted to hydriodic acid.

Uses. Phenolated Iodine Solution is used in undiluted form as an antiseptic for application to wounds. Diluted with an equal volume of water, it has been used as a mouthwash.

Sulfurated Lime Solution, N.F.

Vleminckx' Lotion

Sulfurated Lime Solution is an aqueous solution prepared by boiling sublimed sulfur with lime in water. The resulting solution contains calcium disulfide, calcium pentasulfide and calcium thiosulfate, produced by the following reactions:

(1) $\quad 6CaO + 6H_2O \rightarrow 6Ca(OH)_2$

(2) $\quad 3Ca(OH)_2 + 6S \rightarrow 2CaS_2$
$\qquad\qquad\qquad\qquad +CaS_2O_3 + 3H_2O$

(3) $\quad 3Ca(OH)_2 + 12S \rightarrow 2CaS_5$
$\qquad\qquad\qquad\qquad +CaS_2O_3 + 3H_2O$

The finished product is a clear, orange liquid with a slight odor of hydrogen sulfide. It must be preserved in completely filled, tight containers; otherwise carbon dioxide will precipitate the calcium as the carbonate, and free sulfur will be liberated. The solution is incompatible with mineral acids, and the objective evidences of the incompatibility are the liberation of hydrogen sulfide and elemental sulfur.

Uses. Sulfurated Lime Solution, diluted with 9 volumes of water, is most frequently used as a scabicide. It is commonly prescribed as an ingredient in dermatologic lotions and creams, particularly in combination with zinc sulfate with which it reacts to form polysulfides of zinc.

Magnesium Citrate Solution, N.F.

Magnesium Citrate Solution is a sweetened, flavored, carbonated solution of magnesium citrate containing, in each 100 ml., an amount of this salt equivalent to not less than 1.55 Gm. and not more than 1.9 Gm. of MgO.

Magnesium Citrate Solution was introduced as an official preparation in 1850 and was recognized continuously by the *U.S.P.* until it was dropped by the Fifteenth Revision. Through the successive revisions of the pharmacopeia, the amount of citric acid in the formula was varied in the several attempts that were made to develop a stable, yet palatable, product.

The solution is prepared by reacting magnesium carbonate with citric acid, sweetening and flavoring the liquid, and carbonating it with potassium or sodium bicarbonate and, further, by the use of carbon dioxide under pressure.

The preparation has always shown a tendency to deposit a precipitate on standing. This instability has been attributed to several factors. The official magnesium carbonate is not a definite compound; rather, it is a basic hydrated magnesium carbonate or a normal hydrated magnesium carbonate which contains the equivalent of 40 to 43.5 per cent of magnesium oxide. It has been shown that solutions of magnesium citrate made from samples of magnesium carbonate containing the lower equivalent were more stable than those made from samples containing the higher limit of magnesium oxide. It has also been reported that sterilization of the finished product retards precipitation and that sucrose and carbon dioxide contribute to the instability of the product. Further, experimental evidence indicates that solutions which were calculated to contain dibasic magnesium citrate showed a lesser tendency to precipitate than did solutions in which the normal magnesium citrate was formed. The following equation represents the reaction in which dibasic magnesium citrate is formed:

$$(MgCO_3)_4 \cdot Mg(OH)_2 + 5H_3C_6H_5O_7 \longrightarrow$$
$$5MgHC_6H_5O_7 + 4CO_2 + 6H_2O$$

Since the solution offers a fairly good medium for mold growth, precautionary measures are taken in its preparation to retard this growth. During the manufacture, the solution is heated to boiling before filtration, the bottle into which it is to be filtered is rinsed with boiling purified water, and the filled bottle is stoppered with purified cotton during the cooling period which precedes the carbonation. These procedures do not produce sterility; however, they contribute to the stability of the solution.

According to the *N.F.* the stability of Magnesium Citrate Solution may be improved by pasteurizing or sterilizing the preparation. For solutions which are not intended to be sterilized, the stability may be improved by employing 30 Gm. of citric acid and a quantity of magnesium carbonate equivalent to 6.0 Gm. of magnesium oxide for each 350 ml. of the solution.

Specially prepared containers usually are used for the bottling of this solution. Most of those in use today are capped with the same type of stopper used in retaining the carbonated beverages on the market. It is directed that these bottles be kept lying on their sides so that the cork liners (or rubber liners) of the caps will be kept moist and swollen and thus be tight enough to retain the gas. The bottles should be stored in a cool place, preferably in a refrigerator, to protect them against spoilage. The *N.F.* directs that these bottles should contain not less than 340 ml. and not more than 360 ml., or not less than 195 ml. and not more than 205 ml.

Uses. Magnesium Citrate Solution long

has been one of the most popular of the saline cathartic preparations. Because of its carbonated, acidulous taste and its lemon flavor, it is pleasant to take, and usually can be administered to persons who object to the bitter taste of other saline cathartics. The magnesium acid citrate is said to be less irritant to the intestinal membrane than magnesium sulfate. The usual dose is 200 ml. (approximately 7 fluidounces).

POTASSIUM ARSENITE SOLUTION, N.F.

Fowler's Solution

Potassium Arsenite Solution contains, in each 100 ml., the equivalent of not less than 950 mg. and not more than 1.05 Gm. of As_2O_3.

Potassium Arsenite Solution was the first modern and generally recognized internal arsenic preparation. It was named Fowler's Solution after the English physician, Thomas Fowler, who first introduced it in the latter part of the 18th century as a substitute for the remedy known as "tasteless ague and fever drops."

The solution is prepared by boiling arsenic trioxide and potassium bicarbonate with a small amount of purified water until solution is effected, cooling the liquid, adding the alcohol, and diluting the product with sufficient purified water to make the desired volume. The arsenic trioxide is dissolved preferably in a concentrated solution of potassium bicarbonate so that the reaction will take place more rapidly. Alcohol is added as a preservative to prevent the development of fungus growths in the solution.

Although the chemical composition of Fowler's Solution is not known definitely, it seems quite likely that potassium meta-arsenite may be formed, as indicated by the following equations:

(1) $As_2O_3 + H_2O \rightarrow 2HAsO_2$
(2) $2HAsO_2 + 2KHCO_3 \rightarrow 2KAsO_2 + 2CO_2 + H_2O$

The solution is alkaline to litmus and shows the incompatibilities of the alkalies. A formerly official preparation, Arsenious Acid Solution or *Valangin's Solution,* contained the same amount of arsenic but was acid in reaction and was indicated in dispensing to overcome the incompatibilities of Fowler's Solution.

Uses. Potassium Arsenite Solution long has been used as an alterative. The *N.F.* classifies it as an antileukemic. It is also useful in certain types of chronic eczema and in psoriasis. The usual dose is 0.2 ml. (approximately 3 minims).

AMMONIACAL SILVER NITRATE SOLUTION, N.F.

Ammoniacal Silver Nitrate, Howe

Ammoniacal Silver Nitrate Solution is a solution of silver diammino nitrate containing, in each 100 Gm., the equivalent of not less than 28.5 Gm. and not more than 30.5 Gm. of Ag and not less than 9.0 Gm. and not more than 9.7 Gm. of NH_3.

The official preparation is made by adding strong ammonia solution to a solution of silver nitrate until all but the last trace of black precipitate is dissolved, and filtering the product. When the two reactants are mixed, a black precipitate of silver oxide is formed. This precipitate dissolves in an excess of ammonium hydroxide to form a silver ammonium complex called silver diammino nitrate, $Ag(NH_3)_2NO_3$. Attention is called to the fact that the term *ammino* used in the naming of this compound refers to ammonia and not to amine as in the case of the *amino* compounds.

The solution should be stored in small, glass-stoppered, light-resistant containers, or in light-resistant ampuls.

Uses. Ammoniacal Silver Nitrate Solution is classified as a dental protective. It is used by dentists to deposit silver on exposed dentin and to fill up minute crevices in the teeth. For topical application, it is mixed with a reducing agent, such as formaldehyde (1 in 10) or eugenol, to deposit the metallic silver, in a state of fine subdivision, in the desired area of the tooth.

COMPOUND SODIUM BORATE SOLUTION, N.F.

Dobell's Solution

Compound Sodium Borate Solution contains, in each 100 ml., not less than 250 mg.

and not more than 310 mg. of phenol (C_6H_6O).

The solution is prepared by dissolving sodium borate and sodium bicarbonate in water, adding the glycerin and the liquefied phenol, allowing the liquid to react until effervescence ceases, and adding sufficient purified water to make the required volume.

The nature of the reaction which takes place during the manufacture of this solution is not known definitely. One explanation assumes that the borax is decomposed by glycerin to form a glyceroboric acid which reacts with the sodium bicarbonate to produce an effervescence. The following equations represent these reactions:

(1) $Na_2B_4O_7 \cdot 10H_2O + 4C_3H_5(OH)_3 \rightarrow 2C_3H_5(OH)NaBO_3 + 2C_3H_5(OH)HBO_3 + 13H_2O$

(2) $2C_3H_5(OH)HBO_3 + 2NaHCO_3 \rightarrow 2C_3H_5(OH)NaBO_3 + 2CO_2 + 2H_2O$

According to another explanation, a concentrated aqueous solution of borax behaves as if it contained sodium metaborate, free boric acid, and a small amount of caustic alkali. Consequently, the reaction might be shown as follows:

(1) $Na_2B_4O_7 \cdot 10H_2O + 2C_3H_5(OH)_3 \rightarrow 2NaBO_2 + 2C_3H_5BO_3 + 3H_2O$

(2) $2C_3H_5BO_3 + 6H_2O \rightarrow 2C_3H_5(OH)_3 + 2H_3BO_3$

(3) $2H_3BO_3 + 2NaHCO_3 \rightarrow 2NaBO_2 + 2CO_2 + 4H_2O$

Uses. Dobell's solution is used as a nonirritant wash for mucous membranes. It has been very popular as a mouthwash and a throat gargle. It is used undiluted on mucous membranes. For the dental spray bottle, it is diluted with 5 volumes of water.

SODIUM HYPOCHLORITE SOLUTION, N.F.

Sodium Hypochlorite Solution contains not less than 4 and not more than 6 per cent of NaClO.

No method of manufacture is described for this solution, but now it is produced in very large quantities by the electrolysis of a cold dilute solution of common salt.

The official preparation has replaced the former chlorinated soda solution which was known as Labarraque's solution. This was prepared from monohydrated sodium carbonate and chlorinated lime. The resulting product was about half the strength of the present solution, and it was much more alkaline in reaction. The *N.F.* directs that, if Labarraque's solution is ordered, Sodium Hypochlorite Solution, diluted with an equal volume of water, is to be dispensed.

Commercially, the solution is available under various trade names, such as Clorox and Hyclorite.

Uses. The solution is a valuable germicide, deodorant and bleaching agent. It is very useful in the disinfection of utensils of all kinds which are not injured by its bleaching action. It may be diluted with 4 parts of water and used as a foot bath for prophylaxis against ringworm, athlete's foot and other skin diseases. *The N.F. cautions that this solution is not suitable for application to wounds.*

DILUTED SODIUM HYPOCHLORITE SOLUTION, N.F.

Modified Dakin's Solution

Diluted Sodium Hypochlorite Solution is a solution of chlorine compounds of sodium containing, in each 100 ml., not less than 450 mg. and not more than 500 mg. of NaClO.

This solution is prepared by diluting Sodium Hypochlorite Solution with purified water until its strength is within the official limitations. Sodium bicarbonate is added during the dilution process in a 5 per cent solution until no red color develops when 20 ml. of the sodium hypochlorite solution is shaken with 20 mg. of powdered phenolphthalein. The sodium bicarbonate reduces the hydroxyl ion concentration of the solution by reacting with the hydroxyl ions to form carbonate ions and un-ionized water ($HCO_3^- + OH^- \rightarrow CO_3^= + H_2O$). The resulting solution is not sufficiently alkaline to color powdered phenolphthalein. Although the alkalinity of the solution must be reduced, the product should possess a faintly alkaline reaction in order that it may best exert its therapeutic action.

The solution formerly was assayed in terms of its available chlorine content. The term "available chlorine" indicates the amount of chlorine that can be liberated from a chlorine-containing compound or solution through its oxidizing action; it does not refer to the amount of chlorine existing in molecular combination. Each molecule of sodium hypochlorite is capable of liberating 1 atom of nascent oxygen, which, in turn, is capable of liberating 2 atoms of chlorine from an acid solution containing a chloride. If acetic acid were used to produce the acid solution, the relationship would be shown by the following equations:

(1) $NaClO \rightarrow NaCl + (O)$

(2) $(O) + 2NaCl + 2CH_3COOH \rightarrow 2(Cl) + 2CH_3COONa + H_2O$

Thus, 1 molecule of sodium hypochlorite is capable of liberating 2 atoms of "available chlorine." This makes the "available chlorine" of sodium hypochlorite about 95.5 per cent and explains why there is little difference in the strength of Dakin's Solution whether it is expressed in terms of sodium hypochlorite or as "available chlorine."

Uses. Diluted Sodium Hypochlorite Solution is used as a surgical disinfectant. It is of greatest value in the irrigation of infected wounds, particularly when they are deep and suppurative. It also is useful in irrigating internal cavities, as the bladder. It may be used undiluted, or diluted with from 1 to 4 parts of water.

SOLUTIONS PREPARED BY SIMPLE SOLUTION WITH STERILIZATION

ANTICOAGULANT AND PHYSIOLOGIC SOLUTIONS

Anticoagulant Acid Citrate Dextrose Solution, U.S.P.

A. C. D. Solution

Anticoagulant Acid Citrate Dextrose Solution is a sterile solution of citric acid, sodium citrate and dextrose in water for injection. It contains not less than 95 per cent and not more than 105 per cent of the labeled amounts of citric acid, sodium citrate and dextrose. It contains no bacteriostatic agents.

Two formulas for the solution are given by the *U.S.P.* Solution A contains 7.3 Gm. of citric acid, 22 Gm. of sodium citrate, 24.5 Gm. of dextrose in sufficient water for injection to make 1,000 ml. Solution B contains 4.4 Gm. of citric acid, 13.2 Gm. of sodium citrate, 14.7 Gm. of dextrose in sufficient water for injection to make 1,000 ml. The solution is made by dissolving the salts in water for injection and filtering the product until it is clear. The prepared solution is immediately placed in suitable containers and sterilized, preferably by autoclaving.

The *U.S.P.* states that either 15 ml. of Solution A or 25 ml. of Solution B will provide the several ingredients in approximately the same ratio when added to 100 ml. of blood. An intermediate volume of anticoagulant solution may be used, provided that the formula is adjusted so as to maintain the same ratio between the components and each 100 ml. of blood. The preparation must be labeled to indicate the number of milliliters of it required per 100 ml. of blood.

Uses. A.C.D. Solution is used as an anticoagulant for the storage of whole blood. It maintains the functional capacity of whole blood for a longer period of time than does Anticoagulant Sodium Citrate Solution. The dextrose in the formula aids in preventing hemolysis of red blood cells.

Anticoagulant Sodium Citrate Solution, U.S.P.

Anticoagulant Sodium Citrate Solution is a sterile solution of sodium citrate in water for injection and contains, in each 100 ml., not less than 3.80 Gm. and not more than 4.20 Gm. of sodium citrate. It contains no bacteriostatic agents.

The solution is prepared by dissolving 4 per cent of sodium citrate in water for injection and filtering until clear. Then it should be placed in suitable containers and sterilized, preferably by autoclaving.

Uses. The solution is used as an anticoagulant for plasma and for blood for fractionation. It prevents the clotting of blood by combining with serum calcium ions to form nonionizing calcium citrate. It is used in the proportion of 50 ml. to 500 ml. of normal plasma of blood.

Ringer's Solution, N.F.

Ringer's Solution No. 1 (U.S.P. XIV)

Ringer's Solution is an isotonic solution of 3 chlorides containing, in each 100 ml., not less than 820 mg. and not more than 900 mg. of sodium chloride, not less than 25 mg. and not more than 35 mg. of potassium chloride, and not less than 30 mg. and not more than 36 mg. of calcium chloride.

The solution is prepared by dissolving the 3 salts in recently boiled purified water and filtering the product until it is clear. Although the preparation of this solution does not include sterilization, it is discussed here because it is classified as a physiologic solution, and, as such, it is frequently sterilized when used for irrigating purposes.

Three forms of Ringer's Solution—nonsterile; sterile, but not for parenteral use; and sterile for parenteral use—were officially recognized in the *U.S.P. XIV.* Since the sterile form is now classified as an injection, and since the presently official form is not required to be a sterile preparation, the following caution appears in the *N.F.* monograph: *"Do not use Ringer's Solution for parenteral administration or in preparations to be used parenterally. For such purposes use Ringer's Injection, U.S.P. XVI."*

Uses. Ringer's Solution is a physiologic salt solution and is used as a solvent for medicinal substances which are to be applied topically to delicate tissues. It is also employed for the irrigation of body cavities and, when used for this purpose, a sterile, but not a pyrogen-free, solution would be preferred.

Sodium Chloride Solution, U.S.P.

Sodium Chloride Solution is a sterile solution of sodium chloride in purified water. It contains, in each 100 ml., not less than 850 mg. and not more than 950 mg. of sodium chloride.

The solution is prepared by dissolving 9 Gm. of sodium chloride in sufficient purified water to make 1,000 ml. Then it is filtered until clear, placed in suitable containers and sterilized. Although no process is specified for sterilizing the solution, autoclaving is the preferred method.

Since the solution is not suitable for use by injection, the *U.S.P.* gives the following caution: *"Do not use Sodium Chloride Solution for parenteral administration or in preparations to be used parenterally. For such purposes use Sodium Chloride Injection."*

Uses. The *U.S.P.* categorizes this preparation as a physiologic salt solution. It is an isotonic solution frequently employed as a wash for delicate membranes or for exposed tissue. It is used commonly as a solvent for medications that are intended to be applied topically.

OPHTHALMIC SOLUTIONS

Antazoline Phosphate Ophthalmic Solution, N.F.

Antazoline Phosphate Ophthalmic Solution contains not less than 95 per cent and not more than 105 per cent of the labeled amount of antazoline phosphate.

A 0.5 per cent sterile, isotonic solution of antazoline phosphate is marketed under the name Antistine Ophthalmic Solution.

Uses. It is an antihistaminic ophthalmic solution intended for the symptomatic relief of certain conditions of the eye resulting from allergies.

Benoxinate Hydrochloride Ophthalmic Solution, U.S.P.

Benoxinate Hydrochloride Ophthalmic Solution is a sterile solution of benoxinate hydrochloride in water rendered isotonic by the addition of sodium chloride. It contains not less than 0.38 per cent and not more than 0.42 per cent of benoxinate hydrochloride, calculated on the dried basis. It may contain a small proportion of alcohol.

Benoxinate hydrochloride, a benzoic acid ester related to procaine, is an effective surface anesthetic useful in ophthalmology. It also has bacteriostatic properties. The commercial counterpart of the official product is marketed as a 0.4 per cent solution under the trade-mark name Dorsacaine Hydrochloride Ophthalmic Solution.

Uses. The solution is administered by topical instillation into the eye as a prompt-acting corneal anesthetic of short duration. It is useful in certain short operative procedures involving the eye and the conjunctiva.

Cyclopentolate Hydrochloride Ophthalmic Solution, U.S.P.

Cyclopentolate Hydrochloride Ophthalmic Solution is a solution of cyclopentolate hydrochloride in a buffered, isotonic, aqueous medium. It contains not less than 95 per cent and not more than 105 per cent of the labeled amount of cyclopentolate hydrochloride.

The official product is available commercially under the name Cyclogyl as a sterile solution containing 0.5 or 1.0 per cent of cyclopentolate hydrochloride, Gifford's Buffer and benzalkonium chloride. The solution is stable at room temperature and does not require refrigeration.

Uses. The preparation is a cycloplegic and mydriatic ophthalmic solution. It has been suggested for routine office use to prepare the eye for refraction when fitting glasses. It may be used in certain pathologic conditions of the eye, such as iritis and keratitis.

Epinephrine Bitartrate Ophthalmic Solution, N.F.

Epinephrine Bitartrate Ophthalmic Solution is a solution containing 2 Gm. each of epinephrine bitartrate and boric acid in a sufficient quantity of purified water to make 100 ml. The *N.F.* directs that the solution should be freshly prepared as required.

As an ophthalmic solution, this preparation must be sterile and should contain a preservative if dispensed in multiple-dose containers. Although no specific method is recommended for its sterilization, bacterial filtration is the method of choice because of the instability of the epinephrine. Phenylethyl alcohol or chlorobutanol are suitable preservatives.

Uses. Epinephrine Bitartrate Ophthalmic Solution is a mydriatic. It may be used in the treatment of chronic simple glaucoma because of the ability of epinephrine bitartrate to reduce intra-ocular tension.

Fluorescein Sodium Ophthalmic Solution U.S.P.

Fluorescein Sodium Ophthalmic Solution is a sterile, buffered solution containing, in each 100 ml., not less than 1.86 Gm. and not more than 2.10 Gm. of fluorescein sodium. It contains a suitable antibacterial agent, and it may contain 3 per cent of sodium bicarbonate.

The solution may be prepared by dissolving 2 Gm. of fluorescein sodium, 3 Gm. of sodium bicarbonate and a suitable antibacterial agent in sufficient sterile distilled water to make 100 ml. The sodium bicarbonate is added to buffer the solution at an alkaline pH, at which the fluorescein is more stable. Fluorescein Sodium Ophthalmic Solution must be dispensed in sterile, single-use containers or be used in the form of sterile, impregnated paper strips which release a sufficient amount of the drug for diagnostic purposes when touched to the eye (see monograph on Ophthalmic Solutions in the *U.S.P.*).

Uses. The preparation is used as an ophthalmologic diagnostic solution for the purpose of disclosing corneal injuries and ulcers. The dye will penetrate any ruptures of the cornea and outline them with a distinctly green color so that they can be identified and studied more easily.

Isoflurophate Ophthalmic Solution, U.S.P.

Isoflurophate Ophthalmic Solution is a sterile solution of isoflurophate in a suitable oil. It contains not less than 0.09 per cent and not more than 0.11 per cent of isoflurophate.

The label of the solution must bear the expiration date which is not more than 2 years after the date of manufacture. Isoflurophate or di-isopropyl flurophosphate is sometimes referred to as DFP and is marketed under the name Floropryl as a 0.1 per cent sterile solution in peanut oil.

Uses. This solution is a powerful parasympathomimetic cholinergic and is used primarily in the treatment of glaucoma.

PHENIRAMINE MALEATE OPHTHALMIC SOLUTION, N.F.

Prophenpyridamine Maleate Ophthalmic Solution

Pheniramine Maleate Ophthalmic Solution contains not less than 90 per cent and not more than 110 per cent of the labeled amount of pheniramine maleate.

This solution is a clear, colorless liquid having a pH range between 4.5 and 5.2.

Trimeton Maleate Ophthalmic Solution, the commercial counterpart of the official preparation, is available as a 0.5 per cent aqueous solution.

Uses. Pheniramine Maleate Ophthalmic Solution is used for the relief of ocular symptoms of an allergic origin, such as occur with hay fever.

SILVER NITRATE OPHTHALMIC SOLUTION, U.S.P.

Liquor Argenti Nitratis Ophthalmicus

Silver Nitrate Ophthalmic Solution is a solution of silver nitrate in a buffered water medium. It contains, in each 100 ml., not less than 0.95 Gm. and not more than 1.05 Gm. of silver nitrate. It may contain sodium acetate as a buffer.

Although this preparation should be classified more properly with those made by simple solution without sterilization, it is discussed here because of its use.

The U.S.P. directs that the solution be protected from light and preserved in single-dose inert wax-composition capsules or in other suitable containers. It is usually available in wax containers, formerly known as wax ampuls, containing about five drops of the solution.

Uses. Silver Nitrate Ophthalmic Solution is used primarily for the prevention of gonococcic infections in the eyes of newborn infants. For this purpose, a few drops of the 1 per cent solution are placed in the conjunctival sac of the newborn. The solution is washed out immediately with isotonic saline solution. Failure to use an anti-infective in the eyes of the newborn infant may allow the transmission of gonococci from an infected mother. Since there is some inherent danger in the improper use of silver nitrate solution, it is probable that other anti-infective agents, such as the antibiotics, would be employed for this purpose if state laws would permit their use.

SULFACETAMIDE SODIUM OPHTHALMIC SOLUTION, U.S.P.

Sulfacetamide Sodium Solution (U.S.P. XV); Liquor Sulfacetamidi Sodici Ophthalmicus

Sulfacetamide Sodium Ophthalmic Solution is a sterile solution containing, in each 100 ml., not less than 28.5 Gm. and not more than 31.5 Gm. of sulfacetamide sodium. It may contain suitable buffers, stabilizers and preservatives.

The preparation is available commercially under the trade-mark name Sulamyd Sodium Solution. Since sulfacetamide sodium is highly soluble at a slightly alkaline pH, the official product represents a highly concentrated solution of sulfonamide, having a pH of about 7.4. The solution should be refrigerated and protected from light. On long standing, solutions may darken in color and should be discarded.

Uses. It is used topically in the eye for bacterial infections that are susceptible to sulfonamide therapy.

SULFISOXAZOLE DIETHANOLAMINE OPHTHALMIC SOLUTION, U.S.P.

Sulfisoxazole Diethanolamine Ophthalmic Solution is a sterile solution of sulfisoxazole diethanolamine in a suitable, aqueous medium. It contains, in each 100 ml., an amount of sulfisoxazole diethanolamine equivalent to not less than 3.6 Gm. and not more than 4.4 Gm. of sulfisoxazole.

The official preparation is available under the trade-mark name Gantrisin Ophthalmic Solution. It is a sterile, isotonic solution, having a physiologic pH and containing 4 per cent of Gantrisin, a brand of sulfisoxazole, in the form of its diethanolamine salt. The solution should not be used with silver preparations.

Uses. Sulfisoxazole Diethanolamine Ophthalmic Solution is a sulfonamide preparation having a wide antibacterial spectrum.

It is used in external eye infections that are due to susceptible micro-organisms. The usual precautions in sulfonamide therapy should be observed.

OPHTHALMIC SOLUTIONS PREPARED FROM STERILE OPHTHALMIC POWDERS

Chloramphenicol for Ophthalmic Solution, U.S.P.

Chloramphenicol for Ophthalmic Solution is a sterile, dry mixture of chloramphenicol with a suitable buffer. It contains not less than 85 per cent of the labeled amount of chloramphenicol.

The official powder is commercially available as Chloromycetin Ophthalmic. It contains 25 mg. of chloramphenicol, together with a borate buffer equivalent to 100 mg. of boric acid. The solution is prepared extemporaneously by adding sterile distilled water to the powder in sufficient quantity to make a product containing 0.16, 0.25, or 0.5 per cent of chloramphenicol. A solution prepared in this manner remains stable at room temperature for 10 days.

Uses. Chloramphenicol Ophthalmic Solution is an antibiotic preparation for topical use in the treatment of bacterial conjunctivitis.

Ophthalmic Chlortetracycline Hydrochloride, N.F.

Ophthalmic Chlortetracycline Hydrochloride is a sterile, dry mixture of chlortetracycline with a suitable buffer. It contains not less than 85 per cent of the labeled amount of chlortetracycline hydrochloride. It may contain suitable bacteriostatic agents and diluents.

The commercial counterpart of the official preparation is available as Aureomycin Ophthalmic Powder, Sterilized, and contains 25 mg. of chlortetracycline hydrochloride combined with sodium chloride and sodium borate. The powder is dissolved, under aseptic conditions, in 5 ml. of sterile distilled water, and the resulting solution is dispensed with the sterilized dropper that is provided. When stored under refrigeration, the solution remains stable for 2 days.

Uses. Chlortetracycline hydrochloride is an antibiotic. In a buffered aqueous solution it is used locally in the eye for the treatment of a variety of ocular viral and bacterial infections.

Ophthalmic Oxytetracycline Hydrochloride, N.F.

Ophthalmic Oxytetracycline Hydrochloride is a sterile mixture of oxytetracycline hydrochloride with a suitable buffer and/or bacteriostatic agent. It contains not less than 90 per cent of the labeled amount of oxytetracycline hydrochloride.

Commercially, this ophthalmic powder is marketed as Terramycin Hydrochloride Ophthalmic. It is a dry mixture containing 25 mg. of oxytetracycline hydrochloride and a sodium borate–sodium chloride buffer. The dry powder may be stored at room temperature for 12 months without a significant loss of potency. The solution which is prepared by dissolving the powder in 5 ml. of sterile distilled water is isotonic with tear fluid and is buffered to a pH of 8.2. It remains stable for 48 hours if stored in a refrigerator.

Uses. Oxytetracycline Hydrochloride Ophthalmic Solution may be used locally in the eye for the treatment of ocular infections caused by a wide range of pathogens.

Tetracycline Hydrochloride for Ophthalmic Solution, U.S.P.

Tetracycline Hydrochloride for Ophthalmic Solution is a sterile, dry mixture of tetracycline hydrochloride and one or more suitable buffers. It may contain one or more suitable preservatives and diluents. It contains not less than 85 per cent of the labeled amount of tetracycline hydrochloride.

The official product is available under the trade-mark name Achromycin Ophthalmic Powder, Sterilized. It contains 25 mg. of tetracycline hydrochloride mixed with sodium chloride and sodium borate. The commercial package consists of a bottle of powder and a sterilized dropper bottle. The solution is prepared just before using by dissolving the powder aseptically in 5 ml. of sterile distilled water and is dispensed with the sterilized dropper. If stored in a refrigerator, the solution remains stable for 2 days.

Uses. Tetracycline Hydrochloride Ophthalmic Solution is an antibiotic preparation for topical application in the treatment of ocular infections caused by certain gram-positive and gram-negative organisms.

SOLUTIONS PREPARED BY EXTRACTION

EPINEPHRINE SOLUTION, U.S.P.

Epinephrine Solution 1:1,000; Liquor Epinephrinae

Epinephrine Solution is a solution of epinephrine in purified water prepared with the aid of hydrochloric acid. It contains in each 100 ml., not less than 90 mg. and not more than 115 mg. of epinephrine.

No official method is given for the preparation of this solution, because the method used is highly technical and is not adapted to small-scale production. The solution may be prepared directly from the suprarenal glands of animals, or prepared by simple solution of synthetic epinephrine hydrochloride.

The preparation from adrenal glands involves maceration, at about 70°, of the finely chopped glands with acidulated water. After the resulting solution is heated to about 90° to coagulate albuminoids, it is expressed. Then the expressed liquid is freed from fat, concentrated *in vacuo* and further purified by the addition of alcohol, which precipitates inert constituents. Ammonia then is added to precipitate the epinephrine, which is purified and dissolved in a dilute hydrochloric acid solution. The final solution is adjusted to the official strength.

When the epinephrine is prepared synthetically, it is simply dissolved in water in the form of the hydrochloride.

Epinephrine Solution was first marketed and is still distributed widely under the trade-mark name Adrenalin Chloride Solution. Commercial samples of the solution usually contain an antioxidant such as sodium bisulfite and a preservative such as chlorobutanol.

The solution must be protected from light and air and from contact with metals and oxidizing agents. It should be preserved in small, well-filled, light-resistant, tight containers. The *U.S.P.* notes that it should not be dispensed if it becomes brown in color or if it contains a precipitate.

Uses. Epinephrine is used as a vasoconstrictor to increase blood pressure, to prevent hemorrhage and to prolong the action of local anesthetics. It is a heart stimulant. The solution is used as a stimulant to smooth muscles in the relief of asthma, catarrh and other congestive conditions by local application. It frequently is diluted to concentrations of 1:5,000 to 1:10,000.

LIVER SOLUTION, N.F.

Liquid Liver Extract

Liver Solution is a brownish liquid containing that soluble thermostable fraction of mammalian livers which increases the number of red blood corpuscles in the blood of persons affected with pernicious anemia. Liver Solution contains folic acid and vitamin B_{12} activity. The approximate antianemia potency of Liver Solution in pernicious anemia is expressed in N.F. units (oral). The solution conforms to all other requirements under *Antianemia Preparations*. It customarily contains a suitable preservative, which must be identified on the label.

Since the solution does not lend itself to production on a small scale and in view of the different modifications of the fundamental extraction process that may be used commercially, no official method is given for its manufacture. Briefly, its preparation involves the extraction of fresh liver with a suitable aqueous solvent and purification of the resultant extract. The purified extract must be preserved by the addition of not more than 25 per cent, by volume, of alcohol, or not more than 40 per cent, by volume, of glycerin. The solution should be stored in tight, light-resistant containers.

Uses. Liver Solution is used in the treatment of pernicious anemia. It is intended for the oral administration of liver and should not be confused with the purified solution which is official as Liver Injection.

UNOFFICIAL SOLUTIONS

Title	Description, Preparation and Use
Chloroazodin Solution, N.F. X	A clear, yellow, somewhat oily liquid having a slightly fatty odor and a bitter taste. It is prepared by dissolving 2.6 Gm. of chloroazodin in sufficient glyceryl triacetate (triacetin) to make 1,000 ml. **Use.** Surgical antiseptic.
Compound Dimethyl Phthalate Solution, U.S.P. XV *622 Mixture*	A solution containing 20 per cent by weight each of ethohexadiol and butopyronoxyl in 60 per cent by weight of dimethyl phthalate. **Use.** Topically, to skin and clothing, as an insect repellant.
Diluted Lead Subacetate Solution, N.F. X *Lead Water*	A colorless, slightly turbid liquid having a sweet, astringent taste. It is prepared by diluting 35 ml. of lead subacetate solution with sufficient recently boiled purified water to make 1,000 ml. **Use.** Topically, as an astringent.
Ammonium Acetate Solution, N.F. X *Spirit of Mindererus*	A clear, colorless liquid having a mildly saline, acidulous taste. It is prepared by dissolving 50 Gm. of ammonium carbonate, in hard, translucent pieces, in sufficient diluted acetic acid to make 1,000 ml. The solution should be recently prepared. **Uses.** Diuretic and diaphoretic.
Iron and Ammonium Acetate Solution, N.F. X *Basham's Mixture*	A clear, reddish-brown liquid having an aromatic odor and an acid reaction. It is prepared by adding to 500 ml. of ammonium acetate solution, 60 ml. of diluted acetic acid, 40 ml. of ferric chloride tincture, 120 ml. each of aromatic elixir and glycerin, and sufficient purified water to make 1,000 ml. The preparation must not be dispensed unless it has been recently prepared or previously stabilized by the addition of 1 Gm. of tartaric acid to each liter. **Use.** Hematinic.
Lead Subacetate Solution, N.F. X *Goulard's Extract*	A clear, colorless, odorless liquid, having a very sweet, astringent taste. It is prepared by reacting lead acetate and lead monoxide to form lead subacetate. **Use.** Astringent, usually diluted with 4 volumes of recently boiled purified water.

BIBLIOGRAPHY

American Medical Association, Council on Drugs: New and Nonofficial Drugs, Philadelphia, Lippincott, 1959.

Amsden, J. P.: Physical Chemistry for Premedical Students, New York, McGraw-Hill, 1950.

Burger, A.: Medicinal Chemistry, New York, Interscience, 1951.

Goodman, L., and Gilman, A.: The Pharmacological Basis of Therapeutics, New York, Macmillan, 1958.

Jenkins, G. L., Hartung, W. H., Hamlin, K. E., Jr., and Data, J. B.: The Chemistry of Organic Medicinal Products, ed. 4, New York, Wiley, 1957.

Osol, A., and Farrar, G. E., Jr.: The Dispensatory of the United States of America, ed. 25, Philadelphia, Lippincott, 1955.

Polano, M. K.: Skin Therapeutics Prescription and Preparation, New York, Elsevier, 1952.

Soine, T. O., and Wilson, C. O.: Rogers' Inorganic Pharmaceutical Chemistry, Philadelphia, Lea and Febiger, 1957.

Wooton, A. C.: Chronicles of Pharmacy, Vol. II, London, Macmillan, 1910.

JOSEPH BARNETT SPROWLS, Jr., Ph.D.
Dean, Temple University School of Pharmacy

12

Parenteral Preparations

HISTORICAL
ADVANTAGES AND USES OF PARENTERALS
GENERAL CONSIDERATIONS
PREPARATION OF INJECTIONS
LIST OF OFFICIAL PARENTERALS

Parenteral preparations (also called simply *parenterals*) are those sterile drugs, solutions, or suspensions which are packaged in a manner suitable for administration by hypodermic injection either in the form in which prepared or after addition of a suitable solvent or suspending agent. While the term "parenteral" may be interpreted literally as meaning administration by any means other than through the intestine (from para, "beside," and enteron, "bowel"), common usage has limited it to those methods of administration which involve the use of the hypodermic needle: i.e., intracutaneous, subcutaneous, intramuscular, intraspinal, intravenous, etc. These avenues of drug administration have become so widely accepted that a numerous and varied list of preparations for such purpose are now included in the official compendia. Five forms are recognized, as follows:

1. Injections—solutions of medicaments prepared in a form suitable for injection. Example, Morphine Injection.
2. Sterile suspensions—solids suspended in a suitable medium which are intended for use other than by intravenous or intraspinal injection. Example, Sterile Epinephrine Suspension.
3. Sterile emulsions—fluids suspended in a suitable fluid medium and not intended for intraspinal administration. Example, Sterile Phytonadione Emulsion.
4. Dry solids which, upon the addition of suitable solvents, yield solutions conforming in all respects to the requirements for Injections. Example, Tetracycline Hydrochloride for Injection.
5. Dry solids which, upon the addition of suitable vehicles, yield preparations conforming in all respects to the requirements for Sterile Suspensions. Example, Sterile Penicillin-Dihydrostreptomycin for Suspension.

The subject matter relating to parenteral preparations has become so voluminous as to defy adequate review in a single introductory chapter; hence, this discussion will be confined to a consideration of general technics utilized in the preparation of parenterals, a listing of official injections and sterile suspensions, and brief notes regarding special technics or requirements which are of significance.

HISTORICAL

Although the concept of administering medicines by injection through the skin has existed for centuries, the successful utilization of such a principle resulted primarily from the following 3 developments:

(1) Proof of the germ theory of disease and discovery of methods of producing

sterility (Pasteur, Koch, Lister et al. in the latter half of the 19th century);

(2) Introduction of the hypodermic syringe (invented by C. G. Pravez 1853, popularized by Drs. Alexander Wood and Charles Hunter 1853-55, and improved by Luer 1894*);

(3) Invention of the sealed-glass container for injections called the ampul (S. Limousin, 1886).

Thus, we find that the essential knowledge and technics necessary for the successful production of injectable dosage forms were available before the turn of the century; nevertheless, their adoption as acceptable forms of medication by books of standards has been quite recent. The *United States Dispensatory* of 1877 reported the class of Injections as "a new class of preparations which was, we think, very foolishly introduced among the addenda to the British Pharmacopoeia. On what grounds it was separated from the Liquors is hard to perceive." The *British Pharmacopoeia* of 1885 included monographs for injections which described their preparation by dissolving the active constituent in recently boiled distilled water. They were intended to be used immediately after preparation, and no instructions were included for preservation in sealed containers. Continental pharmacopoeias were much slower in giving even this degree of recognition to the new dosage form.

Parenteral preparations received first official acceptance in this country through the *National Formulary, Fifth Edition* (1926). Monographs were included in that standard for 7 ampuls (ampullae) which were described as "hermetically sealed containers which are filled with a medicinal liquid in a sterile condition, intended for parenteral use." The *Tenth Revision* of the *United States Pharmacopoeia* of the same date included a chapter on sterilization but no monographs for individual ampuls. The monograph for Physiological Saline Solution in the same revision required that the product be sterilized by autoclaving. Quite obviously, the preparation was intended for parenteral use even though its title does not

* As reported in *Source Book of Medical History*, Clendenning, Paul B. Hoeber, Inc., New York, 1942.

suggest such purpose. By contrast, the *Sixteenth Revision* of the *Pharmacopeia* includes 135 injections, sterile suspensions, sterile emulsions and sterile products for injection. The only preparation for which the title "Ampul" has been retained is Iodine Ampuls, N.F., which contains Iodine Tincture in sealed containers. These are intended to be broken and the liquid applied topically for the emergency disinfection of cuts or wounds.

Early in the 20th century, physicians began to complain of undesirable reactions which were often observed following use of the then crudely prepared injections. The following statement is abstracted from an article appearing in the *British Medical Journal* of 1911: Hort and Peafold of the Lister Institute have shown that distilled water which is allowed to stand in sealed sterile containers and subsequently used as an infusion gives rise to toxic symptoms, the cause of which has not been fully explained. Similar symptoms are not observed if recently freshly distilled water is employed.[1] This is an early observation of the existence of *pyrogens,* or fever-producing substances, which are carefully guarded against in modern preparations. While their existence has not yet been explained fully, it is commonly accepted that pyrogens are polysaccharides which result from bacterial growth and may remain in a solution after the bacteria have been filtered off.[2] They may be related to bacterial antigens, even though there seems to be no direct relationship between their development and the pathogenicity of contaminating organisms.

The use of preservatives in injectable forms began at an early date. Dr. E. R. Squibb recommended in 1873 that parenteral solutions be preserved by the addition of 1/6 of 1 per cent of carbolic acid. Other writers suggested the use of salicylic acid or chloroform. The latter was to be included by substituting chloroform water for distilled water as the solvent.[3]

ADVANTAGES AND USES OF PARENTERALS

Parenteral therapy offers several notable advantages over other modes of administration, and many of the special uses are related to these same features. Because the gastrointestinal tract is avoided, it is possible to introduce by this means drugs which might not survive exposure to the digestive fluids. Hormonal and antibiotic drugs are prominent in this group, as will be found by examining the list of official preparations. Since there is very little loss of time for absorption, when intravenous or subcutaneous injections are involved, these routes are generally selected for emergency drugs. Injections such as Levarteranol Bitartrate and Epinephrine are merely two of the examples which might be selected from this group. On the other hand, the routes of administration are so flexible that it is possible to use the parenteral route for long-acting medication. In such a case, oil solutions or suspensions are given by deep intramuscular injection. Thickening agents may be added to further prolong the time of action. Examples of such preparations are Repository Corticotropin Injection, Sterile Procaine Penicillin Suspension and Procaine Penicillin in Oil Injection.

The parenteral routes of administration are available even though the patient be unconscious or otherwise incapable of cooperating. A rather familiar sight today is the patient who has been seriously injured in an accident or has undergone surgery recently and is receiving plasma or other physiologic fluid by intravenous drip or hypodermoclysis. These procedures are used to restore fluid, glucose, and electrolyte balance which have been lost to the blood stream as a result of shock or severe bleeding. Such injections as Dextrose, Dextrose and Sodium Chloride and Ringer's are only a few of the many preparations of this type which are official.

It is possible, in some instances, to localize the action of a drug by injecting it adjacent to the tissue with which it is expected to react. This is the principle which is used in producing a nerve block by use of a local anesthetic drug. The solution is injected near the trunk of a nerve in order to produce a nerve "block," as in dental surgery.

Finally, injection procedures lend themselves to exact regulation of dosage because essentially all of the drug must enter the circulatory system in order to be eliminated. This provides an avenue for the administration of diagnostic agents such as those used in the estimation of blood volume, kidney function or other physiologic "rates."

Parenteral forms are not without disadvantage. Perhaps chief of these is the psychic fear which most people have of the hypodermic needle. Increased cost of medication is another factor. It is considerably more expensive to market a drug in the form of an injection rather than as a tablet or a capsule. Obviously, injectables require much more care in handling than do the simpler dosage forms. Finally, they may not be administered without the use of specialized equipment, and the methods of administration require specialized training.

GENERAL CONSIDERATIONS

It is apparent that substances which are to be introduced beneath the protective epidermis of the body must be free from sources of irritation as well as from infective organisms. For this reason, the preparation of parenterals involves not only a high degree of skill but also the exercise of constant supervision and the application of every practicable method of control. Consideration must be given to the following major factors:

1. **Solubility and compatibility of ingredients** so that no particulate matter or irritant by-products will be present or develop during storage.

2. **Hydrogen-ion concentration and osmotic pressure** so that the material will be biologically compatible with the tissue into which it is to be injected. In small volume injections, these considerations may be of minor importance; in large volume injections, they are critical. The blood can easily neutralize small volumes of injection which are not isotonic or isohydronic, but large volumes of such injections may cause fatal reactions.

3. **Complete freedom from particulate matter**, except in the case of sterile suspensions or emulsions. In sterile emulsions and injections, the condition and the size of particles must be controlled carefully so that they will not agglomerate. Such prepa-

rations generally may not be injected intravenously because of the danger of causing intravascular clotting, and they may not be injected into the spinal canal.

4. **Complete sterility** as nearly as can be determined by adequate control methods. Where sterility cannot be assured by adequate use of heat, maximum safeguards against development of bacterial growth (chemical disinfectants) must be added.

5. **Freedom from pyrogens**

6. **Compatibility of medication with container** (ampul glass) and, in the case of vials, with closure (usually rubber or plastic).

Control of these factors has made it increasingly difficult to manufacture injectables on a small scale. For this reason, their preparation is now carried out in the United States primarily by large manufacturing concerns, a few specialty manufacturers, and a limited number of adequately staffed and equipped hospital pharmacies.

PREPARATION OF INJECTIONS

In the discussion to follow, descriptions of procedures, and statements of requirements will conform as nearly as possible with standards or recommendations set forth in the *Sixteenth Revision* of the *United States Pharmacopeia* and the *Eleventh Edition* of the *National Formulary*.

The stock solution is generally prepared by dissolving carefully weighed or measured quantities of drug in Water for Injection. Since the method of preparation and qualities of Water for Injection are described in Chapter 9, it is not necessary to duplicate them at this point. It is sufficient to say that this is a form of pyrogen-free distilled water which has been distilled recently and is reasonably free from bacterial contamination at the time of collection. Schedules are usually arranged so that the solution can be prepared, and ampuls or vials filled and ultimately sterilized within a few hours. This does not give enough time for pyrogens to be formed within the solution. If the Water for Injection cannot be used at once, it should be stored at temperatures above or below that at which bacterial growth occurs. Since the water coming from the still is quite warm, it is often convenient to keep it heated almost to the boiling point until the time comes for it to be used. Sodium Chloride may be added to the Water for Injection to render the resulting solution isotonic, or Sodium Chloride Injection or Ringer's Injection may be substituted in whole or in part for the Water for Injection unless an individual monograph does not permit.

In some instances, the official books permit other solvents than water to be used. For example, this is true of the barbiturate salt injections where the solvent is not specified. Sixty per cent of propylene glycol is the solvent generally used because this delays hydrolysis of the barbiturate. Every precaution is taken during the preparation period to avoid bacterial contamination of the solution; for, even though these would be removed during the sterilization process, their endotoxins, exotoxins and cellular proteins would remain in the solution and would be a possible cause of pyrogenic reaction. In most manufacturing laboratories, the entire parenteral area is separated from the other operative areas and is kept bacteria-free by use of ultraviolet lights, filtered air supplied under positive pressure, baffled doors and other measures. Employees working in these areas usually wear face masks, sterile gowns and hair covers.

When the ingredients have been dissolved, the solution is filtered carefully. This may be accomplished by using sintered glass, porcelain, or hard filter paper. It is considered that a pore diameter of less than 10 microns is required to give a high polish to a mobile aqueous liquid.[4] Then the filtered solution is placed in ampuls or vials as quickly as possible and before sufficient time has passed for the development of pyrogens (within one working day). If a preservative agent has been added, the solution may be stored under refrigeration for a brief period of time before ampulling.

In some companies, the container of solution is never taken from the preparation room to the filling room. In such instances, the liquid is conveyed through plastic or stainless steel lines directly from the preparation room to ampul-filling machines in the filling area. This reduces the amount of traffic between the preparation and the filling areas and helps to control the sterility of the filling room.

In the preparation of solutions for parenteral packaging, the same general principles apply as in preparing ordinary solutions with the following additional considerations:

1. Added substances must not be used in such quantity that they would produce irritation or excessive toxicity.

2. Many substances which could be added with safety to an oral preparation would be too toxic or irritant for hypodermic use.

The official compendia place limitations upon added substances as follows:

Other substances may be added to preparations for injection to increase stability or usefulness unless otherwise specified in the individual monograph. The added substance must be harmless in the amounts administered, and must not interfere with the therapeutic efficiency or the specified assays and tests. No coloring agent may be added solely for the purpose of coloring the finished preparation.

Specific limits are placed upon certain substances where not otherwise provided: Agents containing mercury and cationic surface-active compounds 0.01 per cent; chlorobutanol, cresol and phenol type 0.5 per cent; sulfur dioxide or an equivalent amount of sodium bisulfite or sodium sulfite 0.2 per cent.

Suitable preservative agents are added to preparations packaged in multi-dose containers, regardless of the method of sterilization and unless prohibited by a monograph or unless the active agent is itself bacteriostatic. Such substances, when added, must be in sufficient concentration to prevent the growth of, or kill micro-organisms. Sterilization procedures are employed even though such agents are present. Preservatives are specifically excluded in the large volume injections which are used to replace fluid, nutrients, or electrolytes, such as Dextrose and Sodium Chloride Injection, Dextrose Injection, Ringer's Injection, Lactated Ringer's Injection and Sodium Chloride Injection. Bacteriostatic agents may be added to Dextrose and Sodium Chloride Injection when it is labeled for use as a sclerosing agent, because when used for such purpose the amount of injection is small, and the quantity of germicide present would not be harmful to the patient.

Examples of substances added to official injections are presented in Table 9. In most instances the materials added are buffers or suitable bacteriostatic agents; however, some of the notable exceptions will be discussed. Epinephrine is often added to injections containing local anesthetic drugs in order to slow the absorption of the drug and prolong the anesthetic effect. Stabilizers are added to such injections as Calcium Gluconate Injection, U.S.P., in which the solution is supersaturated and crystallization must be prevented. Monocalcium disodium ethylenediaminetetra-acetate is the stabilizer used in such radiopaque injections as Sodium Acetrizoate Injection, U.S.P. In this instance the stabilizer is a chelating agent which exchanges its calcium ion for traces of heavy metal which may be present and thus hasten deterioration of the active ingredient.

Injections containing water-insoluble materials may be prepared by dissolving the drug in oil (if it is oil-soluble) or by reducing it to a very fine powder and suspending in a suitable liquid. The traditional fluid for use in suspensions is vegetable oil; however, aqueous suspensions are becoming increasingly popular. Generally speaking, suspensions are administered by deep intramuscular injection so that the material may be absorbed gradually. In preparing such suspensions, the drug may be reduced to a suitable degree of fineness by the use of a ball mill or more modern equipment such as the Micronizer, various colloid mills, or ultrasonic vibration. (See also Chap. 7, Colloids, Emulsions and Suspensions, and Chap. 15, Emulsions.) In the case of aqueous suspensions, it is sometimes possible to regulate the size of crystals which are formed so that they are microcrystalline and suitable for injection. Dispersing agents, such as alcohol or chloroform, may be useful in preparing suspensions in oil.

Aqueous suspensions or emulsions usually include a stabilizing agent. Such materials as partially hydrolyzed gelatin, lecithin,

TABLE 9. EXAMPLES OF OFFICIAL PARENTERALS CONTAINING ADDED SUBSTANCES

PREPARATION	ADDED SUBSTANCE/S	PURPOSE
Aminophylline Injection, U.S.P.	Freshly distilled ethylenediamine solution 60 mg. for each Gm. of aminophylline (optional)	Stabilize the solution
Ascorbic Acid Injection, U.S.P.	Sodium hydroxide, carbonate or bicarbonate	Convert ascorbic acid to soluble salt
Calcium Gluconate Injection, U.S.P.	Calcium D-saccharate or other suitable Ca salts. Ca content not to exceed 5% of Ca in gluconate. Sodium hydroxide to produce pH not above 8.2 (all optional)	Stabilize solution which is supersaturated with respect to Ca gluconate
Repository Corticotropin Injection, U.S.P.	Partially hydrolyzed gelatin; suitable antibacterial agent (latter optional)	To delay absorption of corticotropin
Digitoxin Injection, U.S.P.	5 to 50% alcohol; glycerin or other suitable solubilizing agent (latter optional). See also other injections of Digitalis glycosides	Solvent for glycoside
Lidocaine Hydrochloride Injection, U.S.P.	Epinephrine 1:100,000 (optional)	Prolong activity of local anesthetic
Methylglucamine Diatrizoate Injection, U.S.P.	Methylglucamine	Solubilize diatrizoate
Sterile Procaine Penicillin G Suspension, U.S.P.	Suitable suspending or dispersing agents, buffers, and preservatives (if multiple-dose); procaine hydrochloride not exceeding 2% (optional)	Procaine to relieve pain of injection; other reasons obvious
Reserpine Injection, U.S.P.	Suitable acid	Dissolve alkaloid (convert to soluble salt)
Sodium Acetrizoate Injection, U.S.P.	Sodium hydroxide; monocalcium disodium ethylenediaminetetraacetate (not over 0.012%); sodium biphosphate (not more than 0.015 %)	Convert drug to soluble form; chelating agent to stabilize; buffer
Aurothioglucose Injection, N.F.	Suitable thickening agent (optional)	Maintain dispersion
Chlortetracycline Hydrochloride for Injection, N.F.	Suitable buffer (usually consisting of an amino acid)	Stabilize drug
Mercurophylline Injection, N.F.	Additional theophylline	Stabilizer
Picrotoxin Injection, N.F.	Alcohol or chlorobutanol (optional)	Preservative
Quinidine Gluconate Injection, N.F.	Phenol, 0.25 per cent (optional)	Preservative
Sodium Psylliate Injection, N.F.	Benzyl alcohol, 3 per cent (optional)	Preservative

and nonionic surfactants have been mentioned for this purpose. Of the surfactants, the most commonly used types are the Tweens and the Pluronics.[5] A commercial preparation containing phytonadione in a sterile emulsion form (Mephyton, Merck Sharp and Dohme) is reported to contain 1 per cent of lecithin as the emulsifying agent. A cottonseed oil emulsion suitable for intravenous use (Lipomul I.V., Upjohn) is prepared by using lecithin and a Pluronic. Oil suspensions may have a thickening agent added. An example is found in Sterile Procaine Penicillin G with

Aluminum Stearate Suspension, U.S.P., in which aluminum monostearate is used to gel the oil suspension. The particle size in injectable emulsions should be no larger than 4 microns.[6]

The sterilization of emulsions or suspensions may constitute a major problem, and it is important that the ingredients be sterilized separately before combining and that aseptic technics be used throughout. Heat sterilization may be used upon the packaged product only if the nature of the suspension is not altered appreciably.

Fixed oils which are used as vehicles in parenteral products are subjected to rigid controls with respect to hardness and absorbability. They must have a saponification value of not less than 185 or more than 200 and an iodine value not less than 79 or more than 128. The free fatty acids in 10 Gm. of oil require not more than 2 ml. of 0.02 N. sodium hydroxide for neutralization. The oils must not contain mineral oil or paraffin, since these materials are not absorbed from body tissues.

Filling of Ampuls and Vials

When the stock solution has been prepared and filtered or the suspension properly dispersed, the liquid is ready for filling into containers. In the case of suspensions, provision must be made to keep the liquid agitated in order to ensure a uniform distribution of active constituent. Containers are of two general types—ampuls and vials. The first are cylindrical glass containers sealed at one end and drawn to an elongated neck at the other (Fig. 135). After filling, the neck is sealed by the use of heat. Vials are small bottle-shaped containers of glass which are sealed with rubber or plastic closures (the diaphragm), the latter usually being fastened in place by a metal seal (Fig. 136). In all cases the glass must be clear or lightly colored in order to permit visual inspection of the product.

All grades of glass are not suitable for the manufacture of ampuls and multiple-dose vials. On long-standing in contact with aqueous solutions, soft glass will yield a sufficient amount of soluble silicate to permit the separation of fine crystals. This process, which is known as "silication," is regarded as highly undesirable in injectable preparations. Other types of glass will yield traces of iron or other elements which may cause discoloration or precipitation of active constituents. For this reason, both the *United States Pharmacopeia* and the *National Formulary* have agreed upon standards for 4 types of glass, known as Types I to IV. For each official sterile preparation, the type of container is recommended. Type I glass is of the best quality and may be used for any parenteral preparation. Type II glass containers may not be more than

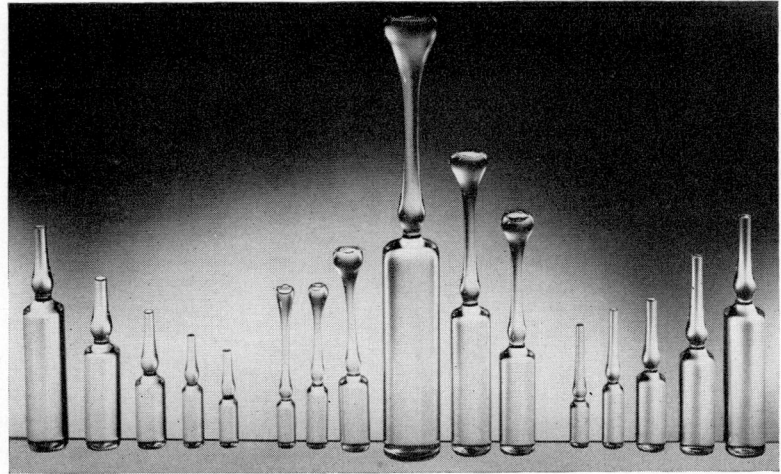

Fig. 135. Different sizes and styles of the most commonly used type of ampul. (Kimble Glass Co., Subsidiary of Owens Illinois, Toledo, Ohio)

Preparation of Injections

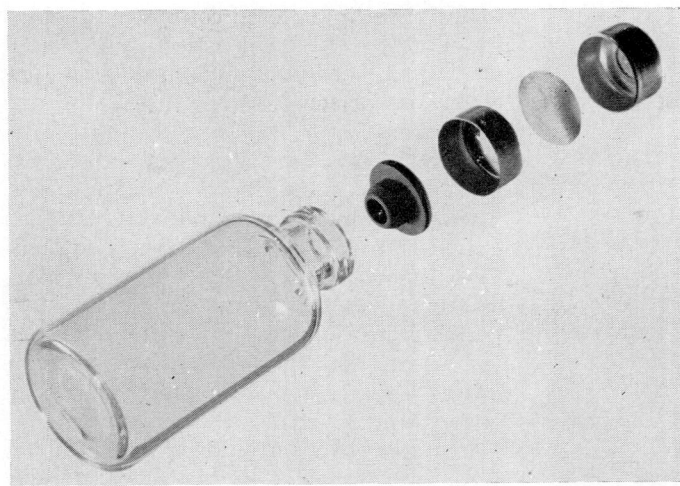

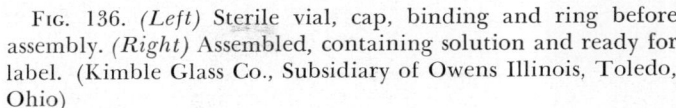

Fig. 136. *(Left)* Sterile vial, cap, binding and ring before assembly. *(Right)* Assembled, containing solution and ready for label. (Kimble Glass Co., Subsidiary of Owens Illinois, Toledo, Ohio)

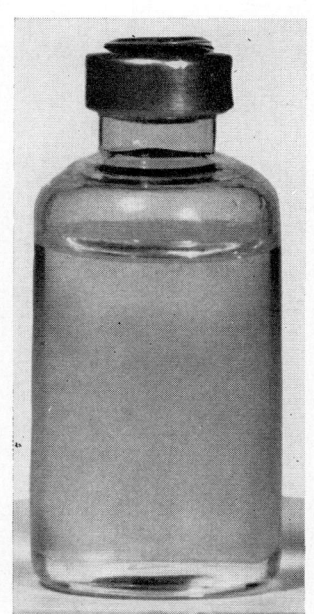

100 ml. in capacity and cannot be sterilized by heat after filling. Type III containers may be of any size, but they may not be sterilized by heat after filling. Type IV containers are made of soda-lime glass and are over 100 ml. in capacity. They are usually used for bulk fluids. Thus, Type I and Type IV containers should be used where a product is to be autoclaved. Type IV will withstand only one or a few autoclavings. Type I containers may be subjected to repeated autoclavings.

All types of containers should be cleaned before filling. This is accomplished by washing with a detergent solution, rinsing with freshly distilled water, and drying. Where possible, it is convenient to dry and sterilize in a single operation by using dry heat at 180° C. Soap solution should not be used for the washing because of the possibilty of precipitating insoluble magnesium or calcium soaps on the inside surfaces of the containers. Machines are available which mechanically inject the washing and rinsing liquids through the neck of the ampuls and partially dry by blowing in compressed air.

Rubber diaphragms are cleaned by boiling for 15 minutes in a 2 per cent solution of sodium carbonate containing 0.1 per cent of an anionic detergent. This process removes excess sulfur or other impurities. The diaphragms are rinsed thoroughly with tap water, then recently distilled water, after

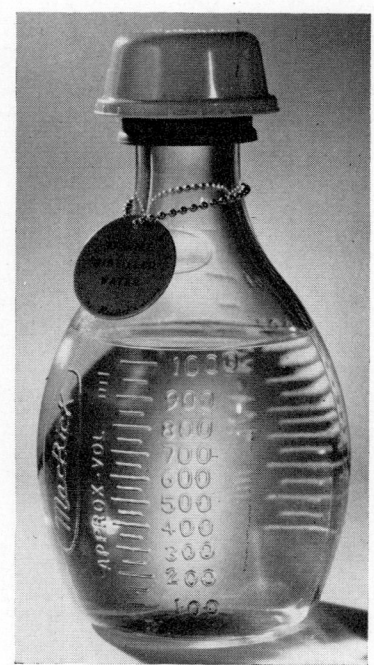

Fig. 137. The Pour-O-Vac container. (Macbick Company, Cambridge, Mass.)

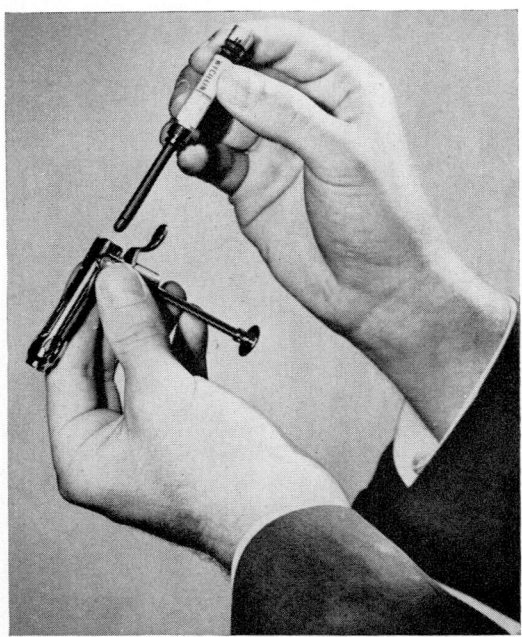

Fig. 138. Inserting a Tubex cartridge in a specially-designed holder for injection. Covering which maintains needle in sterile condition will be removed just before use. (Wyeth Lab. Inc., Philadelphia)

which they are dried and used. If they are not to be used immediately, it is possible to keep them free of contamination by storing them in a closed container in which they are covered by a 1 per cent phenol solution. This solution should be rinsed off by the use of sterile water before the diaphragms are used in sealing vials.

Ordinary pyrex or other screw-cap bottles are utilized as containers by some hospitals. When the solution is to be used within a limited period of time and there is no possibility that the seal will be broken before use, this method seems to give satisfactory results. The Pour-O-Vac container (Fig. 137), is regarded by some hospital pharmacists as a convenient all-purpose container for medium or small-scale operations.

A comparatively new trend in parenteral packaging is that of letting the disposable glass containers serve as a part or all of the syringe. Examples are (1) the rubber-stoppered glass tube with attached needle (Tubex, Wyeth) which is intended for use in a specially designed syringe carriage and disposed of after use (Fig. 138) and (2) glass-disposable syringes, such as the Hypak unit of Becton, Dickinson and Company, in which the entire unit syringe (containing medication and sterile needle) is designed for disposal after a single use (Fig. 139). Various plastic containers have also been studied, but as yet they have not been found suitable for most preparations.

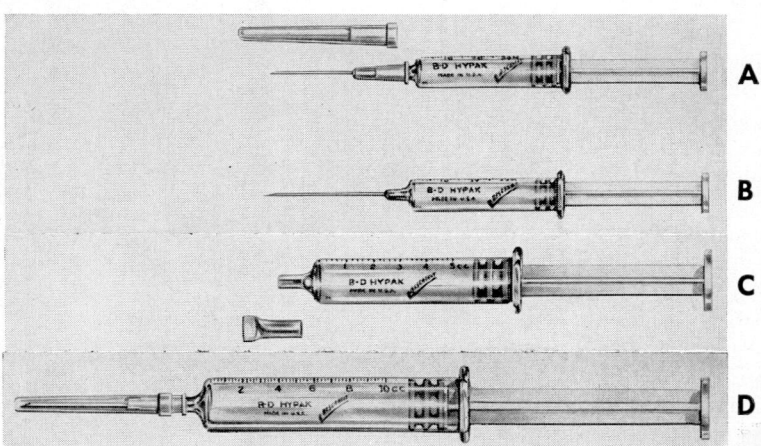

Fig. 139. Illustrating some of the types and sizes of Hypak syringes which are available: (A) Disposable glass syringe (2 cc.) with B-D Yale sterile disposable needle attached; (B) Combination syringe-needle unit; (C) Syringe only (5 cc.); and, (D) Glass syringe (10 cc.) with attached needle. (Becton, Dickinson and Co., Rutherford, N. J.)

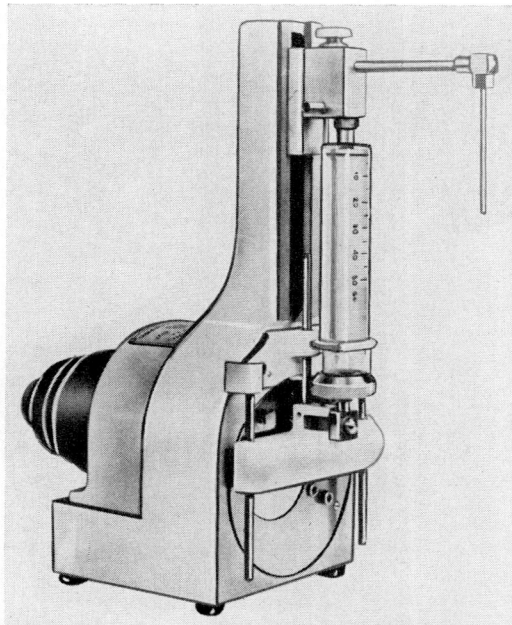

Fig. 140. A simple but efficient ampul-filling machine which measures one volume at a time. (Popper and Sons, Inc., 300 Fourth Avenue, New York)

The filling of ampuls or vials is accomplished by means of mechanical devices which have been designed for this purpose. Regardless of their form, they represent a measuring device attached to a hypodermic needle or a similar small metal tube by which the liquid may be introduced into containers through the neck. Some of these devices consist of a Luer-type syringe attached to a 2-way valve and an injection needle. As the plunger of the syringe is withdrawn, the barrel fills with liquid drawn from a bulk container. When the plunger changes direction, the valve leading to the stock solution closes, and the liquid is forced through a filling tube into the waiting ampul (Fig 140).

Sealing Ampuls

Although ampuls may be sealed by rotating the elongated neck in an ordinary Bunsen flame, the method is slow and does not offer an attractive seal. The rate of sealing can be increased by applying a blast burner or blow torch burner at a point slightly below the tip and pulling off the extra tip of glass with a forceps or by touching it with a glass rod and pulling it away. The fine string of glass which results will melt down to a round bead and form a seal.

Automatic sealers make use of both principles. Fine jets of flame play upon the glass tip from several directions, melting the glass uniformly and permitting it to draw together into a beadlike seal. In some models, the tip of the ampul is touched by heated wires which break the surface of the glass just long enough to encourage the formation of a seal. In all instances, the contents of the ampul must have been introduced with such care that no droplets remain in the neck of the ampul during sealing. Such materials would carbonize and discolor the ampul at the point of sealing. Such accidents do not usually occur when automatic filling devices are used, since these can be adjusted with great accuracy as to depth and position of fill. Machines are available which fill and seal ampuls continuously at a rapid rate with very little supervision (Fig. 141).

Because it is obviously impossible to withdraw the entire content of an ampul, a slight excess of liquid is placed in the container. The necessary amount of excess varies with the size of container and the viscosity of the liquid; hence, the official compendia present tables indicating the excess volumes which are usually sufficient. For mobile liquids, the recommended excess varies from 20 per cent for a dose of 0.5 ml. to a 2 per cent excess for a dose of 50 ml. For viscous liquids, the variation is from 24 to 8 per cent for the same volume.

The filling operation is carried out under aseptic conditions in order to reduce the possibility of bacterial contamination. When final heat sterilization of the product is not possible, this becomes a critical problem, and special precautions may be used. The degree of contamination of the filling room may be determined by exposing petri plates containing nutrient broth and incubating them to find both the numbers and the types of bacteria which are present. For small batches, the filling operation may be conducted in a sterile hood which per-

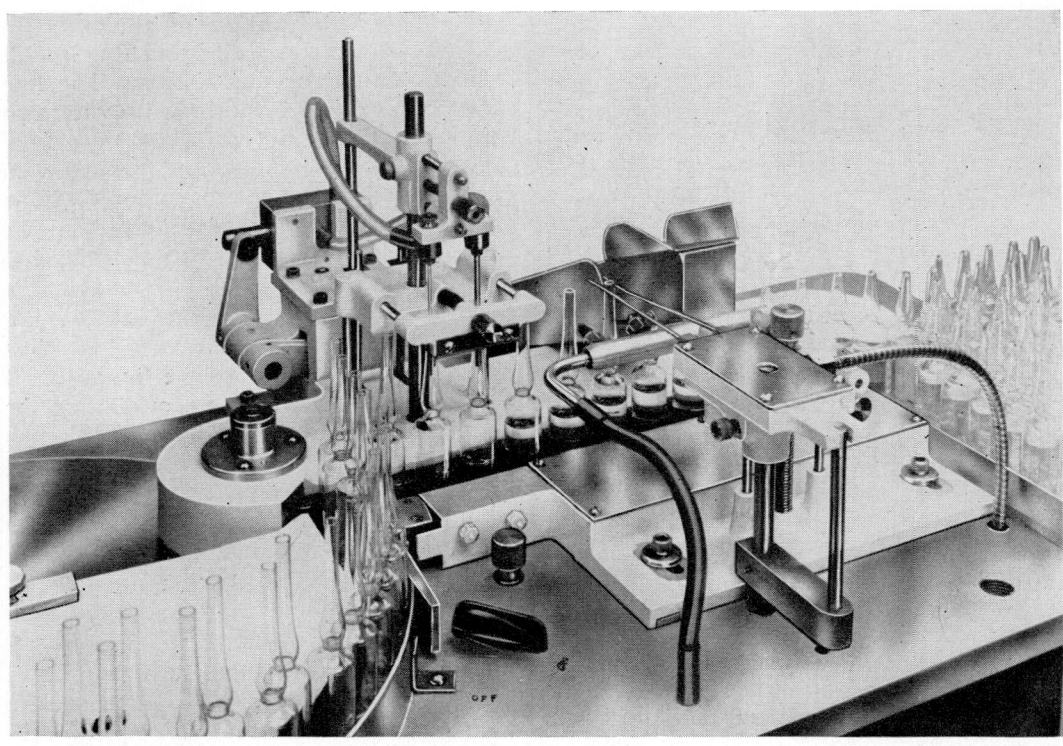

Fig. 141. Automatic ampul-filling and -sealing machine which mechanically fills, flushes with inert gas, pull-seals and ejects the ampuls. (Popper and Sons, Inc., 300 Fourth Avenue, New York)

mits access of the operator's gloved hands through a narrow opening (Fig. 142).

As a rule when it is desirable to replace the air in an ampul by inert gas, this is done by injecting the gas (usually nitrogen) into the ampul immediately before the medication is introduced. The medication then displaces some of the nitrogen, and the sealing operation takes place before the gas is lost to the surrounding atmosphere. Where necessary, the operation can be carried out in a hood of the type mentioned before in which an atmosphere of nitrogen is maintained under positive pressure.

The introduction of powders and vials is carried out by apparatus resembling that used for liquids. Special problems involved are the maintenance of a completely dry area (to prevent clogging of the powder) and a satisfactory method of forced feeding. In one type of apparatus, the forced feeding is maintained by use of an auger worm screw which delivers the powder from a hopper to the filling tube.*

Sterilization

The term "sterilization" refers to those methods which are used to render a preparation free of viable micro-organisms. As applied to parenteral manufacture, it is not a process which is applied at one stage of the manufacture; rather, it is applied continuously. Thus, Water for Injection is sterile at the moment of collection because it has been rendered so by the process of distillation if the still has been cleaned and is operating properly. In some instances, the stock solution is sterilized before packaging in ampuls. The filling operation is usually carried out in an area which has been rendered as sterile as practicable by the use of ultraviolet light, chemical agents and air-

* Chase Manufacturing Company. 47 E. 19th St., N. Y. 3, N. Y.

control methods. Wherever possible, the final container, filled and sealed, is subjected to a process of sterilization which will offer maximum security.

Moist heat is the preferred agent of sterilization because it is the most efficient. It is used in the form of steam under pressure in an apparatus known as the *autoclave* or *steam sterilizer* (Fig. 143). Sterilizers vary in size from a small apparatus, suitable only for sterilizing a few instruments or a small batch of ampuls, to a walk-in size capable of handling cart-loads of material in a single operation. They are equipped with gauges which record the pressure of steam and always should be equipped to record this at the point of exhaust. Since the absolute temperature varies directly as pressure, the temperature within a sterilizer may be calculated from the pressure of steam recorded. Dials commonly show both pressure and temperature readings. These are calculated for the pressure-temperature relationship of water vapor (saturated steam) at the pressure recorded and will be erroneous if the air has not been replaced by steam. Consequently, it is important that steam be allowed to flow through the sterilizer for some minutes in order to achieve thorough replacement of the air before the pressure valve is closed.

Various minimal periods of exposure have been presented in the literature for the most resistant bacterial spores; however, a recent

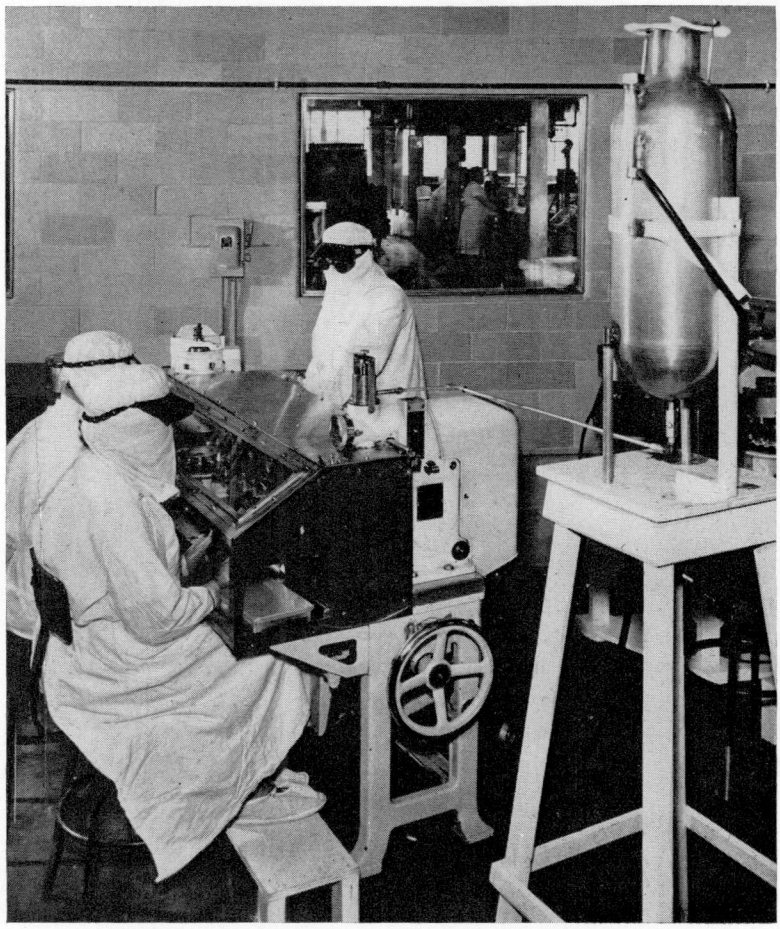

Fig. 142. Aseptic filling using a hood in a sterile area.
(Wyeth Lab. Inc., Philadelphia)

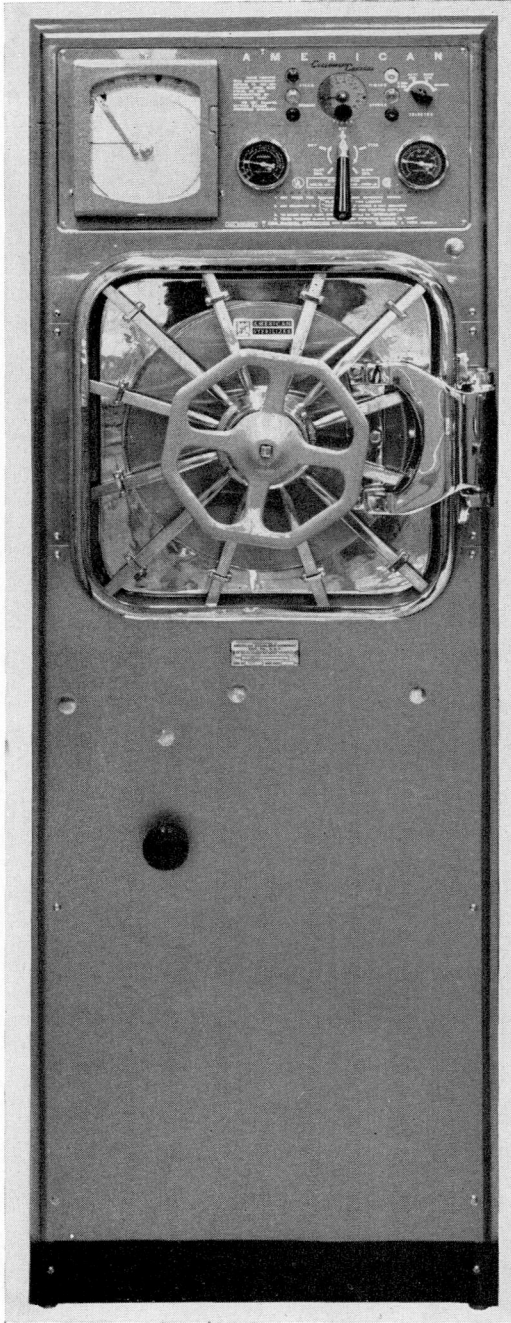

Fig. 143. A modern autoclave. (American Sterilizer Co., Erie, Pa.)

publication[7] indicates that all viable forms are destroyed by an exposure of 12 minutes at 15 pounds of pressure (121° C.). The time is minimal and does not include the period necessary for thoroughly heating materials included in a given load. The time required for preliminary heating will vary with the mass of material and the ease with which steam may penetrate to all parts of the load. Consideration should be given to the size and the thickness of containers and the type of materials in determining the actual time of exposure to use. It is also possible to include temperature detectors within a load which will indicate that a suitable maximum temperature has been used. Where these are utilized, it must be realized that they record maximum temperature but do not record time of exposure; therefore, they are not infallible. Manufacturing companies usually utilize recording thermometers and keep a record of the sterilization procedure used for a given batch. A common rule-of-thumb procedure which is used for ordinary materials is an exposure of 15 pounds for 20 minutes. This provides some margin for safety.

The time of exposure required to kill bacteria varies inversely with the temperature and it may be helpful to know the following relationships between pressure and temperature for pure steam:*

$$5 \text{ lbs. pressure} = 109° \text{ (228° F.)}$$
$$10 \text{ lbs. pressure} = 115° \text{ (240° F.)}$$
$$15 \text{ lbs. pressure} = 121° \text{ (250° F.)}$$
$$20 \text{ lbs. pressure} = 126° \text{ (259° F.)}$$

In some instances where drugs are unstable to heat, it is better to use exposure at a higher temperature for a shorter period of time. Higuchi and Busse[8] studied the possibility of sterilizing a heat-labile drug, procaine, at various temperatures and measured the destructive effect of heat in terms of the half-life of the drug. They concluded that for this compound, it is more desirable to use high temperature sterilization for a brief period of time rather than sterilization at 100° for a prolonged period. The desirability of applying such a technic to the study of other drug sterilization problems is obvious.

Some drugs are self-sterilizing and will

* From Underwood Textbook of Sterilization, Chicago, Lakeside Press, 1941.

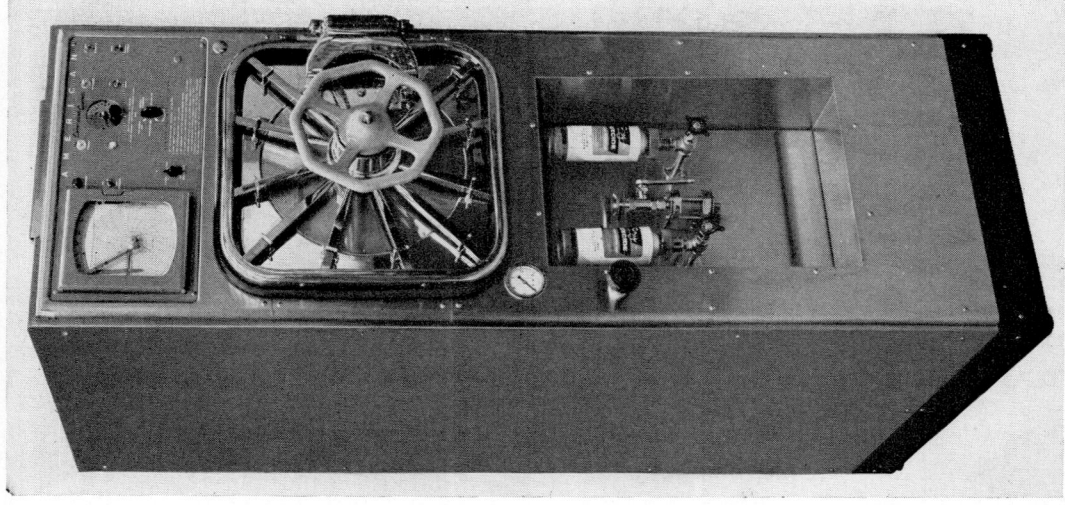
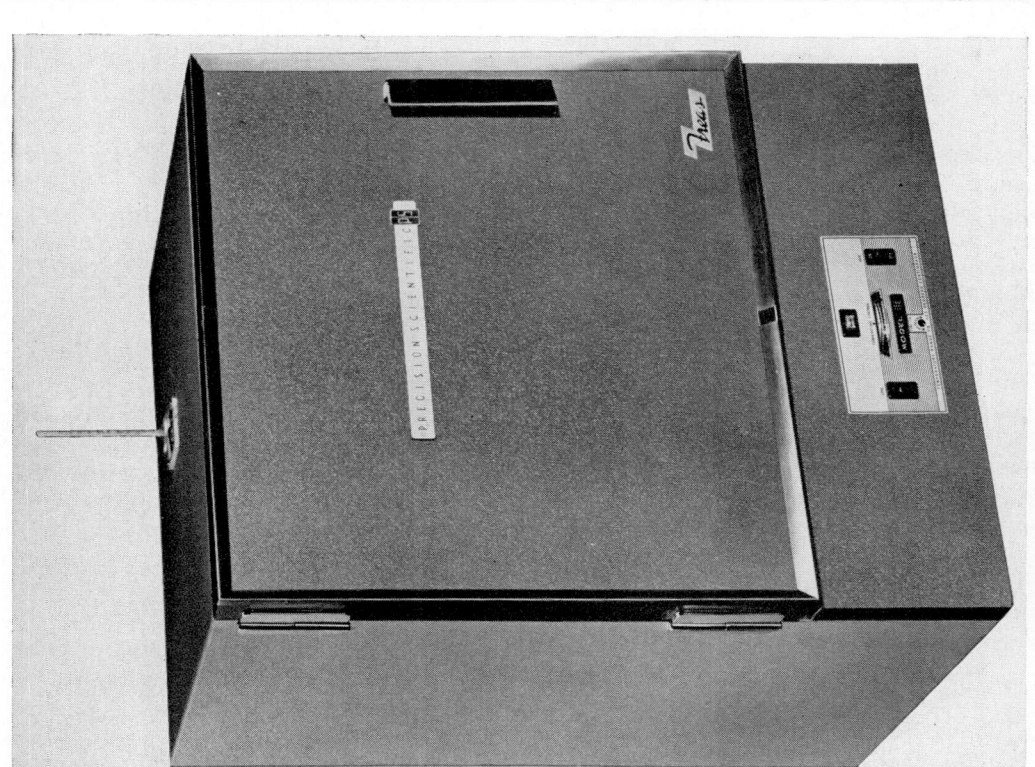

Fig. 144. (*Left*) Hot air sterilizer. Used to sterilize glassware, empty ampuls, and other equipment which can withstand high temperatures. (*Right*) "Cold sterilizer which uses Cryoxcide Gas as a sterilizing agent. Cryoxcide is a nonflammable mixture of ethylene oxide and freon. (American Sterilizer Co., Erie, Pa.)

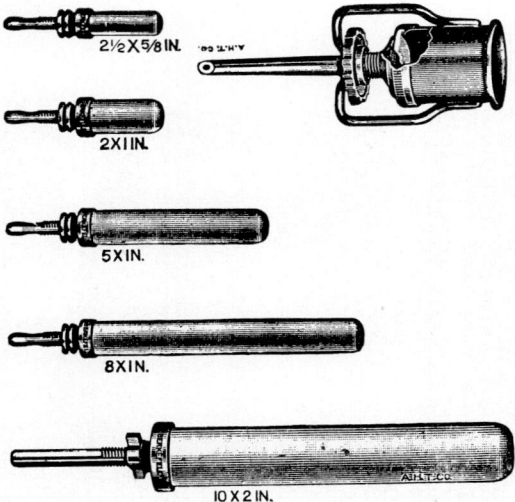

Fig. 145. Bacterial filters. (*Top*) Seitz filter. (*Bottom*) Different sizes of Berkefeld filters.

not require the application of heat; others are not capable of producing sterility in the concentration used but will reduce the time or the temperature required. Added substances, particularly preservatives, will have a similar affect. For this reason, the official compendia do not attempt to specify the process of sterilization to be used; rather, it is assumed that procedures will be used which ensure safety of the product. The official sterility test serves as a final check on the reliability of the method.

Intermittent sterilization, also known as *tyndallization* or *fractional sterilization*, which involves a minimum of 3 exposures to open steam at 24-hour intervals, is now regarded as being unreliable. This method was based upon the presumption that spores would undergo change to vegetative forms following the first exposure and would be destroyed by a subsequent exposure; however, it has been found that spores may not germinate in the absence of nutritive material. The *Pharmacopeia* recommends that such processes be employed only if the efficacy of the procedure has been demonstrated experimentally with thermal-resistant spores in the specified product.

Glassware, such as empty ampuls, is usually sterilized by the use of dry heat at 170° for 2 hours (Fig. 144). Rubber tubing and other equipment is usually prepared by autoclaving. Plastic materials which are not resistant to heat are subjected to gaseous sterilization, usually using ethylene oxide.

Nonaqueous injections and dry powders present a difficult sterilization problem. No water is present; therefore, the powerful killing effect of steam may not be utilized. Furthermore, the usual chemical disinfectants do not appear to be effective in such media.[9] Such preparations are often sterilized by heating to 170° for an hour or more; but the procedure is not universally applicable. In some instances, the active constituent or solvent would be seriously harmed by exposure to such temperatures, and other procedures must be devised. A combination of low heat and aseptic manipulation may be the most practicable solution.

Sterilization by filtration is used for solutions which cannot tolerate even mild heat. A number of filtering media have been devised for this purpose (Fig. 145). Candles of unglazed porcelain were perhaps the first such filters to be used and have the advantage of being easily sterilized by heat. Filters of the Seitz type make use of replaceable asbestos pads. In practical applications, the fluid is caused to flow through the filtering media by the application of pressure. One of the newer types of filters is the ceramic filter of controlled porosity such as those manufactured by the Selas Corporation.* (Fig. 146). A new type of filter which is of the membrane type is the Millipore† disk. This offers the advantages of greater filtering speed and ease of assembly. The membranes are claimed to operate on the principle of straining rather than entrapment or adsorption and are graded with respect to pore size. They are discarded after use (Fig. 147).

The effectiveness of a filter is influenced by such factors as pH of liquid, surface tension of liquid, and pressure applied. Filters must be cleaned, sterilized and tested regularly in order to make certain that they are operating efficiently. Testing is usually performed by using living nonpathogenic strains of organisms and determining

---

* Selas Corporation of America, Drescher, Pa.
† Millipore Filter Corporation, Bedford, Mass.

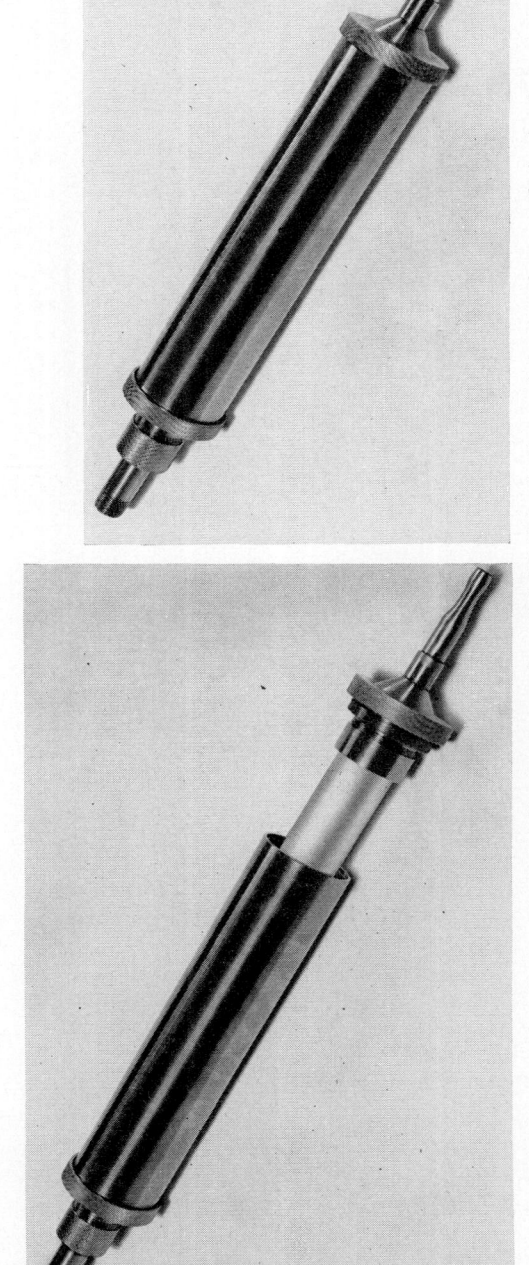

Fig. 146. (*Left*) Cross-sectional view gives detail of construction. (*Right*) Selas in-line stainless steel encased single element microfilter. (Selas Corporation of America, Dresher, Pa.)

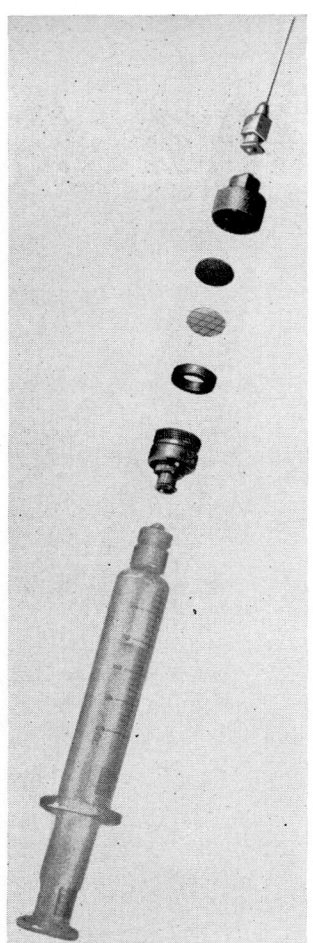
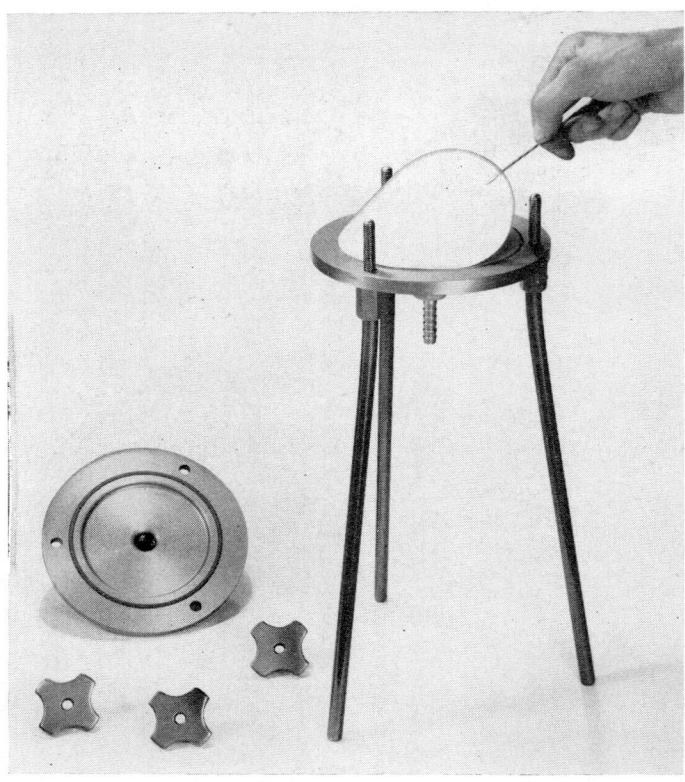

Fig. 147. Two methods of using Millipore filters. *(Left)* Swinny Adapter utilizing hypodermic syringe and Millipore disk. *(Right)* A partially assembled bench-type filter with Millipore disk raised so that it can be seen. (Millipore Filter Corp., Bedford, Mass.)

whether they are effectively removed from the liquid which is to be packaged. They may also be tested with respect to porosity. It has been stated that to be completely reliable for sterilization purposes, a filter should remove all particles down to a size of approximately 3/10 of a micron.[10]

Sterility Testing

Complete and detailed instructions are presented by the *Pharmacopeia* and the *National Formulary* for the testing of sterile products. These will be reviewed here very briefly.

In the case of liquids which have been sterilized with steam under pressure, a sample of 10 or more units (ampuls or vials) must be tested from each batch. For other products, a sample of at least 20 units must be selected. If the product has been filled aseptically, the samples are selected at regular intervals throughout the filling operation.

The samples are removed aseptically from their containers and cultured in Fluid Thioglycollate Medium and Fluid Sabouraud Medium. The first medium is incubated at 30° to 32° for at least 7 days and is expected to detect the presence of bacterial forms. The Sabouraud Medium is incubated at 22° to 25° for not less than 10 days and is intended to reveal contamination with molds or fungi. If the product is bacteriostatic or fungistatic, a neutralizer is added before the sample is transferred to the culture medium.

If no evidence of growth occurs in the culture medium, the product may be re-

List of Official Parenterals

N.B.

TABLE 10. COLOR CODE USED IN LABELING OF INSULINS*

Unitage	Type of Insulin					
Units per ml.	Regular Insulin	Crystalline Insulin	Globin Zinc Insulin	Isophane Insulin	Protamine Zinc Insulin	Lente Insulin
40	Red	Red and gray	Red and brown	Red and blue	Red and white	Red and lavender
80	Green	Green and gray	Green and brown	Green and blue	Green and white	Green and lavender
100	Orange		*Inter-mediate*			
500	Brown and white stripes (diagonal)					

* See Federal Register July 4, 1957 22 F.R. 4721.

garded as sterile. If evidence of growth occurs, the test may be repeated to rule out laboratory contamination, using twice the number of samples.

An interesting statistical evaluation of sterility testing has been presented by Knudsen.[11] These statistical data are most significant to anyone who is attempting to evaluate the reliability of the sterility test for a given batch of ampuls.

Pyrogen test. This test is conducted by using healthy rabbits having a minimum weight of 1,500 Gm. and injecting into them 10 ml. per Kg. of body weight of the material to be tested. Three rabbits are used, and if the temperature rise of one or more is 0.6° or if the sum of temperature elevations exceeds 1.4°, the test is to be repeated using 5 rabbits. The test is positive if 4 or more of the 8 rabbits show a temperature rise of 0.6 or if the sum of the temperature rises exceeds 3.7°.

The official compendia should be consulted for complete details regarding the method of selecting and of housing the animals and other details.

Other tests. Injections are inspected visually to determine the presence of any foreign particles; however, it has not been possible to agree upon a suitable method for standardizing this inspection. The *Pharmacopeia* states that each injection should be subjected individually to a physical inspection when the construction of the container permits.

Labeling

The label of all injections must indicate the name of the preparation, the percentage content or amount of drug contained in a volume of a liquid, and the amount of drug present if a solid. The name of the manufacturer and the manufacturer's identifying lot number must also be present. If the injection is liquid and the solvent is not Water for Injection, the solvent must be identified. In the case of insulin injections, a uniform color code for labels has been adopted by the Food and Drug Administration. This may be presented in table form as shown above.

LIST OF OFFICIAL PARENTERALS

United States Pharmacopeia

Injections

Aminophylline
Amphetamine Sulfate
Ascorbic Acid
Atropine Sulfate
Betazole Hydrochloride
Bethanecol Chloride
Caffeine and Sodium Benzoate
Calcium Chloride
Calcium Gluconate
Calcium Leucovorin
Chlorpheniramine Maleate
Chlorpromazine Hydrochloride
Codeine Phosphate
Corticotropin
Corticotropin, Repository

Parenteral Preparations

Cyanocobalamine
Deslanoside
Desoxycorticosterone Acetate
Dextrose
Dextrose and Sodium Chloride
Dibucaine Hydrochloride
Digitoxin
Digoxin
Dihydromorphinone Hydrochloride
Dihydrostreptomycin Sulfate
Dimercaprol
Diphenhydramine Hydrochloride
Edrophonium Chloride
Emetine Hydrochloride
Ephedrine Sulfate
Epinephrine
Ergonovine Maleate
Ergotamine Tartrate
Estradiol Benzoate
Estradiol Dipropionate
Estrone
Evans Blue
Folic Acid
Heparin Sodium
Histamine Phosphate
Insulin
Insulin, Globin Zinc
Iophendylate
Levallorphan Tartrate
Levarterenol Bitartrate
Lidocaine Hydrochloride
Menadiol Sodium Diphosphate
Menadione Sodium Bisulfite
Meperidine Hydrochloride
Mephentermine Sulfate
Meralluride
Methadone Hydrochloride
Methoxamine Hydrochloride
Methylene Blue
Methylglucamine Diatrizoate
Methylglucamine Iodipamide
Morphine
Nalorphine Hydrochloride
Neostigmine Methylsulfate
Nicotinamide
Nicotinic Acid
Ouabain
Oxytocin
Papaverine Hydrochloride
Parathyroid
Pentobarbital Sodium
Phenolsulfonphthalein
Phenylephrine Hydrochloride
Piperocaine Hydrochloride

Pituitary, Posterior
Potassic Saline, Lactated
Potassium Chloride
Procainamide Hydrochloride
Procaine Hydrochloride
Prochlorperazine Ethanedisulfonate
Progesterone
Promethazine Hydrochloride
Protamine Sulfate
Protein Hydrolysate
Pyridoxine Hydrochloride
Reserpine
Riboflavin
Ringer's
Ringer's, Lactated
Scopolamine Hydrobromide
Sodium Acetrizoate
Sodium Chloride
Sodium Diatrizoate
Sodium Diprotrizoate
Sodium Glucosulfone
Sodium Indigotindisulfonate
Sodium Lactate
Sodium Morrhuate
Sodium Radiochromate
Sodium Thiosulfate
Stibophen
Streptomycin Sulfate
Succinylcholine Chloride
Sulfadiazine Sodium
Sulfisoxazole Diethanolamine
Sulfobromophthalein Sodium
Testosterone Propionate
Tetracaine Hydrochloride
Thiamine Hydrochloride
Tolazoline Hydrochloride
Trimethaphan Camphorsulfonate
Tubocurarine Chloride
Vasopressin

Sterile Suspensions

Bismuth Subsalicylate
Corticotropin Zinc Hydroxide
Cortisone Acetate
Desoxycorticosterone Trimethylacetate
Epinephrine
Hydrocortisone Acetate
*Insulin, Isophane
*Insulin, Protamine Zinc
*Insulin Zinc
Penicillin G, Benzathine
Penicillin G, Procaine

* Listed as suspension by titles, but described as sterile suspensions in *U.S.P. XVI.*

Penicillin G, Procaine, with Aluminum Stearate
Propyliodone
Propyliodone Oil

Sterile Emulsion

Phytonadione

Miscellaneous Products for Injection or Suspension

Sterile Chloramphenicol for Suspension
Erythromycin for Injection
Hyaluronidase for Injection
Mechlorethamine Hydrochloride for Injection
Penicillin G Buffered for Injection
Phentolamine Methylsulfate for Injection
Streptoduocin for Injection
Tetracycline Hydrochloride for Injection
Thiamylal Sodium for Injection
Thiopental Sodium for Injection
Warfarin Sodium for Injection

NATIONAL FORMULARY

Injections

Adrenal Cortex
Amphetamine Phosphate
Aurothioglucose
Benzpyrinium Bromide
Butethamine Hydrochloride and Epinephrine
Cyclopentamine Hydrochloride
Diethylstilbestrol Dipropionate
Dimethyl-Tubocurarine Iodide
Diphemanil Methylsulfate
Estradiol, Aqueous
Estradiol Cyclopentylpropionate
Fructose
Fructose and Sodium Chloride
Gold Sodium Thiomalate
Hexestrol
Hexylcaine Hydrochloride
Hydralazine Hydrochloride
Iodipamide Sodium
Iodopyracet
Levorphanol Tartrate
Liver
Liver, Crude
Magnesium Sulfate
Mannitol
Menadione
Meprylcaine Hydrochloride and Epinephrine
Mercurophylline
Mersalyl and Theophylline
Metabutethamine Hydrochloride and Epinephrine
Metabutoxycaine Hydrochloride and Epinephrine
Metaraminol Bitartrate
Methiodal Sodium
Methylergonovine Maleate
Nikethamide
Nylidrin Hydrochloride
Penicillin, Procaine in Oil
Pentylenetetrazol
Phenobarbital Sodium
Picrotoxin
Procaine, Tetracaine and Nordefrin Hydrochlorides
Propoxycaine Hydrochloride
Propoxycaine and Procaine Hydrochlorides and Levonordefrin
Quinidine Gluconate
Quinine and Urea Hydrochloride
Quinine Dihydrochloride
Sodium Dehydrocholate
Sodium Iodide
Sodium Iodomethamate
Sodium Para-Aminohippurate
Sodium Psylliate
Sodium Salicylate
Sodium Salicylate and Iodide
Sodium Salicylate and Iodide with Colchicine
Sulfamerazine Sodium
Sulfathiazole Sodium
Vinbarbital Sodium

Sterile Suspension

Progesterone
Testosterone

Miscellaneous Products for Injection or Suspension

Chlortetracycline Hydrochloride for Injection
Oleandomycin Phosphate for Injection
Oxytetracycline Hydrochloride for Injection
Sterile Hexobarbital Sodium
Sterile Methacholine Chloride
Sterile Penicillin (Penicillin-Streptomycin) for Suspension
Sterile Procaine Penicillin G and Buffered Crystalline Penicillin G for Suspension
Sterile Sulfathiazole Sodium

BIBLIOGRAPHY

Bogash, R. C.: Compatibilities and incompatibilities of some parenteral medications, Bull. Am. Soc. Hosp. Pharm. **12**:445-448, 1955.

Gershenfeld, L.: The hospital pharmacists's responsibilities in the production of parenterals, Am. J. Pharm. **129**:163-171, 1957.

Graham, W. D., Chalten, L. G., Pernaroski, M., Cox, C. E., and Airth, J. M.: A collaborative study on the detection of particles in ampuled solutions, Drug Standards **27**:61-67, 1959.

Larsen, Frank; Considerations in the preparation of parenteral solutions, Bull. Am. Soc. Hosp. Pharm. **10**:210-219, 1953.

Murphy, J. T.: Practical formulas for use in hospitals, Bull. Am. Soc. Hosp. Pharm. **11**:284-285, 1954.

Olynyk, I., Belcastro, P., and Sperandio, G. J.: A study of parenteral solutions made in hospitals, Bull. Am. Soc. Hosp. Pharm. **14**:573-577, 1957.

Sagen, H. E.: Ethylene Oxide as a sterilizing agent, Am. Pharm. Manuf. A., Sci. Conf. Proc., p. 87, 1954.

Schraub, E. F.: The case for cartridge therapy, Bull. Am. Soc. Hosp. Pharm. **12**:144, 1955.

Skolaut, N. W.: Preparation of small volume injections, Bull. Am. Soc. Hosp. Pharm. **13**:109, 1956.

REFERENCES

1. Hort and Peafold: Brit. Med. J. No. 2659, 1911.
2. Ginger, L. G., Nesset, N. M., Riegel, B. and Fitzsimmons, E. J.: J Am. Pharm. A. (Sci. Ed.) **40**:42, 1951.
3. Bull. Nat. Inst. of Nut., The Nion Corporation, July, 1953.
4. Avis, K. E.: Am. J. Pharm. **129**:410-414, 1957.
5. Charnicki, W. F.: Am. J. Pharm. **130**:409-418, 1958.
6. Markowitz, C., and Mann, F. C.: Am. J. Physiol. **93**:521, 1930.
7. Garrod, L. P.: First Annual Series of Becton-Dickinson Lecture, Published by Becton-Dickinson and Co., Rutherford, N. J., 1957.
8. Higuchi, T. and Busse, L. W.: J. Am. Pharm. A. (Sci. Ed.) **39**:411-413, 1950.
9. Lieberman, M. and Newmark, H.: Bull. Parent. Drug A. **12**:1-6, 1958.
10. Jordan, G. V., Jr.: Bull. Parent. Drug A. **13**:21-23, 1959.
11. Knudsen, L. F.: J. Am. Pharm. A. (Sci. Ed.) **38**:332-337, 1949.

WILLIAM ARTHUR PURDUM, Ph.D.

Vice President in charge of Production and Development, Burrough Brothers Manufacturing Co.; Professor of Hospital Pharmacy, University of Maryland, Baltimore, Maryland

13

Infusions and Decoctions

INFUSIONS
NONOFFICIAL INFUSIONS

DECOCTIONS

INFUSIONS

General. Infusions are aqueous preparations made by extracting vegetable (or animal) drugs by maceration or percolation with hot or cold water.

History. Perhaps the first of various classes of extractive preparations to come into existence, infusions are older than civilization itself. When prehistoric man found need for medication, he gathered a quantity of leaf, root or other plant part, soaked it in water and thereby produced a tea or infusion. Although these preparations seldom are ordered today in prescription practice, they are discussed here because a few are popular as household remedies. The last to remain official was that of digitalis, which appeared in *N.F. IX*, whereas a half century ago the *U.S.P.* and the *N.F.* recognized a total of 5. Three still are found in the *British Pharmacopoeia* of 1953.

Preparation. Since water is employed as the menstruum, it should be obvious that only those drugs whose desired constituents are soluble in water are adapted to use in the form of infusions. For example, satisfactory products can be prepared from drugs which contain glycosides or tannins, whereas infusions cannot be prepared from drugs whose activity resides in resinous material.

The crude drugs used should be in a state of coarse comminution, either cut into thin slices or bruised or ground to a coarse powder. Drugs of a tough, woody character should be in a moderately fine comminution. Fine powders have been used but are objectionable on the grounds that the removal of the insoluble portion of the drug from the infusion is difficult.

Although hot water is capable of extracting the desired constituents more quickly than cold, its use has 3 distinct disadvantages. There is the likelihood that hot water will extract an appreciable amount of inert material which may precipitate from the solution after it has cooled and has been dispensed. Another objection lies in the fact that certain desired principles may be either volatilized or destroyed at high temperatures. In addition, if boiling water is poured over drugs which contain albumin, this albuminous matter will be coagulated almost instantaneously within the drug cells and thereby impede the extraction of the desirable principles. Therefore, it follows that in the preparation of infusions of drugs such as wild cherry, the activity of which depends on the production of volatile substances by enzyme action, cold water must be employed. Heat in this case would not only hasten evaporation of volatile constituents but might destroy the enzyme partially or completely. Purified water is to be preferred, although tap water may be satisfactory in certain instances. If the tap water is appreciably alkaline, the resulting infusion may have a color somewhat different from that of a product made with purified water.

Most infusions are prepared by maceration. For the process of hot maceration, any convenient nonmetallic covered vessel of suitable size may be used. In general, the use of metallic utensils should be avoided because certain plant principles, notably tannins, react with metals and produce discolored products. Earthenware containers are preferred because usually they are thicker than glass or porcelain vessels and therefore retain the heat of the water for a longer period of time. Several types of infusion mugs or pots are available. These are usually earthenware containers having a finely perforated diaphragm which separates the upper and the lower portions of the pot. This diaphragm may either take the form of a flat plate or it may be cup-shaped. The drug to be extracted is placed on the diaphragm, sufficient water is added to cover the drug, and then the pot is closed. As soluble constituents dissolve in the solvent, the resulting solution, having become more dense than the solvent, drops to the bottom of the vessel, bringing less concentrated portions of the menstruum into contact with the drug. In effect, a circulation is set up which continues until the drug is exhausted. The completed infusion, freed from the marc, then may be removed from the vessel by pouring from a spout connected below the level of the perforated plate. If an infusion pot is not available and it is desired that circulatory maceration be employed, the crude drug can be tied up in a cheesecloth or muslin bag and suspended near the surface of the water contained in an ordinary vessel. A hook attached to the under side of the lid facilitates this suspension.

Percolation may be employed advantageously when cold water is to be used as the menstruum. Ordinarily, the volume of water used is large when compared with the quantity of drug to be extracted, and complete extraction will result if the percolation is conducted at a reasonable rate. Percolation is advantageous in that the percolate leaves the percolator free from insoluble matter, whereas the preparation of an infusion by maceration involves subsequent straining. Compound Infusion of Gentian, N.F. VII, was an example of an infusion prepared by percolation and presents an additional exception in that diluted alcohol is prescribed as the menstruum.

N.F. IX provided a general chapter on infusions which included a general formula and procedure for the preparation of all infusions other than one, that of digitalis, for which a specific formula was given. This section carried the warning statement that *"the drug concentration of an infusion representing a potent drug should be specified by the physician."* Furthermore, it stated that an infusion should be prepared by the following formula unless a different strength of product is specified:

THE DRUG, coarsely comminuted   50 Gm.
WATER, a sufficient quantity

To make .... 1,000 ml.

Moisten the drug in a suitable vessel, preferably of earthenware and provided with a cover, with 50 ml. of cold water, and allow it to stand during 15 minutes. Then add 900 ml. of boiling water, cover the vessel tightly and allow it to macerate during 30 minutes. Then strain the mixture and pass enough water through the strainer to make the Infusion measure 1,000 ml. If the activity of the Infusion is affected by the temperature of boiling water, cold water should be used.

The moistening of the drug with cold water permits the permeation of the drug cells by the menstruum and prevents, in part at least, the coagulation of albumin that otherwise would result on application of the hot water.

Infusions have been prepared from more concentrated preparations such as tinctures and fluidextracts, but this is an unethical practice which cannot be condoned. An infusion so prepared differs in composition, taste, odor and appearance from one prepared by the formerly official process. Tinctures and fluidextracts represent the alcohol-soluble as well as the water-soluble principles of the drugs, whereas infusions should contain only the water-soluble constituents. The presence of alcohol-soluble principles may result in the introduction of medicinal properties wholly undesired by the prescriber and may account for the different flavor. Chlorophyll, the green coloring matter of the vegetable world, is insoluble in water but is freely soluble in alcohol, and an alcoholic preparation of a drug diluted with water would differ markedly in appearance from an infusion prepared by the usual process.

Infusions prepared by the general formula contain no preservative and, therefore, deteriorate rapidly. Because of this fact, they must have been prepared recently and dispensed to the patient in amounts intended to last for not more than a few days. Digitalis Infusion and Compound Infusion of Gentian contain a limited quantity of alcohol and will keep for a somewhat longer period than the products having no preservative. Attempts have been made to preserve infusions by sterilizing them and the containers in which they are sealed, but even then, as soon as the container is opened, contamination with bacteria, fungi or other micro-organisms occurs, and the infusion soon spoils.

To obviate the necessity of preparing infusions when called for, the *British Pharmacopœia* recognizes preparations, 2 in number, called **Concentrated Infusions**. These concentrated products contain sufficient alcohol to preserve them for an indefinite period of time. They are not intended to be dispensed in the concentrated state but, when called for, are diluted with 7 times their volume of water However, after dilution, their content of alcohol has been so reduced as to render it ineffective as a preservative.

NONOFFICIAL INFUSIONS

Digitalis Infusion, N.F. IX

Digitalis was introduced into medical practice during the latter part of the 18th century by Dr. William Withering of Birmingham, England, and Digitalis Infusion still is called Withering's Infusion.

It is important to note that the *U.S.P.* recognizes both digitalis and powdered digitalis. The former is standardized biologically only for minimum activity, while the activity of the latter must fall between prescribed minimum and maximum limits. Because of its definite potency, powdered digitalis must be used in the preparation of the infusion. Attention is called to the fact that only 15 Gm. of drug is employed, whereas the general formula in *N.F. IX* calls for 50 Gm. of drug when preparing 1,000 ml. of infusion. Another deviation from the general procedure is the direction that the drug be infused for a full hour. Cinnamon spirit imparts its flavor, and the approximately 10 per cent of alcohol preserves the preparation for a limited time.

Because of its poor keeping quality, the preparation has fallen into relative disuse when compared with other digitalis preparations. However, some physicians still prefer the infusion over other dosage forms as a diuretic.

Infusion of Senna with Magnesium Sulfate, N.F. VII

Compound Infusion of Senna

Formerly recognized under the title Infusum Sennæ Compositum and popularly called Black Draught, this preparation is similar to a "patent" medicine in which the mixed drugs are packaged in dry form and intended to be made into an infusion in the home.

It is used as a laxative.

DECOCTIONS

Decoctions are solutions representing the water-soluble constituents of plant drugs prepared by boiling the drugs in water. While quite similar to infusions, decoctions differ only in that the temperature of boiling water is maintained during the period of extraction, whereas lower temperatures are employed in the manufacture of infusions.

Decoctions are employed to an even smaller degree than infusions, since fewer drugs are suited to the process of decoction. The process is restricted to those whose active principles are soluble in water, are nonvolatile and are not destroyed or injured by ebullition.

Decoctions no longer are given official recognition. As in the case of infusions, the strength of a decoction made from a potent drug should be indicated by the physician. If the strength is not directed otherwise, the product should be prepared according to the following formula, which is taken from the *U.S.P. XII* general chapter on decoctions.

The Drug, coarsely comminuted   50 Gm.
Distilled Water, a sufficient
   quantity   ———
      To make ....1,000 ml.

Place the drug in a suitable vessel provided with a cover, pour upon it 1,000 ml. of cold water, cover it well and boil the mixture for 15 minutes. Then allow it to cool to about 40° C., express, strain the expressed liquid and pass enough cold water through the strainer to make the product measure 1,000 ml.

By pouring cold water on the drug, solution of much of the albuminous matter, if present, is effected, and as the temperature is gradually elevated to the boiling point, the extracted albumin is precipitated. On the other hand, if the drug were placed in boiling water, the albuminous material would be coagulated within the drug cells and interfere with the removal of the desired constituents. During the boiling period, the vessel should be covered loosely to reduce vaporization of the water. Under no circumstance, however, should the product be permitted to boil to dryness; if too much water is lost and there is danger of charring the drug, more water should be added. The requirement that the decoction be strained only after it has cooled to about 40° allows for precipitation of principles dissolved at the boiling temperature but which are not soluble at lower temperatures. Even then, it is not uncommon for a decoction, strained at about 40°, to deposit solid matter after cooling to room temperature. This deposition may be prevented by permitting the product to reach room temperature before straining.

An ordinary pyrex beaker covered by a glass plate is entirely satisfactory for the manufacture of decoctions. In Germany, where decoctions still are employed, frequently the preparations are made in covered vessels of block tin. Iron utensils are not satisfactory because a discolored product will be produced if tannin is present in the drug.

Decoctions should not be prepared by diluting more concentrated preparations (tinctures and fluidextracts) for reasons already discussed under Infusions.

Like infusions, the keeping quality of decoctions is very poor. They contain no alcohol or other preservative and, for this reason, should be prepared freshly. Moreover, they should be dispensed in reasonably small quantities, i.e., quantities intended to last the patient not more than several days. Their storage by the patient in a cold place will retard deterioration caused by the growth of micro-organisms, although low temperatures are very likely to cause precipitation of dissolved material.

BIBLIOGRAPHY

Anonymous: Am. Drug. 14:45, 1885.
Martindale, W.: Pharm. J. 55:415, 1895.

ELMER MICHAEL PLEIN, Ph.D.

Professor of Pharmacy, University of Washington

14

Mucilages, Creams, Glycerogelatins, Glycerites and Collodions

MUCILAGES
    HISTORY
    GENERAL CONSIDERATIONS
    ACACIA MUCILAGE, N.F.
    TRAGACANTH MUCILAGE, N.F.
    CHONDRUS MUCILAGE, N.F.
    MISCELLANEOUS MUCILAGINOUS SUB-
        STANCES
    PECTIN, N.F.
    METHYLCELLULOSE, U.S.P.
    SODIUM CARBOXYMETHYLCELLULOSE,
        U.S.P.
    PROPERTIES AND USES OF MUCILAGES
CREAMS
    HISTORY
    GENERAL CONSIDERATIONS
    PROPERTIES AND USES OF CREAMS
GLYCEROGELATINS
    HISTORY
    GENERAL CONSIDERATIONS
    ZINC GELATIN, U.S.P.
    STORAGE
GLYCERITES
    HISTORY
    GLYCERITES OF THE N.F.
    GENERAL CONSIDERATIONS
    STORAGE
COLLODIONS
    HISTORY
    COLLODIONS OF THE U.S.P.
    GENERAL CONSIDERATIONS
    STORAGE

MUCILAGES

Mucilages are viscid, adhesive preparations made by dissolving or suspending gummy or mucilaginous substances in water. These gummy substances or gums are carbohydrate derivatives obtained as exudates from trees or shrubs. They are more or less soluble in water but generally insoluble in alcohol. Sometimes the gum is not entirely soluble in water but merely swells to form a thick liquid or gel by the absorption of water.

Mucilaginous substances contained within drugs and the dried, mucilaginous exudates obtained from those drugs are referred to as natural mucilages. Natural mucilages and the liquid pharmaceutical products prepared from them should not be confused. The former are merely constituents of drugs or are dried substances prepared from plants (for example, agar), whereas the pharmaceutical products are aqueous preparations.

A clear distinction between gums and natural mucilages has not been made. Some physical properties and various methods of formation of the material within the plants have been considered in attempts to distinguish between them, but none has proved to be satisfactory. Chemically, gums and mucilages are probably of identical nature. Both are mixed polysaccharides which, upon hydrolysis, yield chiefly the sugars galactose and arabinose. They contain galacturonic, glucuronic and methoxylated uronic acids.

History

Gums and mucilage-containing drugs have been used since the time of the ancient Egyptians. The use of this type of drug in medicine was mentioned in several Egyptian papyri. The use of acacia is recorded in writings credited to Hippocrates, the so-called father of medicine (460–377 B.C.) and to the Greek historian, Herodotus (484–425 B.C.). One of the species of acacia, *Acacia seyal,* is considered to be identical with the shittah tree of the Bible. From this tree came the shittim wood said to have been used in making the Ark of the Covenant. Theophrastus, the father of botany, described tragacanth in the 3rd century B.C. The Roman Pliny (23–79) reported that the Egyptian gum was the most expensive one, and stated that gum obtained from the almond or the cherry tree was bad but that obtained from the plum tree was the worst. The differentiation between gums and resins is of comparatively modern date.

General Considerations

Acacia mucilage was official in the first 15 revisions of the *U.S.P.* It is now official in the *N.F.* Tragacanth mucilage became official in the 2nd revision and was included in every revision up to and including the 13th. It is now official in the *N.F.* Flaxseed, slippery elm, cetraria, barley and sassafras pith all contain mucilaginous principles which were extracted by the process of infusion or decoction, and those aqueous preparations were official in early *U.S.P.*'s as infusions or decoctions. Later, the products prepared from sassafras pith and slippery elm were classified with the mucilages.

Three mucilages—acacia, chondrus and tragacanth—are official in the *N.F.*

Acacia Mucilage, N.F.

Acacia Mucilage is prepared with 0.2 per cent benzoic acid as a preservative. Acacia may be either in lump form or in a granulated or powdered condition. In the former case, the lumps first must be washed with cold water to rid the drug of dust and dirt particles. Solution of the lumps is then effected in warm water, but the process is slow. The mucilage can be made much more rapidly from powdered acacia if all of the water to be used is added at one time to the drug in a mortar and the mixture well stirred. However, if only a small quantity of water is added first to the powdered drug, a gummy mass results which dissolves very slowly, even though the remaining portion of water is then added.

Various substances have been suggested as preservatives of Acacia Mucilage. Sodium benzoate, 5 per cent alcohol and chloroform water have been used effectively. The last, while it is an efficient preservative, is objectionable from the standpoint of the flavor it imparts to the preparation. It has been suggested that preservatives be omitted and the mucilage prepared fresh at the time it is needed.

Acacia Mucilage finds use as an emulsifying agent in preparing emulsions by the English method. It increases the viscosity of solutions and is, therefore, a valuable addition to mixtures to prevent rapid settling of insoluble medicaments. Acacia has demulcent properties and often is added to medicines for that purpose. Acacia Mucilage sometimes is used as an adhesive excipient for pills and troches. Excessive amounts of the mucilage must be avoided in pills, otherwise they may be rendered very hard and less soluble, due to the slow solubility of acacia. Acacia Mucilage can be used as a protective colloid in whose presence certain chemicals such as silver iodide are **precipitated.**

Acacia will not tolerate the presence of more than 20 per cent alcohol, being insoluble in alcohol. The mucilage is also incompatible with lead subacetate solution, ferric chloride solution, ferric chloride tincture, ferric sulfate solution, borax solution and aluminum chloride solution.

In 1953, more than 8,300 tons of acacia, valued at about $1,635,000, were imported. Over 7,500 tons of this quantity came from Sudan.

Tragacanth Mucilage, N.F.

Tragacanth Mucilage also is prepared with preservatives, 0.2 per cent benzoic acid and 18 per cent glycerin. This mucilage is more viscous than that of acacia; therefore, it is necessary to force it through muslin to homogenize it. Only a part of the tragacanth actually is soluble in water; the remainder merely absorbs water and swells, thereby producing a thick preparation. The swelling is slow, and, for that reason, the tragacanth undergoes a 24-hour maceration period in preparing the mucilage. Alcohol does not have the precipitating power for tragacanth that it possesses for acacia; therefore, tragacanth can be used effectively to increase the viscosity of mixtures and lotions containing a considerable proportion of alcohol. The *British Pharmacopœia* directs that alcohol be used in the preparation of Tragacanth Mucilage. Alcohol facilitates quick preparation of the product and acts also as a preservative.

Tragacanth Mucilage can be used as an emulsifying agent but does not produce as white an emulsion as acacia. Sometimes it is added to emulsions merely to increase viscosity and to prevent creaming. It is ideally suited to this purpose, since alcohol then can be added to the emulsion as a preservative. Tragacanth Mucilage finds use as an excipient in making troches and pills and as a base for many hand lotions and other cosmetic products. Tragacanth is the gum employed in making Ephedrine Sulfate Jelly, N.F. (p. 273). It also was used in making the methylrosaniline chloride jelly and the thimerosal jelly of *N.F. IX*. About 5 or 10 per cent of tragacanth in water or Ringer's solution makes a fine base for medicated, water-soluble pastes employed in the treatment of bed-sores and ulcers.

In 1953, about 672 tons of tragacanth, valued at approximately $763,000, were imported, mostly from Iran.

Chondrus Mucilage, N.F.

Chondrus Mucilage, like tragacanth mucilage, is thick and requires forcible straining through muslin to break up the lumps and to make it homogeneous. No preservative is used in this mucilage, so it must be prepared freshly as needed. Like tragacanth, chondrus is not precipitated by a moderate concentration of alcohol and therefore is valuable in stabilizing emulsions, mixtures and lotions. Chondrus Mucilage, with added glycerin as a preservative, is a good base for many cosmetic preparations such as hand lotions and sun-tan lotions.

Miscellaneous Mucilaginous Substances

Flaxseed (containing about 6% mucilage), cetraria, althaea, salep, starch, quince seed, elm bark and sassafras pith sometimes are used in preparing mucilages. Agar, sterculia gum (karaya gum) and plantago seed (psyllium seed) are used internally as mechanical remedies for constipation. Agar and karaya gum are administered dry in small pieces and psyllium seed whole with quantities of water to wash the material into the stomach. In the alimentary canal, these drugs absorb water and swell, producing a mucilage which in turn acts as an emollient to lubricate the intestinal tract. The mucilage adds bulk to the feces and keeps it soft. Some commercial products made from these mucilage-containing drugs are combined with vitamin B_1 or cascara. Plantago ovato coating, prepared from the separated outer mucilaginous layers of *Plantago ovato* seeds and psyllium hydrophilic mucilloid with dextrose, also prepared from the outer epidermis of blond psyllium seeds, are official in *N.N.D. 1960*. These are bulk laxatives.

Pectin, N.F.

Pectin, which is closely related to gums and mucilages, is being used successfully in preparing many water-soluble pastes, lotions and emulsions. Pectin paste and thin pectin paste were official in *N.F. IX*. They are used as bases for medicaments intended to be applied externally where greasy bases are objectionable. When the application has served its purpose, it can be removed easily with water. Internally, pectin is used to control diarrheas.

Methylcellulose, U.S.P.

Methylcellulose,[11] a methyl ether of cellulose, is considered here because of its strong hydrophilic properties and its ability to increase viscosity of solutions and to stabilize dispersions and emulsions. Because of its hydrophilic character, it is used as a bulk laxative. When methylcellulose is taken orally with water, it forms a colloidal solution which later loses water in the colon to produce a gel that increases the bulk and the softness of the stool. Its bulk-producing quality also makes it a valuable constituent of reducing aids intended to satisfy hunger by producing a sense of fullness in the alimentary canal.

Methylcellulose is available in 6 different forms which impart different degrees of viscosity to aqueous solutions of identical concentration. These forms are designated 15, 25, 100, 400, 1,500 and 4,000 centipoises, respectively, and refer to the viscosity of the solution when tested in the proper manner. Different viscosity grades are due to differences in polymerization of the product at the time of manufacture. The greater the degree of polymerization, the greater the viscosity of the solution. When methylcellulose is added to aqueous solutions, it increases the viscosity of the preparation, thereby preventing the settling of suspended substances. This property makes it valuable in stabilizing lotions, mixtures, emulsions and some injectables (such as procaine penicillin). Used in higher concentrations, 10 to 20 per cent, methylcellulose produces a gel consistency, and the preparation is suitable as a nongreasy ointment base.

In spite of the fact that methylcellulose is less soluble in hot water than in cold water, solutions of it are best made by pouring on the product about half the required water at boiling temperature, allowing the mixture to stand for 20 to 30 minutes and then adding the rest of the water as cold water or ice. Hot water wets all portions of the methylcellulose and hastens its solution in water. The presence of wetting agents also hasten its solution in water. Solutions of methylcellulose are not affected by changes in pH from 2 to 12. Lotions stabilized with methylcellulose form tough, flexible, adherent films when they dry on the skin. These films give good protection and do not rub off easily, yet they can be washed off with water.

Sodium Carboxymethylcellulose, U.S.P.

Sodium carboxymethylcellulose has nearly the same properties as methylcellulose and therefore is used for the same purposes—i.e., bulk laxative, suspending agent and nongreasy ointment base. Sodium carboxymethylcellulose possesses acid-neutralizing power. Taken orally, it exchanges sodium ions for hydrogen ions in the stomach. Combinations of sodium carboxymethylcellulose and magnesium oxide are available commercially as antacids for treating peptic ulcer and hyperacidity.

Properties and Uses of Mucilages

Mucilages impart a slippery, lubricating sensation to the touch when a small portion of the preparation is rubbed between the fingers. This property of gums and mucilaginous substances is used to advantage in the preparation of surgeon's lubricating jellies. Several commercial houses manufacture lubricating jellies and market them in collapsible tubes under their own proprietary names. Tannic acid has been incorporated into mucilaginous vehicles and used for the treatment of burns. Various parasiticides now are being placed in mucilaginous bases and the products used as lotions. The mucilage serves as an excellent vehicle for the antiparasitic ingredient and has an emollient action for skin surfaces irritated by the parasite. Tragacanth and chondrus are the chief bases for these lubricating and tannic-acid jellies and antiparasitic preparations. Hair-setting lotions, also called finger-wave lotions and wavesets, are made from vegetable mucilages. These lotions may contain some alkali which softens the cuticle and renders the hair shaft easier to set, although slightly acidic preparations are said to give the hair a more "lustrous" appearance. Hair-setting lotions are made from tragacanth, sterculia gum, quince seeds, acacia, pectin and sodium alginate.

CREAMS

Creams are opaque, soft solids or thick liquids, intended for external application, consisting of medicaments dissolved or suspended in water-soluble or vanishing cream bases.

History

Creams became official when the formula for one cream (N.F. Sun Cream) was introduced into *N.F. VIII*. A class of preparations known as Creams has appeared in the *British Pharmacopœia* as medicated, liquid preparations intended for external use and having for their base a mixture of wool fat, olive oil (or some similar fixed oil) and lime water. These preparations are greasy and resemble the lime liniment of *N.F. VIII* or the ammonia liniment, the calamine liniment and the neocalamine liniment of *N.F. IX*. The word cream is used in the synonyms of several preparations such as ointments and pastes in the *British Pharmacopœia*.

Sun Cream, N.F. IX (called also Sun Tan Ointment, was a soft, creamy preparation intended for application to exposed skin surfaces to protect them from certain elements of the sun's rays. It was designed to prevent erythema or sunburn, but at the same time to permit sun tan. Some chemicals are capable of absorbing those wavelengths of sunlight that are responsible for sunburn. These substances are called chemical screens. Sun Cream, N.F. IX, contained 2 chemical screens—ethylaminobenzoate and phenyl salicylate. However, the latter substance has been shown to possess weak sun-screening power and also to filter out some of the wavelengths desirable for tanning.[5] Some substances prevent the passage of or greatly reduce the intensity of sunlight by shading or reflection. These materials are either opaque or highly reflecting powders and are called physical screens. Sun Cream, N.F. IX, contained 1 per cent each of the physical screens titanium dioxide and neocalamine. The base for Sun Cream, N.F. IX, was composed of white wax, stearyl alcohol, triethanolamine, stearic acid, glycerin and water.

General Considerations

The term "cream" is used loosely in naming many products. Milk of bismuth and milk of magnesia frequently are referred to as creams. Many cosmetic preparations are called creams—for example, cold cream, vanishing cream, hand cream and face cream (see Chap. 18 on ointments)—without regard to the type of base that may have been used in the manufacture of the products. Consistency and appearance undoubtedly have been responsible for the nomenclature of these substances.

The *Pharmaceutical Recipe Book,* ed. 3, has formulas for 7 medicated creams, all for external use. Zinc cream is taken from the *British Pharmaceutical Codex* and 2 others, bismuth cream II and zinc and aluminum cream, have bases of similar nature. Cream for waterproofing the skin and bismuth cream I contain a considerable proportion of petrolatum. Sulfur cream is prepared with a base of rose water ointment. Coal tar cream is made with a vanishing cream base. It is the only one of the 7 that can be called a cream if an exclusive class of pharmaceutical preparations is defined strictly.

Properties and Uses of Creams

Many of the water-soluble pastes, such as those prepared with pectin paste or tragacanth mucilage, are more or less transparent or translucent, whereas creams are opaque and usually white, due to the bases employed. Vanishing creams are composed of stearic acid emulsified with potassium, sodium, ammonium or triethanolamine stearate. A small percentage of glycerin often is added to prevent rapid drying. When they are applied to the skin with rubbing, they disappear. A typical formula for a vanishing cream[6] follows:

Stearic acid, triple pressed	15.000
Potassium hydroxide	0.700
Glycerin	8.000
Purified water	76.300
Methylparaben	0.025
Propylparaben	0.015
Perfume	q.s.

Melt the stearic acid and adjust the melted mixture to 80°. Dissolve the other ingredients (with the exception of perfume) in the water and warm the solution to 80°. Gradually add the aqueous solution to the melted stearic acid and stir briskly until the mixture congeals. Incorporate the perfume.

So-called water-soluble bases may be composed of gums or mucilaginous substances with a small amount of stearic acid and stearates to lend pearliness and opacity to the preparation. Many washable bases are now on the market under various trade names. Some washable bases contain combinations of cetyl alcohol, sodium lauryl sulfate and propylene glycol.

Many antiseptics and antiparasitics of proprietary manufacture are compounded in the form of creams. Some hand creams might be considered in the group because they often contain mild medicaments and are applied for their emollient effect. Brushless shaving creams, composed of stearic acid and stearates, while not medicated, might be included because they are somewhat related to the vanishing creams. Custom has established use of the name "cream" with these preparations, as it has with the soap-type shaving creams.

Formulas for several lotion bases have appeared in various publications. The essential difference between solid creams and these lotion bases is increased percentage of water in the latter, and it is conceivable that a solid cream could be diluted sufficiently with water to produce a lotion. Some of these lotion bases contain stearic acid, but they do not seem to be compatible with as wide a range of medicinals as are some of the other type lotions. The following lotion base has been developed by Ohmart and Stoklosa[10] for extemporaneous compounding of medicated lotions.

Cetyl alcohol	15.0
White wax	1.0
Glycerin	50.0
Sodium lauryl sulfate	5.0
Purified water, q.s. to make	1,000.0

Melt the cetyl alcohol and white wax, and heat the mixture to 80°. Dissolve the sodium lauryl sulfate in a mixture of the glycerin and 300 ml. of water, and heat to 80°. Add the aqueous solution to the oil phase very slowly, stirring constantly until the emulsion forms. Continue to stir until the mixture has cooled to about 40°, add enough purified water to make the product measure 1,000 ml., and mix thoroughly.

GLYCEROGELATINS

Glycerogelatins are soft, medicated masses usually molded into the form of blocks, melting at body temperature, and having as a base a mixture of gelatin, glycerin and water. At the time of application, the blocks are melted, and the liquid is applied to the skin with a soft brush.

HISTORY

Glycerogelatins were introduced into *N.F. III* when formulas for 4 of them were included. These 4—salicylic acid, iodoform, firm zinc and soft zinc—remained official through *N.F. V.* In *N.F. VI, N.F. VII* and *N.F. VIII,* only a general formula for glycerogelatins was included. The general formula has not been admitted to later revisions.

GENERAL CONSIDERATIONS

The general formula for *Glycerogelatins, N.F. VIII,* calls for 10 per cent of medicament. Medicaments suitable for use in glycerogelatins are the antiseptics, the germicides and the parasiticides. The formula may be altered, decreasing the quantity of glycerinated gelatin and increasing the quantity of glycerin and water to produce a mass of softer consistency and lower melting point. In the preparation of the product, the medicament is dissolved in or mixed with glycerin, the water added, and then this mixture added to the previously melted glycerogelatin. Heating is continued until a homogeneous mixture results, and the mass is poured into suitable molds.

ZINC GELATIN, U.S.P.

Zinc Gelatin, U.S.P. (zinc gelatin boot, Unna's boot) is a 10 per cent mixture of zinc oxide in a combination of gelatin, glycerin and water. The net proportion of the ingredients is the same as in the formula for *Firm Zinc Glycerogelatin, N.F. V.* It is used as a protective and supportive dressing for varicose ulcers.

N.N.R. 1951 listed gelatin compound phenolized (jelly bandage). It contained 1.5 per cent phenol and 5.5 per cent zinc oxide and was used in preparing bandages to cover chronic ulcers and in preparing pressure bandages for varicose veins. The melted glycerogelatin was painted on the skin, and a spiral bandage applied on top of this. Another coat of glycerogelatin was applied to the bandage, and the two alternated until 4 coats of glycerogelatin and 3 layers of bandage had been applied.

Storage

Glycerogelatins should be preserved and dispensed in well-stoppered containers to prevent absorption of moisture by the glycerin in the preparation. They should be stored in a cool place since they melt at body temperature.

GLYCERITES

Glycerites are solutions of medicinal substances in glycerin. Glycerin is a valuable solvent and vehicle for this type of preparation. It has a wide range of solvent power, allowing solutions of greater strength to be made than are possible with water or alcohol. These solutions of greater strength are valuable as stock preparations for use in prescription pharmacy. Glycerin does not have an unpleasant taste and does not become rancid as do the vegetable oils. It possesses preservative properties that prevent the growth of bacteria and molds.

History

Glycerites were introduced into *U.S.P. V.*, and several of them were official in the succeeding 10 revisions. None is official in the *U.S.P.* at present. Three glycerites are official in the *N.F.*

Glycerites of the N.F.

Boroglycerin Glycerite. This contains from 47.5 to 52.5 per cent of boroglycerin formed when the product is made. A portion of the glycerin is heated with the boric acid at 140° to 150° until the reaction is complete.

$$\underset{\text{glycerin}}{C_3H_5(OH)_3} + \underset{\text{boric acid}}{H_3BO_3}$$
$$= \underset{\text{boroglycerin}}{C_3H_5BO_3} + \underset{\text{water}}{3H_2O}$$

The boroglycerin, while still hot, is dissolved in an equal weight of glycerin. This glycerite can be used directly as an antiseptic application or can be diluted with glycerin. Boroglycerin Glycerite also is called boroglyceride solution and glyceryl borate glycerite.

Starch Glycerite. Starch Glycerite is a jellylike preparation used as a base for water-soluble ointments and as a pill excipient. It is prepared by heating a mixture of starch, glycerin, water and benzoic acid at a temperature of 140° to 145° until a thick, transparent mass results. Starch Glycerite sometimes is called glycerin ointment.

Tannic Acid Glycerite. This contains 20 per cent of tannic acid with small amounts of sodium citrate and sodium sulfite to prevent discoloration. This glycerite affords an astringent preparation for local use and also can be diluted with water to produce rapidly an aqueous solution of tannic acid for some types of preparations. Tannic Acid Glycerite also is called tannin glycerite.

General Considerations

Tragacanth Glycerite (N.F. IX) was not admitted to later editions. It is a thick paste containing 12.5 per cent tragacanth and 77.5 per cent glycerin. It is used as a pill excipient and water-soluble base.

Two glycerites last recognized by *N.F. VIII* are iodine and zinc iodide glycerite and phenol glycerite.

Iodine and zinc iodide glycerite is a solution of iodine rendered soluble by the presence of a soluble iodide, zinc iodide. The zinc iodide acts also as an astringent. This glycerite is called diluted Talbot's solution and is applied topically for germicidal and astringent purposes. It is reported to be of questionable value.

A similar preparation of importance, iodine disclosing solution, *Accepted Dental Remedies, 1959,* is composed of zinc iodide 2.3 per cent, potassium iodide 2.3 per cent, iodine 7.7 per cent, glycerin 49 per cent and water. It is used as a disclosing stain to reveal the presence of plaques.

Phenol glycerite contains 19 per cent of phenol and is intended to provide a convenient method of preparing weaker dilutions of phenol by the addition of glycerin or water. It contains 1 per cent of sodium citrate to prevent darkening. This glycerite is also known as carbolic acid glycerite.

Three glycerites last official in *N.F. VII* are bismuth glycerite, a soluble form of bismuth tartrate used in preparing bismuth elixir and pepsin and bismuth elixir; egg yolk glycerite, containing 45 per cent of strained egg yolk; and pepsin glycerite, containing 10 per cent of pepsin.

Some other unofficial glycerites are: iron quinine and strychnine phosphate *(U.S.P. VIII)*, guaiac *(N.F. IV)*, pine tar *(N.F. V)*, hydrastis *(U.S.P. IX)*, alum and borax. The last two are official in the *British Pharmacopœia*. The *Pharmaceutical Recipe Book* contains formulas for 8 glycerites of such drugs as starch, borax, guaiac, iodine, zinc iodide, lead subacetate, pancreatin and strong silver protein.

Magnesium sulfate glycerite, containing 40 per cent of magnesium sulfate, is used as a lymphagogue. The preparation, applied locally, removes from damaged tissues lymph devoid of antibacterial properties and brings about replacement with fresh lymph. The glycerite is also valuable in treatment of poisoning by poison ivy. Compound ichthyol glycerite is valuable as an antiseptic and produces relief in certain inflammations. Glycerin solutions of the active constituents of some drugs such as cascara sagrada are marketed as glycerites and afford some advantage over tinctures and fluidextracts when the presence of alcohol is not desired.

Glycerite of hydrogen peroxide[2, 13] is prepared by mixing 1.5 to 2.5 per cent of hydrogen peroxide (92%) with anhydrous glycerin. Glycerite of hydrogen peroxide with carbamide is prepared by dissolving urea peroxide 4 Gm. and 8-hydroxyquinoline 0.1 Gm. in sufficient anhydrous glycerin to make 100 ml. The 8-hydroxyquinoline combines with the heavy metals that usually occur as impurities in glycerin. Although harmless in themselves, these trace elements tend to inactivate hydrogen peroxide. Glycerin serves as a stabilizer for the urea peroxide and prolongs its action. The use of anhydrous glycerin produces a more stable product than Glycerin, U.S.P., which may contain as much as 5 per cent water. These glycerites are effective in treating gas gangrene, tetanus, infections of the middle ear, Vincent's disease and some fungus and viral infections.

Storage

Glycerites are all hygroscopic and therefore should be preserved and dispensed in well-stoppered bottles.

COLLODIONS

Collodions are liquid preparations intended for external use, having as their base a solution of pyroxylin in a mixture of alcohol and ethyl oxide, or in other suitable solvents such as acetone, methanol, etc. They are applied to the skin by means of a camel's-hair brush or a glass applicator, whereupon the solvent evaporates, leaving a protective film of pyroxylin over the area. Frequently, medicaments are added to collodions, in which event the protective film holds the medicine in contact with the skin. Any medicament soluble in the solvent may be used in these preparations.

History

In 1846, Professor Schönbein discovered guncotton, and within a few years physicians were preparing ethereal solutions of the substance for use in surgery to hold the edges of wounds and incisions together. Collodions became official with *U.S.P. IV*. Every edition of the *N.F.* has carried formulas for one or more collodions.

Collodions of the U.S.P.

Three collodions are official in *U.S.P.*:

Collodion. This is a simple solution of pyroxylin in a mixture of alcohol and ethyl oxide and produces a film capable of contracting considerably. Such a film is valuable in drawing the edges of an incised wound together or applying pressure to a swollen area. It is not a comfortable film for movable parts of the body, is apt to crack and it is not waterproof.

Flexible Collodion. For movable parts of the body and where a contracting film is not desired, flexible collodion is used. Flexibility is accomplished by the addition of castor oil. Camphor also is added to make it waterproof. Flexible collodion sometimes is called elastic collodion.

Salicylic Collodion. A 10 per cent solution of salicylic acid in flexible collodion is called salicylic collodion. It is intended as an application for its keratolytic effect, especially in treating corns.

GENERAL CONSIDERATIONS

Styptic Collodion, N.F. VII, was not admitted to succeeding editions of the *N.F.* This collodion is a 16 per cent solution of tannic acid in flexible collodion, intended as an application for wounds to stop bleeding by the styptic action of tannin and to seal the wound with a film of pyroxylin.

Other medicaments and combinations of medicaments used in collodions and official at some time are: Salicylic Acid and Fluidextract of Cannabis in Compound Salicylic Collodion, N.F. VI; Sulfonated Bitumen, N.F. V; Cantharides, U.S.P. IV; Iodine, Iodoform and Croton Oil, N.F. IV.

Several proprietary corn remedies are forms of medicated collodions. Appearing on the market now are medicated solutions of synthetic resins in volatile solvents. These preparations are applied to the skin in the same manner as collodions, whereupon the solvent evaporates, and a protective film is left covering the area.

Film-producing solutions are also marketed in aerosol dispenser cans. Vibesate, N.N.D., 1960, contains a modified polyvinyl plastic in ethyl acetate and acetone with a fluoro-chloro hydrocarbon as a propellant. The material is applied by spraying the area to be dressed from a distance of 15 to 30 cm. When the solvents evaporate, a transparent, pliable, occlusive film resembling flexible collodion is left. Vibesate film retards the loss of fluids and electrolytes from injured areas. It is useful as a surgical dressing for burns, operative wounds and surface lesions, especially when gauze dressings are not desirable.

Surgical Spray Dressing, Rezifilm® (Squibb) contains a methacrylate resin with tetramethylthiuram disulfide as an antibacterial and antifungal agent in ethyl acetate. Fluoro-chloro hydrocarbons are used as propellants. Upon evaporation of the solvent, an adherent, flexible, transparent film covers the sprayed area. Surgical Spray Dressing is used as a dressing for minor cuts, abrasions and bruises, as a protective against tape burns and pressure sores and in surgery. Since it contains an antibacterial and antifungal agent, it is used several hours preoperatively for the preparation of the surgical area. The incision may be made directly through the film; and following surgery after the wound is dried, the area may be resprayed.

Inhalation of the vapors of these aerosols should be avoided. Since they are inflammable, they should not be used near an open flame. Needless to say, the containers should not be punctured, or incinerated.

STORAGE

In making and handling collodions, special precautions should be taken to prevent evaporation of the highly volatile solvents. The preparations should be dispensed in well-stoppered bottles equipped with either an applicator or a brush attached to the cap or stopper. Applicator or brush attachments eliminate waste. In the case of the brush, the bristles do not have an opportunity to dry out. Collodions should be kept in a cool place at a temperature not above 30° and remote from fire. They are very inflammable and explosive.

REFERENCES

1. Accepted Dental Remedies, ed. 24, Chicago, American Dental Association, 1959.
2. Brown, E. A., Krabek, W. and Skiffington, R.: New England J. Med. **234**:468, 1946.
3. DeNavarre, M. G.: The Chemistry and Manufacture of Cosmetics. New York, Van Nostrand, 1947.
4. Goodman, Louis, and Gilman, Alfred: The Pharmacological Basis of Therapeutics, ed. 2. New York, Macmillan, 1955.
5. Hammarlund, E. R.: J. Am. Pharm. A. (Pract. Ed.) **15**:226, 1954.
6. Harry, R. G.: Cosmetics: Their Principles and Practices. New York, Chemical Pub. Co., 1956.
7. Jenkins, Glenn L., *et al.*: Scoville's The Art of Compounding, ed. 9. Philadelphia, Blakiston, 1957.

8. Martin, Eric W.: Husa's Pharmaceutical Dispensing, ed. 5. Easton, Pa., Mack Publishing Co., 1959.
9. Martindale, The Extra Pharmacopoeia, Vol. 1. ed. 24. London, Pharmaceutical Press, 1958.
10. Ohmart, L. M., and Stoklosa, M. J.: J. Am. Pharm. A. (Pract. Ed.) **11**:104, 1950.
11. Osol, Arthur, and Farrar, G. E., Jr.: The Dispensatory of the United States of America, ed. 25. Philadelphia, Lippincott, 1955.
12. Ruddiman, E. A., and Nicholas, A. B.: Incompatibilities in Prescriptions. New York, Wiley, 1936.
13. Weaver, E. S.: Bull. Am. Soc. Hosp. Pharm. **4**:240, 1947.

ALFRED N. MARTIN, Ph.D.
Professor of Physical Pharmacy, Purdue University

15

Mixtures, Suspensions, Magmas, Gels and Jellies

MIXTURES
    OFFICIAL MIXTURES
    SOLUBILIZING AGENTS IN MIXTURES
SUSPENSIONS
    PROPERTIES OF SUSPENSIONS
    DISPERSION STABILIZERS AND OTHER
        CONSTITUENTS
    FORMULATION AND PREPARATION
        OF SUSPENSIONS

OFFICIAL SUSPENSIONS
MAGMAS, GELS AND JELLIES
    INORGANIC GELS: OFFICIAL MAGMAS AND
        GELS
    RECENT INVESTIGATIONS OF ANTACIDS
    ORGANIC GELS: OFFICIAL JELLIES AND
        RECENT INVESTIGATIONS

The several classes of preparations in this chapter may be considered as colloidal or coarse dispersions for internal use or for application to mucous membranes. Mixtures and most suspensions, magmas and gels are used internally; jellies are applied to mucous membranes for local action; para-nitrosulfathiazole suspension is administered intrarectally; while bentonite magma may be used either internally or externally for stabilizing suspensions and emulsions. Sterile suspensions, which are intended for parenteral use, are described in Chapter 12.

Nomenclature. Many of the terms employed in pharmacy have evolved from popular usage and in some cases do not have exact meanings. The difficulties of pharmaceutical nomenclature are particularly evident among the preparations of this chapter. The terminology of colloid science is also obscure in some instances, owing to the fact that colloidal classes are complex and cannot always be defined in unambiguous terms.

A comparison of the nomenclature of pharmacy and colloid science as applied to the preparations under discussion is included in Table 11, together with some distinguishing characteristics of each class.

MIXTURES

Mixtures are aqueous or hydroalcoholic liquid preparations containing matter in colloidal suspension intended for oral administration.

The term mixture generally is used in science to refer to a combination of substances in which the constituents retain their separate identities. A mixture is distinguished from a compound in that the constituents of a mixture are not always present in the same proportions. Solutions are defined as *homogeneous mixtures* of two or more substances; colloidal systems, on the other hand, may be either *homogeneous or heterogeneous mixtures*. The word "mixture" was used in pharmacy in the past to refer to any combination of ingredients in

TABLE 11

Pharmacy Title	Colloid Class	Particle Size Range*	Dispersion Stabilizer Required	"Shake Well" Label Required	Appearance and Consistency
Mixture	Colloidal solution, dispersion, or sol	Less than 1 micron	A solubilizer may be added to improve the product	Yes	Clear, colored liquid of water-like consistency
Suspension	Suspension	About 0.5 to 3 microns and aggregates of 5 to 50 microns	Suspending agent	Yes	Creamy liquid with a relatively high viscosity provided by the suspending agent
Magma and gel	Inorganic gel	Particles of about 1 micron or less distributed throughout a gelatinous mass	None	Yes	White, opaque, viscous product
Jelly	Organic gel or jelly	Submicroscopic particles	Gelling agent	No	Translucent semisolid

* Particle sizes in the colloidal and coarse dispersion range are usually expressed in microns (μ). A micron is one 10,000th of a centimeter (10^{-4} cm.).

a liquid medium for internal use, and it included true solutions, colloidal dispersions and coarse suspensions of liquid and solid materials. Since many of these preparations are now grouped with other pharmaceutical classes, the restricted definition as used here is more appropriate.

The official mixtures, with several exceptions that will be discussed later, are colloidal dispersions of plant extractives, together with salts and flavoring agents. They are prepared by simple admixture of the ingredients. The extractive matter of the fluidextracts, the tinctures and the spirits are dispersed as colloidal particles when these alcoholic preparations are mixed with water and syrups.

OFFICIAL MIXTURES

There are no mixtures in U.S.P. XVI. The mixtures of N.F. XI, exclusive of Chalk Mixture and Kaolin Mixture with Pectin, are found in Table 12. The chalk and kaolin products do not conform to the definition of a mixture as given above; accordingly, they are classified with the suspensions, where they logically belong.

SOLUBILIZING AGENTS IN MIXTURES

Official mixtures are not a particularly popular class of preparations; however, the practicing pharmacist sometimes is confronted with the problem of combining alcoholic and hydroalcoholic solutions of vegetable extractives with aqueous solutions in such a way that the matter which is thrown out of solution does not clump and settle to the bottom of the container. In recent years, nontoxic solubilizing agents have been introduced into pharmacy to disperse the alcohol-soluble extractive matter in aqueous mixtures.

The action of certain surface-active agents in dissolving organic compounds, which are only slightly soluble in water, is referred to as *solubilization;* and these surface-active agents are known as *solubilizing agents*. Solubilization is brought about by adsorption or solution of the water-insoluble organic substance within the clusters or *micelles* of solubilizer molecules that exist in the solutions. The mixing of cresol with soap solution to yield saponated cresol solution is an example of solubilization. The nonpolar cresol is taken up in the hydrocarbon part of the soap clusters and

TABLE 12. PREPARATIONS OF THE N.F. PROPERLY CLASSIFIED AS MIXTURES*

English Title and Synonym	Ingredients	Category and Usual Dose
Compound opium and glycyrrhiza mixture (brown mixture)	Glycyrrhiza fluidextract, antimony potassium tartrate, camphorated opium tincture, ethyl nitrite spirit, glycerin and purified water	Expectorant, 4 ml.
Rhubarb and soda mixture	Rhubarb fluidextract, ipecac fluidextract, sodium bicarbonate, peppermint spirit, glycerin and purified water	Cathartic, 4 ml.

* See p. 268 for Chalk Mixture and Kaolin Mixture with Pectin.

is solubilized effectively in an aqueous solution in which it is normally soluble to only a slight extent.

A solubilizing agent such as Polysorbate 80, U.S.P. (Tween 80*) or polyoxyethylene sorbitan monolaurate (Tween 20*) may be used to prevent precipitation when tinctures, fluidextracts, spirits and similar solutions are added to water. The use of Tween 20 as a solubilizing agent has been described by Stoklosa and Ohmart[1] for the formula:

Nux vomica tincture..................	15 ml.
Compound gentian tincture...........	30 ml.
Purified water, enough to make.......	120 ml.

The product may be improved by mixing 5 ml. of Tween 20 with the tinctures. To this solution, water is added in divided portions, shaking after each addition to produce a clear dispersion.

Several problems arise in the use of solubilizing agents as pharmaceutical adjuncts: the agent may impart a disagreeable taste and odor to the mixture; it may cause the solution to foam excessively when agitated; it may lead to increased mold growth in liquid preparations; it may interact (complex) with the constituents of the mixture to yield precipitates, gelatinous masses and other forms of incompatibility; it may result in untoward physiologic effects.

The first of these difficulties was considered by Bogash[2] in a report describing the solubilization of phenobarbital in aqueous solutions. Bogash, and later Applewhite and his associates,[3] suggested glycerin, citric acid, fruit flavors and sodium Sucaryl† as masking agents for disguising the undesirable taste and odor of Polysorbate 80. Banker and Lee[4] found that a polyoxyethylene stearate (Myrj 51*) served as an effective solubilizing agent for the volatile oils in aromatic elixir and did not impart a disagreeable taste or odor to the final product. These investigators reduced the foaming of the product by the use of several drops of a 1:200 aqueous suspension of Dow-Corning antifoam A. F. Emulsion.

Reports in the foreign literature have referred for some time to the increased tendency toward mold growth in solutions of sorbitan derivatives. In this country, Steen, Marcus and Benton[5] observed mold growth after 1 month in aromatic waters containing polyoxyethylene sorbitan esters (Tweens) and no mold formation in the controls. Barr and Tice[6] showed that microorganisms can grow in nonionic surfactants of the polyoxyethylene sorbitan ester type and can split the ester linkage of the surfactant.

Bolle and Mirimanoff[7] first reported on the inactivation of certain preservatives by nonionic surface active agents. DeNavarre[8] has dealt with the problem in a recent series of papers, and he has concluded that the inactivation of preservatives by nonionic agents can be minimized by the addition of 5 to 10 per cent ethanol or hexylene glycol, or by the addition of about 20 per cent of certain quaternary germicides. Barr and Tice[6] investigated the preservative action of a series of agents in a 5 per cent aqueous solution of polyoxyethylene 20 sorbitan monostearate (Tween 60*) and in an oil-in-water ointment base. They found that sorbic acid (an essentially nontoxic agent) and

* Atlas Powder Co., Wilmington 99, Del.
† Abbott Laboratories, North Chicago, Ill.

combinations of sorbic acid and hexylene glycol were the most effective preservatives against a number of common microorganisms. The parabens (para-hydroxybenzoic acid esters) were found to be ineffective in preserving the 5 per cent solution of the surface-active agent.

The parabens are tied up and rendered ineffective by nonionic surface-active agents, and this interaction may explain the failure of the parabens to preserve various mixtures, creams and lotions which contain nonionic agents. Lach et al.[9] have shown that the parabens combine with polyethylene glycol, whereas sorbic acid complexes with glycols only to a limited extent. Kostenbauder et al.[10] have shown that the parabens are tied up to a great extent by polyoxyethylene 20 sorbitan monooleate (Tween 80*). At a concentration of 5 per cent of Tween 80, only 22 per cent of the methyl and 4.5 per cent of the propyl paraben are present as unbound preservative.

Barkley[11] suggested that in the presence of macromolecules which tend to render the parabens ineffective by binding, the following procedures may be used to re-establish their activity: add sufficient preservative to compensate for the amount of paraben tied up by the surface-active agent or macromolecule; add a glycol (e.g., propylene or hexylene glycol) which apparently minimizes the binding; use a macromolecule which is found not to bind with the preservative; combine several preservatives to increase the antibacterial action.

Polyoxyethylene compounds have also been known to lead to the formation of oily droplets, precipitates and gelatinous masses when used as solubilizing and emulsifying agents in various pharmaceutical preparations.

The final consideration in the use of solubilizing agents for mixtures involves possible untoward physiologic action. Polysorbate 80 (Tween 80) produced no evidence of toxicity when ingested daily by animals and human subjects over a period of several months.[2, 12] Tween 80 increases the absorption of fat and fat-soluble vitamins and is available in capsule form for cases of faulty fat assimilation. However, one might conceive of an undesirable situation arising through the use of sorbitan derivatives where the physician desires that the solubilized drug be unabsorbed and remain in the intestinal tract.

SUSPENSIONS

Suspensions represent a class of official preparations which include both powders in dry form to be placed in suspension and drugs suspended in liquid vehicles by means of appropriate suspending agents.

Accordingly, a pharmaceutical suspension may be defined as a dispersion containing finely divided insoluble material suspended in a liquid medium, or available in dry form to be distributed in the liquid when desired. Some suspensions are sterile and are intended for injection or for ophthalmic use; they are discussed in the chapter on solutions.

An acceptable suspension for oral use should possess certain qualities, among which are the following: the material must be composed of small, uniformly sized particles which do not settle rapidly; the particles which do settle to the bottom of the container should not pack into a hard cake, but instead should be redispersed completely and evenly with a minimum amount of agitation; the suspension should not be too viscous to pour freely from the orifice of the bottle; the product should have an agreeable odor, color and taste, and must not decompose or exhibit mold growth during storage. In short, the suspension must provide the patient with a uniform, therapeutically active dosage of the drug in a preparation which is pleasant and convenient to take.

Properties of Suspensions

The particles in a suspension have diameters for the most part greater than 0.5 micron. The individual particles range in size from about 0.5 micron to 3 microns; flocculates or aggregates of particles may attain sizes of 50 microns or larger.

Particles having diameters less than approximately 5 microns show brownian movement (see p. 116), and remain distributed uniformly throughout the suspension, provided that the collisions do not result

---

* Atlas Powder Co., Wilmington 99, Del.

Table 13. Gerding and Sperandio[13] have prepared a table which summarizes the important properties of pharmaceutical suspending agents to which the reader may refer for additional information. The suspending properties of natural gums and suspending agents are also discussed in a number of reports.[14]

Other Constituents. In addition to the medicinal agents and the various dispersion stabilizers, a pharmaceutical suspension may contain colors, sweetening agents, flavors and masking agents, preservatives and humectants. These will be referred to in the discussion of the official and the nonofficial suspensions.

FORMULATION AND PREPARATION OF SUSPENSIONS

The formulation, the preparation and the stabilization of pharmaceutical suspensions is a difficult task, calling for considerable knowledge and skill on the part of the pharmacist.

Formulation. The choice of wetting and suspending agents is of highest importance and should be made only after careful study and experimentation. The concentration of the suspending agent depends on the desired consistency of the product. The agent should supply a viscosity which minimizes sedimentation but is not so great as to prevent easy redistribution of any sediment and rapid flow of the liquid from the container.

The dispersion stabilizer must not interfere with the therapeutic activity of the drugs contained in the product. Some examples of incompatibilities which may occur are the following. Hydrophilic colloids, such as tragacanth, alginates, pectin, carboxymethylcellulose and bentonite are negatively charged and tend to form semisolid gels or claylike sediments when used to suspend bismuth subnitrate and bismuth subsalicylate.[15] Synthetic stabilizers containing polyoxyethylene groups (Tweens and Myrjs) and polyethylene glycol groups are incompatible with phenols. According to Goldstein[16] zirconium oxide can be suspended in methylcellulose solution but forms a precipitate with sodium carboxymethylcellulose; while phenol, resorcinol and tannic acid form clear solutions with sodium carboxymethylcellulose and precipitate with methylcellulose. Possible incompatibilities between drugs and suspending agents and other adjuncts are best ascertained by mixing the ingredients in proper concentrations and observing the samples under various conditions for a sufficient period of time.

Preparation. The suspending agent may be incorporated into the suspension in the form of a mucilage which, for most natural and synthetic gums, may be prepared as follows. The water, containing an effective preservative, is placed in a high-speed mixing apparatus, and the powdered gum is sifted onto the surface of the liquid.

A second method involves wetting the powder with a liquid that the gum does not absorb readily. Alcohol, glycerin and propylene glycol commonly are used for this purpose. Then when water is added, it penetrates between the individual particles of gum and wets them thoroughly without producing lumps.

Methylcellulose is unique in that it is soluble in cold water but insoluble in hot water. A mucilage of methylcellulose is prepared by adding hot water to distribute the particles of the powder without producing lumps, and then cooling the mixture or adding very cold water to dissolve the substance and bring the mucilage to the final volume. If the product is allowed to remain in the refrigerator for some time, a sparkling clear mucilage results.

On the small scale, suspensions are prepared in a mortar or a mechanical mixing apparatus. The insoluble drugs are levigated with part of the mucilage or with a levigating agent such as glycerin, propylene glycol or a suitable nontoxic surface-active agent. When the powders have been reduced to a smooth paste, the vehicle in which any soluble drugs, colors and flavors may be dissolved is added in divided portions. Instead of preparing a mucilage of the suspending agent, the stabilizer may be mixed with the other powders of the formula and rubbed to a smooth paste with small portions of water or the vehicle. Then the suspension is transferred to a graduate, and final portions of the vehicle are used to rinse the mixing vessel and equipment, and the product is brought to the desired volume.

On the industrial scale, insoluble powders are dispersed in liquids by the use of ball, roller and colloid mills. Dough mixers and similar blending machinery may also be employed in the process.

OFFICIAL SUSPENSIONS

The suspensions which have been introduced into *U.S.P. XVI* and *N.F. XI* represent 2 types: dry powder mixtures consisting of the drug, the suspending agent and other adjuncts to be dispersed in water when required, and suspensions of the drugs together with other agents in a liquid medium. The former class includes those drugs which are unstable when stored in the form of a liquid suspension but maintain their therapeutic activity for a reasonable period of time when kept in the dry powdered form.

Acetyl Sulfisoxazole Oral Suspension, U.S.P., contains the antibacterial agent in a suspension having a pH of 5.0 to 5.5.

Chloramphenicol Palmitate Oral Suspension, U.S.P., consists of a suspension of chloramphenicol palmitate in a mixture of dispersing and flavoring agents. It serves as a convenient administration of the antibiotic, the dose of which is 500 mg. 4 times a day.

Cortisone Acetate Ophthalmic Suspension, N.F., is a sterile suspension of cortisone acetate in an aqueous medium with a suitable bacteriostatic agent. It is intended for use in those instances in which the anti-inflammatory action of cortisone is deemed advisable. Because it is possible to transmit infections by the application of nonsterile ophthalmic preparations, the *U.S.P.* and the *N.F.* require that all preparations intended for such use be sterile (cf. Discussion of ophthalmic solutions in Chap. 11. For a discussion of the methods used in preparing sterile suspensions and possible preservatives to be used, see Chap. 12, Parenteral Preparations). The suspension is applied in concentrations of 0.5 or 2.5 per cent and is commercially available in these strengths. It should be preserved in tight containers.

Diphenylhydantoin Oral Suspension, U.S.P., is a suspension of diphenylhydantoin in a suitable medium containing 2.25 to 2.75 Gm. of the drug in each 100 ml. of suspension. Diphenylhydantoin is used as an anticonvulsant. The dose of the suspension is stated as that amount which is equivalent to 100 mg. of the drug to be repeated as many as 4 times a day.

Erythromycin Oral Suspension, U.S.P., is a suspension of erythromycin ethylcarbonate or other suitable salt or ester of erythromycin, together with suitable suspending and dispersing agents. The preparation also may contain suitable colors, flavors, buffers and preservatives. It may be packaged as a dry powder for suspension. In the liquid form the suspension usually is available in the concentration of 200 mg. of the drug per 5 ml.; in the dry form it is packaged in the amount of 2.4 Gm. of erythromycin in 60 ml. containers. Erythromycin is used as an antibiotic and antiamebic.

Nitrofurantoin Oral Suspension, U.S.P., contains 460 to 540 mg. of nitrofurantoin in each 100 ml. and has a pH of about 4.5. The suspension must not come in contact with metals other than stainless steel and aluminum. The drug is used as a urinary tract antibacterial agent, and the suspension is taken in sufficient amount to provide a usual dose of 100 mg. 4 times a day.

Novobiocin Calcium Oral Suspension, U.S.P., is an antibiotic preparation of the drug suspended by appropriate agents in an aqueous vehicle containing colors, flavors and preservatives and having a pH of about 6.5. The dose of the preparation is sufficient to supply 250 mg. of novobiocin calcium every 6 hours.

Nystatin for Oral Suspension, U.S.P., is a dry mixture of the drug combined with suitable suspending, dispersing, flavoring and preserving agents. Nystatin is an antifungal antibiotic and is administered as an aqueous suspension in the concentration of 500,000 U.S.P. units 3 times a day. The preparation is ordinarily available in the concentration of 2,400,000 U.S.P. units in 24-ml. containers.

Oral Oxytetracycline for Suspension, N.F., is a dry powder containing oxytetracycline, together with harmless dispersing and flavoring agents, and is preserved in tight containers protected from light. Oxytetracycline is a broad-spectrum antibiotic; the usual dose corresponds to 250 mg. of the antibiotic 4 times a day.

Para-nitrosulfathiazole Suspension, N.F., is a liquid suspension of the drug together with appropriate suspending and preserving agents. This antibacterial agent is used intrarectally; the usual dose of the 10 per cent suspension is 10 ml.

Phenoxymethyl Penicillin for Oral Suspension, U.S.P., is a dry mixture of the drug, together with suitable suspending, coloring, flavoring, buffering and preserving agents. The powder must not contain more than 1 per cent of moisture. The usual dose of the antibiotic is 200,000 U.S.P. units (approximately 130 mg. of phenoxymethyl penicillin) 4 times a day.

Other oral suspensions of penicillin have been introduced as pharmaceutical specialties and deserve mention at this point. Sabatini and Gulesich[17] reported on the formulation of a stable oral aqueous suspension of procaine penicillin G. The suspension consisted of 85,000 units per milliliter of procaine penicillin in a vehicle containing sodium gluconate, sodium citrate, sorbitol, and suitable flavors, colors and preservatives. Tragacanth in 0.2 per cent concentration was found to afford the best suspending qualities and allowed free resuspension of the product without caking. A mixture of mint, imitation chocolate and imitation custard flavor were found to provide the best flavor when clinically tested. A combination of insoluble saccharin and saccharin sodium together with D-sorbitol further improved the taste. Finally, the addition of 5 per cent kaolin was found to eliminate the grittiness of the formula and produce a creamy product. The smoothness of the suspension was further improved by using procaine penicillin G with a particle size of 40 to 60 microns. Although a smaller particle size produced greater smoothness, such a product was found to be quite bitter. No loss in penicillin potency occurred after a storage period of 13 months at room temperature in this vehicle. Color, odor, taste and resuspendability also remained satisfactory after this time.

Charnicki and Kober[18] studied the effects of flavors on the stability of penicillin in concentrations of 100,000 to 250,000 units in oral penicillin-triple sulfonamide powders for suspension. These authors reported that the stability of the penicillin depended greatly on the flavor used. Accelerated tests were conducted in which the flavored powders were kept at 100° C. or 4 days and then suspended and assayed for penicillin content. Long-term stability tests at room temperature were also carried out as a final criterion. Since the structure and the composition of most flavoring agents and mixtures are not known, and since reliable predictions of stability cannot be based on structural considerations alone, the authors found it necessary to study the stability of each flavoring agent individually. It was concluded that satisfactory flavored powders, which maintained the labeled amounts of penicillin and sulfonamides in storage, for as long as 43 months, could be prepared by this method.

Selenium Sulfide Detergent Suspension, U.S.P., is an aqueous suspension of selenium sulfide stabilized at pH 3.6 to 4.5 and containing 2.25 to 2.75 Gm. of SeS_2 in each 100 ml. of the suspension. It is used as an antiseborrheic topically on the scalp in the amount of 5 to 10 ml. for 5 minutes, then removed by thorough rinsing.

Sulfacetamide, Sulfadiazine and Sulfamerazine Suspension, N.F., is a combination of the 3 sulfonamides in a buffered aqueous suspension, together with suitable suspending, flavoring, coloring and preserving agents. The preparation is administered orally as an antibacterial agent, and the concentration is adjusted so that each dose contains 2 Gm. of the combination of sulfonamides.

Sulfamethiazole Suspension, N.F., is an aqueous suspension of the antibacterial agent, together with buffering and suitable flavoring, suspending, preserving and coloring agents. The dose of the suspension corresponds to 0.5 Gm. of the drug and is administered from 4 to 6 times daily.

Tetracycline Oral Suspension, U.S.P., is a liquid suspension of tetracycline, tetracycline hydrochloride or another suitable salt of tetracycline, which is stabilized with harmless suspending and dispersing agents and contains the desired flavoring agents. This product may also be packaged as a dry powder. It is administered 4 times a day in a dosage corresponding to 500 mg. of tetracycline hydrochloride.

Trisulfapyrimidines Oral Suspension, U.S.P., is a liquid suspension containing 3.0 to 3.7 Gm. each of sulfadiazine, sulfamerazine and sulfamethazine in 100 ml. of suspension. Suspensions that are commercially available usually contain 33 mg. each of the 3 sulfonamides in 1 ml. of the suspension. The preparation also may contain sodium citrate or lactate as a stabilizer and a suitable antibacterial agent.

The product should be stored in light-resistant containers at a temperature above freezing. It is administered initially in a dose of 40 ml. followed by a 4 ml. maintenance dose every 4 hours.

Kerr and Zopf[19] studied the suitability of various suspending and flavoring agents for use with a combination of these 3 sulfonamides. The dispersion stabilizer of choice was sodium alginate (Kelgin LV) in 1.5 per cent concentration. Other agents in the order of preference were bentonite magma, tragacanth and pectin. Of the 2 flavoring agents used, cacao syrup presented a problem because of the theobroma oil; cinnamon syrup proved to be more acceptable. Glycerin and sodium saccharin assisted in masking the bitter taste of the sulfonamides. Mold developed in the samples early in the investigation and was eliminated by the addition of a combination of methylparaben and propylparaben.

Chalk Mixture, N.F., belongs with the new class of pharmaceutical suspensions, since it contains particles of sizes beyond the colloidal range, which are maintained in uniform distribution by means of a suspending agent.

This preparation contains prepared chalk ($CaCO_3$) suspended in bentonite magma and sweetened and flavored with saccharin sodium and cinnamon water. The chalk and the soluble saccharin are levigated with a mixture of bentonite magma and cinnamon water to form a smooth paste. The remaining magma and sufficient purified water are added finally to complete the preparation.

Chalk mixture is used as an antacid and is administered in a dose of 15 ml.

Huyck[20] found that when a 4 per cent magma of colloidal aluminum magnesium silicate (Veegum HV) was used in Chalk Mixture, a better preparation was obtained than when bentonite magma was employed as the suspending agent.

Pienta, Marcus and Benton[21] reported that Veegum HV, in concentrations of 1.5 to 3 per cent, produced a better suspension of prepared chalk than was possible with bentonite, sodium alginate or methylcellulose 15 centipoises.

Lesshafft and DeKay[22] found that Veegum HV in 3.5 per cent concentration and tragacanth, 0.63 per cent by weight, were the most acceptable for suspending prepared chalk. Samples containing these suspending agents required a minimum of shaking for resuspension of the drug.

Kaolin Mixture with Pectin, N.F. This product is an aqueous suspension of kaolin and pectin combined with tragacanth, flavoring and sweetening agents and containing the preservative, benzoic acid. The preparation is used as an adsorbent and demulcent principally in cases of diarrhea and is administered in doses of 30 ml. In addition to its demulcent action, pectin assists tragacanth as a suspending stabilizer for kaolin.

Swafford and Nobles[23] suggested the use of a finely divided acid polymer, Carbopol 934,* as a suspending agent for use in kaolin-pectin suspensions. The acid polymer is brought to a pH of about 7 with sodium carbonate to form the mucilage of Carbopol, according to directions in the Goodrich Co. bulletin. The following formula demonstrates the use of this suspending agent.

Kaolin	11.66
Pectin	0.26
Carbopol 934	0.18
Sucaryl sodium	0.60
Peppermint oil	0.35
Methyl salicylate	0.35
Sodium carbonate	
Purified water, of each enough to make..	60

* B. F. Goodrich Chemical Co., Cleveland 15, Ohio.

All ingredients except the water are mixed together in a mortar. Water is added slowly with trituration until the desired volume is reached.

Pienta et al.[21] reported that Veegum HV, 3 per cent, yielded a satisfactory suspension of kaolin. Guth and his associates[24] investigated various kaolin-pectin formulas. They found that, when sufficient pectin was used to prevent rapid settling and caking of the kaolin, the suspension had a jellylike consistency. The addition of a surface-active agent, sorbitan monooleate (Span 80), broke the gel structure and permitted the suspension to flow without altering the suspending properties of the pectin. (See the section Surfactants and Deflocculating Agents, p. 263.)

MAGMAS, GELS AND JELLIES

Official magmas, gels and jellies belong to the colloid class known as gels, which include both inorganic and organic substances. A gel is a semisolid system consisting of hydrated threads or granules of the dispersed phase intimately associated with the dispersion medium. It may be formed by rapid precipitation from highly supersaturated solutions to form a gelatinous mass, by altering the temperature or by adding a second solvent to a lyophilic sol, and by other means. The methods of preparing official gels and jellies are discussed with the various preparations.

Confusion has arisen through the establishment of 2 separate pharmaceutical classes, *magmas* and *gels,* to represent preparations that belong to a single colloid class known as inorganic gels. Differentiation between official magmas and gels on the basis of particle size is not possible since modern manufacturing procedures, involving passage of the final product through a colloid mill, render the difference in particle size of these products indistinguishable. The sizes of the particles of commercial samples of Magnesia Magma are the same and sometimes appear smaller than those of Aluminum Hydroxide Gel and Aluminum Phosphate Gel. The particles of bentonite in the magma, for the most part, are considerably smaller than those in the official gels.

Difficulties also arise when one attempts to differentiate between Ephedrine Sulfate Jelly and pectin paste,* which fall into the single colloid class of organic jellies.

Consequently, it is useful to consider

---

* Pastes are discussed in the chapter on ointments.

TABLE 14. GEL CLASSES AND OFFICIAL PREPARATIONS WHICH BELONG WITH EACH GROUP

Gel Class	Preparation of the Gel and Nature of the Structure	Official Preparations
Inorganic Gels		
Gelatinous precipitate	Produced by rapid precipitation and hydration from highly supersaturated solutions to yield a gelatinous mass and a supernatant liquid. The gel in high concentration may exhibit thixotropy*	Bismuth Magma Magnesia Magma Aluminum Hydroxide Gel Aluminum Phosphate Gel Dihydroxyaluminum Aminoacetate Magma
Inorganic jelly	Results from strong sorption of water by highly dispersed particles. The jelly may show thixotropy*	Bentonite Magma
Organic Gels (Organic jellies)	Crystalline or amorphous jellylike network in which both solid and liquid phases are continuous, similar to but probably more complex than inorganic jelly structures	Ephedrine Sulfate Jelly Pramoxine Hydrochloride Jelly Pectin Paste, N.F. X.

---

* Thixotropy refers to the change of a gel into a liquid upon agitation and a return of the liquid to the gel state when the preparation is allowed to stand undisturbed for some time.

both colloid and pharmaceutical classifications. According to Weiser,[25] gels may be divided into (1) inorganic gels including gelatinous precipitates and inorganic jellies and (2) organic gels (or jellies). The characteristics of these gel-types are found in Table 14, together with the pharmaceutical preparations that belong to the various classes.

Gelatinous Precipitates and Jellies. A gelatinous precipitate results from mixing solutions of inorganic chemicals, which react to form insoluble particles that in turn have an affinity for water. A highly supersaturated solution is formed when the concentrated solutions are mixed. Microcrystalline nuclei then develop and rapidly grow to produce the particles that attract water strongly to yield a gelatinous mass. Finally, the gelatinous precipitate settles slowly, leaving a supernatant liquid.

A more uniform gel structure, which results from a slow development of the gelatinous mass and in which both the dispersed phase and the liquid medium are continuous throughout the system, is known as a *jelly* to differentiate it from a gelatinous precipitate.[25] Both inorganic and organic jellies exist, as noted in Table 14.

Theory of Gel Structure. No sharp demarcation can be made between liquid sols and semisolid gels; nor can a definite division be made between crystalline and amorphous regions within a gel structure. The semisolid nature of the structure may result from chemical bonds, weak secondary forces or links between crystalline regions.[26] It is thought to be the result of attachment between the particles which lie in a random brush-heap arrangement.[27]

Barium sulfate usually precipitates as a granular mass, but with high concentrations of reacting solutions the sediment may become gelatinous. Magnesium hydroxide and aluminum hydroxide magmas have a gelatinous character but do not set to semisolid gels. Silica gel is formed by reacting sodium silicate with hydrochloric acid. A sol of silica fibrils and a dilute solution of silicic acid is formed, and then, under suitable conditions of concentration, pH and temperature, the system slowly changes to a rigid gel as the fibrils link together.[28] Thus, these substances as well as others form precipitates with various degrees of gelatinous character.

Inorganic Gels: Official Magmas and Gels

As observed in Table 14, the gels of the *U.S.P.*, together with most of the magmas, belong to the group known in colloid science as gelatinous precipitates. Bentonite magma may be considered as an inorganic thixotropic jelly. Except for the latter preparation, magmas and inorganic gels have about the same consistency and have the same appearance both when observed visibly and when viewed under the microscope. Moreover, the method of preparation of these magmas and gels conforms to that given in Table 14 for gelatinous precipitates. Consequently, they are discussed together in this section.

Magmas and inorganic gels may be defined as viscous aqueous preparations containing finely divided hydrous inorganic matter intended primarily for oral administration. If the product has been prepared properly, the particles remain uniformly dispersed throughout the system; however, a supernatant liquid develops in time. The uniformity of the mixture is re-established easily by shaking the container, and directions to "shake well before using" must be included on the label of magmas and gels. The size and the irregularity of the particles may be reduced by passing the product through a colloid mill (see the chapter on Emulsions, p. 286, for a discussion of the colloid mill).

Bentonite Magma, U.S.P., is a 5 per cent (w/v) dispersion of bentonite in purified water. The bentonite powder is peptized and dispersed to form a sol (liquid dispersion) by sprinkling it on hot water. After the powder has become thoroughly wetted, it is allowed to stand with occasional stirring for 24 hours, and then is stirred until a uniform mixture is obtained.

After the dispersion has cooled and is allowed to stand undisturbed for some time, it sets to a jelly. When the product is shaken, it reverts to the liquid form, but again forms a jelly if allowed to stand. This reversible sol-gel transformation may be repeated indefinitely. The phenomenon is known as *thixotropy*, and bentonite magma is said to be a *thixotropic gel*.* If bentonite magma is diluted until the concentration of bentonite is below about 4 per cent, it no longer exhibits thixotropy but remains instead in the liquid state.[29]

Bentonite magma is used as a suspending agent and as an emulsifying and stabilizing agent for internally as well as externally administered products. However, its tan color sometimes militates against its use in pharmaceutical and cosmetic products. It has an alkaline reaction (pH 9 to 10) which may also be undesirable for some purposes. The gelatinous character of bentonite magma is reduced when it is combined with solutions of about pH 7 and below.

Bismuth Magma (Milk of Bismuth, Bismuth Cream), N.F., is an aqueous dispersion of bismuth hydroxide and bismuth subcarbonate in the form of a gelatinous precipitate. It is prepared by chemical reaction between bismuth subnitrate, nitric acid, ammonium carbonate and diluted ammonia solution. The reactions which occur are indicated in the following equations:

$$Bi(OH)_2NO_3 + 2HNO_3 \rightarrow Bi(NO_3)_3 + 2H_2O$$
$$Bi(NO_3)_3 + 3NH_4OH \rightarrow Bi(OH)_3 + 3NH_4NO_3$$
$$4Bi(NO_3)_3 + 6(NH_4)_2CO_3 + H_2O \rightarrow$$
$$(BiO)_2CO_3 \cdot H_2O + 12NH_4NO_3 + 4CO_2$$

The excess alkalinity produced by the ammonia water and the ammonium carbonate is removed along with the soluble ammonium nitrate by washing with water until the washings cease to give a pink color with phenolphthalein test solution. The method of preparation is described in detail in the *N.F.*

Bismuth Magma is an astringent and an antacid, and a protectant and adsorbent for coating the lining of the intestines and ulcer craters. It is used in enteritis, diarrhea, dysentery and ulcerative colitis. The usual dose is 4 ml. The magma should be preserved in tight containers and protected from freezing. The product separates somewhat on standing, and requires a "shake well" label.

Magnesia Magma (Milk of Magnesia), U.S.P., is a white, viscous liquid containing 7 to 8.5 per cent of $Mg(OH)_2$ in the form of a gelatinous precipitate. No formula is given in *U.S.P.* for its manufacture; however, it may be prepared by double decomposition according to the equation,

$$2NaOH + MgSO_4 \rightarrow Mg(OH)_2 + Na_2SO_4$$

or by the hydration of freshly calcined magnesium oxide:

$$MgO + H_2O \rightarrow Mg(OH)_2$$

the latter process being more convenient on the industrial scale.

The product may react with glass containers in which it is stored; accordingly, 0.1 per cent of citric acid may be added to minimize this action. Magnesia magma also reacts with cork to produce an off-color in the preparation; therefore, cork liners should not be used in the caps of the bottles. Milk of magnesia should be stored in tight containers in a cool place, but it should not be exposed to extremely low temperatures since freezing produces a coarsening of the particles.

A volatile oil or blend of oils may be added in a concentration of 0.05 per cent by volume for flavoring purposes.

Magnesia magma is used as an antacid in a dose of 4 ml. for hyperacidity of the stomach and as a cathartic in a dose of 15 ml.

Aluminum Hydroxide Gel (Colloidal Aluminum Hydroxide), U.S.P., is a gelatinous precipitate containing hydrated aluminum oxide and aluminum hydroxide to which sweetening, flavoring and preserving agents may be added. In one of the methods of preparation, a solution of aluminum chloride and a solution containing sodium carbonate and sodium bicarbonate are reacted to form a highly supersaturated solution from which the gelatinous aluminum hydroxide precipitates. The magma is dialyzed and then passed through a colloid mill.

---

* Gelatin and agar jellies change into sols when heated and revert to the gel state when cooled. However, the reversible sol-gel transformation of thixotropy occurs at constant (room) temperature and is thus said to be an isothermal process. It is brought about by mechanical agitation rather than by heat changes. Thixotropy is of Greek origin and means "to change by touching."

Aluminum hydroxide gel is used as a gastric antacid, particularly in the treatment of peptic ulcers, and acts by absorbing and neutralizing the hydrochloric acid of the stomach and by supplying a protective coating to the inflamed and ulcerated areas. Since it is not absorbed from the intestinal tract, it produces no toxicity; since it buffers the gastric juice at about pH 3.5 while absorbing excess hydrochloric acid, it does not produce alkalosis and does not disturb the digestive enzymes which function normally in acid solution. The disadvantages of aluminum hydroxide gel are the absorption of phosphates from the intestinal tract and the constipation action.

The dose of the gel is 8 ml., which may be repeated 4 times during the day.

Dried Aluminum Hydroxide Gel, U.S.P., is an amorphous powder prepared by drying the liquid gel at a moderate temperature. It is used frequently in the form of tablets for the same purpose as the liquid gel. The usual dose is 300 mg. administered 4 times a day, or hourly if necessary.

Some writers state that the product is not particularly useful since the particles become enlarged during the drying process. However, Dale and Booth[30] found that a tablet consisting of dried aluminum hydroxide gel and magnesium trisilicate showed prolonged antacid action at pH 3 to 4 and was equally as effective as a comparable liquid gel.

In 1949 and again in 1952, Hammarlund and Rising[31] studied the buffering capacities of various gastric antacids and, like Dale and Booth, concluded that a mixture of two parts of aluminum hydroxide and one part of magnesium trisilicate exhibited the features of a good antacid. These workers pointed out that the ideal antacid is not necessarily one that most nearly neutralizes the gastric acidity (i.e., elevates the pH of the gastric fluid from about 1.5 to 7), but rather one that buffers the gastric contents at a pH at which the hydrochloric acid is absorbed while the gastric enzymes continue to function properly in digestion. The pH should be maintained at about 3 to 5 in order to bring about the desired compromise between these two effects.

Dale and Booth[30] refer to the lack of agreement among investigators on the pH range which is required for effective antacid action. The pH may vary considerably, depending on the clinical purpose for which the drug is used. According to these investigators, when a pH as high as 6.8 is desired, a tablet containing magnesium trisilicate, calcium carbonate and magnesium carbonate is the product of choice. It holds the pH above 4 for 1 hour with a 1-tablet dose and for more than 2 hours with a 2-tablet dose.

Aluminum Phosphate Gel, N.F., is used for the same purpose as aluminum hydroxide gel but has the advantage of not interfering with phosphate absorption from the intestines. The phosphate gel has also been found to be superior for the treatment of peptic ulcers in patients with chronic diarrhea or with a deficiency in bile and pancreatic juice. Aluminum phosphate gel possesses about one half the acid absorptive power of the hydroxide.

This gel may be prepared by reacting aluminum chloride and sodium phosphate under carefully controlled conditions so as to form a gelatinous precipitate of finely divided particles. The product is dialyzed, mixed with sweetening, flavoring and preserving agents, and may then be passed through a colloid mill.

The dose is 15 ml. 6 times a day.

Dihydroxyaluminum Aminoacetate Magma, N.F., serves the same purpose as the aluminum gels which have just been discussed, and compares favorably on the basis of buffering capacity. Because it contains a lower percentage of aluminum than the aluminum hydroxide preparations, it is claimed to be less astringent to the intestines, hence less constipating. The drug may be flavored with suitable flavoring agents and stabilized by the use of suitable stabilizing agents and preservatives. The usual dose is equivalent to 500 mg. of the drug. This antacid compound is also available in tablet form.

RECENT INVESTIGATIONS OF ANTACIDS

Schleif[32] reviewed the *in vitro* methods for evaluating antacids and developed a new method, based on that of Rossett and Flexner,[33] which more nearly simulated the conditions found in the stomach in the presence of excess acid. The apparatus employed by Schleif continuously recorded the pH of the preparation as hydrochloric acid was added to the antacid. The speed of the action of an antacid was taken as the time required for it to raise the pH of the medium to a definite value. Schleif also determined the buffering range of the antacid and the duration of antacid action. Hinkel et al.[34] tested a new aluminum hydroxide polymer in tablet form and found it to be superior to other aluminum hydroxide tablets with respect to the speed of neutralization and the duration of buffer action when tested by the *in vitro* method of Rossett and Flexner.[33]

Grote et al.[35] investigated the antacid properties of dihydroxy aluminum sodium carbonate (DASC), a new antacid. DASC was found to produce a rapid neutralization of acidity to pH 4 and the maintenance of pH above pH 3 for at least 2 hours, thus affording prompt and prolonged buffering of gastric fluid. In 1956, Packman, Harrison et al.[36] began a comparative *in vivo* and *in vitro* study of 4 antacids, DASC, aluminum hydroxide, calcium carbonate and sodium bicarbonate. They concluded that the *in vivo* method was superior and that the *in vitro* method should be used only as a rough screening technic. Since antacids are used for gastric hyperacidity and for peptic ulcers, the authors evaluated the antisecretory and antipeptic activity of the antacids in addition to maintenance of pH and acid neutralizing power. Packman, Harrison, Abbott and Trabin[36] combined these various factors into an "index of antacid effectiveness" which was found to be greatest for DASC and lowest for aluminum hydroxide.

ORGANIC GELS: OFFICIAL JELLIES AND RECENT INVESTIGATIONS

Pharmaceutical jellies belong in the colloid class of organic gels. They are soft, translucent, semisolid preparations containing medicinal agents, aromatic odorous ingredients, preservatives, a humectant* such as glycerin or propylene glycol, a gelling

---

* A humectant has an affinity for water and protects the product against the rapid loss of moisture.

agent and water. Other stabilizers and adjuncts, such as buffers, also may be included.

Ephedrine Sulfate Jelly, N.F., is used for the application of ephedrine to the nasal passages. The use of tragacanth as the gelling agent results in great variation of viscosity of the product; however, no standards have been established to assure uniformity in consistency.

The ingredients are mixed together, and the product is stored in a closed container for about a week to allow complete hydration of the tragacanth. The product is then strained and placed in collapsible tubes.

In 1949, Huston and his associates[37] in Canada reported on the use of sodium alginate for the preparation of ephedrine sulfate jelly. Later, Fiedler and Lee[38] suggested the formula:

Ephedrine sulfate	10
Sodium alginate	40
Methyl salicylate	0.1
Eucalyptol	1
Sodium benzoate	2
Glycerin	100
Purified water	857
To make about	1,000

The sodium alginate is triturated with glycerin in a mortar to form a smooth paste, the ephedrine sulfate and the sodium benzoate are dissolved in the water, and the solution is added in divided portions to the first mixture. The oils are added, and the mixture is allowed to stand for about 3 hours to permit the formation of a smooth jelly.

Since sodium alginate may be obtained commercially in standard viscosity grades, this product does not have the disadvantage of the official tragacanth jelly.

According to Schwarz and Levy[39] the variation of Ephedrine Sulfate Jelly depends on the type of tragacanth used. Although the jelly may have a uniform initial viscosity, it may change markedly on aging. In another study,[40] these authors showed that both homogenization and the temperature employed during manufacture could alter the rapidity and extent of hydration and thus affect the viscosity of the final tragacanth preparation. The viscosity remained at a maximum during storage when the pH was kept near 5.0. The proposal of the National Formulary to add sodium phosphate as a stabilizer to Ephedrine Sulfate Jelly was studied by Schwarz and Levy[39] and was found actually to decrease the stability of the jelly. However, these authors found that the addition of Sodium Biphosphate, U.S.P., had a stabilizing effect on tragacanth preparations. According to Schwarz and Levy, sodium phosphate should be replaced by sodium biphosphate if a stabilizer is to be used.

Pramoxine Hydrochloride Jelly, N.F., is a 1 per cent preparation of the drug in a suitable jelly base and is used topically as a local anesthetic.

Recent Investigations

Hutchins and Singiser[41] investigated a number of natural and synthetic gums for use in pharmaceutical jellies, among which were Aqualized Tragacanth Gum, Kelgin LV, Methocel 400 cps., CMC-70 MV, Jaguar Gum and Veegum.* Sodium alginate (Kelgin LV) was found to be one of the best gelling agents for a number of commonly used drugs. The authors suggested the formula: Kelgin LV 7 per cent, glycerin 7 per cent, methylparaben, 0.2 per cent, calcium gluconate 0.05 per cent and purified water 86.25 per cent. Calcium ions were added to produce a firm gel. Fiedler and Lee[38] eliminated calcium ions from their product, since they observed that the jelly lost water on standing when the salt was incorporated.

Kaufman, Burlage and Lloyd[42] used another approach to the formulation of a jelly base. They developed a product containing 2 per cent tragacanth, and a small amount of liquid petrolatum, which was emulsified in the base. The mineral oil was added to produce an emollient effect on the skin. Sorbitan monolaurate was used to improve the emulsifying properties of tragacanth (cf. the section on mixed emulsifying agents in the chapter on Emulsions, p. 282) and benzalkonium chloride was used as the preservative. Sterilization of the product by boiling was also found necessary to protect the gel against fermentation. The base was compatible with a number of dermatologic agents in ordinary concentrations.

Taub, Meer and Clausen[43] studied the pH range and concentration of various preservatives for use with tragacanth jellies. A combination of methyl and propyl parabens was found to provide effective preservative action. However, the possible complexation and inactivation of the parabens by gums should be considered. Eisman, Cooper and Jaconia[44] found that tragacanth reduced the antibacterial properties of preservatives in certain concentrations; and Tillman and Kuramoto[45] demonstrated interaction between methylcellulose and propyl and butyl paraben. Often there is no visible evidence of the tying up of the preservative by the gum, making this form of incompatibility all the more difficult to uncover and guard against.

REFERENCES

1. Stoklosa and Ohmart: J. Am. Pharm. A. (Pract. Ed.) **12**:23, 1951.
2. Bogash: Bull. Am. Soc. Hosp. Pharmacists **10**:365, 1953.
3. Applewhite, Buckley, and Nobles: J. Am. Pharm. A. (Pract. Ed.) **15**:164, 1954.
4. Banker and Lee: J. Am. Pharm. A. (Pract. Ed.) **16**:169, 1955.
5. Steen, Marcus and Benton: J. Am. Pharm. A. (Pract. Ed.) **13**:180, 1952.
6. Barr and Tice: J. Am. Pharm. A. (Sci. Ed.) **46**:442; 445, 1957; J. Soc. Cosm. Chem. **9**:171, 1958; Am. Perfumer Aromat. **73**, No. 1: 20, 1959.
7. Bolle and Mirimanoff: J. Pharm. Pharmacol. **2**:685, 1950.
8. DeNavarre: J. Soc. Cosm. Chem. **7**:427, 1956; ibid. **8**:68, 371, 1957; ibid. **10**:81, 1959; Am. Perfumer Aromat. **73**, No. 1:31, 1959.
9. Lach, Ravel and Blaug: J. Am. Pharm. A. (Sci. Ed.) **46**:615, 1957.
10. Patel and Kostenbauder: J. Am. Pharm. A. (Sci. Ed.) **47**:289, 1958; Pisano and Kostenbauder, ibid. **48**:310, 1959.

---
* See Table 13 for a description of these agents.

one of the experiments, Barton prepared an emulsion containing acacia mucilage, almond oil and water.

The report on the early development of emulsions[3] also refers to an investigation by Fathergill and French. John Fathergill, an English physician of the 18th century, recognized the importance of emulsification for administration of oily medicinals, and requested French, a London apothecary, to experiment with mixtures of oil and water. French's results, published by Fathergill in 1757, referred to the use of acacia, syrups, honey, egg yolk, tragacanth, quince seed mucilage and starch jelly for the emulsification of almond, linseed, olive, anise and clove oils, and for beeswax, benzoin and similar medicinal substances. The oils, the water and the mucilage were triturated in glass or marble mortars, and the ratio of the 3 phases was varied to obtain the most stable product.

The early part of the 19th century witnessed the publication of many formulas for pharmaceutical emulsions, but it was not until the second half of the century that an interest was shown in improving the methods of emulsification. From the time of the early development of pharmaceutical emulsions in the 17th and the 18th centuries, o/w emulsions were prepared by the gradual addition of oil to egg yolk, to acacia and tragacanth mucilages or to an aqueous suspension of crushed almond seeds. Mohr's *Lehrbuch der Pharmazeutischen Technik,* which was translated into English by Redwood in 1849, described this process. The method, being particularly popular with the British pharmacists, became known as the British method or, as Remington called it in 1886, in the first edition of *The Practice of Pharmacy,* the *English method.* Since a number of pharmacists in this country assisted in establishing the most desirable proportions of oil, water and gum acacia, the procedure is referred to sometimes as the *American method.* However, some writers seem to favor the term *wet gum method,* since the process involves wetting and dispersing the emulsifying agent, usually gum acacia, with water to form a mucilage and adding oil gradually to the aqueous phase with trituration.

In 1874, Hans Wilder[4] described the method which was developed by Hager and Mohr and was favored by pharmacists in Germany and elsewhere on the Continent. According to this method, acacia was dispersed in the oil contained in a dry mortar, after which the water was added all in one portion and the mixture triturated until emulsification had occurred. Remington's *Practice of Pharmacy* referred to this procedure as the *continental method;* it has become known also as the *dry gum method.*

In 1872, Forbes[5] introduced the *bottle method* for the preparation of volatile oil emulsions. The procedure followed the dry gum method: acacia and the oil were placed in a dry bottle and mixed by agitation, the aqueous phase was added all at one time, and the bottle was shaken until emulsification had occurred.

The theory of emulsions, which was discussed in Chapter 7, has evolved for the most part during the present century. The synthesis of a large number of surface-active agents in recent years and the development of many new cosmetic and medicinal emulsions, resulting from an alcohol shortage during World War II, have led to the popularity of emulsified lotions and creams and have greatly stimulated research in this field.

Thus evolved a science and technology which for more than 300 years has intrigued not only the pharmacist and the physician but also the physicist, the chemist and the technologist.

PURPOSE OF EMULSIFICATION

Primarily, the reason for emulsification centers around the desirability of administering both aqueous and oil-soluble substances in the same mixture. Based on the use to which they may be put, emulsions are divided into two groups: emulsions for internal use and emulsions for external application.

EMULSIONS FOR INTERNAL USE

Emulsions for internal use may be administered orally or given by intravenous injection.

Orally Administered Emulsions. Pharmaceutical emulsions which are given orally are of the oil-in-water type. Enveloping the medicinal oil in a film of emulsifying agent aids in masking the disagreeable taste and the "oily" sensation which often accompanies the oral administration of a drug. Flavoring agents may be added to the external aqueous phase of the emulsion to increase the palatability.

Water-soluble drugs that are distasteful cause more difficulty than oils, since they remain in the external phase of an o/w emulsion. It is sometimes possible to disguise water-soluble drugs by the method of *dual emulsification*. Husa[6] refers to the masking of a bitter-tasting water-soluble drug by this method: the drug is incorporated in the internal phase of a water-in-oil emulsion; then, by the use of a hydrophilic emulsifying agent, the oily product is made the internal phase of an oil-in-water emulsion. Thus the bitter substance is masked effectively by placing it in the innermost phase of a dual water-in-oil-in-water emulsion. Such multiple emulsions in which the internal phase contains globules of the opposite phase are not uncommon; Seifritz[7] discussed the preparation of a quinque-multiple emulsion and included a microphotograph in his report in which one may discern 5 stages of phase alternation.

The distribution of drugs and flavors between the oil and the water phases is an important consideration in disguising unpleasant tastes. According to the distribution principle, a substance will be found in both phases of an emulsion but will concentrate predominantly in the liquid in which it is more soluble. The attempt to mask a distasteful drug by oil-in-water emulsification may be defeated if the drug possesses some water-solubility and passes partially into the external phase, and if the flavor and the masking agent are predominantly oil-soluble and concentrate primarily in the internal phase.

Emulsification is also useful for increasing the absorption of fats through the intestinal walls. It is first necessary to consider briefly the stages of fat digestion and assimilation. When fats and oils are ingested, they are emulsified in the duodenum by the bile salts. Then the emulsified fats are partially hydrolyzed by the pancreatic juice and are finally absorbed through the intestinal wall. That portion of fat which is not broken down to fatty acids and lower glycerides may be absorbed in the emulsified form, and passed into the blood stream if the emulsion globules are less than about 1 micron in diameter.

Olive oil and mineral oil in emulsified form are assimilated rapidly when the particles are sufficiently small.[8] Consequently, the most efficient absorption is attained by dispersing the oil by homogenization into globules preferably of about 0.5 micron diameter.

Intravenous Injection of Emulsions. Parenteral emulsions have been studied in recent years for administration of food and medicinal oils in both animals and human beings. Vitamin A is taken up rapidly by the tissues when injected in the form of an emulsion.[9] Emulsified chaulmoogra oil, vitamin K and some sex hormones have also been injected, and rats have been protected from rickets by injections of a cod-liver oil emulsion.[10] Emulsified oils also have been injected as diagnostic aids in the study of the function of liver and other organs. Hom *et al.*[11] recently reported a study of a radiopaque to be administered intravenously for visualization of the liver and the spleen.

Parenterally administered emulsions require special care during manufacture. The choice of the emulsifying agent and the size and the uniformity of the globules are critical in preparations for intravenous use. Egg lecithin was used in the early work, but recent investigations have shown it to be hemolytic. More recently, a sterile form of gelatin, serum albumin, purified soybean phosphatides and combinations of sorbitan esters of fatty acids* and their polyoxyethylene derivatives† have been used. However, as a result of preliminary clinical trials, Lambert, Miller and Frost[12] showed untoward physiologic effects in man

---

* Available as Spans from the Atlas Powder Co.
† **Available as Tweens from the Atlas Powder Co.**

which militated against the widespread use of such emulsifiers.

The preparation of emulsions for injection involves the formation of a coarse emulsion, which is then homogenized, collected and sealed in sterile flasks and autoclaved. Finally, the product is tested for sterility and for globule size.

Emulsions for External Application

Both o/w and w/o emulsions may be applied to the surface of the skin and the mucous membranes. By the process of emulsification, it is possible to produce a lotion or a cream that has the proper consistency, spreads well over an affected area, is washed from the surface easily, does not stain clothing and is appealing to the patient from the standpoint of general appearance, odor, color and "feel." When one contrasts the well-formulated emulsion base of today with the greasy product of earlier times, it is not difficult to realize why the physician and the patient demand the modern dermatologic preparation.

Emulsification of a drug in a base usually leads to a decrease in the rate and the extent of absorption through the skin and the mucous membranes. This principle is employed in the use of an o/w emulsion of ephedrine which, when applied to the nasal mucosa, is absorbed more slowly than an oil solution of the drug. The presence of the medication is thus prolonged in the desired area.

However, emulsification sometimes increases the rate of *percutaneous absorption* (i.e., absorption into and through the skin). Water-soluble antiseptics are absorbed through the skin more readily when incorporated in the aqueous phase of o/w bases than when administered in greasy vehicles. Coal tar is absorbed more effectively from an emulsified base; the physician should reduce the concentration of coal tar below that which ordinarily is specified when the drug is administered in a grease base. The degree to which the concentration of coal tar should be reduced has not yet been established, but usually it is safe to lower it to about one half of the original strength.

COMPOSITION OF AN EMULSION

As previously noted in the definition of an emulsion, the principal ingredients consist of two immiscible liquids, usually water and oil, and a third phase, the emulsifying agent.

The Aqueous Phase

In addition to water, the aqueous phase may contain water-soluble drugs, preservatives and coloring and flavoring agents. Distilled water, or pure water which has been deionized effectively, is often used in emulsions, since calcium and magnesium ions of hard water and other electrolytes may have an adverse effect on the stability of some emulsions, particularly those containing soaps as emulsifying agents.

Examples of drugs which sometimes are added to the aqueous phase of an emulsion are potassium iodide, ammonium chloride and chloral hydrate. They should be dissolved in the diluting vehicle and added carefully to the emulsion to minimize their effect on the stability of the product. Flavoring agents also are added to the aqueous phase, where they serve to mask disagreeable tastes and odors and provide a pleasant flavor to the product. Although they may be partly oil-soluble, the flavors must possess sufficient water-solubility to remain primarily in the aqueous phase. Preservatives also may dissolve to some extent in the oil as well as in the water phase of an emulsion, and enough preservative must be used so that, after equilibrium has been established, sufficient agent remains in the water to preserve it against attack by microorganisms. The efficiency of preservatives in emulsions may be tested by the method of Rdzok et al.[13]

The Oil Phase

The oil phase of an emulsion consists of fixed or volatile oils, resins, gum resins, waxes and fats; it may contain oil-soluble drugs such as phenyl salicylate, camphor and oil-soluble vitamins and antiseptics.

Sometimes an antioxidant is added to prevent rancidity of the oil and destruction of the vitamins. α-Tocopherol serves as an antioxidant for liquid petrolatum; when added to the oil in a concentration of 10 parts per million, it prevents the development of a disagreeable odor and taste. Dodecyl and propyl gallate and nordihydroguaiaretic acid (N.D.G.A.) are also effective antioxidants, and are recognized by the Food and Drug Administration for this purpose.[14]

Fats and oils should be kept free of micro-organisms since these bring about rancidity. Eisman, Jaconia and Mayer[15] found that, while nonsporulating organisms succumbed within 24 hours when added to sesame oil, the spores of *B. subtilis* were destroyed only slowly and incompletely by antiseptics such as thimerosal, ethyl alcohol and benzyl alcohol. Of a number of agents tested by these investigators, only hexylresorcinol, carvacrol, epichlorhydrin and ethylene oxide were effective against the spores in anhydrous sesame oil. It is apparent from these results that oils normally found in emulsions may become contaminated only from the use of highly impure water; the use of clean equipment and containers, a good grade of oil and distilled or pure deionized water containing an effective preservative should ensure freedom from micro-organisms.

The Emulsifying Agent

In the absence of an emulsifying agent, oil can be dispersed in water to the maximum extent of about 2 per cent. The average particle size in such dilute o/w emulsions, which are properly called *oil hydrosols,* is on the order of 0.1 micron, although it may be as large as 10 microns.

Emulsifying agents are required for the preparation and the stabilization of the more concentrated emulsions, containing about 10 to 80 per cent of internal phase, which are commonly used in pharmacy. Until recently, natural emulsifying agents were used almost exclusively in pharmacy. However, for the past several decades, the newer synthetic agents have been employed in the preparation of emulsified lotions, creams, ointments and other pharmaceutical and cosmetic products.

Surface-active agents, which are now often referred to as *surfactants,* are substances that concentrate at a surface or an interface and lower the surface or interfacial tension. Included in this group are wetting agents, deflocculating agents, detergents, suspending agents, emulsifying agents and others. Emulsifying agents differ from other surfactants in that they not only reduce interfacial tension but also form films around the dispersed globules. An emulsifying agent, then, is a particular type of surfactant that (1) reduces interfacial tension between oil and water and thus aids in the dispersion of one liquid in the other and (2) envelops the globules in a sheath to prevent coalescence and separation of the dispersed liquid as a distinct layer. The first of these properties represents the emulsifying action, and the second expresses the stabilizing property of the emulsifying agent.

Properties of Emulsifying Agents. Each surface-active agent has certain characteristic physical and chemical properties which determine the effectiveness of the agent under various conditions of use. These properties may be expressed as the *hydrophil-lipophil balance,* and the *chemical nature* of the surfactant.[16]

The hydrophil-lipophil balance of a molecule determines the type of activity which the agent is expected to manifest. It will serve primarily as a wetting agent, a detergent, a solubilizing agent, an o/w or w/o emulsifying agent or some other type, depending on its hydrophil-lipophil balance.

For example, when an emulsifying agent is dispersed in one of the phases of an oil-and-water mixture, it is adsorbed for the most part at the interface. Each emulsifying agent contains a water-attracting or *hydrophilic* and an oil-attracting or *lipophilic* part. If the agent is too hydrophilic, it dissolves completely in the body of the aqueous phase and exerts no effect at the interface. If it is too lipophilic, it dissolves completely in the oil and does not concentrate at the interface. The molecule of a well-balanced emulsifying agent is so constituted that, when it is dispersed initially in the oil or the aqueous phase, it will migrate to, and concentrate predominantly at, the interface, where it is oriented with the hydrophilic group in the water phase and the lipophilic group in the oil. An

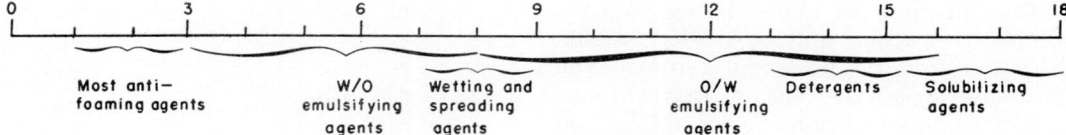

emulsifying agent which displays these properties is said to have the proper hydrophil-lipophil balance.

If an emulsifying agent is predominantly hydrophilic, it will tend to form an o/w emulsion; if it is predominantly lipophilic, it will favor the formation of a w/o emulsion. Sodium oleate has the characteristics of a good o/w emulsifying agent, since it possesses a hydrophilic carboxyl group (—COONa) that predominates over the lipophilic hydrocarbon group ($C_{17}H_{33}$—):

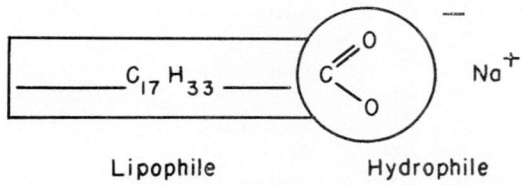

On the other hand, calcium oleate and other polyvalent soaps are predominantly lipophilic and form w/o emulsions.

The hydrophil-lipophil balance of surface-active agents has been expressed empirically by Griffin[17] in terms of a numerical "HLB" scale that extends from about 1 to 50. An agent with a low HLB (i.e., with a value of about 1 to 10) is primarily lipophilic, while a surfactant having a higher HLB is hydrophilic.

For the preparation of a w/o emulsion, the emulsifying agent should have an HLB of about 3 to 8. An o/w emulsion, on the other hand, is favored by an emulsifying agent with an HLB of about 8 to 16. The HLB values for a number of synthetic emulsifying agents are found in Table 16. The most favorable range for various classes of surfactants is shown in the HLB scale illustrated at the top of this page.

The optimum HLB ranges for the formation of stable w/o and o/w emulsions depend, in part, on the particular oil or mixture of oils involved. That is to say, each oil requires an emulsifying agent of a specific HLB value for the formation of an o/w emulsion and another value for the formation of a w/o product. These are known as the "required HLB" values of the oil. The "required HLB" values for a number of oil-phase ingredients, which have been taken from the reports of Griffin,[17] are found in Table 15.

The *chemical nature* of a surface-active agent determines how efficiently it functions for any particular purpose. It may be a soap, a sulfated alcohol, or an ester; the hydrocarbon portion may be saturated or unsaturated; the molecule may be ionic or nonionic in character, or it may be a complex hydrophilic colloid of natural origin. The relationship between action and chemical identity is not well understood, and no generalizations can be formulated.

The hydrophil-lipophil balance and other properties which depend on the physical and the chemical natures of the emulsifying agent will be discussed in more detail under the heading of mixed emulsifying agents (p. 282).

TABLE 15. "REQUIRED HLB" VALUES FOR OIL-PHASE INGREDIENTS*

	W/O EMULSION	O/W EMULSION†
Acid, stearic	–	17
Alcohol, cetyl	–	13
Lanolin, anhydrous	8	15
Oil, cottonseed	–	7.5
essential	–	9–16
mineral, heavy	4	10.5
mineral, light	4	10–12
vegetable	–	7–12
Petrolatum	4	10.5
Wax, bees	5	10–16
paraffin	4	9

*Griffin: J. Soc. Cosmet. Chem. 256; "Atlas Surface Active Agents," Atlas Powder Co., p. 18, Wilmington, Del.

† Refers to fluid o/w emulsions. O/W emulsions of a thicker texture or creaminess require a somewhat lower HLB.

Classification of Emulsifying Agents. Emulsifying agents may be divided roughly into 2 groups: synthetic and natural. The synthetic agents are classified as anionic, cationic and nonionic, depending on whether the anion (negative portion), the cation (positive portion) or the entire undissociated molecule provides the emulsifying action. Ampholyte emulsifying agents, containing both anionic and cationic groups in a single molecule, are now also known, an example being triethanolamine lauryl alanine. Synthetic emulsifying agents, together with their HLB values, are found in Table 16, and emulsifying agents obtained from natural sources are found in Table 17.

It is convenient to make a distinction

TABLE 16. SYNTHETIC EMULSIFYING AGENTS

IONIC CLASSES AND CHEMICAL COMPOUNDS	HLB*
Anionic	
Glyceryl monostearate—self emulsifying (Tegin) [a]	5.5
Triethanolamine oleate	12
Sodium oleate	18
Potassium oleate	20
Sodium lauryl sulfate	40 (approx.)
Cationic	
N-cetyl N-ethyl morpholinium ethosulfate (Atlas G-263) [b]	25–30
Benzalkonium chloride (Zephiran Chloride) [c]	....
Nonionic	
Sorbitan monooleate (Span 80) [b]	4.3
Sorbitan monolaurate (Span 20) [b]	8.6
Polyoxyethylene monostearate (Myrj 45) [b]	11.1
Polyoxyethylene monolaurate (Atlas G-2127) [b]	12.8
Polyethyleneglycol 400 monolaurate [d]	13.1
Polyoxyethylene vegetable oil (Emulphor El-719) [e]	13.3
Polyoxyethylene sorbitan monooleate (Tween 80) [b]	15.0
Polyoxyethylene sorbitan monolaurate (Tween 20) [b]	16.7

* Griffin: J. Soc. Cosmet. Chem. 5:249.
[a] Goldschmidt Chemical Corporation, New York, N. Y.
[b] Atlas Powder Company, Wilmington, Del.
[c] Winthrop-Stearns, Inc., New York, N. Y.
[d] Kessler Chemical Co., Philadelphia, Pa.
[e] General Aniline and Film Corporation, New York, N. Y.

TABLE 17. EMULSIFYING AGENTS OF NATURAL ORIGIN

NAME	SOURCE AND COMPOSITION	EMULSION TYPE
Acacia	Potassium, calcium, and magnesium salts of *d*-glucuronic acid	O/W
Egg yolk	Lecithin, cholesterol, proteins	O/W
Gelatin	Polypeptides, aminoacids	O/W
Malt extract	Proteins, dextrin	O/W
Lecithin	Phospholipid from egg yolk, soya bean and nerve tissue	O/W
Saponin	Nitrogen-free glycoside from quillaja and senega root	O/W
Cholesterol	A sterol found in nerve tissue and wool fat	W/O
Wool fat	A complex mixture of alcohols fatty and acids from the wool of the sheep	W

between *true* or *primary* emulsifying agents, which are capable of forming and stabilizing emulsions, and *stabilizers* or *auxiliary* agents,* which, although not forming acceptable emulsions when used alone, assist the primary emulsifier in stabilizing the product. A number of auxiliary emulsifying agents are included in Table 18.

Mixed Emulsifying Agents. An emulsifying agent frequently consists of a blend of emulsifiers rather than a single agent. As mentioned in the last paragraph, auxiliary agents may be mixed with primary emulsifiers for various purposes. Furthermore, primary emulsifying agents that tend to form water-in-oil emulsions may be combined with true oil-in-water emulsifying agents to provide a blend which is more efficient than either agent alone.

The mixture contributes one or several actions, which may be enumerated as follows: (1) it provides the proper hydrophil-lipophil nature; (2) it establishes a stable film at the interface; and (3) it supplies the

* Stabilizers are also known as quasi-emulsifiers, secondary emulsifying agents and emulsifying aids or adjuncts.

TABLE 18. AUXILIARY EMULSIFYING AGENTS

Product	Source and Composition	Principal Use
Agar	Dried colloid substance from certain algae containing a polygalactose sulfate and other constituents	Hydrophilic thickening agent and stabilizer for o/w emulsions
Bentonite	Colloidal hydrated aluminum silicate	Hydrophilic thickening agent and stabilizer for o/w and w/o lotions and creams
Cetyl alcohol	Chiefly $C_{16}H_{33}OH$	Lipophilic thickening agent and stabilizer for o/w lotions and ointments
Chondrus	Dried bleached seaweed	Hydrophilic thickening agent and stabilizer for o/w emulsions; weak o/w emulsifier
Glyceryl monostearate	$C_{17}H_{35}COOCH_2CHOHCH_2OH$	Lipophilic thickening agent and stabilizer for o/w lotions and ointments
Magnesium hydroxide	$Mg(OH)_2$	Hydrophilic stabilizer for o/w emulsions
Methylcellulose	Series of methyl esters of cellulose	Hydrophilic thickening agent and stabilizer for o/w emulsions; weak o/w emulsifier
Pectin	Purified carbohydrate extracted from the inner rind of citrus fruits and apple pomace	Hydrophilic thickening agent and stabilizer for o/w emulsions; weak o/w emulsifier
Silica gel	Hydrous oxide of silica	Hydrophilic stabilizer used in the preparation of ointments
Sodium alginate	The sodium salt of alginic acid, a purified carbohydrate extracted from giant kelp	Hydrophilic thickening agent and stabilizer for o/w emulsions
Sodium carboxymethylcellulose	Sodium salt of the carboxymethyl esters of cellulose	Hydrophilic thickening agent and stabilizer for o/w emulsions
Spermaceti	Waxy substance from the head of the sperm whale, containing cetyl palmitate	Lipophilic thickening agent and stabilizer for o/w and w/o ointments
Stearic acid	A mixture of solid acids from fats, chiefly stearic and palmitic	Lipophilic thickening agent and stabilizer for o/w lotions and ointments. Forms a true emulsifier when reacted with an alkali
Stearyl alcohol	Chiefly $C_{17}H_{35}OH$	Lipophilic thickening agent and stabilizer for o/w lotions and ointments
Tragacanth	Dried gummy exudation from species of *Astragalus* containing a soluble portion, and an insoluble portion that swells in water	Hydrophilic thickening agent and stabilizer for o/w emulsions; weak o/w emulsifier
Veegum	Colloidal magnesium aluminum silicate	Hydrophilic thickening agent and stabilizer for o/w lotions and creams

TABLE 19. EFFECT OF LECITHIN: CHOLESTEROL RATIOS ON THE TYPE OF EMULSION FORMED*

Volume of Oil Phase in ml.	Volume of Aqueous Phase in ml.	% Lecithin	% Cholesterol	Ratio of Lecithin: Cholesterol	Type of Emulsion Formed
5	6.0	0.33	0.017	19.4 : 1	O/W
5	5.5	0.18	0.018	10 : 1	O/W
5	5.4	0.148	0.0185	8 : 1	Indefinite
5	5.3	0.113	0.019	6 : 1	W/O
5	5.2	0.077	0.019	4.1 : 1	W/O
5	5.1	0.04	0.02	2 : 1	W/O

* Corran and Lewis: Biochem. J. 18:1368, 1924.

desired consistency to the product and contributes certain other properties such as emolliency, spreading and deflocculating.

1. As explained in a previous section (p. 281), the type of emulsion which is formed depends on the relative proportion of hydrophilic and lipophilic character that the emulsifying agent or mixture of agents exhibits.

Lecithin is an o/w emulsifying agent, and cholesterol is a w/o emulsifier. However, when mixed together in the proper proportions, they are capable of forming a stable emulsion of either type. The data in Table 19 show that, when the ratio of lecithin to cholesterol is greater than 10 to 1, an o/w emulsion is produced; when the ratio is less than 6 to 1, a w/o emulsion is formed; and, finally, when an intermediate proportion of about 8 to 1 is chosen, an unstable product results.[18] These findings are corroborated by investigations with egg oil,[19] which contains phospholipids (lecithin) and sterols (cholesterol) in the proportion of about 6 or 7 to 1 and has a tendency to form w/o emulsions. On the other hand, egg yolk contains lecithin, cholesterol and a protein fraction in the proper proportion and of sufficient hydrophilic character to form stable o/w emulsions.

The HLB system of Griffin[17] is based on a similar principle. When Span 80, which is lipophilic (HLB = 4.3), is combined with Tween 80, which is hydrophilic (HLB = 15.0), the emulsifier mixture is capable of producing either an o/w or a w/o emulsion, depending on the ratio of the two agents. Chun et al.[21] attribute the action of tragacanth in acacia emulsions to HLB. They found the HLB of acacia to be 8.0 and that of tragacanth 13.2. A mixture of the 2 agents in the proper proportion yields the desired HLB for the formation of a stable o/w emulsion.

2. According to Schulman and Cockbain,[20] some emulsifying agents tend to form weak compounds or "interfacial complexes" at the surface of the globules. For example, the o/w emulsifying action of sodium oleate is improved by combination with cetyl alcohol, cholesterol and similar lipophilic agents through a tendency of the molecules to form a complex. The emulsifying power of gelatin is also increased by combining it with cholesterol, oleic acid, stearic acid and cetyl alcohol, with which it is known to form compounds.

Schulman and Cockbain suggest that a complex favors the formation and the stabilization of an o/w emulsion by lowering the interfacial tension to a greater extent than is accomplished by either agent alone; by forming a compact yet flexible film at the interface; and by increasing the electric charge on the surface of the globules owing to the increased concentration of emulsifier ions at the interface. On the other hand, a complex that promotes a w/o emulsion forms a rigid, electrically uncharged interfacial film, according to these investigators.

3. Tragacanth, agar and chondrus frequently are combined with acacia to thicken the external phase of an o/w emulsion and to reduce the rate of creaming. Pectin, alginates and cellulose esters also are used for this purpose. Cetyl alcohol, stearyl alcohol, glyceryl monostearate and certain waxes such as spermaceti and beeswax serve as "bodying agents" to improve the consistency of the oil phase of lotions, creams and ointments, and to supply emollient properties to these bases.

Serrallach, Jones and Owen[22] proposed another hypothesis to explain the exceptional efficiency of mixtures of emulsifying agents. They observed that tragacanth tended to increase the rapidity of film formation, acacia imparted strength to the film, and agar increased the consistency of a cod-liver oil emulsion that was stabilized with a combination of these 3 agents.

Antagonistic Emulsifying Agents. It should be noted that some emulsifying agents are incompatible and cannot be used in combination. For example, colloids that possess electric charges of opposite sign are likely to coagulate when combined.

The older view holds that all lipophilic and hydrophilic emulsifiers are necessarily "antagonistic" because they tend to form emulsions of opposite types. However, in light of the arguments presented above in the paragraph labeled (1), this idea gradually is being replaced by the principle of hydrophil-lipophil balance. The findings of Schulman and Cockbain as discussed above in the paragraph labeled (2) and those of Serrallach *et al.* under (3) also justify the practice of mixing emulsifiers of opposite types.

PREPARATION OF EMULSIONS

The preparation of an emulsion is often a difficult task involving more art than science. Cobb[23] observed that "to master emulsion manufacture, it often seems that one must be smarter than the emulsion, get up earlier in the morning, work harder, and study more."

The process of emulsification involves violent agitation and disruption of the liquid phases. When a number of factors, including viscosity, ratio of the volume of the two phases, densities and interfacial tension are favorable, one liquid is broken into particles and the other liquid reaggregates to form the continuous phase. The emulsifying agent is adsorbed at the surface of the globules during mixing, and the system is stabilized by the emulsifier film.

A number of methods of preparation have been employed, depending primarily on the emulsifying machinery, the order in which the ingredients are mixed and the emulsifying agents which are employed. These factors are discussed in the following sections.

Devices and Machines for Emulsification

A number of hand-operated devices and power-driven machines are used for the preparation of emulsions. In the pharmacy laboratory and prescription department, small lots are prepared in a mortar or a bottle; in industry, large tanks and kettles are employed.

Mortar and Pestle. The Wedgwood or porcelain mortar and pestle are used most frequently in the laboratory for emulsifying fixed oils and sometimes volatile oils. A porcelain mortar with a flat bottom and vertical sides and a matching cylindrical pestle has been developed by Cooper to provide more efficient shearing action during trituration. The glass mortar and pestle should not be used for emulsification since they do not provide surfaces of sufficient roughness to divide the internal phase into fine globules.

The Bottle. Volatile oils and other volatile liquids of low viscosity may be emulsified by agitating the ingredients in a bottle. The use of the bottle first suggested by Forbes (loc. cit.), was studied extensively by Briggs,[24] in 1920. Briggs found that intermittent shaking was superior to continuous agitation for the preparation of an emulsion of benzene in sodium oleate solution. In one experiment, he prepared emulsions containing 90 volumes of benzene in 10 volumes of a 1 per cent sodium oleate solution, and found that continuous agitation required 9,900 shakes and a period of more than 1 hour to form the emulsion. When employing the intermittent method of shaking once, allowing the container to remain at rest for 30 seconds, again shaking once, and following this by a 30-second rest period, and so on, Briggs was able to emulsify the same product with 18 shakings in a period of 10 minutes.

Briggs attributed the superiority of intermittent agitation to shearing of the internal phase without unduly disturbing the external phase; whereas he maintained that continuous agitation tends to disrupt both phases and retard emulsification. Woodman[25] later investigated this method and attributed the success of interrupted shaking to the fact that the rest periods allow sufficient time for adsorption and orientation of the emulsifying agent at the interface before the globules are disintegrated again by the next agitation.

High-Speed Impeller-type Mixers. The hand-operated egg beater, the electric kitchen-type mixer and milkshake mixers (including the Waring Blendor) sometimes are used in the prescription department and in the laboratory for the preparation of small lots of emulsions. When these devices are used in a manner so that air is not whipped into the product, good results may be obtained. Husa and Becker[26] compared the efficiency of various mechanical stirrers and found that the hand-operated egg beater produced emulsions which compared favorably with those made in the mortar. The automatic soda-fountain mixer produced excellent emulsions when a mucilage of the emulsifying agent was placed in the container and the oil was added in a fine stream.

On the industrial scale, emulsifying machinery consists of a suitable-sized vessel provided with a jacket that permits heating and cooling of the contents, and a high-speed stirring device such as a propeller or turbine mixer. The coarse emulsion which is formed with this equipment finally is passed through a homogenizer or a colloid mill.

Homogenizers. The hand-operated homogenizer, which is shown in Figure 148, is a worthwhile addition to any pharmacy laboratory or prescription department. The small model has a capacity of about 1 pint and operates on a principle similar to that of the large motor-driven homogenizers. On the small scale, the emulsion is preformed in the mortar or the bottle and is then transferred to the bowl of the homogenizer. The operator uses a pumping action on the lever arm to force the emulsion through an orifice in the bottom of the bowl and against a spring-loaded plate. The internal phase is broken into small globules of uniform size as it passes through the orifice and is dashed against the plate. Husa and Becker[26] found that a linseed-oil emulsion prepared in the mortar contained particles with an average diameter of greater than 6 microns. When the product was passed through a hand homogenizer, the diameters of the particles were less than 2.5 microns and considerably more uniform in size.

The homogenizer for large-scale manufacture of emulsions is operated by an electric motor; the preformed emulsion is forced successively through 2 chambers or "stages of homogenization." When emulsions, particularly those containing protein emulsifying agents, are forced through a small orifice under high pressure, the globules that are produced tend to clump together so as to form *floccules*. It has been observed that, if the emulsion is passed through a second valve and chamber at a lower pressure before it is discharged from the homogenizer, the floccules are dispersed effectively and the globules remain in the desired *deflocculated* state. Because of this phenomenon, 2-stage homogenizers are employed in present-day practice. The emulsion is forced through the first valve under a gauge pressure of 2,500 to 5,000 pounds per square inch (p.s.i.) and then is passed through a second stage at 500 to 1,000 p.s.i.

The homogenizer is used extensively to prepare ice cream and homogenized milk, as well as pharmaceutical and cosmetic emulsions.

A second type of homogenizer is now commercially available in the form of ultrasonic machines. The principle involves the use of high frequency ultrasonic radiation which disrupts the liquids and distributes one liquid as globules in the other. The apparatus can operate at a frequency of about 20,000 cycles per second, which is equivalent to a homogenization pressure of 30,000 p.s.i.

Colloid Mill. The colloid mill is used sometimes for pilot plant and industrial-scale emulsification, particularly when suspended solids are present in the mixture or when the emulsion is too viscous for homogenization. The mill consists of a cone-shaped disk that rotates at a high velocity and at a small adjustable distance from a stationary cone. The coarsely formed emulsion is introduced into the hopper of the machine and is fed by gravity into the space between the rotor and the stator, where it is sheared into fine globules and forced out below the stator. The product

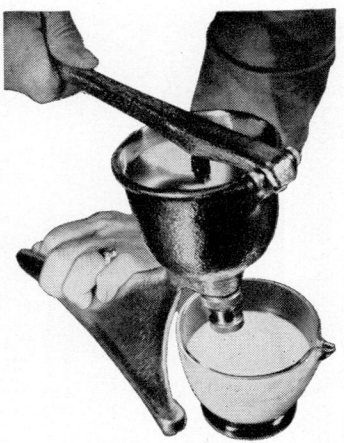

Fig. 148. Small hand homogenizer.

may be recycled through the machine until the desired globule size and uniformity are obtained. The colloid mill is shown in Figure 149. The operation of impellers, homogenizers and colloid mills is reviewed by Kempson-Jones.[27]

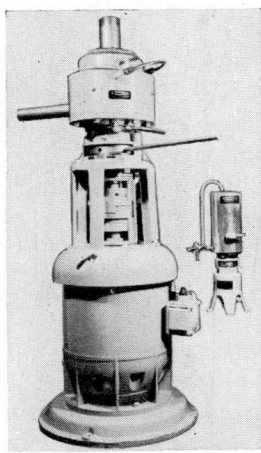

Fig. 149. Electric colloid mill.

Methods of Emulsification

Based on the order of mixing and the phase in which the emulsifying agent is dispersed initially, emulsification may be divided into two distinct methods: addition of the external phase to the internal phase containing the emulsifying agent and addition of the internal phase to the external phase containing the emulsifying agent. The first procedure has been known traditionally as the continental method and the second as the English method. Other emulsification procedures which are employed usually involve some modification of the two basic methods. One of these, the bottle method, is used for the preparation of small lots and may involve either the continental or the English procedure.

Addition of the External to the Internal Phase Containing the Emulsifying Agent (The Continental or Dry Gum Method). This method is favored by most American pharmacists for the preparation of o/w emulsions in the prescription laboratory. It involves mixing the oil and the powdered acacia in a dry Wedgwood or porcelain mortar, triturating the mixture until the powder is distributed uniformly throughout the oil, adding a measured portion of water all at one time, followed by rapid trituration to form the *nucleus* or *primary emulsion,* and finally adding water and other ingredients to complete the product. The primary emulsion is formed with 4 parts by volume of fixed oil, 2 parts by volume of water, and 1 part by weight of acacia.

Suppose that the pharmacist is required to prepare 60 ml. of a 50 per cent cod-liver oil emulsion. (A 50% emulsion is one in which the oil constitutes 50% of the total volume.)

Cod-liver oil .... 30 ml.
Acacia, powdered,
Purified water, enough to make..... 60 ml.

The 4 parts of oil (30 ml.) are mixed in a dry Wedgwood mortar with 1 part of powdered acacia (7.5 Gm.). One or 2 minutes may be required to distribute the gum evenly throughout the mixture. Some pharmacists have warned against excessive trituration at this stage, because acacia contains constituents which become soluble in the oil with continued trituration; and this may lead to the formation of a w/o emulsion instead of the desired o/w type. However, Husa and Becker[26] discovered no adverse effect by triturating oil and acacia for as long as 5 minutes. The writer has found that students sometimes make poor emulsions through a failure to mix the 2 ingredients adequately rather than through triturating for an excessive period of time.

To the oil and the well-dispersed emulsifying agent, 2 parts of purified water (15 ml.) are added *all at once,* and the primary emulsion is formed by light rapid trituration. If insufficient water is added at this stage or if the water is added slowly, the oil is present in a large enough excess at any moment to favor a water-in-oil emulsion, despite the presence of the predominantly hydrophilic emulsifying agent. When more water is added to recover the o/w product, the emulsion usually breaks. An excessive amount of water at this stage will also result in a poor or a broken emulsion, since the viscosity of the continuous phase is reduced to a point where the oil is no longer sheared into small globules. Although a w/o emulsion may be favored momentarily when 2 parts of water are added as required in this procedure, the well-dispersed acacia particles leave the bulk of the oil phase and are adsorbed rapidly at the interface, and, being wetted and hydrated by the water, tend to produce a stable o/w emulsion. In a few seconds after the addition of the 2 volumes of water, a creamy, white, primary emulsion is formed, and a crackling sound is heard as the oil is extended into filaments and dispersed as globules in the viscous mucilage by the rapid movement of the pestle.

The primary emulsion should be triturated for at least 5 minutes before dilution in order to produce a fine-grained product. Additional water, containing flavoring ingredients, preservatives and water-soluble drugs, may then be incorporated. Oil-soluble ingredients should be added to the oil phase before emulsification is begun. The emulsion is transferred to a graduate, and portions of water are used to rinse the mortar and the pestle and to bring the product to the final volume.

If apothecaries' weights and measures are used, the proper quantities for 4 fluidounces of a 50 per cent emulsion are 2 fluidounces of oil, 1 fluidounce of water and 4 drams of acacia.

The continental method may be employed also for the manufacture of emulsions on the industrial scale. In the preparation of an o/w emulsion, the oil-phase ingredients containing an o/w emulsifying agent are placed in a tank of suitable size; and a small amount of water is added and stirred into a mixture of the oil and the emulsifier to form a smooth w/o emulsion. Then a sufficient quantity of water is added quickly and agitated vigorously to invert the emulsion and form an o/w product. Finally, additional water and other ingredients are added to complete the emulsion.

If the oil phase contains waxy materials, a steam-jacketed tank is used, and the mixture is heated to a temperature sufficient to melt the ingredients. The aqueous phase is heated a few degrees higher so that it has the same temperature as that of the oil mixture when added to the tank. The emulsion is allowed to cool slowly with stirring. Phase reversal during emulsification, as practiced in this procedure, is sometimes difficult to control; but it usually leads to a fine-grained emulsion of such uniformity that it may require no homogenization.

Addition of the Internal to the External Phase Containing the Emulsifying Agent (English, American or Wet Gum Method). In the preparation of an o/w emulsion, this procedure involves the addition of oil to an aqueous solution of the emulsifying agent. In this way, the external phase, water, is always in excess, and the ratio of the volumes of the two liquids is such as to favor the formation of an o/w emulsion.

The mortar and pestle are employed for small lots, and acacia frequently is used as the emulsifying agent. The proportion of fixed oil, water and acacia that has been found to be the most successful for preparing the primary emulsion is 4 : 2 : 1—the same ratio that is used in the continental method. However, some pharmacists prefer to mix 1 part of acacia with an equal quantity of water and then dilute this mucilage with a little more water before adding the 4 parts of oil, which results in a ratio that is somewhat different from 4 : 2 : 1.

Using the same example given under the small-scale continental method, let us consider the various steps of the English method. To make 60 ml. of a 50 per cent cod-liver oil emulsion, 2 parts of water (15 ml.) are added *all at once* to 1 part of powdered, or preferably granular, acacia (7.5 Gm.) in a Wedgwood or porcelain mortar and the mixture is triturated by light rapid movement of the pestle until a smooth mucilage is formed. By using granular rather than powdered acacia, it is easier to obtain a smooth mucilage which is free of lumps. When powdered acacia is used, it is advisable to wet it with a small amount of glycerin before adding water in order to obtain a uniform mucilage. As previously noted, some pharmacists prefer to add about 1 part of water (7.5 ml.) rather than 2 parts to the 1 part of acacia;

either quantity of water at this stage results in a good emulsion.

The oil is added slowly in small increments (1 to 5 ml.) with continuous trituration so that each portion is distributed and emulsified in the mucilage before the next quantity is added. If the emulsion becomes too thick to absorb the oil rapidly before the nucleus is completed, a small amount of water may be added to re-establish the proper consistency and to produce a homogeneous mixture. This is usually necessary when only 1 part of water has been used to prepare the mucilage.

The primary emulsion is triturated for at least 5 minutes to ensure complete dispersion of the oil, and then it is diluted with water as described under the continental method.

In most cases, the English method has no advantages over the continental method for the preparation of small lots, and, in fact, is less satisfactory because of the additional time involved in making a good product. However, it may be necessary to use the English method when the emulsifying agent, such as fresh egg yolk, is not available in the dry powdered form or when the oil phase, such as copaiba, is too viscous to distribute the emulsifying agent properly.

On the industrial scale, the English method is carried out according to the following procedure. The various oils and oil-soluble ingredients that constitute the nonaqueous materials are blended together with the application of heat if necessary. The aqueous phase is prepared in a similar manner. If heat has been used to melt the oil-phase ingredients, the aqueous phase is heated to about the same temperature. The liquid that is to become the internal phase is added slowly to the external phase in a tank or steam-jacketed kettle. Vigorous agitation is maintained with a propeller-type agitator or high-speed turbine mixer. Then the product may be passed through a **homogenizer** or a **colloid mill** to obtain a **product** with small globules of uniform **size**.

In order to ensure success in the preparation of emulsions by the above two methods, certain precautions must be taken:

1. For the preparation of small lots, a Wedgwood or porcelain mortar and pestle should be used to provide the rough surfaces necessary for shearing the particles of the internal phase. Husa and Becker[28] obtained unusual success by using a Wedgwood mortar in conjunction with a porcelain pestle.

2. The vessel in which the emulsion is to be prepared must be clean and dry, the container in which the oil is measured must be moisture-free, and the graduate for measuring the water must be oil-free to ensure successful emulsification.

3. The order and the method of mixing, as described under the two procedures, must be followed carefully, and the ingredients must be measured or weighed accurately. The 4 : 2 : 1 ratio is adequate for most fixed oils; however, for linseed and mineral oils, better results are obtained when 3 parts of oil are mixed with 2 parts of water and 1 part of acacia. Although acacia is used most frequently in the two methods, particularly for the small-scale preparation of emulsions, other primary and auxiliary emulsifying agents such as egg yolk, gelatin, pectin, tragacanth and chondrus may be employed. The 4 : 2 : 1 ratio is applicable only to emulsions pre-

TABLE 20

Emulsifying Agent	Proportions of Oil : Water : Emulsifier	
	Fixed Oils, Except Liquid Petrolatum and Linseed Oil	Liquid Petrolatum, Linseed Oil and Volatile Oils
Acacia.........	4 : 2 : 1	3 : 2 : 1 or 2 : 2 : 1
Tragacanth....	40 : 20 : 1	30 : 20 : 1 or 20 : 20 : 1

pared with acacia. When tragacanth* is used as the emulsifying agent, for example, the ratio is 40 : 20 : 1, since only about one tenth as much tragacanth as acacia is necessary in either method. The proportions are summarized in Table 20.

* Although tragacanth is recognized generally as an auxiliary agent, it may be used sometimes as a primary emulsifier.

Variations of the Principal Methods. A number of modifications of the two fundamental procedures are employed in the manufacture of emulsions.

One such variation involves the use of a bottle for small-scale emulsification of volatile oils and other liquids of low viscosity. The ratio of volatile oil, water and acacia employed in the bottle method is 3:2:1 or 2:2:1, the proportion of acacia being greater than that used for fixed oils because of the lower viscosity of the essential oils.

The original bottle method, as introduced by Forbes,[5] involved a continental-type procedure; however, either the continental or the English method may be followed. For the preparation of a volatile oil emulsion, 2 parts by volume of oil are mixed with 1 part by weight of powdered acacia in a dry bottle of ample capacity. After the acacia has become well dispersed in the oil, 2 parts by volume of water are added all at one time, and the mixture is shaken vigorously until the primary emulsion is formed. Then water and water-soluble ingredients may be added in divided portions, agitating the container after each addition.

If the English method is followed, small portions of oil are incorporated into a mucilage of acacia by shaking the bottle after each addition. Alternatively, all of the oil is added at once and the bottle is shaken intermittently according to Briggs' method, which was discussed in a previous section of this chapter (p. 285).

The formulas for various turpentine liniments employing egg yolk as the emulsifying agent have appeared through the years in pharmaceutical literature. The products contain about 1 part of egg yolk for each 4 parts of turpentine oil and are prepared by a modification of the English method. For example, 50 ml. of well-strained egg yolk, 200 ml. of purified water and 50 ml. of acetic acid are placed in a bottle, 200 ml. of turpentine oil is added in small portions, and the bottle is shaken after each addition to form the emulsion.

Sometimes the bottle is used for the preparation of fixed oil emulsions. For example, to 50 ml. of a 1 per cent aqueous solution of sodium oleate contained in a bottle of suitable size, 50 ml. of cottonseed oil may be added in divided portions with intermittent shaking to form an o/w emulsion. The product, Cod Liver Oil Emulsion with Malt, may be prepared in a bottle according to the method given in the N.F. X.

Liniments and lotions may be prepared in a bottle by the *nascent soap method*. According to this procedure, an oil, such as linseed or olive oil, containing sufficient free fatty acid is placed in a bottle, and an equal volume of alkali, such as calcium hydroxide solution, is added. When the mixture is shaken, the fatty acid of the oil reacts with the alkali to form a calcium soap, which in turn promotes a w/o emulsion. Lime Liniment, which was official in N.F. VIII, was prepared extemporaneously in this manner. The soap is formed *in situ* (i.e., at the time of mixing); when formed in this manner, it is said to be a "nascent soap," and the emulsification procedure is often called the *nascent soap method* of emulsification. It may be used to prepare either o/w or w/o emulsions, depending on whether sodium hydroxide or calcium hydroxide solution is used. Other monovalent and polyvalent hydroxides also may be employed.

A modified nascent soap method was used by Dorey[29] for the emulsification of arachis oil. The oil, containing oleic acid, and the aqueous phase, containing potassium hydroxide, were fed as separate streams into a homogenizer. The soap was formed *in situ,* and the emulsion that was produced contained globules of oil of which 97.3 per cent had diameters of less than 1 micron.

Goldner[30] suggested a method for preparing a cod-liver oil emulsion using pectin as the emulsifying agent and employing a combination of the continental and the English methods. The formula for a 50 per cent emulsion is:

Cod-liver oil	50.0 ml.
Pectin	1.0 Gm.
Syrup	10.0 ml.
Methyl salicylate	0.4 ml.
Purified water	40.0 ml.

The primary emulsion, containing one half of the oil, is prepared by a continental-type procedure as follows. The pectin is triturated in a mortar with 25 ml. of cod-liver oil, 25 ml. of water are added, and rapid light trituration is continued until the emulsion begins to form. The mixture is set aside for 10 minutes to allow for adequate hydration of the pectin, then the product is triturated until a thick creamy emulsion is formed.

The methyl salicylate, the syrup and the additional purified water are added slowly with stirring, and the remaining 25 ml. of oil are incorporated into the primary emulsion in small portions according to the English method.

EMULSIFYING AGENTS FOR INTERNALLY USED PRODUCTS

The official emulsions are intended for oral and parenteral administration; therefore, they require the use of edible or non-toxic o/w emulsifying agents. Liniments, lotions, creams and ointments, on the other hand, usually employ agents which need not be edible. These latter emulsifiers belong largely to the synthetic class; they will be discussed in the next section.

Acacia is probably the only true emulsifying agent of the natural gum class; the other gums produce viscous but coarse emulsions, and are used principally as stabilizers. Acacia is particularly useful for preparing emulsions in the mortar, since it provides a mucilage of ample consistency to allow the oil to be sheared into finely divided particles. However, acacia is not viscous enough to prevent rapid rise of the globules with subsequent formation of a cream layer on the surface of the emulsion. Thickening agents such as agar and tragacanth sometimes are added to acacia emulsions to minimize the creaming effect.

According to Krantz and Gordon,[31] emulsions prepared with acacia are stable over a pH range of 2 to 10. However, preparations containing acacia are not resistant to attack by micro-organisms and require the presence of a preservative. About 6 per cent by volume of alcohol, 0.2 per cent benzoic acid or 0.2 per cent methyl parahydroxybenzoate may be used for this purpose.

Egg Yolk. This is an excellent o/w emulsifying agent and is used extensively in the home and in industry for the preparation of food emulsions. Egg yolk itself is an o/w emulsion, consisting of a fat and a water phase which are emulsified by a combination of lecithin, cholesterol and a protein fraction.

As previously noted in the preparation of turpentine liniments, egg yolk may be used in the presence of acids without loss of efficiency; it is also resistant to the action of electrolytes. Because of resistance to moderate amounts of acids and salts, egg yolk is also used extensively in food emulsions such as mayonnaise. In the preparation of pharmaceutical emulsions, the yolk is separated from the albumin and strained to remove clumps. Then it is placed in a mortar or a bottle, the oil is incorporated into the yolk, and water and other ingredients are added. The yolk of an average-sized egg weighs about 15 Gm., a quantity sufficient to emulsify 60 ml. of a volatile oil or 120 ml. of a fixed oil.

The main disadvantage of egg yolk is its tendency to decompose; unless the emulsion is used in a short period of time, it should be preserved with 0.2 per cent benzoic acid, 10 per cent alcohol or 0.2 per cent methyl parahydroxybenzoate. The emulsion should be stored in the refrigerator and should be consumed within several days.

Some pharmacists use the whole egg for emulsifying purposes; however, it is generally agreed that egg albumin is somewhat inferior to the yolk as an emulsifying agent.

Gelatin. Briggs and Schmidt,[32] in 1915, and Holmes and Child,[33] in 1920, made detailed studies of gelatin. However, it was not until Limburg[34] showed the effect of pH on the efficiency of gelatin as a protective colloid that it was used successfully as an emulsifying agent. Gelatin is a negatively charged colloid at pH values above its iso-electric point and is positively charged at pH values below the iso-electric point.* Since the oil globules in an o/w emulsion are negatively charged, gelatin is readily adsorbed on the surface of the particles if the pH is below the iso-electric point.

The iso-electric point of gelatin varies with the origin of the product. Gelatin that is obtained from an acid-treated precursor has an iso-electric point of pH 8 and acts best as an emulsifying agent at about pH 3 where it is positively charged. Gelatin from an alkali-treated precursor has an iso-electric point of 4.7 and is used at about pH 8 where it is negatively charged.

Since gums such as acacia, tragacanth and agar are negatively charged, they cannot be combined with a positively charged gelatin; two oppositely charged hydrophilic colloids, such as acid-treated gelatin and acacia, may be incompatible in certain proportions, since they tend to form a coacervate. However, gelatin having an iso-electric point of 4.7 may be combined with gums if maintained at a high pH value where the gelatin has a negative charge.

Gelatin is commercially available as Pharmagel A† for use in acid solution and as Pharmagel B† for use in the alkaline range. The characteristics of the Pharmagels are summarized in Table 21.

The application of Pharmagel A and B for preparing pharmaceutical emulsions has been developed by Tice,[35] and is discussed in the *U.S.P.* The following formula demonstrates the use of Pharmagel A:

Oil	500 ml.
Gelatin (Pharmagel A)	8 Gm.
Tartaric acid	0.6 Gm.
Alcohol	60 ml.
Flavors as desired	
Syrup	100 ml.
Purified water, a sufficient quantity to make	1,000 ml.

Add the Pharmagel A and the tartaric acid to 300 ml. of water, allow to stand for a few minutes, then heat until the gelatin is dissolved. Raise the temperature to about 98° C. and main-

---

* Iso-electric point is discussed in Chapter 5, pp. 93–94 and the charge on colloid particles is discussed in Chapter 7, p. 118 et seq.

† Pharmagel Corporation, 55 W. 42nd St., New York 18, N. Y.

TABLE 21

Product	Iso-electric Point	Optimum pH for Use	Electric Charge in the Useful pH Range
Pharmagel A	8	3	+
Pharmagel B	4.7	8	−

tain at this temperature for about 20 minutes. Cool to 50°, then add the syrup, the flavor dissolved in the alcohol and, finally, enough water to make 500 ml. Add the oil, agitate the mixture thoroughly and then pass through a homogenizer until the oil is dispersed completely and uniformly. Finally, place the product in bottles and shake well after it cools.

Pharmagel B is compatible with gums in alkaline solution and may be used with or without auxiliary emulsifying agents such as tragacanth and agar. The use of Pharmagel B in the alkaline range is demonstrated in the following formula:

Oil	500 ml.
Gelatin (Pharmagel B)	5 Gm.
Sodium bicarbonate	2.5 Gm.
Alcohol	60 ml.
Flavor as desired	
Syrup	100 ml.
Agar	2.5 Gm.
Purified water, a sufficient quantity to make	1,000 ml.

Dissolve the gelatin in 200 ml. of water, using moderate heat, cool the solution and add sodium bicarbonate and agar previously dissolved by boiling with 100 ml. of water. Then add the syrup, the flavor dissolved in alcohol, and finally enough water to make 500 ml. Add the oil and mix vigorously, then pass through a homogenizer until the globules of oil are finely and uniformly dispersed. Mix the product thoroughly when cool; place in bottles.

Although gelatin emulsions cannot be formed in a mortar, fine-grained products are prepared by use of the homogenizer. Flavor emulsions, which are prepared from oils such as lemon and orange, usually contain low concentrations of oil, and, when prepared with gelatin, require the addition of a viscous gum to prevent rapid creaming. However, a thickening agent is not required for an emulsion containing 40 to 60 per cent of oil, since the high concentration of internal phase provides sufficient consistency.

Malt Extract. This viscous brown liquid contains dextrin and a protein fraction in addition to other substances which causes it to function as an emulsifying agent. It is used together with auxiliary agents to emulsify and mask the taste of cod-liver oil.

Synthetic Emulsifying Agents. Only a limited number of synthetic agents are safe for internal use. Among these are the sorbitan esters (Spans), the polyoxyethylene sorbitan esters (Tweens) and purified glyceryl monostearate. These will be discussed in the section devoted to nonionic emulsifying agents.

Auxiliary Emulsifying Agents for Internal Use. Agar, carrageenin,[36] chondrus, pectin, tragacanth, sodium alginate and the synthetic cellulose derivatives are used as stabilizers or quasi-emulsifiers according to the actions enumerated under the section on mixed emulsifying agents.

Although most of these agents are used as auxiliary emulsifiers, some are also capable of performing as true emulsifying agents. Goldner[30] has demonstrated the use of pectin as a primary emulsifier. Osborn and DeKay[37] reported that methylcellulose, 15 cps.* in 5 and 10 per cent concentrations was capable of producing good emulsions of cod-liver oil and mineral oil when the coarse emulsions were passed through a hand homogenizer. However, methylcellulose 1,500 cps., when used alone in 1 and 5 per cent concentrations, was not a suitable emulsifying agent.

The methods of preparing and preserving these agents may be found in Chapter 15 where they are discussed in relation to their role as suspending agents. Most of the auxiliary emulsifiers are used in about 1 per cent concentration, based on the total volume of the emulsion.

Finely divided solids which are used as auxiliary agents, and sometimes as primary emulsifiers, are discussed in a later section (p. 297).

---

* The designation cps. is an abbreviation for centipoises, the unit in which absolute viscosity is expressed. See the footnote to Table 13, p. 264.

EMULSIFYING AGENTS FOR EXTERNALLY USED PRODUCTS

Synthetic emulsifying agents are superior to natural gums and proteins in that the former are not so susceptible to decomposition by micro-organisms. Furthermore, being of synthetic origin, the ratio of hydrophilic and lipophilic groups in the molecule may be altered to supply a wide range of emulsifying agents. This versatility is advantageous for externally applied emulsions where the w/o type shares equal importance with the o/w class. However, some natural agents of vegetable and animal origin are still used in the manufacture of externally applied emulsions. The anionic, the cationic and the nonionic synthetic agents and some of the natural emulsifiers will be discussed in this section.

Anionic Emulsifying Agents. This class includes monovalent, polyvalent and organic soaps, sulfates and sulfonates, as found in Table 16.

Soaps have a disagreeable taste and produce an irritating and laxative action in the intestinal tract; consequently, they are not used in orally administered emulsions. Soaps are used widely in industry as emulsifying agents for the processing of rubber and leather, for the manufacture of lubricants, in the preparation of asphalt emulsions for road building, for the formation of o/w emulsion paints and for insecticidal emulsion sprays, auto waxes, floor polishes and cosmetic and pharmaceutical emulsions. Soaps are used also for their *solubilizing* action on organic substances that are only sparingly soluble in water. Saponated Cresol Solution, N.F., contains 50 per cent cresol solubilized in a potassium or sodium soap.

The alkali soaps, including sodium, potassium and ammonium salts of lauric, myristic, palmitic, stearic and oleic acids, are hydrophilic and form o/w emulsions. The metallic soaps, including calcium, magnesium, zinc, lead and aluminum salts of fatty acids, are water-insoluble and tend to promote w/o emulsions. Both types are used for the preparation of some pharmaceutical liniments and cosmetic creams.

Donnan[38] was the first investigator to

show that the lowering of interfacial tension by an emulsifying agent is influential in emulsification insofar as it results in adsorption of the agent at the interface. Working with the sodium salts of various fatty acids, Donnan and Potts[39] found that sodium caprylate (C_8) was the first member of the series to bring about a lowering of interfacial tension. The fatty acid salts (soaps) of higher molecular weight reduced the interfacial tension to a proportionately greater extent, as shown in Figure 150. Donnan and Potts then showed conclusively that the reduction in interfacial tension was directly related to the emulsifying power of the various soaps. The sodium soaps of lower fatty acids gave no emulsions, sodium caprate and nonylate gave poor emulsions, while the higher fatty acid salts (laurate and myristate), which showed a marked effect in lowering of interfacial tension, produced fairly satisfactory emulsions. These investigators also found that soaps show an optimum concentration at which emulsifying power is a maximum.

Bancroft[40] and later Clowes[41] and Bhatnagar[42] extended Donnan's theory to explain why monovalent soaps tend to form o/w emulsions while polyvalent soaps form the w/o type. They considered the soap film around the globules as a separate phase, with an interfacial tension between both the oil and the water phases. A monovalent soap is wetted by water and not by oil, so that the interfacial tension is lower on the water side than on the oil side of the membrane. Consequently, the soap film curves in a manner so as to surround and envelop the oil phase. On the other hand, a polyvalent soap is wetted more easily by the oil, and the consequent lowering of interfacial tension on that side of the film causes the emulsifying agent to enclose the globules of water in the oil phase, thereby forming a w/o emulsion.

The manufacture of soap emulsions was discussed under the heading of methods. The nascent soap method is used frequently; about 2 to 10 per cent of soap is required to prepare the emulsion. In an emulsion prepared by reacting the fatty acids of the oil with an alkali, sufficient fatty acid should be present so that some remains unneutralized after the soap is formed. The excess free fatty acid improves the hydrophil-lipophil balance of the soap and acts as an auxiliary emulsifier. Although a soap alone forms a fairly stable emulsion, usually the product is improved by the addition of an auxiliary stabilizing agent such as cetyl alcohol, stearyl alcohol or glyceryl monostearate.

Organic soaps, which are known also as amino soaps, are prepared by reacting aminohydroxy compounds with fatty acids. Triethanolamine oleate is prepared according to the following reaction:

$$(HOCH_2CH_2)_3N + C_{17}H_{33}COOH =$$
triethanolamine $\quad$ oleic acid

$$(HOCH_2CH_2)_3NH\text{---}OOC(C_{17}H_{33})$$
triethanolamine oleate

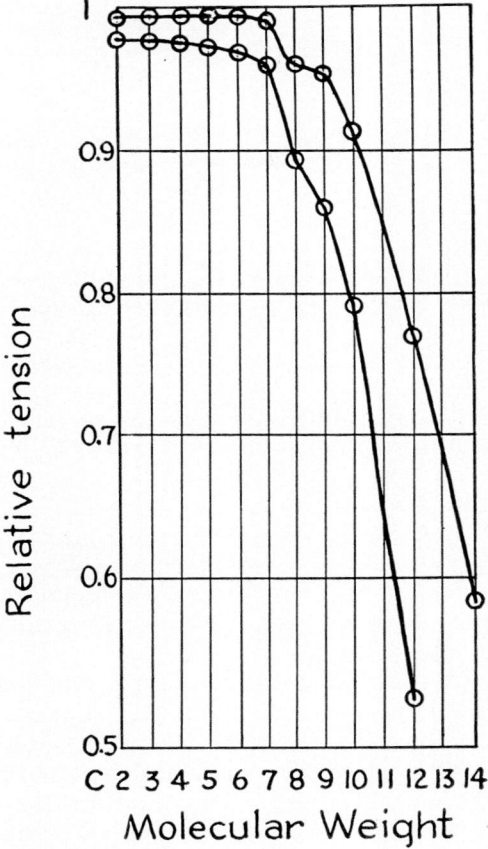

FIG. 150. Graph showing the relation of interfacial tension and molecular weight. The upper curve represents the relative interfacial tension of 0.0025 N solutions and the lower curve 0.0050 N solutions of the fatty acid salts.

Soaps formed from 2-methyl-2-amino-1,3-propanediol also have been suggested for pharmaceutical emulsions.[43] The formula of the stearate is:

$$(HOCH_2-\underset{\underset{CH_3}{|}}{\overset{\overset{NH_2}{|}}{C}}-CH_2)-OOC(C_{17}H_{35})$$

2-methyl-2-amino-1,3-propanediol stearate

Organic soaps produce o/w emulsions. They have the advantage over inorganic soaps in that they represent a better balance between hydrophilic and lipophilic groups and are practically neutral in reaction (pH 8). The soap ordinarily is formed *in situ* during mixing and emulsification, and the final emulsion is fine-grained and stable.

Some amines, such as morpholine, are

$$HN\begin{matrix}CH_2-CH_2\\ \\CH_2-CH_2\end{matrix}O$$

volatile and consequently are useful for preparing horticultural sprays and polishing waxes.

The volatile amine evaporates after the emulsion is applied, leaving a water-resistant film of oil or wax.

The following formulas illustrate the use of organic soaps in emulsions.

Liquid petrolatum	20 Gm.
Stearic acid	3 Gm.
Triethanolamine	1 Gm.
Purified water	76 Gm.

The stearic acid and the mineral oil are heated on a water bath to 75° C. to melt the acid. The triethanolamine is dissolved in the water, and the solution is heated to 78° C. and added slowly with stirring to the oil phase. The emulsion is allowed to cool with occasional mixing. The cream has a pH of about 8.

Liquid petrolatum, heavy	30 Gm.
Paraffin	7 Gm.
Ceresin	2 Gm.
Stearic acid	8 Gm.
2-Amino-2-methyl-1,3-propanediol	3 Gm.
Purified water	50 Gm.

The first 4 ingredients, constituting the oil phase, are heated at 75° C. until fused; the last 2 ingredients are mixed and heated to 78° C. and then are added slowly with stirring to the oil phase. The mixture is agitated until it has cooled.

Soaps, both inorganic and organic, have two major disadvantages, a low resistance of organic and alkali soaps to reaction with calcium and other polyvalent ions, and a marked sensitivity of all the soaps to acids. These incompatibilities deserve further discussion.

The alkali and the amino soaps are converted to water-insoluble metallic soaps in the presence of polyvalent ions. Since metallic soaps tend to form w/o emulsions, the presence of polyvalent ions in o/w soap emulsions causes a precipitation of the emulsifying agent as an insoluble soap and breaks the emulsion or promotes the w/o type.

Sensitivity of soaps and other surface-active agents to polyvalent ions commonly is measured by adding a 0.5 per cent calcium chloride solution to the surfactant until a definite turbidity is produced; the ability of the agent to withstand the effect of calcium ions is known as the *calcium tolerance*. Alkali soaps have a very low calcium tolerance; amino soaps are slightly more resistant, but they also have a low order of stability in the presence of polyvalent ions.

Sequestering agents sometimes are incorporated in soap emulsions to improve the calcium tolerance. These chemicals tie up the polyvalent ions in the form of soluble complexes and prevent the reaction with monovalent soaps. The water softener, sodium hexametaphosphate (Calgon), and the organic chemical, ethylenediamine tetraacetic acid (EDTA), are examples of sequestering agents.

Inorganic soaps are stable only at high pH values—greater than about pH 10—while organic soaps may remain in aqueous solution in the neutral range—about pH 8. However, the addition of an excess of acid to either type of soap liberates the free water-insoluble fatty acid:

$$C_{17}H_{35}COONa + H^+ \rightleftharpoons C_{17}H_{35}COOH + Na^+$$

The addition of an acid to an emulsion stabilized with a soap destroys the emulsion, since the free fatty acid that is produced is only a weak auxiliary emulsifier. Even weak acids such as salicylic, benzoic and boric may reduce the pH sufficiently to precipitate the free acid and break the emulsion.

The trend in dermatologic practice is toward the use of acidic lotions and creams with pH values corresponding to the normal reaction of the skin. The surface of the skin is coated with a layer of fatty acids and other acid substances which protect it against infection by micro-organisms. This protective film, known as the "acid mantle," provides the surface of the skin with a pH value of about 4 to 6. Consequently, soap emulsions are finding less use because of their alkaline reaction, particularly since the advent of the newer surface-active agents, which are stable in acid media.

Sulfated oils are more tolerant than are soaps to polyvalent ions, for, although they may react with calcium ions, the calcium compounds are water-soluble. Sulfated oils are also stable in the presence of small amounts of acids. Sulfated hydrogenated castor oil was official in *N.F. IX* as Hydroxystearin Sulfate.

Sulfated fatty alcohols include such compounds as sodium cetyl sulfate, sodium lauryl sulfate and triethanolamine lauryl sulfate; these alcohols are used extensively in cosmetic and pharmaceutical lotions and creams. They are capable alone of forming stable o/w emulsions but are improved by the presence of auxiliary stabilizers. For this purpose, cetyl alcohol, steryl alcohol and glyceryl monostearate, being weak emulsifiers, may be added. Moreover, the auxiliary emulsifier improves the consistency of the product and forms a softer cream which is said to have better spreading, penetrating and emollient properties. The sulfated fatty alcohols are incompatible with iodine, mercuric salts, relatively high concentrations of acids and cationic agents, and are hydrolyzed by prolonged heating.

Emulsions may be formed by melting the waxy auxiliary agents in the oil phase at an elevated temperature, dissolving the sulfated fatty alcohol in the water which is heated to a temperature slightly above that of the oil phase, slowly adding the aqueous solution to the oil with agitation, and finally allowing the product to cool with occasional stirring. The following formula illustrates the use of the primary emulsifier, sodium lauryl sulfate, in combination with 2 quasi-emulsifiers, cetyl alcohol and stearyl alcohol.

White petrolatum	15 Gm.
Cetyl alcohol	5 Gm.
Stearyl alcohol	5 Gm.
Sodium lauryl sulfate	1 Gm.
Purified water	74 Gm.

Sulfonated compounds are used as wetting agents and only infrequently as emulsifying agents. One of the best known compounds of this class is Dioctyl Sodium Sulfosuccinate, N.F., which is marketed as Aerosol OT.*

Cationic Agents. Cationic surface-active agents are those chemicals the action of which is dependent on the cationic or positively charged group. Benzalkonium Chloride, U.S.P.,† is an important member of this class and has the formula $C_6H_5CH_2\text{-}N(CH_3)_2RCl$, in which R represents a mixture of alkyl radicals from C_8H_{17} to $C_{18}H_{37}$.

Cationic agents have marked bactericidal properties and are used primarily as local antiinfectives rather than as emulsifying agents. They must not come in contact with anionic chemicals such as soaps since the two types are incompatible. The active group of the cationic agent combines with the anion, and, although precipitation may not be evident immediately when the substances are used in low concentration, the germicidal action of the cationic agent is destroyed; and the emulsifying property of the anionic emulsifier may be impaired or nullified.

Nonionic Emulsifying Agents. The entire undissociated molecule of certain chemicals, containing hydrophilic and lipophilic groups in proper balance, may act

---

* A product of the American Cyanamid Company, New York, N. Y.

† Zephiran Chloride, Winthrop-Stearns, New York, N. Y.

as an emulsifying agent. Included in this group are glyceryl esters, fatty acid esters of sorbitan and their polyoxyethylene derivatives, and polyethylene glycol esters and ethers.

By combining hydrophilic radicals such as hydroxyl (—OH) and polyoxyethylene (—CH_2CH_2O)$_n$ groups with lipophilic substances such as straight chain hydrocarbons, a wide range of hydrophil-lipophil nature may be obtained in any series of nonionic emulsifying agents.

Glyceryl monostearate, $C_{17}H_{35}COOCH_2$-$CHOHCH_2OH$, is too lipophilic to serve as an effective emulsifier, but it may be used as an auxiliary agent. When mixed with a small amount of an o/w emulsifier such as sodium stearate or sodium lauryl sulfate, it possesses the desired characteristics of an emulsifying mixture and is known as "glyceryl monostearate—self-emulsifying."

An important group of nonionic agents are obtained by partially esterifying the anhydrides, derived from sorbitol and other sugar alcohols, with various fatty acids. Sorbitan laurate, palmitate, stearate and oleate constitute the series of Spans.* Since they are lipophilic in nature, they tend to form w/o emulsions and to stabilize o/w emulsions. The polyoxyethylene derivatives of the Spans, known as the Tweens,* are water-soluble or dispersible and favor o/w emulsions. In practice, a Span and a Tween usually are mixed to provide an emulsifier combination that has the HLB necessary to produce a stable emulsion of the desired type. Knowing the required HLB of the oil phase as listed in Table 15, one may calculate the quantities of any Span and Tween, several of which are found in Table 16, that are necessary to produce the proper balance for a stable emulsion. For example, if one desired to prepare 100 ml. of a mineral oil emulsion (required HLB-12) emulsified with a 5-Gm. mixture of Span 20 (HLB-8.6) and Tween 20 (HLB-16.7), the product would require about 60 per cent or 3 Gm. of Span 20 and 40 per cent or 2 Gm. of Tween 20 in the emulsifier phase. These figures are easily checked, since the percentage contributions of the 2 emulsifiers to the over-all HLB must be additive, or:

$$(8.6 \times 0.6) + (16.7 \times 0.4) = 11.8$$

The details of the method are given in the booklet of the Atlas Powder Co.[16]

Polyethylene glycol esters, such as the monostearate, may be used to prepare emulsified lotions and creams. The formula for a representative member of this class is:

$C_{17}H_{35}COO(CH_2CH_2O)_nH$
polyethylene glycol 400 monostearate
in which n varies from 8 to 10

Natural Emulsifying Agents. Cholesterol, wool fat and certain wool-fat concentrates and derivatives form stable w/o emulsions and are used primarily for the preparation of ointments;[44] the reader is referred to the chapter on Ointments for a detailed discussion of this group.

Bandelin and Tuschhoff[19] have reported on the use of *egg oil** for the stabilization of cosmetic and pharmaceutical emulsions. Egg oil is an amber to brown liquid extracted by a new solvent process from the egg, and consists principally of fats, phospholipids and sterols. A cosmetic product that utilizes egg oil as a stabilizer and emollient is:

Egg Oil Hand Lotion

Glyceryl monostearate	18
Stearic acid	13
Propylene glycol	25
Alcohol	50
Triethanolamine	2.5
Egg oil	10
Perfume	5
Water	376.5

FINELY DIVIDED SOLIDS AS EMULSIFYING AGENTS

Colloidal clays such as bentonite, Veegum,† Pharmasorb Colloidal,‡ magnesium hydroxide, aluminum hydroxide, magnesium oxide and silica gel are among those

---

* Atlas Powder Co., Wilmington, Del.

* Available from the Vio Bin Corporation of Monticello, Ill.

† Colloidal magnesium aluminum silicate, Vanderbilt Co., New York, N. Y.

‡ A hydrous magnesium aluminum silicate, Mineral and Chemical Corporation of America, Menlo Park, N. J.

insoluble substances that have been used as emulsifying agents. As early as 1907, Pickering[45] undertook an extensive study of insoluble emulsifying agents and showed that powders which were easily wetted by water formed o/w emulsions, while those which were wetted preferentially by oil tended to produce w/o emulsions. The clays represent the first type, and carbon black the second type of solid emulsifiers. It is believed that the finely divided solids, like other emulsifying agents, form and stabilize emulsions by concentrating at the interface, where they produce a coherent film around the globules and prevent coalescence of the internal phase.

Bentonite may be used to form either an o/w or a w/o emulsion, depending on the order of mixing. If a bentonite magma is placed in a mortar and the oil phase is added gradually with trituration, an o/w emulsion is produced, since the aqueous phase is always in excess during the preparation. However, if bentonite is dispersed in oil and water is added gradually, it is possible to form a w/o emulsion. The following formula, which was suggested by Hubbard and Freeman,[46] demonstrates the use of bentonite in o/w and w/o emulsions.

Camphor ⎱ aa	0.6
Menthol ⎰	
Phenol	1.2
Calamine ⎱ aa	7.2
Zinc oxide ⎰	
Boric acid	3.6
Olive oil	48.0
Bentonite (6%) in lime water, q.s. ad.....	120.0

The bentonite suspension is placed in an electric mixing apparatus, a uniform mixture of camphor, menthol, phenol, calamine, zinc oxide and boric acid is added, and the olive oil finally incorporated. An oil-in-water emulsion is formed.

If a water-in-oil product is wanted, the oil containing the menthol, the camphor and the phenol is placed in the mixer, and the mixture of powders is added. The bentonite in lime water is added last.

Veegum may be used to prepare stable o/w emulsions of mineral and vegetable oils; however, it is employed more frequently as a stabilizer for lotions and creams, containing soap or nonionic emulsifying agents. Pharmasorb Colloidal serves as a secondary emulsifier. Magnesia magma and kaolin are sometimes added to mineral-oil emulsions to serve as stabilizing agents. Silica gel has been recommended as a solid emulsifier for the preparation of ointments.[47]

DETERIORATION AND PRESERVATION OF EMULSIONS

One of the most important properties of pharmaceutical and cosmetic emulsions is the stability of the finished product. A stable emulsion is characterized by absence of flocculation and creaming; absence of coalescence of the globules and separation of the internal phase from the emulsion; absence of deterioration by micro-organisms; and maintenance of elegance with respect to general appearance, odor, color and consistency. Accordingly, the types of instability in a pharmaceutical emulsion may be classified as follows: (1) flocculation and creaming, (2) coalescence and breaking, (3) deterioration by micro-organisms and (4) miscellaneous physical and chemical changes.

The factors contributing to these forms of instability, and the methods of stabilizing and preserving emulsions against degradation, are discussed in this section.

Flocculation and Creaming. Flocculation is the joining together of globules to form large clumps or floccules, which rise or settle in the emulsion more rapidly than do the individual particles. As previously mentioned under homogenization, the passage of an emulsion through an orifice at a high pressure sometimes results in flocculation.

Creaming is the rising ("upward creaming") or settling ("downward creaming") of globules or floccules to form a concentrated layer at the surface or at the bottom of the emulsion. The term has been derived from the well-known process of cream formation, which occurs in milk when it is allowed to stand for some time.

Although the formation of a thick cream layer is often desirable in milk, it is regarded as a mark of *instability* in pharmaceutical emulsions. Creaming results in a lack of uniformity of the product, and unless the container is agitated thoroughly before each dosage is removed, may lead to variations in the amount of drug which is administered. Furthermore, the appearance of the emulsion is affected by creaming, and this is as real a problem to the pharmaceutical compounder as is separation of the internal phase.

Stokes' equation includes the various factors concerned in the creaming process:

$$V = \frac{2r^2 (d_i - d_e) g}{9\eta}$$

V is the velocity of sedimentation, r is the radius of the globules of the internal phase, d_i is the density of the internal phase, d_e is the density of the external phase, g is the gravity constant, and η is the viscosity of the external phase.

The equation shows first that the radius of the globules is a major consideration; doubling the radius increases the velocity of settling or creaming by a factor of 4. Reducing the particle size by passing the emulsion through a homogenizer decreases the velocity of creaming considerably. The result of homogenization of milk is well known. However, as previously noted, homogenization under high pressure sometimes leads to flocculation, and the large clumps which are formed may cream more rapidly than the individual globules in the unhomogenized emulsion.

The density difference $(d_i - d_e)$ in the above equation shows that, when the density of the internal and the external phases are equal (i.e., when d_i equals d_e), the velocity of creaming is zero. When the internal phase is less dense than the continuous liquid, which generally is the case in o/w emulsions, $(d_i - d_e)$ takes on a negative value and thus V is also negative. A negative velocity expresses the fact that creaming occurs in an *upward* direction. When the dispersed liquid is denser than the dispersion medium, the density difference $(d_i - d_e)$ is positive and V likewise is positive. This condition, which generally occurs in w/o emulsions, results in a settling of the globules, or, as it is sometimes expressed, in *downward* creaming.

The gravity factor in the numerator of the equation is essentially constant under ordinary circumstances. However, creaming may be accelerated, as is often done in the dairy industry, by centrifugation.

The velocity of creaming is inversely proportional to the viscosity of the external phase of the emulsion; that is, the creaming velocity is reduced by an increase in viscosity of the continuous medium. Auxiliary emulsifiers, such as agar and methylcellulose, sometimes are added to improve the consistency of the emulsion for this purpose. However, one must guard against flocculation, since the use of an unsuitable thickening agent may result in clumping, with subsequent increase in effective particle size and a corresponding increased rate of creaming.

Coalescence and Breaking. Unlike creaming, the coalescence of globules and the subsequent breaking of an emulsion are irreversible processes. Under the conditions of creaming, the globules are still surrounded by a protective sheath of emulsifying agent and may be redispersed simply by agitating the product. However, in an emulsion which has broken, i.e., in which the phases have separated as distinct layers, simple mixing fails to re-establish the stable emulsion. The emulsion may be reconstituted only by incorporating more emulsifying agent and passing the product through the proper emulsifying machinery.

Any system containing finely divided particles is unstable, owing to the excess energy of the dispersed phase. Accordingly, the conditions of equilibrium in an emulsion are satisfied only when the immiscible liquids have separated into 2 layers. The globules coalesce slowly or rapidly, depending on the strength of the emulsifier film and to a less extent on other factors, until the product is completely "cracked." Although many properties, such as electric charges on the particles, low interfacial tension and increased viscosity, have been suggested as stabilizing factors, it generally is agreed today that the most significant element in stabilizing an emulsion against breaking is the emulsifier film surrounding the dispersed particles. If the emulsifying agent or combination of agents is adsorbed and oriented at the interface in a manner such as to form a tough, coherent barrier, the film will withstand the tendency of the globules to coalesce, and the emulsion will remain stable for the desired period of time.

According to King,[48] the only precise method for estimating the stability against breaking involves a microscopic analysis in which the average globule size is determined from time to time as the emulsion ages. The degree of coarsening of the emulsion at each time indicates the rate of breaking. In the case of rapidly breaking emulsions, of course, visual observation of the separation is carried out easily. Microscopic methods, while more nearly accurate, require the measurement of several hundred to several thousand globules for each analysis, and, therefore, are tedious and time-consuming.

Deterioration by Micro-organisms. Molds, yeasts and bacteria may bring about the decomposition of the emulsifying agents, contaminate the aqueous phase, produce rancidity in the oil and destroy oil-soluble vitamins. Spalton[49] states that a preservative should be a powerful fungistatic rather than bacteriostatic agent, since it is more likely that fungi (molds and yeasts) may contaminate emulsions. The presence of certain drugs, such as benzoic and salicylic acid or high concentrations of alcoholic solutions, may provide adequate protection against micro-organisms; however, it is usually desirable to add an agent which will act specifically as a preservative. Combinations of parahydroxybenzoates—0.1 to 0.2 per cent of the methyl ester and 0.02 to 0.05 per cent of the propyl ester—frequently are used; the combination is particularly effective against molds, yeasts and bacteria, so long as the emulsifying agent and other ingredients do not complex with the preservative agents to nullify their action.

Since most preservatives are partially soluble in oil, some of the agent tends to pass into the oil, where it becomes ineffective as a protective agent for the aqueous phase. Consequently, one must be certain that the preservative is added in adequate amounts to protect the product.

Miscellaneous Physical and Chemical Changes. Care must be taken to protect emulsions against deterioration by light, extreme temperatures and oxidative and hydrolytic rancidity of the oil. Freezing and thawing result in a coarsening and sometimes in the breaking of an emulsion; high temperatures produce the same effects. However, some emulsions, particularly those that are stabilized with synthetic emulsifying agents, are unusually resistant to extreme heat and cold. Benerito and Singleton[50] reviewed the effect of heat on the stability of emulsions. Hom, et al.[11] employed heat tests in the evaluation of the stability of emulsions for injection. Light and rancidity affect the color and the odor of oils and may destroy their vitamin activity. Antioxidants are necessary if the oils are likely to become rancid. Emulsions should be kept in tight containers and stored at moderate temperatures; and if affected by light, they should be stored in dark bottles.

OFFICIAL PRODUCTS

N.F. XI contains 2 emulsions, both of them being administered orally. U.S.P. XVI recognizes 1 preparation in the official class of Emulsion.

Liquid Petrolatum Emulsion (Mineral Oil Emulsion, N.F.). This emulsion is prepared by the continental method with acacia as the emulsifying agent. Other emulsifying agents and adjuncts may be used, and the method may be altered in conformity with the requirements of large-scale production. Vanillin, the flavoring agent in this emulsion, may be replaced by other flavors or mixtures of flavoring substances. The 60 ml. of alcohol per 1,000 ml. of emulsion may be replaced by 60 ml. of sweet orange peel tincture or 2 Gm. of benzoic acid as the preservative.

The product is used as a laxative in doses of 30 ml. and is considerably more palatable than liquid petrolatum in the unemulsified form.

Phenolphthalein in Liquid Petrolatum Emulsion, N.F. Both agar and acacia are used to prepare this laxative emulsion. Part of the oil is emulsified with the acacia by the continental method. Then the remaining liquid petrolatum is added in portions alternately with the agar solution; this procedure maintains the proper consistency.

Vanillin and saccharin are used as flavoring and sweetening agents, but they may be replaced by other official flavors. Preservatives also may be added if desired. Official permission is given to replace the acacia or agar, or both, with other emulsifying agents; and other methods may be employed for making the emulsion. Phenolphthalein is added to this product to increase the laxative properties.

Each 15-ml. dose of the emulsion contains 7.5 ml. of liquid petrolatum and 60 mg. of phenolphthalein.

Sterile Phytonadione Emulsion, U.S.P., is a sterile emulsion of phytonadione or vitamin K_1. It is an o/w emulsion and contains a suitable emulsifying agent of this type. The emulsion has a pH between 5 and 7 and is usually available in the concentration of 50 mg. of phytonadione in 1 ml. The emulsion is injected intravenously in the dose of approximately 0.5 ml. and is used for its prothrombogenic vitamin activity.

REFERENCES

1. Lee: Pharm. Arch. **7**:53, 1936.
2. Cotgrave: A Dictionary of the French and English Languages, 1611, as reported by Lee *in* Introduction to Pharmacy, ed. 3, p. 458, New York, McGraw-Hill, 1954. Also see: Chemist & Druggist **132**:475, 1940.
3. Anonymous: Chemist & Druggist **132**:475, 1940.
4. Wilder: Druggist Circ., December 1874.
5. Forbes: Am. J. Pharm. p. 61, 1872.
6. Husa: Pharmaceutical Dispensing, ed. 4, p. 249, Iowa City, Husa, 1951.
7. Seifritz: J. Phys. Chem. **29**:738, 1925.
8. Ann. Int. Med. **29**:1, 1948; Stare: Proc. Soc. Exp. Biol. Med. **75**:680, 1950; Stare: J. Am. Dietetic Assoc. **27**:191, 1951.
9. Groth and Skurnik: Acta. med. scandinav. **101**:333, 1939.
10. Koehne and Mendel: J. Nutrition **1**:399, 1929.
11. Hom, Autian, Martin, Berk and Teplick: J. Am. Pharm. A. (Sci. Ed.) **46**:255, 1957.
12. Lambert, Miller and Frost: J. Am. Pharm. A. (Sci. Ed.) **45**:685, 1956.
13. Rdzok, Grundy, Kirchmeyer and Sylvester: J. Am. Pharm. A. (Sci. Ed.) **44**:613, 1955.
14. Peereboom: Am. Perfumer Aromat. No. 2, **73**:27, 1959; Williams: *ibid.* **73**:39, 1959. The other articles on antioxidants in this issue should also be consulted.
15. Eisman, Jaconia and Mayer: J. Am. Pharm. A. (Sci. Ed.) **42**:659, 1953.
16. Atlas Surface Active Agents: Wilmington, Del., Atlas Powder Company, 1950.
17. Griffin: J. Soc. Cosmetic Chem. **1**:311, 1949; *ibid.* **5**:1, 1954.
18. Corran and Lewis: Biochem. J. **18**:1368, 1924.
19. Bandelin and Tuschhoff: J. Am. Pharm. A. (Pract. Ed.) **14**:106, 1953.
20. Schulman and Cockbain: Tr. Faraday Soc. **36**:651, 661, 960, 1940.
21. Chun, Joslin and Martin: Drug & Cosmetic Ind. **82**:164, 1958.
22. Serrallach, Jones and Owen: Ind. Eng. Chem. **25**:816, 1933.
23. Cobb: *in* Emulsion Technology, p. 7, Brooklyn, Chemical Pub. Co., 1946.
24. Briggs: J. Phys. Chem. **24**:120, 1920.
25. Woodman: J. Pomol. Hort. Sci. **4**:95, 1925.
26. Husa and Becker: J. Am. Pharm. A. (Sci. Ed.) **30**:141, 1941.
27. Kempson-Jones: Am. Perfumer Aromat. **71**:88, 1958.
28. Husa and Becker: J. Am. Pharm. A. (Sci. Ed.) **30**:83, 1941.
29. Dorey: *in* Emulsion Technology, sect. 7, Brooklyn, Chem. Pub. Co., 1946.
30. Goldner: J. Am. Pharm. A. (Pract. Ed.) **3**:324, 1942.
31. Krantz and Gordon: J. Am. Pharm. A. **15**:93, 1956.
32. Briggs and Schmidt: J. Phys. Chem. **19**:478, 1915.
33. Holmes and Child: J. Am. Chem. Soc. **42**:2049, 1920.
34. Limburg: Rec. trav. Chem. **45**:875, 1926.
35. Tice: J. Am. Pharm. A. (Sci. Ed.) **24**:1062, 1935.
36. Fitzgerald and Skauen: J. Am. Pharm. A. (Sci. Ed.) **44**:358, 1955.
37. Osborn and DeKay: J. Am. Pharm. A. (Pract. Ed.) **2**:420, 1941.

38. Donnan: Z. phys. chem. **31**:42, 1899.
39. Donnan and Potts: Kolloid Z. **4**:208, 1910.
40. Bancroft: J. Phys. Chem. **17**:514, 1913; *ibid.* **19**:275, 1915.
41. Clowes: J. Phys. Chem. **20**:407, 1916.
42. Bhatnagar: J. Chem. Soc. **120**:1768, 1921.
43. Bergy: J. Am. Pharm. A. (Pract. Ed.) **3**:358, 1942.
44. Conrad: Am. Perfumer Aromat: **71**:70, 1958.
45. Pickering: J. Chem. Soc. **91**:2001, 1907.
46. Hubbard and Freeman: J. Am. Pharm. A. (Pract. Ed.) **2**:78, 1941.
47. Prout and Harris: J. Am. Pharm. A. (Pract. Ed.) **2**:432, 1941.
48. King: Tr. Faraday Soc. **37**:168, 1941.
49. Spalton: Pharmaceutical Emulsions and Emulsifying Agents, p. 98, London, Chemist and Druggist, 1948.
50. Benerito and Singleton: Drug & Cosmetic Ind. **79**:381, 1956; Am. Perfumer Aromat. **69**:37, 1957; J. Am. Oil Chem. Soc. **33**:364, 1956.

BIBLIOGRAPHY

Becher: Emulsions: Theory and Practice, New York, Reinhold, 1957.

Berkman and Egloff: Emulsions and Foams, New York, Reinhold, 1941.

Carter: Basic emulsion technology, Am. Perfumer Aromat. **71**:43, 1958.

Chen, Cyr and Langlykke: Pharmaceutical emulsions, Drug & Cosmetic Ind. **81**:596, 1957.

Emulsion Technology, ed. 2, Brooklyn, Chemical Pub. Co., 1946.

Spalton: Pharmaceutical Emulsions and Emulsifying Agents, Chemist & Druggist, London, 1950.

Sumner: Clayton's Theory of Emulsions and Their Technical Treatment, ed. 5, New York, Blakiston, 1954.

Sutheim: Introduction to Emulsions, Chemical Pub. Co., Brooklyn, 1946.

ALLEN I. WHITE, Ph.D.
Dean, School of Pharmacy,
Washington State University

17

Soaps, Liniments, Lotions, Oleates and Sprays

SOAPS
    DEFINITION
    HISTORY
    MANUFACTURE
    PROPERTIES
    USES
    OFFICIAL SOAPS

LINIMENTS
    CLASSIFICATION
    DENTILINIMENTS
    PETROXOLINS
LOTIONS
OLEATES
SPRAYS

SOAPS

DEFINITION

The term soap refers to a class of chemical substances which are salts of certain fatty acids. Because of traditions growing out of the long history of soap manufacture and the common use of this substance, certain limitations usually are placed on a definition of soap. Ordinarily, the definition is limited to that material produced by the reaction of raw ingredients in the soap kettle. When at equilibrium, this reaction produces a mixture of relatively constant composition containing approximately 70 per cent true soap and 30 per cent water, to which may be added a very small amount of salt. This mass commonly is known as *neat soap, pure soap* or *genuine soap.* In addition, because the common uses of soap rely on its ability to exhibit properties such as detergency and lowering of surface tension, the ordinary concept of soap includes only those compounds which are water-soluble. In a strictly chemical sense, water-insoluble salts of fatty acids are also soaps.

The chemical structure of soap may be represented as:

$$R\text{---}COOM$$

R is any saturated or unsaturated straight-chain hydrocarbon ranging from 7 to 21 carbon atoms. M is any atom or group of atoms, inorganic or organic, which has a positive charge and is capable of neutralizing the acid carboxyl group to form the desired compound. Sodium, potassium and ammonium ions are examples of inorganic substances used; the ethanolamines are examples of organic bases used.

HISTORY

As far as is known, it was not soap but an alkaline lye that was used for washing in the ancient civilizations. The word "soap" used in the King James translation of the Bible is misleading. It is understood to mean the lye from wood ashes.

The first authentic record of soap is found in the *Historia Naturalis* (VIII, 51) of Pliny the Elder (A.D. 1st century). According to Pliny, the Romans learned the preparation of soap from the Germans, who used a soft soap prepared from the fat or tallow of goats and the whiteburned or calcined ashes of beechwood as a kind of pomade rather than as soap. In his *History of Inventions, Discoveries and Origins*, Beckman states that the Latin word *sapo* is derived from the German *sepe*, which has been retained in the Low German. The Latin poet, Martial (A.D. 1st century), probably was the first to use the word *sapo*.

The knowledge that the formation of soap from fat and alkali is a definite chemical reaction was not gained until the early 19th century, when the French chemist, M. E. Chevreul (1787–1889), published the first reports on his classical studies on the chemical constitution of fats.

Modern developments in the field of surface-active agents resulting in the production of many competing products have given rise to the impression that soap gradually is becoming an obsolete material. This is not true, although the relative importance of soap has changed. In recent years, newer and different surface-active agents have been found to be superior to soap in instances where only a short time ago soap was the best, if not the only, product available. Nevertheless, there are still many situations calling for a surface-active agent in which soap does a superior job and is likely to remain a substance of choice. In addition, the economy of soap is likely to continue to make it a highly competitive product.

MANUFACTURE

Soap may be made from a large variety of fats and oils. Animal fats obtained from the meat-packing industry furnish a comparatively cheap source of material. Tallow from cattle and mutton tallow from sheep have been used commonly as raw materials. Lard from hogs may be used, but other uses for this substance make it more expensive. Whale and seal oils also have been employed. Many vegetable oils are common starting materials for soap. Among the more common vegetable oils used are: coconut, corn, cottonseed, olive, palm, palm kernel, peanut, rapeseed, sesame, soybean, sunflower and tung. Due to the quantity of supply and the competition with other markets for some of these oils, only a few of them are employed widely as raw materials.

The first step in the manufacture of a soap consists of hydrolyzing the fat molecule, a glyceride of various fatty acids (1). This may be accomplished as a separate process with the resulting fatty acids purified and later neutralized (2) or as a combined procedure in which the fatty acids immediately are neutralized by alkali present in the reaction mixture (3).

(1) $\begin{array}{l} R_1COOCH_2 \\ | \\ R_2COOCH \\ | \\ R_3COOCH_2 \end{array} + H_2O \xrightarrow[\text{catalyst}]{\text{heat, pressure}}$

$R_1COOH + R_2COOH + R_3COOH + C_3H_5(OH)_3$

(2) $R_1COOH + R_2COOH + R_3COOH + 3NaOH \rightarrow$
$R_1COONa + R_2COONa + R_3COONa + 3H_2O$

(3) $\begin{array}{l} R_1COOCH_2 \\ | \\ R_2COOCH \\ | \\ R_3COOCH_2 \end{array} + 3NaOH \rightarrow$

$R_1COONa + R_2COONa + R_3COONa + C_3H_5(OH)_3$

Three different applications of these reactions are employed industrially: the *kettle process*, the *cold process* and the *continuous saponification process*. The kettle process as used today is a complex refinement of the old traditional method of boiling fat and alkali (leached wood ashes) together in a large kettle. More soap is still produced by this process than by the others. In the modern soap factory, the "kettle" is a huge, especially equipped tank capable of handling 25 to 50 tons of oil at a time. Heat is supplied by admitting steam into the bottom of the tank. Other inlets provide for the controlled admission of alkali, water and brine solution. Outlets make possible the withdrawal of the by-products, the washings and the soap itself.

The simple cold process requires only

sufficient heat to liquefy the fats (95° F.) when the alkali solution is added and mixed with it. After addition of perfume or other substances, the mixture is placed in a "cooling frame" where the saponification process proceeds for several hours, considerable heat being evolved from the reaction. After standing for several days, during which time the mass cools and solidifies, the sides of the frame are removed, and then the soap may be cut into bars, stamped and wrapped by special machinery. This relatively low-cost process is not used very much at the present time since it is not possible to remove either the desirable by-product, glycerin, or the undesirable impurities derived from the fat used.

The continuous saponification process is a more modern development growing out of research to overcome the disadvantages of the large amount of time and plant space required by the kettle process. A high-temperature (450° F.) autoclave (600 lbs./sq. in.) has hot fat and catalyst entering at its bottom and hot water entering at its top. The oil is split into its component fatty acids and glycerin. Since the fatty acids are water-insoluble and lighter than water, they float out on top and may be withdrawn continuously from the autoclave. The glycerin, being water-soluble, drops to the bottom of the autoclave with the water and is withdrawn continuously there. The fatty acids produced may be used directly or separated by fractional distillation. Soap is formed by neutralizing the acids with proper alkali. By this process, large quantities of soap can be produced in a relatively small amount of space in a period of a few hours. In addition, a wide variety of soaps can be prepared easily by selection of fatty acids and alkalies and by variation in water content.

PROPERTIES

Since ordinary soap is usually a mixture of salts of various fatty acids, and since many different mixtures rightfully may be called soap, only general physical and chemical properties may be applied to it.

It usually is said that soap is soluble in water. When soap is mixed with water, it forms colloidal solutions or gels, depending on the concentration. This accounts for the faint cloudy appearance of water-soap mixtures. Dilute solutions of soap in water have a surface tension less than that of water, with the result that such solutions have a slippery feel, form suds or lather when agitated and are capable of emulsifying oil and dirt. The latter property, together with the ability of its solutions to wet material to which they may be applied, causes soap to be called a detergent. Soap is soluble in alcohol, forming true, clear solutions.

When mixed with water, soap undergoes ionization (4).

$$(4) \quad RCOOM \underset{}{\overset{HOH}{\rightleftharpoons}} RCOO^- + M^+$$

The anions formed are capable of combining with undissociated soap molecules, forming highly charged colloidal aggregates. Soap also partially hydrolyzes in the presence of water (5).

$$(5) \quad 2RCOOM + HOH \rightleftharpoons (RCOO)_2MH + M^+ + OH^-$$

In addition to the acid soap formed, this reaction produces small amounts of alkali at equilibrium. Thus, even when soaps are prepared from exact equivalent amounts of fatty acids and alkali, a slight alkalinity is produced in aqueous soap solutions.

Soap will react with ions of the alkaline earth metals and the heavy metals if they are present in water, forming salts which are insoluble in water and therefore precipitate out. Such ions as magnesium and calcium which are found in hard water thus remove soap from solution and decrease its ability to perform desired functions. If an excess of soap is used, then the precipitated material will be emulsified, and the desired function may be obtained at a higher cost.

Frequently, soaps are classified as either soft soaps or hard soaps. Soft soaps are made with potassium alkali and usually contain a relatively high proportion of potassium oleate. Hard soaps are made with sodium alkali and usually contain a relative low proportion of potassium oleate. The ratio of stearate to oleate (and salts of other unsaturated acids) affects the firmness of a soap. This explains the *U.S.P.* requirement that medicinal soft soap be made from oils whose liberated fatty acids have an iodine number of not less than 85. (The higher the iodine number, the greater the amount of unsaturated acids present in an oil.)

USES

In addition to its common use as a cleansing agent and for industrial uses, soap is used in pharmacy and medicine for a variety of purposes.

As a surface-active agent, soap is capable of reducing interfacial tension between liquid-solid, liquid-liquid and liquid-gas phases. Because of this fact, soap is used as an emulsifying agent. Such preparations as benzyl benzoate lotion and rose water ointment exemplify this use. The ability of soap to aid in emulsification can be judged by comparing the surface tension of pure water, 73 dynes/cm. at 22°, with that of a $0.03N$ solution of sodium oleate, 27 dynes/cm. in the 2-phase system. This same solution of sodium oleate will reduce the interfacial tension between water and benzene from 35.0 to 2.22 ergs.

As a wetting agent, soap is capable of dispersing materials that otherwise would form aggregates and separate from an aqueous mixture. This dispersing property is used in saponated cresol solution, in which the large quantity of cresol present (50%) is prevented from separating from the water (in which it is soluble to the extent of about 2%) by the presence of a potassium soap.

Over the years, soaps have been employed in medical practice for a variety of purposes. In most of these, the cleansing power of soap is the basis for its medical use. Soap has the ability to remove not only the clearly evident dirt on the skin but also micro-organisms and other microscopic material. However, it should not be concluded that soap is germicidal. It removes rather than destroys skin bacteria. Thus, when the surgeon performs the ritualistic preoperative scrubbing, a considerable amount of time is spent in accomplishing a very thorough cleansing. The ordinary handwashing of most people removes little of the microscopic material on the skin.

In addition to the scrubbing of the surgeon's hands, soap is used preoperatively to cleanse the skin of the patient at and around the area of an incision. Soap also has been used to cleanse wounds caused by either trauma or surgery. It is employed either as a treatment in itself or to prepare the area for further treatment in dermatologic conditions such as scabies.

Although it seldom is thought of as such, soap is probably the most important prophylactic agent in use today. It is well known that there is a relationship between disease rates and sanitary practices. Frequent and intelligent use of soap can reduce so-called "hand-to-mouth" infections as well as some other kinds of diseases easily transmitted by either direct or indirect contact.

OFFICIAL SOAPS

By definition, a number of compounds which are salts of relatively pure fatty acids may be included as official soaps as well as the mixtures traditionally known as soaps and bearing that word in their titles. Thus, the official salts of stearic acid, magnesium stearate, sodium stearate and zinc stearate, as well as zinc undecylenate, may be classified correctly as soaps. However, it is the author's purpose here to discuss only those mixtures properly classified as pharmaceutical preparations. (The sterile solution of the mixture of sodium salts of unsaturated fatty acids that occur in cod-liver oil, sodium morrhuate injection, is discussed in Chapter 12, dealing with injections.)

MEDICINAL SOFT SOAP, U.S.P.
Sapo Mollis Medicinalis; Green Soap; Soft Soap

Medicinal Soft Soap is made by the saponification of vegetable oils with potassium hydroxide. Only those vegetable oils whose liberated fatty acids have a saponification value not greater than 205 and an iodine value not less than 85 may be used. Oils formerly suggested by the *U.S.P.* included corn, cottonseed, linseed, olive and soybean. Excluded are coconut and palm kernel oils. The addition of the free oleic acid ensures a high ratio of unsaturated fatty acid salts and, therefore, a soft consistency of soap.

In making this soap, a small amount of glycerin is added to the aqueous alkali solution in order to promote the emulsification of the hot oil with the alkali solution. This brings the alkali and the fat into more intimate contact and increases the rate of saponification. The glycerin also aids in forming a clear soap and prevents the formation of soap crystals. When saponification is complete, the mixture will give a clear solution when added to water. Any unsaponified oil present would cause a turbidity in the solution.

The product is a soft, unctuous and slightly alkaline yellowish brown mass. The color will vary according to the color of the oil used. Years ago, hemp seed oil and olive oil having considerable chlorophyll present in them were used to make soft soap. The resulting product was green in color—hence the still-used synonym, Green Soap. This soap should be stored in well-closed containers because it is quite hygroscopic due to the amount of glycerin present. Medicinal Soft Soap is the preferred soap for the medical uses of soap mentioned earlier in this chapter. It is the principal constituent of soft soap liniment which is essentially a liquid soap. It and other liquid soaps are now popular for toilet, surgical and shampoo purposes.

Hard Soap, N.F.
Sapo Durus; Soap

Hard soap, defined by the *N.F.* as a "sodium soap," is made by the saponification of a hard fat with sodium hydroxide. To obtain the desired consistency, usually animal fats (tallow) which are rich in stearin content and relatively low in palmitin and olein content are used. However, vegetable oils such as olive oil also are used. The name "Castile soap," by which it is often known, arose out of the fact that a hard soap made from olive oil was produced in the ancient kingdom of Castile, Spain. Thus, true Castile soap is primarily sodium oleate, but contains some sodium palmitate and sodium stearate. So-called Castile soaps found on the market today often have a small amount of coconut oil soap added to them to increase their lathering quality. Sometimes the outer surface of Castile soap is colored a light brown by the oxidation of ferrous oxide added to the soap mass to give it a mottled appearance.

Hard Soap has been used internally to promote biliary and intestinal secretions. It has been combined with laxative and so-called alteratives in pills. It also has been shaped into rectal suppositories and used in enemas to promote evacuation of the lower bowel. Its surface-active properties account for its pharmaceutical uses such as an emulsifying agent in lotions, a detergent in toothpowders and a "slipping agent" in liniments.

Hexachlorophene Liquid Soap, U.S.P.

Hexachlorophene Liquid Soap is a solution of hexachlorophene in a liquid potassium soap. The *U.S.P.* provides that the amount of hexachlorophene should be not less than 225 mg. and not more than 260 mg. in each 100 Gm. of liquid soap. The soap base should contain 10 to 13 per cent of a potassium soap such as medicinal soft soap. The remainder of the mixture is water. If a manufacturer desires, substances that act as water softeners may be added to the mixture. The resulting liquid is clear and amber-colored, having a characteristic soapy odor, and is alkaline in reaction.

The *U.S.P.* makes provision for a more concentrated preparation that may be diluted according to suitable directions carried on the label. Such a preparation is more economical when large quantities of the soap are used. When properly diluted, such a preparation should conform to the requirements of the official Hexachlorophene Liquid Soap. Because it has been found experimentally that some nonionic detergents, such as Polysorbate 80, apparently inactivate hexachlorophene, the *U.S.P.* includes a note suggesting that no more than 8 per cent by weight of such agents be added to the liquid soap.

The addition of the germicidal hexachlorophene presents a liquid soap which is a bacteriostatic detergent very effective for preoperative scrubbing. A residue of hexachlorophene remains on the skin and exerts a prolonged antiseptic action. In addition to the liquid soap, a number of toilet bar soaps containing hexachlorophene are available and are recommended for their ability to reduce the number of the bacteria on the skin responsible in part for the putrefaction of sebaceous secretions. At the same time, these soaps will reduce the number of other micro-organisms on the skin mantle that cause dermatologic troubles.

LINIMENTS

Liniments are oily or alcoholic liquids and semisolids for external application, usually applied with friction. This class of pharmaceuticals sometimes is referred to as *embrocations* because of the method of application.

Liniments belong to the oldest modes of application known, and from early time until the 19th century often they were nothing more than plasters and ointments brought into a semisolid form. The original term for these preparations used by the Romans, Aurelius Cornelius Celsus and Pliny (A.D. 1st century), was *litus*, derived from the verb *linere*, meaning to besmear, to spread or rub over. The term *linamentum* was used by Celsus for a sort of lint. In its present meaning, the word *linamentum* did not come into general use until the end of the 16th century. Jean de Renou, in *Institutionum Pharmaceuticarum, Libri Quinque*, Paris, 1608, tells in a short chapter, "De Linimento, seu Litu" (Of the Liniments or Litus), that "linimentum mediae est consistentiae inter unguentum et oleum" (the consistency of a liniment lies between an ointment and an oil), and Joh. C. Schröder in his *Pharmacopoeia Medico-Physica (Chymica)*, the first edition of which appeared in 1641 at Frankfurt, states that "in praxi plerumque Linimenti ac Unguenti nomina confundi" (in practice the terms Liniment and Ointment are frequently confounded).

A few decades ago, liniments were a popular form of medication and many formulas were devised, a large number of them being patented. In *U.S.P. XVI*, 1 liniment is recognized; in *N.F. XI*, 3 are recognized.

CLASSIFICATION

Liniments may be studied best by dividing them into 3 classes: (1) alcoholic solutions, (2) oily solutions and (3) emulsions and suspensions.

Class 1. Alcoholic Solutions. Alcohol and hydroalcoholic mixtures are employed widely as vehicles for liniments, not only because alcohol is a good solvent for many of the drugs employed but also because of its ability to penetrate the skin and because it is itself a mild rubefacient, counterirritant and astringent. Frequently, soap and oils are added to alcoholic liniments to make them slippery and thus facilitate the rubbing action involved in their application. The official liniments falling into this class should be clear solutions.

CAMPHOR AND SOAP LINIMENT, N.F.

Soap Liniment

Camphor and Soap Liniment is prepared by effecting a solution of camphor, rosemary oil and hard soap in the hydroalcoholic solvent. The preparation should stand in a cool place for at least 24 hours before filtering. The hard soap contains some sodium palmitate which will precipitate out because it is insoluble in the solvent at cool temperatures. The removal of this precipitate will eliminate the dispensing of a solution which may become turbid. Extreme cold should be avoided or much of the soap may be removed by filtration.

This liniment makes an excellent base for other liniments and frequently is used as such. It may be used as a solvent for many substances, the high percentage of alcohol present (62 to 66%) aiding in this respect. The small amount of camphor present imparts only a mild rubefacient action.

This liniment has also been called Camphorated Tincture of Soap and Liquid Opodeldoc.

CHLOROFORM LINIMENT, N.F.

Chloroform Liniment is made by mixing chloroform with camphor and soap liniment. The addition of chloroform makes this liniment a strong, quick-acting rubefacient and counterirritant. If, on addition of chloroform to the camphor and soap liniment, a cloudy product results, it is probable that the liniment contains an excess of water. Because of the volatility of the chloroform, it is best to prepare this preparation as needed to avoid dispensing an inferior product. When it is necessary to store it, Chloroform Liniment should be kept at a low temperature in a tightly closed container.

Medicinal Soft Soap Liniment, U.S.P.

Soft Soap Liniment, Tincture of Green Soap   *Alcoholic*

The widely used synonym for this preparation, Tincture of Green Soap, goes back to the days when some of the oils used in the manufacture of soft soap contained chlorophyll and thus imparted a green color to the product. The official preparation is now a pale brown in color. It is made by dissolving lavender oil and medicinal soft soap in alcohol. Then this solution is permitted to stand for 24 hours before filtering and making up to volume. This standing period is to permit the precipitation of the alcohol-insoluble portions of the soap. Medicinal Soft Soap Liniment is an excellent detergent but is very strongly alkaline and, therefore, undesirable for many purposes. It is employed as a shampoo and to cleanse the skin preoperatively. It seldom is used as a liniment.

Class 2. Oily Solutions. Solutions of medicinal agents in fixed or volatile oils often are used as liniments. Fixed oils are good solvents for some rubefacient and irritant drugs and they furnish the necessary lubricant action for the rubbing of a liniment. Their ability to penetrate the skin is not so great as those having an alcoholic base and, consequently, their action is milder. Cottonseed, olive, sesame, almond and other oils may be used. Some volatile oils such as methyl salicylate and turpentine oil are rubefacient and irritant in themselves and so are employed alone, used as solvents for other drugs of similar action or combined with fixed oils to reduce their effect. Like the liniments of Class 1, these should be free from insoluble material and bear the label, *"For External Use Only."*

Camphor Liniment, N.F.

Camphorated Oil

Camphor Liniment is a 20 per cent solution of camphor in cottonseed oil. Cottonseed oil is preferred for making this liniment because of its lower cost as compared with olive oil, which is generally the solvent for camphor injections. This preparation must not be used for injection purposes because it is not sterile, and the cottonseed oil is not a suitable solvent for parenteral use.

To facilitate solution, the cottonseed oil is warmed on a water bath before the addition of the camphor. Because of the volatility of camphor, the heating should not be continued after the addition of the camphor, and the container should be stoppered tightly. Unless the camphor is powdered, solution takes place very slowly. If alcohol has been used in powdering the camphor, it must be removed completely, as traces of it will produce a cloudy product. Likewise, a wet container will cause the solution to be turbid. Camphorated oil is a very popular counterirritant for minor sprains, chest colds and neuralgias.

Class 3. Emulsions and Suspensions. Liniments may contain insoluble materials or consist of mixtures of immiscible liquids. When such conditions exist, it is best that an emulsion be formed, if possible, to prevent rapid separation of the ingredients and to improve the product's appearance.

Emulsification of liniments usually is accomplished by the formation of a soap which acts as the emulsifying agent. When an alkaline material such as ammonia water or lime water is added to a liniment base containing a fixed oil, soap is formed from the ensuing reaction. Then, by vigorous agitation, the oil and the water present may be formed into an emulsion. In addition to the usual label, *"For External Use Only,"* liniments which are emulsions or suspensions should bear the label, *"Shake Well,"* to ensure equal distribution of all constituents. Ammonia liniment and calamine liniment, formerly recognized by the N.F., are examples of such liniments.

DENTILINIMENTS

Dentiliniments are solutions of medicinal agents to be rubbed into the gums. These preparations were developed through co-operation of members of the pharmaceutical and the dental associations and were first introduced in *N.F. V. N.F. VII* recognized Compound Aconite and Iodine Dental Liniment, but this preparation is no longer official. This type of preparation is used very seldom in dental practice and practically never is called for in a pharmacy.

PETROXOLINS

Petroxolins are perfumed preparations containing medicinal substances in a saponated oily base to be applied externally with friction. It is claimed that the combination of the soft ammonium soap and the light mineral oil presents a good vehicle for medicines which are to penetrate the skin. Other trade names for parallel preparations are: Linogen, Linoliniment, Linoval, Parogens, Penetrol, Petrogen, Petroliment, Valselol, Valsol, Vaseloxyne, Vasenolum, Vaseosan, Vasogen, Vasol, Vasopolent, Vasopon, Vasoval.

Two types of petroxolins have been developed, *liquid* and *solid*. For the liquid type, former editions of the *N.F.* gave a recipe for the manufacture of a "liquid petroxolin" which had a soapy mineral-oil base resembling an oily liniment in consistency. The addition of medicinal agents to this base produces preparations which may be applied externally for either local or systemic action. Such preparations seldom are used in this country at the present time.

Solid petroxolins differ from liquid petroxolins principally because of the addition of yellow wax, which produces a product of firm consistency. The *N.F. IX* recipe for solid petroxolin is as follows:

Yellow wax	350 Gm.
Light liquid petrolatum	200 Gm.
Oleic acid	320 Gm.
Lavender oil	30 cc.
Alcohol	50 cc.
Strong ammonia solution	60 cc.
To make about	1,000 Gm.

Melt the yellow wax with the liquid petrolatum on a water bath, incorporate the oleic acid and transfer the mixture at once to a warm mortar; when nearly congealed, add the alcohol and the strong ammonia solution which previously have been mixed and warmed, and stir continuously until cool. Finally, incorporate the lavender oil.

In the manufacture of solid petrox, the mortar should be warmed to a temperature above the congealing point of yellow wax before the wax mixture is transferred to it. This will prevent a separation of the wax in small lumps. Likewise, the alcohol and the strong ammonia solution should be warmed sufficiently before adding them. This preparation is particularly recommended as a base for ointments containing Peruvian balsam because the usual granular separation of resinous material does not take place when it is used.

LOTIONS

Lotions are aqueous preparations containing insoluble material for external application without friction. The Latin term *lotio* is derived from the verb *lavare*, meaning to wash. Lotions usually contain antiseptic or germicidal substances useful in the treatment of skin diseases or substances that are cooling and sedative to an irritated skin. Although some lotions may be solutions, most of them are either suspensions or emulsions.

The modern development of dermatology has demanded a lotion that is cosmetic in character as well as one that contains the necessary medicinal substance. Lotions sometimes are preferred to ointments because they require less rubbing for their application and they leave a smaller amount of residue on the skin. This has led to the development of the emulsion-type lotion which many pharmacists now are called on to prepare. Schobel and Lichtin have recommended the following formula as one producing an oil-in-water emulsion capable of efficiently carrying medication into the skin and possessing wide compatibility:

Methylparaben	0.25
Propylparaben	0.15
Sodium lauryl sulfate	10.00
Propylene glycol	120.00

Stearyl alcohol	25.00
Light liquid petrolatum	250.00
Purified water	595.00
To make about	1,000.00

Melt the stearyl alcohol on a water bath, add the liquid petrolatum, and heat to 70°. Dissolve the methylparaben and the propylparaben in hot water, add the sodium lauryl sulfate and the propylene glycol. Adjust the aqueous solution to 70°. Pour the mixture containing the water into the oil phase, in a fine stream, with continuous stirring. Continue to stir until the temperature is below 45°.

Other modern developments have introduced thickening or suspending agents for those lotions consisting of finely divided precipitates carried in suspensions. Mucilages of gums, such as acacia and quince seed, and tragacanth are being replaced by nonfermentable substances such as bentonite and methylcellulose. Many lotions are now packaged in convenient plastic squeeze bottles that permit the dispensing of these thick liquids in convenient quantities. Pressurized containers that dispense lotions through action of a "push button" are also being introduced on the market.

Since lotions contain insoluble or immiscible material in suspension, they always should be labeled *"Shake Well"* and *"For External Use Only."*

Benzyl Benzoate Lotion, N.F.

Benzyl Benzoate Lotion consists of an emulsion of benzyl benzoate, an oily substance, in water and prepared by mixing the benzyl benzoate with triethanolamine and oleic acid and then shaking with water and making to volume. The triethanolamine reacts with the oleic acid to form a soap which functions as the emulsifying agent.

$$CH_3(CH_2)_7CH:CH(CH_2)_7COOH + N(C_2H_4OH)_3 \rightarrow$$
$$CH_3(CH_2)_7CH:CH(CH_2)_7COONH(C_2H_4OH)_3$$

For the extemporaneous preparation of a benzyl benzoate lotion, the *N.F.* offers a formula for saponated benzyl benzoate. This consists of a mixture of benzyl benzoate with oleic acid and triethanolamine. When a lotion is desired, this mixture may be diluted with water and then agitated vigorously.

This water-miscible lotion does not stain clothing and is removed readily by washing. The *N.F.* lotion contains 26 to 30 per cent by weight of benzyl benzoate, the concentration usually employed in the treatment of scabies, head lice and nits.

Calamine Lotion, U.S.P.

Over the years, Calamine Lotion has been employed more popularly than any other lotion. Many suggestions have been made to improve old formulas in order to obtain a more satisfactory product. In order to reduce sedimentation rates, to keep the fine insoluble particles in a dispersed state and to promote adhesion to the skin, many different suspending agents and vehicles have been investigated. Differences in opinion as to what is most satisfactory have not been resolved, and, as a result, a number of manufacturers produce calamine lotions from formulas different from that of the *U.S.P.* Many different formulas have been considered for inclusion in the *U.S.P.* The *U.S.P. XVI* formula for Calamine Lotion is very much like the *U.S.P. XIII* formula and makes use of bentonite magma as the suspending agent in place of the polyethylene glycols used in the *U.S.P. XIV* formula.

To prepare Calamine Lotion, prepared calamine and zinc oxide are triturated into a smooth paste with glycerin and a portion of the bentonite magma that has been diluted with an equal part of lime water. Then the remainder of the diluted magma is added gradually, and the lotion made to volume with lime water. Care should be exercised to get a uniform paste of finely divided particles, which may be dispersed readily by shaking.

Calamine Lotion is used extensively as a mildly astringent and protective coating for inflammatory skin diseases. Its pink color has made it popular as a base for other lotions.

Phenolated Calamine Lotion, U.S.P.
Compound Calamine Lotion

Phenolated Calamine Lotion is a 1 per cent solution of liquefied phenol in calamine lotion. It is prepared by mixing the proper amounts of each ingredient. The addition of phenol slightly increases the antiseptic power and contributes local anesthetic and antipruritic properties to calamine lotion.

Dimethisoquin Hydrochloride Lotion, N.F.

Dimethisoquin Hydrochloride is commercially known as Quotane Hydrochloride and is used as a topical local anesthetic. It is recommended for use in the lotion form to treat moist lesions due to a variety of causes such as insect bites, poison ivy and poison oak, pruritus, minor burns and nonspecific irritations.

The N.F. does not present a formula for the preparation of a patented product. The commercially available lotion is prepared as a 0.5 per cent mixture in a water-miscible emulsion base that has a fleshlike color. It also contains 0.1 per cent menthol and 10 per cent zinc oxide. The N.F. requires that the lotion contain not less than 90 per cent and not more than 110 per cent of the labeled amount of dimethisoquin hydrochloride. It is usually dispensed in plastic squeeze bottles.

Monobenzone Lotion, N.F.

Monobenzone Lotion is usually a 5 per cent solution of monobenzone in isopropyl alcohol and propylene glycol. The N.F. does not specify the concentration but requires that the lotion contain not less than 94 per cent and not more than 106 per cent of the labeled amount.

Monobenzone is a hypopigmenting agent that inhibits the formation of melanin in the skin. It appears to do this by inhibiting the enzyme, tyrosinase, that normally functions to convert tyrosine to the precursor of melanin, dihydroxyphenylalanine. Its effect is somewhat uncertain but it has been used successfully in preventing the development of hyperpigmented areas in melasma of pregnancy, Addison's disease, special cases of photosensitization, and severe freckling. It is not recommended for use in the more common and somewhat temporary cases of freckles. It should be noted that monobenzone will not remove pigment already formed. Its action is temporary, and its application must be continued as long as the effect is desired.

The commercially available product of this material is known as Benoquin Lotion.

White Lotion, U.S.P.
Lotio Alba

White Lotion is prepared by mixing slowly and with constant stirring filtered dilute solutions of zinc sulfate and sulfurated potash. It is important to add the sulfurated potash solution *to* the zinc sulfate solution so that a finely divided precipitate will be obtained and the formation of zinc hydroxide and basic zinc salts avoided. The slower the rate of mixing and the greater the amount of agitation, the finer the insoluble material will be as it is formed in the reaction.

$$ZnSO_4 + K_2S \rightarrow K_2SO_4 + ZnS$$

Since sulfurated potash is an indefinite mixture of several substances, the equation given represents only in part what takes place. It is probable that some thiosulfate and some free sulfur as well as polysulfides of zinc also are present. Even though a fine precipitate is formed, it becomes lumpy on standing, and so White Lotion should be prepared freshly and shaken vigorously before dispensing. It has been stated that the beneficial action of White Lotion is dependent on a small amount of hydrogen sulfide formed in its manufacture. Since any H_2S formed would escape from solution rather quickly, the dispensing of freshly prepared mixtures is even more vital if this theory is true. White Lotion is used in the treatment of a number of dermatologic diseases and has been a favorite for the treatment of acne. It is referred to sometimes as Lotio Sulfurata or Sulfurated Lotion.

OLEATES

Technically, an oleate is either a salt or an ester of oleic acid. In pharmaceutical practice, traditionally, the term oleate has been applied to a solution of a metal or an alkaloidal oleate in an excess of oleic acid. There may be exceptions to this definition, such as the obsolete preparation known as lead oleate. These preparations have decreased in popularity during recent years as modern medicinals have replaced them. A few of them, particularly mercury oleate, still are used in the treatment of various dermatologic conditions.

MERCURY OLEATE, N.F.
Oleatum Hydrargyri

Mercury Oleate is prepared by the action of mercuric oxide on oleic acid.

$$2C_{17}H_{33}COOH + HgO \rightarrow (C_{17}H_{33}COO)_2Hg + H_2O$$

The 2 ingredients are mixed together and warmed to a temperature not to exceed 60°. Higher temperatures should be avoided to prevent decomposition of the oleic acid. Using finely divided mercuric oxide and avoiding the formation of lumps by sifting the oxide into the oleic acid accelerates the reaction. The use of alcohol as a means of bringing the 2 reactants into more intimate contact has been recommended but is not included in the official formula. Contacts with metal utensils should be avoided so that the mercury ions will not be reduced and amalgamate with the metal. The finished product should contain the equivalent of 24 to 26 per cent of mercuric oxide.

Mercury Oleate is used in dermatology as a parasiticide, as against pediculi, and in the treatment of various other skin diseases. It has been used as a means of applying mercury systemically by inunction. Pharmaceutically, it is used in preparations containing finely divided metallic mercury (mercury ointments, mercury mass) because its consistency is effective in preventing the coalescence of the finely divided mercury globules. In this connection, it is spoken of as an "extinguishing agent."

The preparation has been called Oleated Mercury.

SPRAYS
(Inhalations and Inhalants)

Sprays may be defined as aqueous or light mineral oil solutions of drugs to be sprayed or dropped in the nose and the throat. Modern packaging makes use of plastic squeeze bottles that deliver the solutions into the nasal passage more effectively than can be accomplished by the use of droppers. Only one spray is retained by the official texts (Tyrothricin Spray), although closely related preparations are included under the titles Inhalations and Inhalants.

Inhalations are solutions of drugs that may be administered by the use of suitable devices to reach the respiratory tree in the form of fine mists. They usually contain bronchodilating agents which relieve congestion due to asthma or hay fever. Nebulizers capable of producing droplets no more than a few microns in size are most commonly used for their administration.

Inhalants are drugs or combinations of drugs possessing a sufficiently high vapor pressure that they may be carried into the upper respiratory passages with inspired air. Usually, inhalants are packaged in plastic or metal devices called inhalens that contain the drugs impregnated on paper strips or other suitable material; through them the inspired air passes as it is drawn into the nasal passage. They also may be packaged as low-pressure aerosols that carry finely powdered drugs into the upper respiratory tract. Inhalants usually contain vasoconstrictor, aromatic, or aromatic substances intended to relieve nasal and pharyngeal congestions.

EPINEPHRINE INHALATION, U.S.P.

This 1:100 solution of epinephrine in purified water contains sufficient hydrochloric acid to keep the epinephrine in solution. Also known as Ephinephrine Hydrochloride Spray, this preparation is used to relieve congestions in the pharynx. Because epinephrine contains phenolic hydroxyl groups that are easily oxidized to colored quinone compounds, contact with air causes discoloration. Such a product is unsuitable for use, and the *U.S.P.* specifies in a note that this inhalation should not be used if it is brown in color or if it contains a precipitate. It is best stored in small, tightly stoppered and well-filled bottles that are light-resistant.

ISOPROTERENOL HYDROCHLORIDE INHALATION, U.S.P.

Isoproterenol hydrochloride is a compound closely related to epinephrine and, like it, may be used to relieve congestions such as bronchial asthma by inhalation from a nebulizer. The *U.S.P.* does not specify a particular concentration for the solution to be used by inhalation but does require that such solutions contain 95 to 105 per cent of the labeled amount. One-half and 1 per cent solutions of isoproterenol hydrochloride are available under the brand name of Isuprel Hydrochloride.

Such solutions are to be made isotonic with sodium chloride so that they will be more compatible with the mucus of the upper respiratory tract. Like epinephrine solutions, isoproterenol solutions will discolor by auto-oxidation and should not be dispensed if the solution has turned brown or if it contains a precipitate.

Isoproterenol Sulfate Inhalation, N.F.

The sulfate salt of Isoproterenol is used in the aqueous isotonic solution sold under the brand name Norisodrine Inhalation. In other respects the sulfate inhalation resembles the hydrochloride inhalation and, similarly, should be stored and handled to protect it against deterioration.

Propylhexedrine Inhalant, U.S.P.

Propylhexedrine is an analog of epinephrine that is sold widely in inhalers under the trade-marked name of Benzedrex. It is used primarily to relieve congestions in the nasal passages due to colds, allergies and other causes. It does not produce some of the undesirable side-effects elicited by desoxyephedrine and some of the other epinephrine analogs. To make the inhalers, a solution of propylhexedrine is used to impregnate some fibrous material such as filter paper, and then this is allowed to dry. Aromatic materials such as menthol may be added to the mixture for the psychological effect they have on the user. When the inhaler is placed in a nostril and air breathed in through the inhaler, the volatile propylhexedrine is carried into the upper respiratory tract, where it will cause a shrinking of congested mucous membrane. The *U.S.P.* requires that propylhexedrine inhalant contain not less than 90 per cent of the labeled amount of $C_{10}H_{21}N$.

Tyrothricin Spray, N.F.

Since tyrothricin is practically insoluble in water, manufacturers of this spray must employ harmless solubilizing and wetting agents in making the aqueous dispersion. The application of tyrothricin in the upper respiratory tract well might be accompanied by use of a vasoconstrictor to reduce the congestion usually present during infections in that area. The use of Tyrothricin Spray should not be indiscriminate, because tyrothricin is toxic when it enters the blood stream; therefore, the area of application must be free of any injury which might permit such entry. Concentrations of tyrothricin usually do not exceed more than 0.5 mg. per milliliter when it is used as a spray.

BIBLIOGRAPHY

Soaps

Berkman, S., and Egloff, G.: Emulsions and Foams, New York, Reinhold, 1941.

Fishbein, M. (ed.): Medical Uses of Soap, Philadelphia, Lippincott, 1945.

Gortner, R. I.: Outlines of Biochemistry, ed. 3, New York, Wiley, 1949.

Jamieson, G. S.: Vegetable Fats and Oils, New York, Reinhold, 1932.

Liniments

Bliss, A. R.: Drug and Cosmetic Ind. **40**: 54, 1937.

Lesser, M. A.: Drug and Cosmetic Ind. **51**: 647, 1942.

Lotions

Schobel, K. L., and Lichtin, J. L.: J. Am. Pharm. A. (Pract. Ed.) **15**:420, 1954.

Sprays

Bliss, A. R.: Drug and Cosmetic Ind. **39**: 588, 1936.

LOUIS C. ZOPF, D.Sc.
Dean, College of Pharmacy,
State University of Iowa

18

Ointments, Cerates, Plasters and Cataplasms

OINTMENTS
    GENERAL CONSIDERATIONS
    APPLICATION
    CLASSIFICATION
    PREPARATION

PACKAGING, STORAGE AND LABELING
CERATES
PASTES
PLASTERS
CATAPLASMS

OINTMENTS
GENERAL CONSIDERATIONS

Ointments are semisolid preparations, for external application, of such consistency that they may be applied to the skin readily by inunction. They should be of such composition that they soften, but not necessarily melt, when applied to the body. They serve as vehicles for the topical application of medicinal substances and also function as protectives and emollients for the skin. An ointment is also known as a salve or chrisma. An ointment for use in the eye is called an ophthalmic ointment or oculentum.

In the past, an ointment has been defined as "a fatty preparation of such a consistency as to be easily applied to the skin by inunction, gradually liquefying when in contact with it." Our present concept of this type of preparation is much broader. Today, in addition to such oleaginous mixtures, we include preparations of greater efficiency possessing the same general consistency but with an entirely different appearance. They may be entirely free of oleaginous substances. In many instances, they are emulsions of fatty or waxlike materials containing comparatively high proportions of water.

HISTORY

The use of fats derived from every source obtainable, and mixtures of these with active and inert materials, belong to the earliest substances employed by man for medicinal purposes. Our earliest records on the use of various fats and oils (Ointments-Unguents) date back to the Babylon-Assyria era, about 3,000–5,000 B.C. The examination of remains of such ointments, found in the excavated tombs of Egyptian kings, supports the view that the fats of ointment bases of olden times were taken almost exclusively from the animal kingdom.

The concept of Ointment in the modern sense is the product of a long development. In ancient times, there was no special terminology differentiating between liquid or semisolid preparations used as an anointment. The Greeks had a list of different terms classifying these anointments: (1) partly according to their use, e.g., "malagma," softening ointment (from *malasso*, soften) and (2) partly according to some important ingredients, e.g., "keroma," wax ointment (from *keros*, wax), which proved to be the predecessors of the later cerates.

The great Greco-Roman physician, Claudius Galenos (A.D. 2nd century), invented a formula for an ointment consisting of olive oil, rose oil, white wax and a small quantity of water. This proved to be the prototype for all the cosmetic ointments which later became known under the name of cold cream. In the form given to it in the book of a mysterious 13th century author, known under the name of Mesue Jr., this cold cream has found its way, with minor modifications, into all of the pharmacopeias of the world up to and including the present. It was about this time (13th century) that the distinctions between oils, ointments and plasters became general; e.g., Olea being liquid oily ointments, Unguenta semisolid smears, and Emplastra masses sticking firmly to the skin.

The above concept of ointments remained unchanged for almost half a millennium. The following definition, given in the first *U.S.P.*, published in 1820, confirms the above position—namely, that the concept of Mesue Jr. still prevailed in the early 19th century: "Ointments are prepared from lard or oil rendered of the consistence of butter by the addition of suet, wax or spermaceti, so as to suspend the dry powders and more ponderous articles, with which they are frequently incorporated. As they are to be applied to the skin, they should be soft or fluid at the temperature of the body. The following formulas are calculated for a temperature not exceeding 60° Fahr. In higher temperature, more suet or wax may be added."

From the middle of the 19th century on, we encounter several attempts at a broadening of the concept of the term ointment. The ointment bases offered by nature were purified, augmented and partly replaced by artificial ones, introduced with special regard for the purposes they were intended to serve. These new ointment bases appeared in the following sequence:

1858: Glycerin and Starch: The apothecary Schacht found that glycerin and starch, if heated in certain proportions and to a certain temperature, combined to a translucent jelly, to which he gave the name plasma and recommended it as a good ointment base. This mixture appeared in continental pharmacopeias as Unguentum Glycerini, in the *English Pharmacopœia* as Glycerinum Amyli and in the *U.S.P.* as Glyceritum Amyli.

1873: Cosmolin and Paraffin Ointment. Dr. A. W. Miller, in 1873, published a paper on "Cosmolin and Paraffin Ointment," which later was to be known as petrolatum.

1876: Stearic Acid. Herman Hager, in 1876, wrote in his handbook that "stearic acid is used as a substitute for white wax in the preparation of ointments to be sold over the counter."

1885: Wool Fat, "Oesypus," Rediscovered. In 1885, the pharmacologist Oscar Liebreich rediscovered the therapeutic value of wool fat, the "œsypus" of the ancient Greeks, which he called "lanolin."

1895–98: Wool Fat Alcohols. In the years 1895–98, the Russian chemist Lifschuetz discovered and proved that the ease with which wool fat (lanolin) is taken up (by water) depends, not as formerly was supposed, on the cholestrin ethers it contains but on the free alcohols which he had isolated as a group.

1907: Eucerin. It was the great dermatologist, Paul G. Unna, who on the basis of his research introduced in 1907 "Eucerin," a new basis for ointments consisting of a part of Lifschuetz's alcohols with 20 parts of paraffin ointment and 20 parts of water. This proved to be the forerunner of the American counterpart, "Aquaphor."

1920–44: Numerous contributions appeared during this period, among which hydrogenated oils, sulfated and sulfonated hydrogenated oils, as well as stearic acid, sodium stearate, glyceryl stearate mixtures possessing self-emulsifying properties and polymers of glycols, such as polyethylene glycol 4,000, and esters of these glycols such as polyethylene glycol monostearate, became of foremost importance.

1945–59: Surface-active agents, Plastibase, (a hydrocarbon base), attapulgite, silicones, Veegum, guar gum, carbopol, etc., were introduced in these years. These substances are useful adjuncts to ointment bases or can be used as bases themselves.

In summary, we may note that the **term** *ointment* has passed from the Greco-Roman times when the term was used in its broadest sense (to include anything used as a "smear," whether it be aqueous or oily) through the more restricted use of the term (from the time of Mesue, Jr.) when it was applied to only soft unctuous preparations, to the modern tendency which seems to be attempting to broaden the use of the term to again include aqueous as well as fatty and hydrocarbon bases under the term of ointment; e.g., the designation of vanishing creams and bentonite pastes as ointments.

APPLICATION

Ointments, pastes, salves, cerates and plasters are grouped together according to their similar pharmaceutical properties, as well as for their similar therapeutic purposes.

These fatty or oily preparations are known as **"emollients"** (from Latin *emollire,* to soften) and as such are used for their local action on the skin. They are employed as: (1) protectives, (2) agents for softening or rendering the skin more pliable and (3) vehicles or carriers for more active drugs. In the latter case, they may serve as vehicles for drugs having as their chief purpose a local action in which it is desirous of maintaining a slow liberation of the drug from the base over a long period of time; or they may serve as vehicles for drugs from which absorption and systemic effects are desired. In this case, the ointment should be rubbed thoroughly into the skin to ensure adequate absorption through the sebaceous glands.

Preparations serving a similar purpose, but of an aqueous nature, such as mucilages, gums, pectin pastes, starch pastes, etc., and applied to mucous membranes, are known as **demulcents** (from Latin *demulcere,* to smooth down). According to Sollman, this corresponds to the natural mechanisms for the protection of the body surfaces. The skin normally possesses a thin layer of emollient oil while the membranes of the interior of the body are moistened with mucus, which is a typical gummy demulcent. Viscid water-miscible solutions (e.g., of the gums) adhere to these moist surfaces better than does oil, while oily and fatty preparations adhere better to the epidermis.

These preparations, together with the oils and the liniments, fulfil the physician's desire for a gradation from the fluid oil bases to the stiffer wax bases and permit the use of mixtures of any desired consistency. When the preparation is to be rubbed into the skin, the liquid or soft fats, the oils and soft ointments are desired, while protection and prolonged contact are obtained best by the use of the stiffer preparations such as the cerates, the plasters and the pastes.

CLASSIFICATION

Ointments can be classified best according to type (based on composition):

I. OLEAGINOUS OINTMENT BASE
1. Anhydrous
2. Does not absorb water readily (hydrophobic)
3. Insoluble in water
4. Not washable

II. ABSORPTION OINTMENT BASE
1. Anhydrous
2. Will absorb water (hydrophilic)
3. Insoluble in water
4. Most are not washable

III. EMULSION OINTMENT BASE
A. Emulsion Ointment Base w/o
 1. Hydrous
 2. Will absorb water
 3. Insoluble in water
 4. Not washable
 5. Water-in-oil emulsion

B. Emulsion Ointment Base o/w
 1. Hydrous
 2. Will absorb water
 3. Insoluble in water
 4. Washable
 5. Oil-in-water emulsion

IV. WATER-SOLUBLE OINTMENT BASE
1. Anhydrous
2. Will absorb water
3. Soluble in water
4. Washable
5. Greaseless

In the past, ointment bases have been classified or divided into 3 types, according to their penetration or penetrability, as follows:

1. **Epidermic ointments** are those which demonstrate no, or at the most very slight, power of penetration into the skin. These are indicated especially when it is intended that a therapeutic effect shall be exerted chiefly on the diseased epithelium. In this group are placed the bases which contain petrolatum, waxes and their combinations.

2. **Endodermic ointments** are those which possess some power of penetration into the deeper layers of the skin. In this group are placed the softer bases which liquefy at body temperature, such as the vegetable oils, lard, wool fat, lanolin and/or combinations of these.

3. **Diadermic ointments** are those which penetrate the skin, thus offering a better opportunity for absorption of the medicament. Ointments of the emulsion type and the water-soluble bases belong to this group.

Comments

In the light of more recent evidence on the processes of absorption through the skin and the liberation of substances from ointment bases, we must look on the above therapeutic classification with some degree of skepticism.

Recent evidence seems to place more importance on the chemical and the physical relationship between the base and the medicament incorporated therein than on the penetrating properties of the base itself. More precisely, then, whether the medicament itself can be absorbed is the important consideration.

This idea apparently was initiated by Sauerland[1] in 1912, when he concluded that the influence of the ointment bases varies according to the substance. In 1918, Sollman[2] gave further proof for this thought when he stated that oils and ointments delay the absorption of fat-soluble substances such as phenol, mustard oil or dichlordiethyl sulfide, analogous to the partition of a substance between a good solvent and a poor solvent in a test tube. In 1934 and 1935, Bliss[3] employed the histology of the skin to explain his conception of absorption and pointed out that site of application, thinness of skin, freedom from hair and richly supplied lymphatics were aids for absorption. He also concluded that the drug itself rather than the vehicle in which it was applied was the determining factor of absorption.

In 1939, Brown and Scott[4] brought further evidence to substantiate the work of Sollman and Sauerland when they reported that a substance must possess both oil and aqueous solubility in order to penetrate the human skin and that an extremely high or low partition coefficient is less conducive to absorption than intermediate values. They found that the type of base had no effect on the quantity of substance absorbed.

In 1942, Fuller, Hawking and Partridge[5] reported on a series of experiments performed in order to determine the effect of media on the absorption of sulfonamide drugs. They concluded from their *in vitro* studies that the differences in rate and amount of absorption between the different "sulfa" compounds apparently depends on their differences in solubility. Their results from an *in vivo* study of absorption and execution of these compounds when applied to wounds show a satisfactory agreement between the results of the *in vitro* and the *in vivo* studies. These men also conclude that the fundamental consideration in the absorption of substances from ointments is "the ratio of the surface of the preparation to its volume." If the surface is relatively large, as in a thin film, the delay from oil preparations is small. This is the case when ointments are smeared over a large surface.

In 1940, the work of Emmens[6] probably demonstrated more effectively than any other the part ointment bases play in absorption. He stated that volatile organic solvents (ether, benzene and 95% alcohol) were more effective carriers of active material from the skin surface than was nut oil or lanolin. In his experiments with rats and mice, inunction in benzene or ether was as effective as, or even more effective than, injection of the same medicament (androgenous estrogens) dissolved in oil. In tests with rabbits, inunction in benzene, but not in ether, was superior to injection in oil. In 1938, Macht[7] in a series of experiments also reported that some drugs incorporated in fat were absorbed less readily than the same drugs applied in aqueous or hydroalcoholic solution.

Polano, Bonsel and Van der Meer[8] have shown that absorption does occur from petrolatum and lard bases, particularly when applied to damaged epithelium. Absorption can and does occur from any ointment base, depending not only on the composition of the base but also on the condition of the skin and on many other factors. Polano concludes that, when it is desired to have a drug penetrate into the skin, this effect probably may be obtained most easily by applying o/w emulsions and hydrogenated fats. The difficulty is in knowing when penetration is desirable. It is obvious that a topical anesthetic must penetrate to the nerve fibers, but should antibiotics for topical use get into the blood stream?

Michelfelder and Peck[9] studied the absorption of pyribenzamine hydrochloride and pyribenzamine base through the damaged and the intact skin under various conditions. Their study showed that, within limits, the greater the concentration of the drug and the longer the period of inunction, the greater was the absorption.

Plein and Plein[10] have shown that penetration and absorption from selected ointment bases varied not only with the drug but also with the condition of the skin at the time of the *in vivo* test. They also concluded that penetration and absorption are not wholly dependent upon the vehicle, that relative penetration and absorption of different drugs from a series of ointment bases are not in the same order for all medicinal agents and that drugs vary greatly in their ability to penetrate through normal intact skin.

Drawing our conclusions from the more recent evidence regarding the part ointment bases play in the absorption of substances through the skin, we can then postulate that:

1. Ointment bases in general tend to slow or delay absorption through the intact epidermis and from mucous surfaces.

2. It is not the penetration of the base in a direct sense which determines whether absorption will occur through the intact skin or not, but the chemical and the physical (solubility) relations between the drug and the base which determine whether absorption will occur and in what amounts it will occur.

3. Petroleum ether, benzene and chloroform are efficient substances for preparing the skin for absorption and they carry substances dissolved in them through the skin much more efficiently than if these same substances were incorporated in ointmnt bases.

4. The amount of damage to the epidermis and the degree of loss of normal skin barriers to absorption are more important than the vehicle in determining penetration through the epidermis.

Much study also has been devoted to the field of ointment bases as carriers for antiseptics. These studies also reveal a conflict of opinion as to the value of aqueous ointment bases and anhydrous bases as carriers for antiseptics. Some authors have reported the increased effectiveness of antiseptics in aqueous bases, while others have reported that the antiseptic action was not greatly increased over that of the anhydrous base. In summarizing and analyzing the results of these reports, one can make the following general conclusions:

1. There is as yet no ointment base reported which can serve as a universal ointment base.

2. The conclusion by G. F. Reddish, "that the antiseptic value of an ointment could not be told by the antiseptic value of its constituents" still holds true.

3. Claims for water-containing ointment bases as vehicles for antiseptics over that of the greasy type bases are not justified unless on an individual basis.

4. The chemical and the physical nature of the antiseptic, which is incorporated in the base, has as much, or perhaps more, to do in determining the final bactericidal action of the product than the composition of the vehicle in which it has been incorporated.

Classification of Bases

According to Beeler,[11] various authors have described an ideal ointment base as possessing the following chemicophysical properties: (1) stable; (2) neutral in reaction; (3) nongreasy; (4) not degreasing in action; (5) nonirritating; (6) nondehydrating; (7) nonhygroscopic; (8) removable by washing with water; (9) compatible with all medication; (10) free from objectionable odor; (11) nonstaining; (12) efficient on dry, oily or moist skins; (13) capable as serving as a medium for chemicals soluble in either fat or water; (14) capable of stock preparation for extemporaneous use; (15) composed of readily available ingredients of known chemical composition; (16) capable of holding at least 50 per cent of water; (17) easily compounded by the pharmacist; (18) melting or softening at body temperature.

The following is a classification of those substances which, at this time, are used to a greater or lesser extent as ointment bases in themselves or contribute some pharmaceutical property to the base as a whole.

I. HYDROCARBONS
Liquid petrolatum
White petrolatum
Yellow petrolatum
Paraffin
Ceresin
Plastibase (Jelene)

II. ALCOHOLS
A. Aliphatic
  1. Monohydroxy
    Lauryl
    Myristyl
    Cetyl
    Oleyl
    Stearyl
  2. Polyhydroxy
    Ethylene glycol
    a. Polyethylene glycols 200 to 700 are liquids
      Polyethylene glycols 1,000 to 6,000 are solids and are known as Carbowaxes
    Diethylene glycol
    Propylene glycol
    Glycerol
B. Cyclic
  Cholesterol
  Isocholesterol
  Oxycholesterol
  Anhydrous wool fat
  Hydrous wool fat
  Parachol
  Protegin
  Falba absorption base

Mixtures, the hydrophilic property of which is due, in part, to these alcohols

III. ALCOHOL-ETHERS (Cellosolves and Carbitols)
Ethylene glycol methyl ether (methyl cellosolve)
Ethylene glycol ethyl ether (cellosolve)
Ethylene glycol butyl ether (butyl cellosolve)
Diethylene glycol methyl ether (methyl carbitol)
Diethylene glycol ethyl ether (carbitol)
Diethylene glycol butyl ether (butyl carbitol)

IV. ACIDS
A. Aliphatic
  Lauric
  Myristic
  Palmitic
  Oleic
  Stearic
B. Cyclic
  No examples commonly used in ointments

V. ESTERS
A. Monohydroxy alcohols
  1. Aliphatic
    Beeswax white
    Beeswax yellow
    Carnauba wax
    Spermaceti
  2. Cyclic
    Cholesterol palmitate
    Cholesterol stearate
B. Polyhydroxy alcohols
  1. Dihydroxy (glycols)
    a. Mono-esters
      Ethylene glycol laurate, oleate, ricinoleate, stearate
      Propylene glycol laurate, oleate, ricinoleate, stearate
      Diethylene glycol laurate, myristate, oleate, palmitate, ricinoleate, stearate
      (1) Polyethylene glycol 400 monolaurate, monostearate

b. Di-esters
Ethylene glycol dilaurate, distearate
Diethylene glycol dilaurate, distearate
(2) Polyethylene glycol 300 di-oleate, polyethylene glycol 1,000 di-oleate

2. Trihydroxy (glycerol)
a. Mono-esters
Glycerol monomyristate, oleate, palmitate, ricinoleate, stearate
b. Di-esters
None commercially prepared
c. Tri-esters (fats)
Synthetic
Glyceryl tristearate
Natural (animal)
Lard
Lard, benzoinated
Mutton suet
Natural (vegetable)
Almond oil, expressed
Cacao butter
Castor oil
Cocoanut oil
Corn oil
Cottonseed oil
Linseed oil
Olive oil
Soybean oil
Modified natural fats
Hydrogenated castor oil
Hydrogenated corn oil
Hydrogenated cottonseed oil
Hydrogenated soybean oil
Sulfated-hydrogenated castor oil
Sulfonated (sulfated) castor oil
Sulfonated (sulfated) olive oil

3. Tetra-hydroxy (erythritols)
a. Mono-esters
Erythritol monostearate
b. Di-esters
Erythritol distearate
c. Tri-esters
Erythritol trioleate
d. Tetra-esters
Erythritol tetrastearate

4. Penta-hydroxy (penterythritols)
a. Mono-esters
b. Di-esters
c. Tri-esters
d. Tetra-esters
e. Penta-esters
} Not available commercially at this time

5. Hexa-hydroxy (mannitol, sorbitol, dulcitol)
a. Mono-esters
Mannitol monolaurate, oleate, stearate
Sorbitol monolaurate, oleate, stearate
b. Di-esters
Sorbitol dilaurate, dioleate, distearate
Mannitol distearate
c. Tri-esters
Mannitol triricinoleate, tristearate
Sorbitol triricinoleate
d. Tetra-esters
e. Penta-esters
f. Hexa-esters
} Not available commercially at this time
6. Hexahydroxy anhydrides (sorbitan and hexitan)
Sorbitan monolaurate, oleate, stearate
Polyoxyethylene sorbitan monooleate (Polysorbate 80, U.S.P.) also known as Tween 80
7. Fatty Acid Esters
Polyoxyethylene stearate (Polyoxyl 40 Stearate, U.S.P.) also known as Myrj 52.

VI. SOAPS
Oleates (sodium, potassium, ammonium, calcium, magnesium)
Stearates (sodium, potassium, ammonium, calcium, magnesium)
Petroxolins
Vanishing creams (sodium, potassium, ammonium, triethanolamine soaps)

VII. MISCELLANEOUS
A. Cold creams
B. Silicon derivatives
Colloidal clays
1. Bentonite
2. Veegum
3. Attapulgite
Silica gel
Silicones
C. Cellulose derivatives (see chapter on Emulsions)
D. Gelatin (see chapter on Emulsions)
E. Sodium Alginate (see chapter on Emulsions)
F. Glycerite of starch (see under History)

VIII. PHYSICAL CLASSIFICATION (BASED ON COMPOSITION)
A. Oleaginous-hydrocarbon (see under chemical classification)

B. Absorption
C. Emulsion
D. Water-soluble

Hydrocarbons

This group represents the most inert of chemical compounds. It comprises a group of substances with a wide range of melting points so that a mixture of any desired consistency and melting point may be prepared with representatives of this group. These substances are stated to possess the least power of penetration and, therefore, are used chiefly as protectives and emollients in topical application.

The liquid paraffins are used chiefly as agents in which powders are incorporated (triturated, rubbed) before they are mixed with the bases of a higher consistency. This aids in reducing the particle size of the powder. These are also mixed with petrolatum to make it less viscous.

The petrolatums, white and yellow, are the most frequently used of our ointment bases. Their advantages lie in their consistency, stability, blandness and chemical inertness, which allows almost any medicinal substance to be incorporated in them. Their disadvantages lie in their greasiness and inability to absorb or mix with water. However, this can be remedied by mixing 15 per cent of wool fat with it; this mixture will absorb up to 50 per cent of water. Dyniewicz has recommended a base composed of petrolatum 3 parts and wool fat 1 part. For further information on the value of combinations of wool fat and petrolatum and oxy and iso cholesterol and petrolatum, one may refer to Dr. Eugen Unna's article on Ointment Bases, cited in the list of references at the end of this chapter.

Paraffin and ceresine are of a higher melting point and are used chiefly as stiffening agents. Paraffin melts between 50° to 57° C. and ceresine melts between 78° to 80° C. Their advantages lie in their homogeneous structure. They do not crystallize on cooling after having been melted, and for this reason are preferred to beeswax in cosmetic ointments. Ceresine is also known as ozokerite, earth wax and mineral wax. It is composed of hydrocarbons of complex composition and frequently is adulterated by the addition of paraffin.

Plastibase (Jelene)* is a combination of mineral oils and heavy hydrocarbon waxes, having a mol. wt. of about 1,300, the large proportion of which are liquid and are retained in what is believed to be a matrix of submicroscopic interstices. The base is a soft, unctuous, colorless, jellylike material which melts at 90° to 91° C. and maintains a desirable consistency over a wide temperature range (−15° to 60°).

Some precautions must be observed in the compounding of Plastibase ointments since such substances as menthol, methyl salicylate and camphor are dissolved by Plastibase, with the result that ointments containing these chemicals become too soft. Likewise, coal tar produces an ointment too soft to prevent separation. Plastibase does not lend itself to the incorporation of waxes as stiffening agents because it is difficult to cool the resulting mixture to a smooth consistency. Plastibase ointments are best prepared by levigating the medicinal agent with a small portion of the base, then incorporating this with the remainder of the base.[12]

Alcohols

Aliphatic: MONOATOMIC. This group is made up of the fatty alcohols chiefly from C_{12} through C_{18}. They are used in some cases as stiffening agents but chiefly for their emollient and emulsion stabilizing properties. They are greaseless, forming water-absorbent emulsions, and render the skin velvety rather than smooth and slippery. Cetyl alcohol is the most commonly used of this group, although stearyl alcohol has been recommended for use in several bases. These may be used as additive in 1 to 5 per cent concentration or from 5 to 20 per cent as the principal wax. Beeler's Base and the University of California Hospital Base illustrate their use:

BEELER'S BASE

Cetyl alcohol	15.0
White wax	1.0
Propylene glycol	10.0
Sodium lauryl sulfate	2.0
Water	72.0

* Product of E. R. Squibb & Co.

U. C. H. BASE

Cetyl alcohol	6.4
Stearyl alcohol	6.4
Sodium lauryl sulfate	1.5
White petrolatum	14.3
Mineral oil	21.4
Water	50.0

Ointments containing these alcohols must be stirred thoroughly in the preparation thereof.

POLYATOMIC. This group, which includes such substances as diethylene glycol, propylene glycol and glycerol, is used chiefly in ointments containing water—particularly when the emulsion is of the oil-in-water type. Due to the hydroscopicity, they absorb and retain moisture from the air, thus acting as humectants in the emulsion. Propylene glycol has been recommended as a substitute for glycerol not only because of shortages during war but also because of assists in obtaining a more intimate dispersion of soap, oils, greases and other such substances in water.

The application of this group of compounds developed greatly with the introduction of polymers of these substances into pharmacy. Various polymers of ethylene glycol of the general formula $HOCH_2(CH_2OCH_2)CH_2OH$ having molecular weights from 200 to 6,000 have been utilized in many formulas. Polyethylene glycols are liquids when the molecular weight is below 700 and are waxlike solids of increasing consistency as the molecular weight increases to 6,000. The compounds from 1,000 on up are unctuous but water-soluble; they are inert and may be recommended as major ingredients of water-removable ointment bases.

Cyclic. Cholesterol and the cholesterol alcohols, oxy, and iso, together with the mixture of these alcohols and of their esters in their natural proportions as in Adeps Lanae or in a purified and concentrated form (Protegin, etc.), are the chief representatives of this group. The latter mixtures are included here because their hydrophilic properties and the beneficial softening effect on the skin are reported to be due to the wool fat alcohols and esters present in these mixtures. Parachol, Protegin X, Falba absorption base, etc., generally are mentioned or discussed under the heading of "Absorption Bases."

While wool fat was used by the Greeks under the name of "Oesypus," its modern use begins with the rediscovery of its properties by the pharmacologist Liebreich in 1885. Hartman, in 1860, and Schulze, in 1872, proved that wool fat contained cholesterol and oxycholesterol, and O. Braun discovered the hydrophilic properties of this same fat. In 1886, Liebreich assigned the hydrophilic properties of wool fat to the cholesterol esters. The Russian chemist Lifschuetz discovered in wool fat the free alcohols isocholesterol and oxycholesterol, to which the capacity of wool fat to absorb water is chiefly due. It was P. G. Unna who realized the medical and the pharmaceutical value of Lifschuetz's discovery and worked to perfect its practical application. In 1907, he introduced Eucerin, a mixture of 5 per cent of Lifschuetz's alcohols in petrolatum. This base possessed the property of absorbing water up to 700 per cent.

The above facts do not necessarily reveal the relentless effort of workers to prepare a satisfactory ointment base. The introduction of wool fat in 1885 was hailed because it was thought that now at last a base was available that did not possess the undesirable propery of the others—namely, immiscibility with water, alcohol and glycerin—and yet possessed the advantages of stability, blandness and unctuousness.

The disadvantages of wool fat, soon to be discovered, are: (1) tendency toward rancidity, (2) disagreeable odor, (3) water-absorbing capacity less than is desirable for cooling ointments, (4) its pitchlike consistency. While the introduction of hydrous wool fat reduced the above objections somewhat, they still remain to a certain degree; therefore, these two bases are generally mixed with the hydrocarbon bases.

Introduction of the purified and concentrated form of wool fat such as Protegin marks another step in the relentless effort to overcome the disadvantages of wool fat and to develop its advantages. With the isolation of the active hydrophilic alcohols and their incorporation into the inert base petrolatum, according to Unna, we have satisfied the desire for a satisfactory ointment base.

According to studies by Johnston and Lee,[13] mixtures of cholesterol and cholesteryl esters have greater emulsifying power than cholesterol alone; of the esters, they believe cholesteryl stearate to be the best.

Hydrophilic Petrolatum, U.S.P. XVI, contains cholesterol. This formula differs from that which was introduced in *U.S.P. XIII* in that the original formula contained less cholesterol and 15 per cent wool fat. Wool fat was deleted because of its potential sensitizing effect on the skin. There has been a decreasing apprehension on the part of practitioners to the use of wool fat in dermatologic preparations. The increase in cholesterol in the *U.S.P. XIV* and *XV* formulas gives a product which is capable of absorbing large quantities of water.

The *British Pharmacopœia* contains an Ointment of Wool Alcohols:

Ointment of Wool Alcohols

Wool alcohols*	60.0
Hard paraffin	240.0
White or yellow soft paraffin	100.0
Liquid paraffin	600.0

Alcohol-Ethers (Cellosolves)

These substances, together with the glycols, are used chiefly for their solvent, wetting and hygroscopic properties in cosmetic ointments. As yet, they have not been introduced in official ointments. They possess the solvent properties of alcohols and ethers and therefore are unique in this field. Their approximate use is as follows: beard softener 5 per cent, hand cream 10 per cent, liquid cleansing cream 10 per cent, astringent lotion 10 per cent. They are used in place of glycerin because they possess its hygroscopic and wetting powers without its stickiness.

Acids

The acids of this group used in the ointment field are generally from 12 to 18 carbon atoms in length. They are used generally as a source of free acid in order to react with alkali and form a soap either in cold or vanishing cream ointment bases. Sometimes stearic acid is used as a stiffening agent, but this use is not general.

As these acids generally are used to form a soap, and this in turn is to act as the emulsifying agent, the acid of choice, of course, is the one which will make the most stable emulsion. In this respect, it has been shown that there is an increase in emulsifying power of soaps from C_{12} to C_{18} and that, above C_{18}, we again have a continual decrease in this property. Therefore, it follows that stearic acid is probably the most frequently used acid of the group and explains why vanishing creams are almost always known as stearate creams. Oleic acid is used to form the oleates of substances to be incorporated into ointments; e.g., mercury oleate, atropine and cocaine oleate. It is used also to prepare the petroxolin ointment bases. (See under Soaps.)

Esters

Esters of Monoatomic Alcohols: ALIPHATIC. This group consists chiefly of beeswax (yellow and white), carnauba 84° to 86° C. wax and spermaceti 42° to 50° C. They have melting point ranges of from 42° to 50° C. for spermaceti to 84° to 86° C. for carnauba wax. Beeswax is intermediate, with a melting point of 62° to 65° C. They are used chiefly to increase the consistency of ointments, particularly those which are distributed in the warmer southern areas. They are used generally in amounts up to 5 per cent.

These compounds consist chiefly of esters of the higher fatty alcohols and acids such as cetyl palmitate, myricil cerotinate and melissyl palmitate. However, beeswax and carnauba wax contain, in addition to the esters, free fatty acids such as cerotic acid, carnaubic acid and melissic acid. It is this free fatty acid content that is desired in beeswax for use in cold creams. For this purpose, beeswax should possess an acid number of 18 to 23 in order that enough soap may be formed by reaction with the alkali to stabilize the emulsion formed. Spermaceti, while chiefly ester, contains a small amount of free cetyl alcohol and very small amounts of free acid. Hence, it is

---

* Wool alcohol is a crude mixture of steroid and triterpene alcohols prepared by treating wool fat with alkali and separating the fraction containing cholesterol and other alcohols.

used only for its hardening effect and the free cetyl alcohol it contains.

While comparatively stable, these substances will turn somewhat rancid on long standing if exposed to air.

CYCLIC. These consist chiefly of the fatty acid esters of cholesterol, oxycholesterol and isocholesterol. They are used for these hydrophilic properties similar to cholesterol itself. They are used chiefly combined with petrolatum in amounts up to 3 and 5 per cent and confer upon it the property of absorbing and emulsifying water, forming water-in-oil emulsions. For more comprehensive information as to preparation and use, see Cyclic Alcohols (p. 323).

Esters of Polyhydric Alcohols. This group is comprised of the fatty acid (C_{12}–C_{18}) esters of the polyhydroxy alcohols from glycol to mannitol. It also includes the esters of such compounds as glycol ethers. Of the many compounds of this type already known, it is interesting to note that, up to the present, the only polyhydric alcohol fatty acid esters occurring naturally have been the triglycerides of various animal, vegetable and fish oil and fats. All of the others are prepared synthetically, generally by reacting the chlorhydrin with the sodium salt of the acid; e.g., glycerochlorhydrin or propylene glycol chlorhydrin and sodium stearate.

Because of their similar properties, all of the synthetically prepared compounds are discussed together, and the following comments hold for all of the groups under Esters of Polyhydric Alcohols, except the naturally occurring triglycerides.

SYNTHETIC COMPOUNDS. It should be made clear that the usual commercial products available are not single chemical compounds but are mixtures of the mono-, the di- and in some cases the tri-fatty acid esters, with perhaps a small percentage of free fatty acids. In addition, because these compounds in themselves are poor emulsifying agents, small amounts of soap, wetting agent or other surface-tension reducing agents are necessary to give these compounds emulsifying properties. Thus, glyceryl monostearate is available as glyceryl monostearate, nonemulsifying and glyceryl monostearate, self-emulsifying. Glyceryl monostearate is admixed with soap (usually sodium stearate), which lends it the self-emulsifying properties.

In themselves, these mixtures do not possess the necessary properties of an ointment base. They do not melt or soften at body temperature. However, they are excellent emulsifying agents and are useful in preparing ointment bases of the cold and vanishing cream types. The type of emulsion formed is determined generally by the ratio of free hydroxy groups to those esterified and the percentage of free fatty acid. Thus, glyceryl monostearate will make an o/w emulsion while glyceryl tristearate will make a w/o emulsion. Sorbitol distearate is used to prepare o/w emulsions and sorbitol tetrastearate to prepare w/o emulsions. The ratio of free hydroxy groups to esterified ones determines whether the agent is more water-miscible or oil-miscible, and this, in turn, determines which phase, oil or water, will be the external phase. (The phase with which the emulsifying agent is most miscible will be the external phase.)

Glyceryl monostearate, glyceryl monostearate self-emulsifying, diglycol stearate and other similar compounds are widely used in the cosmetic and the pharmaceutical industries. The following formula serves as illustration:*

Ointment Base

Mineral Oil	15.0
White Petrolatum	20.0
Glyceryl monostearate S.E.	12.0
Stearic acid	5.0
Lanolin	5.0
Water	43.0

The general procedure for preparing emulsions containing polyhydric alcohol esters is to mix the oil miscible ingredients and warm to 80° C. Heat the water phase to about 85° C. and add the oil phase to the water phase with constant stirring.

Diglycol stearate or polyethylene glycol esters may often be used as the emulsifier in place of glyceryl monostearate, self-emulsifying.

Polyhydric alcohol esters, when mixed with petrolatum, confer upon it the prop-

* Cosmetic & Drug Manual, Glyco Products Co., Inc., 1953.

erty of absorbing or emulsifying water; e.g., petrolatum when incorporated with small amounts of sorbital oleate or laurate will absorb high percentages of water. The following formulae will serve to illustrate the use of these compounds:

Elvin[14]

Glyceryl monostearate	10.00
Liquid petrolatum	35.00
Spermaceti	13.00
Water	38.00

Harry[15]

Diglycol stearate	15.00
Liquid paraffin	5.00
Glycerin	5.00
Water	75.00
Preservative q.s.	
Sorbitol monolaurate	10.00
Liquid paraffin	20.00
Distilled water	70.00
Preservative q.s.	

NATURAL TRIGLYCERIDES OR ESTERS. This group, which comprises the natural animal and vegetable fats, served as the chief source of ointment bases until the middle of the 19th century. Among these fats, mutton suet and lard have played the most important roles. Of the animal fats, lard has always been preferred.

These fats, while similar chemically in that they are mixtures of the glycerides of palmitic, stearic and oleic acids, vary in the percentage of unsaturated acids (oleic, linoleic, linolenic) as esters and, thereby, differ in consistency. The consistency of these fats is in a direct ratio to the iodine number or degree of unsaturation of the glycerides. The glycerides of unsaturated fatty acids have lower melting points than those of the saturated acids. Thus, lard is softer and blander in consistency than mutton suet because of its higher percentage of triolein.

The vegetable and the animal fats have two disadvantages as ointment bases: (1) the water-absorbing capacity is low; (2) a pronounced tendency toward rancidity is present.

The property of water absorption is desirable in order that crystalline substances may be dissolved in water and the solution then incorporated into the base. This makes for smoother and more uniform ointments. Also, high percentages of water are desirable in ointments because of cooling and soothing effects. This property of absorbing water also makes bases easier to wash off the skin.

The development of rancidity in ointments is definitely undesirable because of the irritating properties of the oxidized fats. Rancid fats also possess a nauseating odor which is undesirable from a psychological standpoint. This disadvantage of animal and vegetable fats was recognized very early in the use of these compounds, but it was Deschamps in 1843 who discovered the preservative action of benzoin on lard. Since that time, benzoinated lard has become official in many of the leading pharmacopeias of the world. However, the true mechanism of the preservative action of benzoin on fats was not reported until 1933, when Husa and Riley[16] proved conclusively that coniferyl benzoate was the constituent of Siam benzoin responsible for the preservative effect on lard.

It has also been shown that air, light and metal containers hasten the development of rancidity in these fats.

Benzoinated lard never really became extensively popular with physicians or pharmacists because of its unstability. Unna stated that benzoinated lard was not appreciated by the German dermatologists because of the irritation caused by the benzoin on tender and already irritated skins, and, secondly, because of its lack of complete stability.

Mutton suet, the purified abdominal fat of the sheep, is much firmer than lard and does not become rancid so easily. Its melting point is 45° to 50° C., whereas lard melts between 36° and 42° C.

VEGETABLE OILS. These oils are used chiefly in ointments to lower the melting point or to soften the bases of a higher consistency and also as an adjunct to hydrocarbon bases to increase their emollient effects and to decrease their drying effects. These oils can be used as ointment bases in themselves when a high percentage of powder is incorporated in a small amount of oil so that the resulting consistency is quite viscous. Thus, zinc oxide in castor oil is prescribed frequently.

The use of these oils in cosmetic preparations such as nourishing cream, hand lotions and cold creams for dry skin is very extensive. In cosmetic, use, olive oil seems to be preferred, while expressed almond oil and cacao butter and cocoanut oil follow, respectively. Olive oil and linseed oil formerly were recommended strongly for use on the skin when it was thought vitamin F was the skin vitamin and that it was closely related to the unsaturated acids in these oils. However, this theory lacks confirmation and is no longer applied to these oils.

Castor oil differs from the other oils in that it contains hydroxy fatty acids and, therefore, has slightly different solubility properties. It is soluble in 95 per cent alcohol while the other oils are not. It is miscible with such substances as Peruvian balsam, whereas the other oils are not and will separate on standing.

HYDROGENATED OILS. Two of the three disadvantages of vegetable oils for use in ointment bases, i.e., consistency and development of rancidity, apparently are overcome for the most part through the process of hydrogenation. This is true because consistency and development of rancidity are both directly dependent on the degree of unsaturation. The immiscibility with water still remains as a disadvantage.

By hydrogenation under controlled conditions, such oils as cottonseed, soybean, corn oil and castor oil can be converted into white, semisolid, lardlike fats, or into hard, almost brittle, waxes. A completely hydrogenated oil is brittle and waxlike and is not satisfactory for ointment base use unless mixed with a base of a much softer consistency. Similarly, then, an oil hydrogenated to an ointmentlike consistency is not completely hydrogenated and, therefore, contains unsaturated acids or esters. These are subject to oxidation and the development of rancidity, and, therefore, these bases can never reach the stability of petrolatum bases. However, the hydrogenated oils are much more stable than the natural fats and can be used very satisfactorily in prescription work. They have been the subject of much research as to their value as ointment bases, and it is believed that they will be used much more in the future as their value and properties become established more firmly. For a more extensive treatment of these bases, see the articles by Fiero (Bibliography, p. 346). Hydrogenated peanut oil is now used as an ointment base in the *Swiss Pharmacopœia* for ointments of lead iodide, potassium iodide, mercuric iodide and sulfur.

Hydrogenated Sulfated Oils. With the application of the process of sulfonation to hydrogenated oils, it appears that, for the most part, the disadvantages of vegetable fats as ointment bases have been overcome.

The consistency is satisfactory, the development of rancidity is very slow, the miscibility with liquids of an aqueous nature is sufficient for all pharmaceutical as well as most therapeutical needs.

Up to the present, the only sulfated hydrogenated oil recommended for ointment use has been castor oil. This oil, when hydrogenated to an iodine number of less than 10, is still capable of sulfation, because of the presence of the hydroxyl radical. It has the consistency of an ointment, whereas other sulfated oils are liquid. The consistency varies with the extent of sulfation. It has a pH of 6, and this is considered valuable because this is approximately the pH of the skin. It readily incorporates water, alcohol, glycerin, glycol and liquid petrolatum, as well as other bases such as petrolatum, spermaceti and wax. Hydrogenated sulfated castor oil is not subject to rancidity because it is completely hydrogenated and free from unsaturated acids.

The oil, according to Fiero,[17] possesses a peculiar stickiness which is advantageous when it is desired to produce an ointment which will adhere to the skin. For ointments in which a smooth, less adhesive property is desired, this stickiness can be removed by the addition of substances such as petrolatum, fats, glycerin, glycols or water. If the resulting ointment is too soft, the consistency may be increased by the addition of spermaceti, hydrogenated castor oil, stearic acid and other substances.

POLYSORBATE 80, U.S.P., chemically is polyoxyethylene sorbitan mono-oleate and is one of a series of compounds characterized by the partial fatty acid esterification of the anhydrides of sorbitol, with the addition of a polyalkalene oxide molecule through one of the hydroxy groups. This increases its water miscibility and, therefore, influences these products to form oil-in-water emulsions. This group of compounds is known commercially as Tweens. The Spans compounds are just the partial fatty acid esters of sorbitan with the polyalkalene oxide group. This makes these compounds less water-miscible; therefore, they tend to form water-in-oil emulsions.

These compounds are utilized most effectively when formulated on the basis of their hydrophile-lipophile balance values. These values are available in a pamphlet published by the Atlas Powder Co. The HLB value seems to be an expression of the relative simultaneous attraction of an emulsifier for water and for oil. In this way, the oil-loving spans have low HLB values (1.8 to 8.6) while the water-loving Tweens have high values, 9.6 to 16.7. (For table, graphs and methods of calculating these figures, the student is referred to the brochure of the Atlas Powder Co., "Guide to the Use of Atlas Surfactants and Sorbitol in Pharmaceutical Products," 1958. Polyoxyl 40 Stearate, U.S.P., chemically is polyoxyethylene stearate, a reaction product of stearic acid and ethylene oxide. Polyoxyethylene derivatives of fatty acids are known commercially as Myrjs (Atlas Powder Co.).

Like Polysorbate 80, Polyoxyl 40 Stearate is dispersible in water. This water miscibility influences Polyoxyl 40 Stearate and the other polyoxyethylene fatty acid derivatives to form oil-in-water emulsions. Since the polyoxyethylene fatty acid derivatives are nonionic in nature, they possess the advantages characteristic of this type product. They are particularly useful for emulsification in the presence of astringent salts.

Polyoxyl 40 Stearate was used as the emulsifying agent in Hydrophilic Ointment U.S.P. XV. Certain medicaments, phenolic compounds, carboxylic acids, etc., must be incorporated with care in Hydrophilic Ointment U.S.P. XV, since it as been shown[18] that Polyoxyl 40 Stearate interacts with some pharmaceuticals to form soluble and insoluble molecular complexes. This interaction may be evidenced by a marked softening of the finished product. The formula for Hydrophilic Ointment U.S.P. XVI contains sodium lauryl sulfate as the emulsifying agent in place of Polyoxyl 40 Stearate, thereby eliminating this particular difficulty.

Soaps

While there are many soaps that may be used as ointment bases, the sodium, the ammonium and the potassium salts of oleic or stearic acid are used most commonly. The calcium and the magnesium salts are used sometimes, but not so frequently as the above.

Soaps may be used as such (preformed); e.g., as sodium stearate, and satisfactory ointment bases may be prepared by mixing water with the powdered soap (generally in concentrations of from 20 to 30%) after which other ingredients may be incorporated. They also may be added to other bases, e.g., soft soap in compound sulfur ointment.

Soaps may serve as ointment bases or contribute some property to the base and be formed as a reaction product during the preparation. Ammonium oleate, when formed by the reaction between oleic acid and ammonium hydroxide in light liquid petrolatum and wax, yields the class of bases known as petroxolins. Sodium stearate, when formed by the reaction between stearic acid and a sodium base in the presence of oils, water and waxes, yields the vanishing cream bases. Calcium oleate, when formed by mixing olive oil in correct proportions and adding calamine and zinc oxide, yields the frequently used calamine cream. In slightly different proportions, this mixture yields calamine liniment.

Although soaps are used generally in ointment bases for their emulsifying properties, they were introduced initially into the ointment field to increase the penetrating properties of the preparations in use at that time. For instance, it generally is believed that the class of preparations known as oleates (e.g., mercury oleate), in addition to being introduced for their pharmaceutical value, were advocated also because of their supposedly increased penetrating properties.

The class of preparations known as petroxolins (chiefly ammonium oleate) were introduced because of their miscibility with water and their power of penetration. The following statements were used in introducing a petroxolinlike preparation: "The name Penetrol has been adopted as exceedingly appropriate for this line of preparations to which it applies, on account of the readiness with which they penetrate the tissues carrying the remedies combined with them." "Penetroles offer a great advantage to the physician as a means for the administration of menthol, methyl salicylate, camphor, guaiacol, ichthyol and iodine by absorption through the skin."

Petroxolins were introduced into medical and pharmaceutical practice by E. Pearson and Co. of Hamburg, in 1893, under the generic name Vasogen, which was supposed to consist of a mineral oil impregnated in a secret manner with oxygen. Later investigation showed that the basal preparation Vasogen consists of a mixture of mineral oil, oleic acid and ammonia. Both a liquid and a solid form were offered. The solid differed in that it contained petrolatum in place of petrolatum oil. These preparations appeared in various official books under the names of Parogen (*Pharmaceutical Codex*, 1907), Petrolatum Saponatum (*N.F.*, 1906), Petroxolinum (*N.F.*, 1916). Petroxolins, because of their alkalinity, are recommended as the best bases for Peruvian balsam. This applies in a general way to all balsams or resins. When incorporated in petroxolin, they will not separate out as when incorporated in hydrocarbon or fatty bases.*

The emulsifying properties of soaps are exhibited best in the group of ointment bases classed as vanishing creams. Here we have a comparatively small amount of soap emulsifying up to 80 per cent of water, forming o/w emulsions. Vanishing creams have been in use as a cosmetic for many years. However, only comparatively recently, have these preparations been advocated for use as carriers of medicinal agents.

The advantage of these preparations as carriers of medicinal agents supposedly lies in their high water content. This, it is claimed, leads to more rapid release of the medicament from the base, thereby favoring absorption from the skin and more rapid and satisfactory antiseptic action on the surface of the skin. These claims must be discounted to some extent in the light of more recent evidence (see p. 319).

Soaps formed by the reaction between a fatty acid such as stearic acid and an amine such as triethanolamine are widely used as emulsifying agents in modern dermatologic formulations. In contrast with metallic soaps amine soaps are less alkaline; hence, they are less apt to be irritating to injured epidermis. Emulsions prepared with amine soaps are more stable in the presence of divalent and trivalent metal ions than are those prepared with monovalent metal soaps like sodium oleate.

Vanishing creams usually consist of from 10 to 25 per cent stearic acid, a portion of which (15 to 25%) is saponified and from 60 to 80 per cent water. The following formula is basic:

Stearic acid triple pressed 200.0
Potassium hydroxide 14.0
Water 800.0
Perfume q.s.

In the preparation of vanishing creams, one of the important considerations is the choice of saponifying agent. Each possesses properties which in some cases might be considered an advantage or in others a disadvantage.

Carbonates may be used successfully in the hands of the skilled operator but should not be used by the novice. There is always the possibility of entrapping the CO_2 formed by the interaction of stearic acid and the carbonate. Generally, after the cream has thickened and set, it will be found to be impregnated with numerous bubbles.

Sodium and potassium hydroxides are both good and possess no serious disadvantages. Their chief difference lies in the fact that the potassium soap generally produces a softer cream with a higher degree of pearliness than a sodium soap.

Sodium borate produces a very white

---

* For a complete story of the development of these preparations, see N.F. Petroxolins and Parallel Preparations, Pharmaceutical Experiment Station, University of Wisconsin, Circular No. 5, 1918.

cream. However, it is said to have the disadvantage in that creams emulsified with it have a tendency to grain.

Ammonia water has a tendency to discolor creams made with it. It has also been stated that it is difficult to stabilize the perfume in these creams.

The ethanolamines, di- and tri-, have been recommended as alkalis for creams and are used quite frequently. The advantages claimed are their mild alkalinity, the good texture of the resulting creams and their pearly appearance. The di- or triethanolamine may be reacted with the stearic acid in the preparation of the cream, or di- and triethanolamine stearate may be purchased and used as such.

Glycerin in the past has been a constituent of most vanishing creams. Its chief use is as a hygroscopic agent to prevent the creams from drying through evaporation of water.

When included in the formula, it should not exceed 10 per cent, and generally 5 per cent is sufficient. The objection to too much glycerin is its tendency to absorb moisture after application to the skin. More recently, the glycols, the cellosolves and the carbitols have been replacing glycerin in these formulas.

The general methods of manufacture are as follows: The stearic acid is melted on a water bath and heated up to 85° C. If any other oil-miscible or oil-soluble ingredients are included in the formula, these are added to the stearic acid and heated with it. The water, containing the alkali and any other water-soluble ingredients of the formula, is also heated to 85° C. Then the hot alkaline solution is added to the hot oil solution slowly and with stirring. The temperature should be maintained for 10 to 15 minutes to ensure complete reaction between the stearic acid and the alkali. Then the cream is allowed to cool slowly with stirring. However, the stirring must not be so vigorous as to beat air into the product. After standing for 24 hours, the cream is perfumed and run through an ointment mill. If an ointment mill is not available, it is very important that the temperatures mentioned above be adhered to and that the cream cool very slowly to prevent the crystallizing out of the waxes and the free stearic acid. If these directions are adhered to rigidly, a fairly satisfactory cream can be made without the use of a mill.

When vanishing creams are to be used as ointment bases, one must keep in mind that they are essentially soaps and, therefore, are incompatible with acids or acidic substances. Therefore, their use is limited.

Miscellaneous

Cold Creams

Cold creams are emulsions which are made up of oil (40 to 60%), wax or spermaceti (5 to 15%) and water (20 to 25%). A cooling effect is produced by the slow evaporation of water when these creams are applied to the skin, hence the name **cold cream**. These are emulsions of the water-in-oil type and serve as alternates with vanishing creams when a more emollient effect is desired.

Cold creams frequently have been recommended as ointment bases, particularly as vehicles for antiseptic substances such as thymol, chlorthymol and cinnamon oil. *In vitro* testing by the agar cup plate method shows these agents to yield larger zones of inhibition in cold cream bases than in petrolatum bases. The official Rose Water Ointment frequently is prescribed as a base for many substances, such as thymol, ammoniated mercury, Peruvian balsam and sulfur, zinc oxide, etc.

Manufacture. In the past, cold creams generally were prepared with vegetable oils such as almond oil, olive oil or expressed almond oil and waxes, and spermaceti. In later years, however, a large percentage of the vegetable oil has been replaced by mineral oil because of its greater stability, thereby removing the preservation problem which always accompanies the use of vegetable oils. However, vegetable oils and lanolin are added in small quantities when the drying effects of mineral oil are undesirable.

In preparing cold creams, the same general rule applies as that for vanishing creams, i.e., the oil-miscible or soluble ingredients are mixed and heated to approximately 75° C. The water-miscible or soluble ingredients are added together and heated to the same temperature. Then the water solution is added slowly and with stirring to the oil phase. The temperature should be maintained for about 10 minutes and allowed to decrease slowly to prevent crystallizing of the waxes. Stirring should be slow and continuous, using care not to whip air into the product. The following is a typical formula:

Liquid paraffin	570.0
White wax	140.0
Spermaceti	20.0
Lanolin	50.0
Borax	7.0
Water	200.0
Perfume q.s.	

In most cold cream formulas, the emulsifying agent is the soap formed by the reaction between the alkaline sodium borate and the free acids in the beeswax. Therefore, it is essential that the beeswax be pure and that the acid number be high enough (17 to 23) so that enough soap may be formed to prepare a stable emulsion. The amount of alkali used is dependent on the acid number of the beeswax. If the beeswax has an acid number of 17 to 23, the amount of sodium borate necessary to react is generally about 5 to 7 per cent of the amount of beeswax present in the formula.

These creams are soap emulsions and, therefore, like vanishing creams are incompatible with acids or substances having acidic properties. Acids will destroy the soaps and break the emulsion.

Silicon Derivatives

This group is characterized chiefly by the mineral clays associated with fuller's earth and kaolin. The chief representative of this group is bentonite, admitted to the *N.F.* in 1940. The chemical description of bentonite varies slightly with different investigators. It is described generally as an aluminum and magnesium silicon hydrate (H_2O ($Al_2O_3 \cdot 3MgO) \cdot 4SiO_2 \cdot nH_2O$), a 2 per cent solution which possesses a pH of 9.5 to 9.8. Physically, it has been described as a detergent, colloid, suspensoid and emulsoid.

Therapeutically, Fantus has described it as safe for internal and external preparations. It can be used independently as an evacuant and with insoluble substances. It can be used internally in emulsions with cod-liver oil, castor oil and liquid petrolatum, and externally in lotions, creams and pastes, with or without olive oil.

A base of ointment consistency may be prepared from the following formula:

Bentonite	5 Gm.
Water	20 Gm.

Procedure. Add the water slowly to the bentonite in a mortar, triturating until a smooth paste is obtained.

Homogeneous ointments are prepared best by incorporating the medicinal agents into the already formed base. Mixing the insoluble powders with the bentonite powder and then adding water tends to make a grainy product. This base has few incompatibilities, and most medicinal agents may be incorporated in it. The consistency of the base may be controlled easily by increasing or decreasing the amount of water in the formula. The concentrations of medicinal agents employed in these formulas are the same as those ordinarily employed in other ointment bases.

Much work has been carried out to determine the value of bentonite as an ointment base because an aqueous preparation of it possesses almost all of the qualities a dermatologist desires from a nongreasy base. However, on actual clinical use, several disadvantages have been discovered.

A base of bentonite and water only was found to be slightly drying and unstable on standing. Addition of a humectant in amounts up to 10 per cent will retard this action. Ointments prepared from bentonite do not encourage mold growth.

Darlington and Guth[19] report that the pH of bentonite bases may be adjusted by means of buffer mixtures. The *in vitro* activity of ammoniated mercury was enhanced by incorporation in acid-buffered bentonite bases.

Barr and Guth[20] have prepared 6 bentonite bases using 5 cation saturated bentonites (Na, K, Ca, Mg and H bentonites) and Volclay bentonite (which contains all 5 cations) as major components of the bases. Anti-infective ointments were then prepared using these various bentonite bases as vehicles. These ointments showed greater antibacterial activity, *in vitro*, than their respective *U.S.P.* and *N.F.* ointments. Sulfathiazole, phenol and ammoniated mercury showed greater activity when incorporated in a H bentonite base than when these drugs were incorporated into the other bentonite bases.

Colloidal Magnesium Aluminum Silicate (Veegum)* is an inorganic emulsifier, thickener, suspending agent and film former. It is dispersed readily in water by adding it to the water slowly with continuous agitation. Usually 1 to 4 per cent of Veegum is employed to stabilize emulsions and suspend insoluble material. However, firm preparations of ointment consistency can be prepared, using 10 per cent Veegum. The viscosity of a Veegum Dispersion containing more than 3 per cent solids is decreased by simple agitation. The apparent viscosity increases again when the material is allowed to remain at rest. This increase and decrease in viscosity is known as *thixotropy*.

In addition to being compatible over a wide pH range (1 to 11), Veegum dispersions are compatible with large amounts of most organic solvents.

Attapulgite is a hydrous magnesium aluminum silicate obtained from Attapulgus, Georgia, as well as from other areas. The magnesium content of attapulgite is higher than that of bentonite.

Activated attapulgite, having a higher adsorptive capacity than attapulgite, is prepared by heat-treating attapulgite.

Little work has been reported on the use of activated attapulgite as a suspending agent or ointment base constituent. Aqueous suspensions of activated attapulgite vary in viscosity and sedimentation rate, depending on the method of preparation. Suspensions may be prepared by high-speed stirring, pregelling, presoaking, and a combination of pregelling and presoaking, at room temperature and at elevated temperatures.†

* R. T. Vanderbilt Co.
† Pharmasorb bulletin, Minerals & Chemicals Corp. of America.

Silica Gel. In 1937, Peronnet and Gene[21] reported that silica gel, when mixed with glycerin, possessed certain characteristics which might be used in the manufacture of certain ointments which are official in the *French Pharmacopœia*. Prout, Eddleman and Harris[22] investigated the value of such a base as a carrier for germicidal substances. They found that zinc oxide, boric acid, phenol and ammoniated mercury in a silica gel–glycerin base all had greater zones of inhibition than the *U.S.P.* ointments of these same substances.

Prout and Harris[23] also reported on the emulsifying properties of silica gel and formulated the following base:

Hydrogel	45.00
Hydrous wool fat	5.00
Liquid petrolatum	15.00
White petrolatum q.s.	
To make	100.00

Procedure. Mix the hydrous wool fat with the liquid petrolatum in a mortar and thoroughly levigate the hydrogel (silica gel) with this mixture. Finally, add the white petrolatum and continue the trituration until a creamlike emulsion is produced.

Silicones. Silicones are a series of synthetic polymers in which the basic structure is not carbon but an alternate chain of silicon and oxygen atoms (e.g., —O—Si—O—Si—). Each silicon atom has one or more organic groups, generally a methyl or a phenyl group, attached to it.

The silicone fluids are used in medicine and pharmacy. They are clear, sparkling, oily liquids which vary in viscosity from 0.65 to 1,000,000 centistokes. Water repellency is their outstanding feature, and this property, combined with their resistance to change due to heat or oxidation, makes them very useful in preparations for the management of dermatologic disorders in which protection from moisture is indicated. Lesser[24] has published a review of the applications of the silicones in pharmacy and medicine.

Rochow[25] has reported that the silicone fluids are practically inert physiologically and appear to be essentially nontoxic.

Plein and Plein[26] have prepared a number of silicone ointment bases by modifying official and other recognized ointment formulas. Silicone Gibson Base represents such a formula.

SILICONE GIBSON BASE

Cetyl alcohol	15.0
Sodium lauryl sulfate	1.0
D.C 200,* 1,000 cts.	40.0
Purified water	43.0
Methyl paraben	0.25
Propyl paraben	0.15

Physical Classification

Oleaginous and Hydrocarbon Bases

These are discussed in the sections headed Hydrocarbons, Natural Triglycerides and Vegetable Oils.

Absorption Bases

Absorption bases are usually anhydrous bases which have the property of absorbing several times their weight of water, forming emulsions. The word absorption does not describe the action of these bases when applied to the skin.

Absorption bases vary in their composition, but, for the greater part, they are mixtures of cyclic alcohols (cholesterol and cholesterol alcohols) with petrolatum.

Absorption Base†

Cholesterin	30.0
Cottonseed oil	30.0
White petrolatum	940.0

Absorption bases were developed because it was desirable to have a product to which water or an aqueous solution of medicinal substances could be added easily. They generally have a high degree of compatibility toward the majority of medicaments used topically. As a class, they are relatively heat-stable and can be utilized in their anhydrous form or emulsified with the addition of water. However, absorption bases still possess the undesirable property of greasiness, but they are more readily removable from the skin than the oleaginous bases.

---

* Dow Corning dimethylsiloxane polymer.
† From the Formulary of the University of Iowa Hospitals.

Emulsion Bases

Bases coming under this classification are also known as washable ointment bases. Washable as used here refers to the ease with which these bases can be removed from the skin and the clothing with water. This is one of the outstanding advantages of these bases.

In general, the formula for washable ointment bases contains an aqueous phase, an emulsifying agent and an oleaginous phase. The water phase may vary from 10 to 80 per cent of the total base. Most bases of this group will permit the incorporation of additional water without a loss of ointment consistency.

Many emulsion bases contain cetyl and/or stearyl alcohol. These fatty alcohols add stability to the emulsion, impart a smooth feel to the skin and assist in water retention of emulsion bases. Stearyl alcohol, in particular, causes the greatest potentiation of the water number of petrolatum.[27] The water number[28] is defined as the largest amount of water which 100 Gm. of an ointment base will hold at normal temperature.

The availability of a number of newer organic compounds, the surface-active agents, has given a much greater degree of flexibility to ointment formulation, particularly of emulsion bases. In the field of surface-active agents which perform such functions as wetting, emulsifying, dispersing and solubilizing agents, we have a multiple choice. Surface-active agents may be ionic or nonionic. The ionic types are either anionic or cationic, depending on whether the characteristically surface-active portion of the compound lies in the anion or the cation. For example, in soap the anion (oleate) is the effective portion of the molecule; therefore, soap is classified as anionic.

Nonionic surfactants depend chiefly on hydroxyl groups and ether linkages (polyhydric alcohol anhydrides and polyoxyethylene chains) to create the hydrophilic action. Polysorbate 80* and Polyoxyl 40 Stearate† official in the U.S.P. represent such surface-active agents.

---

* Tween 80, a product of Atlas Powder Co.
† Myrj 52, a product of Atlas Powder Co.

Generally, nonionic agents may be used more widely in ointment formulation. Ionic surface-active agents exhibit a particle charge, hence are sensitive to the presence of other ions. Thus, soaps (anionic agents) are ineffective in hard water and in electrolytes. Cationic agents, on the other hand, are not stable in the presence of anionic agents or soap. Since nonionic agents do not ionize, they are comparatively insensitive to hard water, electrolytes and ionic surface-active agents. Furthermore, nonionic surfactants are generally less toxic and less irritating than ionic agents.

Some of the incompatibilities observed when using Hydrophilic Ointment U.S.P. XV as a vehicle (softening, separation, etc.) may be due to the reported[18] interaction between Polyoxyl 40 Stearate and some pharmaceuticals to form soluble and insoluble complexes. Similar reactions occur with other polyoxyethylene-type surface-active agents. (See p. 328).

There are several factors which must be considered in the preparation of emulsion bases. The quality and the quantity of ingredients, the order of mixing, the speed and the type of mixing, the temperature at which the emulsion is made, the choice of the emulsifier—all are important. The usual method of preparation involves melting the greaselike materials and waxes in one container, heating the water with the water-soluble components in another container and mixing both at the same temperature, 75° C. Stirring is continued until a smooth cream results.

Water-Soluble Bases

Water-soluble ointment bases include those bases prepared from polyethylene glycol polymers known as carbowax compounds. The name "carbowax" is applied to those compounds having a molecular weight above 1,000. They are water-soluble, nonvolatile, unctuous compounds. They do not hydrolyze or deteriorate nor will they support mold growth.*

Carbowax 1,000, 1,500, 1,540, 4,000 and 6,000 are of interest in ointment formulation. Carbowax 1,000 is a soft, unctuous compound while carbowax 1,500 is a soft waxy solid similar in consistency to petrolatum. Carbowaxes 4,000 and 6,000 are hard, translucent solids with melting points of 50° to 55° and 58° to 62°, respectively. They are most useful as components of ointment bases, for, in addition to the general property of being emulsifying and dispersing agents, they also add to the consistency of the base. Carbowax compounds having molecular weights below 1,000 are usually liquids.

Carbowax 1,500 or 1,540, as such, can be used as a vehicle for the topical application of medicinal substances. However, it is usually desirable to blend a higher molecular weight compound with one of the lower molecular weight (200 to 600) liquid polyethylene glycols for ointment formulation.

P.E.G. Ointment, U.S.P. XVI

Polyethylene glycol 4,000 .... 400.0
Polyethylene glycol 400 .... 600.0

The high degree of solubility of this base precludes the addition of aqueous solutions much in excess of 5 per cent of the total formula. The following formula is recommended when larger amounts of aqueous or alcoholic preparations are to be incorporated:

Polyethylene glycol 4,000 .... 47.5
Polyethylene glycol 400 .... 47.5
Cetyl alcohol 5.0

This base is also a good vehicle for the incorporation of salicylic acid and its salts, the cetyl alcohol tending to inhibit the solubilizing effect of the salicylates on polyethylene glycol mixtures.

McClelland and Bateman[29] have reported that the carbowax compounds are no more irritating to the skin than lanolin or petrolatum. Smyth, Carpenter and Weil[30] have reported that the acute oral and dermal toxicity and irritating powers of polyethylene glycols are very low. They report that, in human patch tests, the carbowax compounds were no more irritating than lanolin, petrolatum, simple cerate and simple ointment.

PREPARATION

Since ointments are applied primarily to irritated areas, it is an unbreakable rule

---

* Carbide and Carbon Corp.: "Carbowax" Compounds and Polethylene Glycols, 1946.

that these preparations must not contain granular or gritty particles which might cause further irritation.

It has been shown also that the germicidal activity of many of our antiseptic substances is enhanced greatly by reducing the particle size below that which is generally commercially available.

Therefore, all technics in the preparation of ointments should be carried out with the express purpose of having the substances incorporated therein, in the finest state of subdivision it is possible to achieve.

In compounding ointments, the following rules should be observed:

1. Insoluble substances to be incorporated in ointment bases should always be in the impalpable powder form.

2. Insoluble substances are best incorporated when first levigated with a liquid and then incorporated into the base.

3. Substances to be incorporated into ointments should be dissolved before incorporation when possible.

When substances incorporated into ointment bases must be reduced to a fine state of subdivision, three methods are generally available: (1) use of an ointment slab and spatula or muller, (2) use of the mortar and pestle, (3) use of an ointment mill.

These methods may or may not involve fusion, depending on the nature of the medicament to be incorporated into the base and the base itself. Fusion is generally necessary where resins and waxes are included in the formula. In preparing ointments by fusion, care must be taken not to char the ingredients. The use of the direct flame is not necessary as the temperature of the water bath is sufficient to melt any of the various bases. The substance having the highest melting point is melted first, and so on, until all of the substances have been added. The melted base may be strained if necessary and it must be stirred until congealed to prevent separation and the crystallizing out of the higher melting point ingredients.

Ointment Slab. The usual technic consists of rubbing the powder with a small amount of base until thoroughly distributed in a finely subdivided state, then incorporating this concentrated ointment into the remainder of the base. However, better results are obtained when the powder is first made into a paste with either a vegetable or a mineral oil and then incorporated into the base. Sometimes water may be used to advantage in this way and then the water taken up in a hydrophilic base.

A stainless-steel spatula with a long,

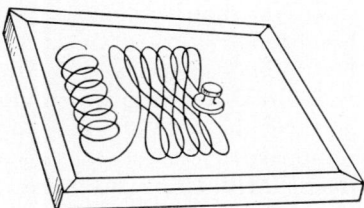

Fig. 151. Slab and muller.

broad flexible blade is essential to the preparation of good ointments. The use of small, less flexible blades does not give one either the pressure or the surface area to do a good job with any quantity of ointment. Where danger of chemical reaction exists, as with iodine and mercury salts, a hard rubber spatula should be used.

The use of a muller in reducing the size of particles is sometimes advantageous. More pressure can be exerted; therefore, more friction is developed which will aid in reducing particle size. The ground-glass surface (slightly roughened) of the muller, when rubbed in a figure-eight motion across the roughened surface of the ointment slab, provides an excellent combination for reducing the size of gritty particles. The ideal technic then would be to: (1) make a paste of the powders with oil or water, (2) rub to a fine particle size with the aid of a muller, (3) incorporate this paste in the base with the aid of a spatula.

Mortar and Pestle. It is the general consensus that the mortar and pestle should be used when large quantities of liquid are to be incorporated into a base or when exceptionally large quantities of ointment are to be made. The use of mortar and pestle is considered not as efficient as the muller or the spatula in reducing the size of particles incorporated in or protected by fat because of the small surface area under levigation at any one time. Then, too, the particles have a tendency to "ride" out from under the pestle, and the grinding effect is limited. Nevertheless, according to experiments by L. Rosenthaler,[31] the products obtained in either way differ very slightly as to their homogeneity, provided that the same accuracy has been employed. In these same experiments, he found that 5 minutes of actual rubbing time was necessary to produce homogeneity in products prepared by either method. However, he does not give any information as to which method is most effective in the breaking down of agglomerate particles.

Ointment Mill. The ointment mill is convenient and ideal for quantities of a pound or more.

When making ointments on a larger scale, generally the powders are sifted into the melted base and stirred slowly until congealed. Then this mixture is placed in the ointment mill and run through the mill until smooth and free from particles. Some ointments such as ammoniated mercury require several millings. In some cases, a concentrated mixture of the base and the powder is run through the mill several times and then mixed with the remainder of the base.

There are two types of ointment mills, one known as the "paint mill" type, which consists essentially of a steel disk revolving on a stationary steel surface, the second generally known as the three-roller ink mill. In this machine, 3 rollers operate at different speeds. The roller having the highest speed takes the ointment off the slower roller, and, since the speed of all 3 rollers is different, a shearing action, which smooths out the ointment, is secured.

However, it should be stated here that the use of the muller and slab is just as efficient for small quantities of ointment as the ointment mill is for large quantities of ointment.

PACKAGING, STORAGE AND LABELING

Ointments should be stored in tightly stoppered glass or porcelain jars and in a cool place. This will prevent separation as

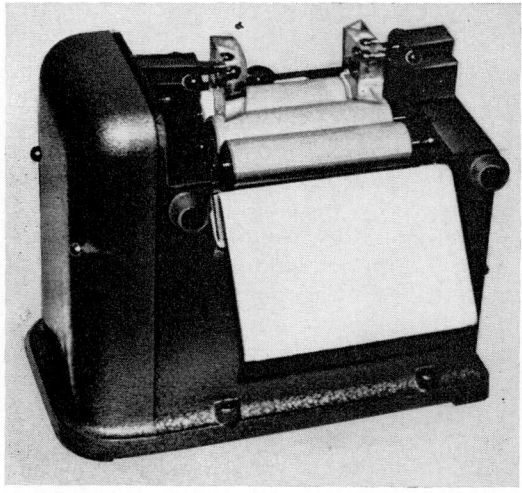

FIG. 152. Type "SMR" 3-roller mill (research and pharmacy model). (Chemical and Pharmaceutical Industry Co., Inc., New York.)

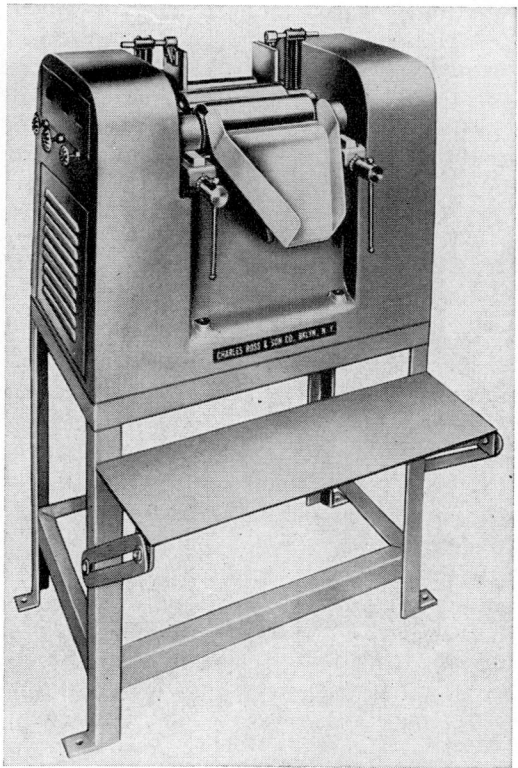

FIG. 153. Ross water-cooled laboratory 3-roller mill.

well as retard the development of rancidity. For dispensing in small quantities in prescription or over-the-counter work, collapsible tubes are the containers of choice. These containers reduce oxidation to a minimum and prevent the loss of water, particularly in those ointments containing large quantities of it, and thus are great aids in prolonging the stability of a preparation. They are also more sanitary, as the ointment is not contaminated by the applicant's fingers as is the case in removing ointments from jars.

One difficulty encountered in the use of collapsible tubes is the labeling of the tubes. If the label is to be attached, the tube may be dipped in compound benzoin tincture or in a regular lacquer and allowed to dry. It is desirable to use the labels in strip form so as to encircle the tube completely, thus helping prevent their coming off. Labels should be attached at the very top of the tube so that they will not be destroyed until the tube is almost empty. At best, labels are not very satisfactory, as the tube is likely to be completely rolled

TABLE 22. OINTMENTS OF THE U.S.P.

Ointment	Percentage of Active Ingredient	Base
Ammoniated Mercury	Ammoniated Mercury 5%	Liquid Petrolatum, White Ointment
Ammoniated Mercury, Ophthalmic	Ammoniated Mercury 3%	Liquid Petrolatum, White Ointment
Anthralin	Anthralin 0.1 to 1.0%	
Bacitracin	500 units/Gm.	Liquid Petrolatum, White Petrolatum
Benzoic and Salicylic Acid	Benzoic Acid 6% Salicylic Acid 3%	Polyethylene Glycol Ointment
Chloramphenicol, Ophthalmic	Chloramphenicol 1 mg./Gm.	
Chrysarobin	Chrysarobin 6%	Yellow Ointment
Coal Tar	Coal Tar 1%	Zinc Oxide Paste, Polysorbate 80
Dibucaine, Ophthalmic	Dibucaine 0.5%	
Epinephrine Bitartrate, Ophthalmic	Epinephrine Bitartrate 1%	Hydrophilic Petrolatum
Hydrocortisone	Hydrocortisone 1%	
Hydrophilic		Methylparaben, Propylparaben. Sodium lauryl Sulfate, Propylene Glycol, Stearyl Alcohol, White Petrolatum, Water
* Hydrophilic Petrolatum		Cholesterol, Stearyl Alcohol, White Wax, White Petrolatum
Iodochlorhydroxyquin	Iodochlorhydroxyquin 3%	
Isoflurophate, Ophthalmic	Isoflurophate 0.0250%	
Neomycin Sulfate	3.5 mg./Gm.	
Nystatin	Nystatin 100,000 units/Gm.	
Petrolatum Rose Water		Spermaceti, White Wax, Liquid Petrolatum, Sodium Borate, Rose Water, Purified Water and Rose Oil
Piperocaine Hydrochloride, Ophthalmic	Piperocaine HCl 4%	Petrolatum
Polyethylene Glycol		Polyethylene Glycol 4,000 and 400
Polymyxin B Sulfate	17,000 units/Gm.	
Prednisolone	Prednisolone 0.50%	
Sulfacetamide Sodium, Ophthalmic	Sulfacetamide Sodium 10%	
Sulfisoxazole Diethanolamine, Ophthalmic	Sulfisoxazole 4%	
Sulfur	Precipitated Sulfur 10%	Liquid Petrolatum, White Ointment
Tetracaine, Ophthalmic	Tetracaine 0.5%	White Petrolatum
White		White Wax, White Petrolatum
Zinc Oxide	Zinc Oxide 20%	Liquid Petrolatum, White Ointment

* Not official as an ointment but classified here for convenience.

Table 23. Ointments of the N.F.

Ointment	Percentage of Active Ingredient	Base
Belladonna	Pilular Extract of Belladonna 10%	Yellow Ointment
Boric Acid	Boric Acid 10%	Liquid Petrolatum, White Ointment
Calamine	Calamine 17%	Yellow Wax, Wool Fat, Petrolatum
Dimethisoquin Hydrochloride		
Ethyl Aminobenzoate	Ethyl Aminobenzoate 5%	White Ointment
Ichthammol	Ichthammol 10%	Wool Fat, Petrolatum
Menthol, Compound	Menthol 10%, Methyl Salicylate 10%	White Wax, Hydrous Wool Fat
Mercurial, Mild	Mercury 10%	White Ointment
Mercuric Oxide, Yellow	Yellow Mercuric Oxide 1%	Liquid Petrolatum, White Ointment
Mercurous Chloride, Mild	Mild Mercurous Chloride 30%	Hydrous Wool Fat, White Petrolatum
Mercury Bichloride, Ophthalmic	Mercury Bichloride 0.03%	White Petrolatum
Monobenzone	Monobenzone 20%	
Nitrofurazone	Nitrofurazone 0.2%	Polyethylene Glycols 1540, 3000, and 300
Penicillin		
Pine Tar	Pine Tar 50%	Yellow Wax, Yellow Ointment
Resorcinol, Compound	Resorcinol 6%, Zinc Oxide 6%, Bismuth Subnitrate 6%, Rectified Birch Tar Oil 6%	Yellow Wax, Petrolatum, Wool Fat, Glycerin
Rose Water		Spermaceti, White Wax, Expressed Almond Oil, or Persic Oil, Sodium Borate, Purified Water, Rose Oil
Thimerosal	Thimerosal 0.1%	Purified Water, Cholesterol, Wool Fat, White Wax, Stearyl Alcohol, White Petrolatum
Undecylenic Acid, Compound	Undecylenic Acid 5%, Zinc Undecylenate 20%	Polyethylene Glycol Ointment
Yellow		Yellow Wax, Petrolatum

upon itself as the last of the ointment is used, and the label soiled or destroyed. Many pharmacists use a pasteboard box (powder box) to hold the tube and carry the label, while the tube itself is stamped in the tin with the prescription number. This will permit the identification of the prescription if the box is lost.

COMMENTS ON SOME U.S.P. AND N.F. OINTMENTS

Chrysarobin Ointment, U.S.P. Chrysarobin Ointment is prepared by first dissolving (triturating) the chrysarobin in the chloroform and then adding the melted yellow ointment slowly with trituration until congealed.

Chrysarobin is extremely irritating to mucous membranes, and particular care must be observed not to get it into the eyes. Chrysarobin and its preparations are classified as dangerous drugs and must be dispensed with prescribed warning statements.

Hydrophilic Ointment, U.S.P. This contains:

Methylparaben	0.25
Propylparaben	0.15
Sodium Lauryl Sulfate	10.0
Propylene glycol	120.0
Stearyl alcohol	250.0
White petrolatum	250.0
Water	370.0
To make about	1,000 Gm.

Directions. The petrolatum and the stearyl alcohol are heated to 75° C., and the other ingredients are dissolved in the water which also is heated to 75° C. These are then mixed and stirred slowly until congealed.

Hydrophilic Ointment is a useful washable ointment base and can be used in place of cold creams and vanishing creams for this purpose. It is compatible with acid or alkali and similarly with most pharmaceutical substances, such as coal tar, Peruvian balsam, ichthyol, naftalan, etc.

Sodium Lauryl Sulfate serves as the emulsifier in Hydrophilic Ointment, while the stearyl alcohol acts as an adjuvant emulsifier and adds to the physical property of hardness.

Antibiotic Ointments. Penicillin Ointment was deleted from *U.S.P. XV* (though admitted to *N.F. X* and continued in *N.F. XI*) since it was found that sensitization occurs in some instances when penicillin is used topically. If penicillin ointment has to be prepared extemporaneously, anhydrous ointment bases should be used wherever possible: first, because water greatly shortens the length of time in which the ointment will remain active, even under refrigeration, and secondly, because of the great water solubility of penicillin it is removed by the tissue fluids very rapidly, making it difficult to maintain a high concentration locally when using a water base. White or yellow petrolatum or Aquaphor are suitable bases for penicillin. If it is necessary to use a hydrous base, the ointment should be stored at 15° C.

Sterilization of these greasy bases must be carried out by using dry heat at 150° to 160° C. for 1 hour. Autoclaving (steam heat) will not accomplish sterilization of oily substances.

It generally is agreed that other antibiotics such as chlortetracycline, chloramphenicol, oxytetracycline and bacitracin are best prepared in anhydrous oleaginous bases for greatest stability at room temperature. If it is desired to dispense them in emulsion type or water-soluble bases, the ointments should be refrigerated. Exceptions to this are neomycin, tyrothricin and polymyxin B, which are stable at room temperature in ointment bases of the water-miscible, greasy and vanishing-cream type. A useful anhydrous oleaginous base for the water-unstable antibiotics is:

Antibiotic	—
Liquid petrolatum	65.0
White petrolatum	925.0
To make about	1,000.0 Gm.

Coal Tar Ointment, U.S.P. The formula for Coal Tar Ointment in *U.S.P. XVI* contains a surface-active agent, Polysorbate 80, which serves a dual purpose. It not only functions as a dispersing agent but also aids in the removal of the ointment from the skin. The coal tar should always be mixed with the Polysorbate 80 before incorporating it into the zinc oxide paste. The *U.S.P. XVI* Coal Tar Ointment contains 1 per cent of coal tar, which is a reduction from the formula offered in the *U.S.P. XV*, which contained 3 per cent coal tar.

Stronger Mercurial Ointment, N.F. X This is prepared by triturating the mercury with the oleate of mercury in a warm mortar, until the mercury is finely dispersed (extinguished) in the oleate. A finely dispersed mercury is accomplished most easily by light and rapid trituration, which coats the mercury globules with a thin film of the oleate and, thereby, prevents their coalescence. Long trituration under heavy pressure is to be avoided, for this will cause the mercury to coalesce again after dispersion. DeKay and Kessler[32] state that the following conditions are necessary for rapid dispersion of mercury by trituration: (1) a protective film must be formed around each globule of mercury, (2) the dispersing mixture must be of the correct consistency or viscosity, (3) the dispersing mixture must be wetted by the mercury.

Stronger Mercurial Ointment, applied by rubbing on the skin, is one of the best means of administering mercury for antisyphilitic purposes. Systemic absorption is desired from the application of this ointment; therefore, great care should be taken to see that the mercury is finely dispersed. If the ointment is prescribed in divided doses, each dose should be weighed and wrapped in waxed paper.

Tannic Acid Ointment, N.F. X. This is prepared by dissolving the tannic acid in glycerin with the aid of gentle heat. Sodium sulfite, 0.2 per cent, is also added to prevent any ions that might be present from discoloring the ointment through the formation of black iron tannate.

Ichthammol Ointment, N.F. XI. This is pared by incorporating 10 per cent of ichthammol with wool fat and yellow petrolatum. Ichthammol becomes granular on heating so that fusion cannot be used in the preparation of ointments containing it.

Iodine Ointment, N.F. X. Approximately 4 per cent iodine is contained in Iodine Ointment. Potassium iodide is used to render the iodine soluble in the glycerin. Then this mixture is added to the ointment base. The use of iron or steel utensils should be avoided during the preparation of this ointment.

Stainless Iodine Ointment, N.F. IX. Stainless Iodine Ointment contains 5 per cent of iodine in combination with oleic acid. The iodine is dissolved in the oleic acid with the aid of heat. Metallic utensils must not be used during the manufacture because of the chemical reactivity of the iodine.

Alkaline Sulfur Ointment, N.F. VIII. Alkaline Sulfur Ointment contains 20 per cent of sublimed sulfur. This is rubbed into a paste with the potassium carbonate and the water; this mixture is incorporated with wool fat and the whole incorporated into the base.

Sulfur preparations often contain alkaline agents to increase the penetrability of the sulfur into the membranes of the parasite.

CERATES

HISTORY

The term "cerates" for a class of unctuous preparations is not new in ointment terminology. For the most part it has been associated with preparations containing high percentages of wax, hence the name cerate (from Latin *cera,* wax). However, there are several cases where the term apparently is used as synonymous with ointment.

In the early translations of the Greek text of Galen into Latin, the title for his formula of an ointment consisting of white wax, rose oil and some water is given as "Ceratum Infrigidans." It is this title under which we find the same preparation in the *Dispensatorium Valerii Cordi* (1546) as the first formula within a special class named "Cerota," which class is placed quite adequately between the still stiffer "Emplastra" and the softer "Unguenta." However, in the *Pharmacopœia Augustana* (1564), this preparation appears as "Unguentum Infrigidans Galeni." This tendency to treat all unctuous preparations as ointments is shown in the last two revisions of the *British Pharmacopœia*, in which the several cerates still retained were transferred to the class of ointments. The *U.S.P.* and the *N.F.*, with the 13th revision and the 9th edition, respectively, deleted all cerate preparations, and, as a result, the class is no longer official.

USE

Cerates are fatty preparations resembling ointments, but of a firmer consistency and of a higher melting point, because of their high wax content. They should be of such consistency as to be spread easily without previous melting on muslin or other cloth, and yet not melt through the cloth when applied to the skin.

Cerates are intended to act locally, chiefly as a protective application for irritated or raw surfaces. They are used generally as vehicles for substances which exert a protective, cooling, astringent or stimulating action, such as rosin, lead subacetate, cantharides and turpentine. Fantus states, "Their importance is derived chiefly from the fact that they form a good dressing for ulcers, chiefly by keeping dressings from sticking to the raw surface, the importance of which may be appreciated when it is realized that each time a dressing that sticks is pulled off, not only does the patient suffer unnecessary pain, but healing is also disturbed."

PREPARATION

The similarity of cerates to ointments makes what has been said regarding the preparation of ointments in which fusion is used apply also to the preparation of cerates. Moreover, the high wax content of these preparations makes it even more essential that the "stirring until congealed" be applied here to prevent the crystallizing out of the waxes with higher melting points.

The cerate formulas are divided in their use of white wax and yellow wax. It seems to be the general consensus that yellow wax is not as subject to rancidity as white wax, and therefore is to be preferred for these preparations. However, yellow wax generally contains mechanical impurities; therefore, the melted mixture always should be strained through a cloth before the medicinal substances are incorporated.

The firm consistency of cerates is not adapted to the mechanical admixture of powdered substances as such. The cerate should always be melted and then the powders finely subdivided therein.

STORAGE AND PACKAGING

Cerates should be preserved in tightly stoppered glass jars at a temperature below 40° C. These preparations are subject to rancidity; therefore, freshly made preparations should not be placed in jars which still contain some of the old cerate. Rancid preparations should never be used. Cerates are best dispensed in ointment jars, because their consistency is too firm to be easily extruded from collapsible tubes. The danger of contamination is not present here, because the cerate is generally spread on the muslin cloth with a knife which does not come into contact with the infected or irritated surface.

Cantharides Cerate. Cantharides Cerate is also known as Blistering Cerate, because of its vesicant activity. Care must be exercised when either cantharides or the cerate is handled so as not to let it come into contact with the skin. Blistering usually can be avoided by washing the area immediately with warm soapsuds.

Cantharidin, the active principle of cantharides, is first extracted by maceration with turpentine oil and glacial acetic acid. Then the macerated mixture is mixed with the previously fused and strained base, and the whole is heated on a water bath until it has been reduced to a specified weight. This assures complete solution of the cantharidin in the fatty base.

In addition to its use as a blistering agent, it is also used in the preparation of Emplastrum Cantharidin.

PASTES

HISTORY

The introduction of the use of so-called pastes into the dermatologic field is comparatively recent when one thinks in terms of the length of time ointments and cerates have been in use. This class or group of preparations was introduced by the noted dermatologists Unna and Lassar about 1900. Up to that time, the term "paste" (Latin, *pasta;* French, *pata*) was used exclusively for internal preparations, the majority of which were of gumlike consistency —e.g., Pasta Althaeae and Pasta Glycyrrhizae. The increase in the popularity of pastes is clearly indicated by Caspari when he says, "Ointments and Cerates have been largely superseded, especially in Europe, by dermatologic pastes and glycerogelatins."

USE

The term "paste" for external medicaments, like the term "ointment," seems to be an all-inclusive term. It has been applied to 2 entirely different types of preparations: (1) to ointmentlike mixtures of starch, zinc oxide or calcium carbonate with light liquid petrolatum, white petrolatum, wool

TABLE 24. UNOFFICIAL CERATES

CERATE	PERCENTAGE OF ACTIVE INGREDIENT	BASE
Cerate, N.F. VIII		White Wax, Benzoinated Lard
Rosin, N.F. VIII	Rosin 35%	Yellow Wax, Lard
Compound Rosin, N.F. VIII	Rosin 23%, Turpentine 12%	Yellow Wax, Prepared Suet, Linseed Oil
Camphor, N.F. V	Camphor Liniment 10%	White Wax, White Petrolatum, Benzoinated Lard
Cantharides, N.F. VIII	Cantharides 35%, Turpentine Oil 15%, Rosin 17.5%	Yellow Wax, Benzoinated Lard
Lead Subacetate, N.F. VIII	Lead Subacetate Solution 20%, Camphor 0.2%	Wool Fat, White Petrolatum

fat, white wax, benzoinated lard and other fats which are medicated with salicylic acid, resorcinol, bismuth subnitrate, acetylsalicylic acid, eugenol and Peruvian balsam, and (2) to jellies containing glycerin with starch, glycerogelatins or other water-soluble gels, such as pectin and tragacanth.

The fatty "pastes" contain as much as 50 per cent of powder with soft fat, or as much as 70 per cent of powder with less viscous oils as the vehicle. Pastes containing these large amounts of powder differ from ointments by having a slight drying action, due to adsorption or capillarity. Medicaments incorporated in these bases are absorbed less readily than from ointments and, therefore, have a more superficial action, but they give better protection. They are used chiefly as vehicles for astringent and antiseptic agents.

Thus Fantus states, "Pastes are especially indicated when it is intended that a therapeutic effect shall be exerted chiefly on the diseased epithelium (epidermatic action)."

Pastes are not suitable for application to hairy parts like the scalp, as they will form a densely matted mass.

The water-soluble gels, such as glycerin with starch and pectins, are useful when fatty bases are undesirable. According to Fantus,[33] fatty preparations are unsuited for application to wet or moist surfaces. He states, "Whenever an ointment does not stick to the site of application it not only does no good, but is liable to do harm by causing the retention of secretion, which forms a culture medium, and thus favors the proliferation of micro-organisms and the consequent irritation of the surface by their poisonous products. In conditions that border on the prohibitive type, pastes, by reason of their slight drying action, may still be useful."

The water-soluble gels of about the consistency of ointments are advantageous when applied to moist surfaces, because of the miscibility with the aqueous fluids. Also, they have the advantage of cleanliness and easy removal from the skin.

Pectin and tragacanth pastes were introduced by Fantus and Dyniewicz[34] for the treatment of ulcers and bedsores. The cavity is first filled with the paste, then is covered with a piece of waterproof cellophane considerably larger than the sore. Adhesive plaster is used to fasten down the edges of the cellophane.

The pastes are made of different consistencies, and to standardize the viscosity a "flow time" test has been devised. The test is carried out by placing 60 ml. of the preparation in square-cornered bottles of 4-ounce capacity. Then the bottles are placed on their sides, and the time necessary for the jelly to assume a horizontal position is noted. Jellies thin enough to assume a horizontal position in 1 hour are known as "horizontal jellies." Those whose surfaces have moved to some extent are classified according to the angle of deviation from the vertical—e.g., 50° in 1 hour. Because the viscosity produced by different lots of pectin and tragacanth may vary, the above test should be applied to a small quantity of paste before large batches are made.

Pastes prepared with glycerogelatin as the base soften at body temperature and may be applied after softening by warming. When harder glycerogelatin pastes are prescribed, generally the jar is placed in warm water to melt the paste, which is then painted on with a brush.

PREPARATION

For all practical purposes, the oily or fatty pastes containing insoluble powder are prepared in the same manner as ointments. The same rules apply to these preparations. Therefore, they do not warrant individual consideration and are merely listed.

The water-soluble gels, such as pectin and tragacanth, generally are prepared by first wetting the pectin or the tragacanth with a small amount of glycerin and then adding a sufficient quantity of hot water. Starch and glycerin are simply mixed and heated together, while starch "paste" is made by mixing starch with cold water and then adding this to boiling water with stirring. For practical purposes, the method of compounding prescribed in *N.F. IX* will serve as a guide in the extemporaneous preparation of this type of preparation.

TABLE 25. PASTES OF THE U.S.P.

PASTE	PERCENTAGE OF ACTIVE INGREDIENT	BASE
Aluminum	Aluminum 10%	Zinc Oxide
Zinc Oxide	Zinc Oxide 25%, Starch 25%	White Petrolatum

TABLE 26. PASTES OF N.F. XI AND UNOFFICIAL PASTES

PASTE	PERCENTAGE OF ACTIVE CONSTITUENT	BASE
Zinc Oxide with Salicylic Acid, N.F. XI	Salicylic Acid 2%	Paste of Zinc Oxide
Pectin, N.F. IX		Pectin, Glycerin, Benzoic Acid, Ringer's Solution
Pectin, Thin, N.F. IX		Pectin, Glycerin, Benzoic Acid, Ringer's Solution
Zinc Oxide, Hard, N.F. IX	Zinc Oxide 25%, Purified Siliceous Earth 5%	Benzoinated Lard
Zinc Oxide, Soft, N.F. IX	Zinc Oxide 25%, Precipitated Calcium Carbonate 25%	Oleic Acid, Linseed Oil, Solution Calc. Hydroxide

STORAGE AND PACKAGING

The oily and the fatty pastes generally are preserved best in tightly stoppered glass or porcelain jars. These should be clean, and new preparations should not be placed in jars containing any of the old preparation. This will help retard rancidity, particularly in those pastes containing linseed oil or benzoinated lard.

The water-soluble gels must also be stored in tightly stoppered containers to prevent the drying which occurs on exposure to air. These must also be freshly prepared because, on standing, for several months, liquefaction generally takes place—particularly with pectin pastes.

These preparations are extremely liable to mold growth, and preservatives must be added to prevent it. Benzoic acid, sodium benzoate or the para-hydroxy-benzoate derivatives are capable of preventing the growth.

Aluminum Paste, U.S.P. This is prepared by levigating the aluminum with liquid petrolatum and then incorporating the mixture with zinc oxide ointment. It is important that the aluminum used be in the form of a very fine powder.

PLASTERS

Plasters (Latin, *emplastrum*) have been defined as semisolid or solid adhesive masses spread on cloth of various sizes and shapes intended for topical application. They may or may not contain medicinal ingredients, depending on the purpose intended.

Like ointments and cerates, plasters are one of our oldest forms of medication. They are listed in *De Medicina* by Celsus (about A.D. 1st century) under the heading of Emplastra and are distinguished from "pastils" by the method used in compounding and from emollients by the materials used. The materials used in the plasters of that day indicate that there has not been much change in the ingredients of these preparations up to the official ones of today. A formula of a soothing white plaster is given as white lead, 128 Gm.; prepared calf's suet and wax, each 192 Gm.; olive oil, 750 ml., with which the white lead is boiled. Another consists of litharge, 168 Gm.; olive oil, 250 ml.; and an equal quantity of sea water, boiled, to which when off the boil, a little wax may be added. This is very similar to our lead plaster of today. This latter mixture is known as a "Diachylon" plaster and has formed an important part in the basis of the official plaster masses in nearly all of the pharmacopeias of the world. Later (1900–20), India rubber was introduced as the preferred basis of plasters and is still used today. In recent years, plasters containing vinyl resin, plasticizers and other chemical additives have been introduced.

USE

Plasters differ from most of this group of preparations in that they are essentially free from fats. They also differ in their therapeutic purpose in that plasters are used for their adhesiveness and the "support" they can give in the immobilization of an area, while cerates and ointments are not but are used rather to prevent the sticking of the dressing to the raw inflamed area.

While plasters are used chiefly for their local mechanical action in immobilizing an area, medicinal agents apparently can be absorbed from this mode of application. Therefore, plasters have been divided into 3 groups with regard to their therapeutic action:

1. **Epidermatic.** Plasters intended to exercise a supportive, protective, antiseptic, counterirritant or vesicant effect—e.g., mustard plasters, adhesive plasters, cantharides plasters.

2. **Diadermatic.** Plasters intended to produce an endermatic effect, such as anodyne, astringent, sedative or stimulant—e.g., such plasters as belladonna, lead oleate, rosin and wax.

3. **Endermatic.** Plasters intended for constitutional and systemic effects. Caspari states that "for this purpose the modern plaster mulls, also known as salve mulls, are now preferred by physicians."

PREPARATION

In the past the plaster bases have consisted chiefly of lead plaster, gum resins, burgundy pitch, etc. However, these have been replaced almost completely by India rubber as a base. The making of an India rubber plaster mass requires the use of extensive apparatus for the preparation of the rubber, the gums, the mixing of the masses and the spreading on the cloth. It is for this reason that the pharmacist of today rarely, if ever, manufactures or prepares plasters.

Of concern to the manufacturers of adhesive plasters are the complaints frequently received regarding the sensitizing nature of the constituents of the mass employed in its preparation. It has been stated that pine rosin, burgundy pitch and para rubber, which are and may still be contained in such preparations, may cause sensitization. The newer adhesive plasters consisting of vinyl resin, plasticizers and other chemical additives possess a very low incidence of irritation and excellent ability to remain adhered to the skin under severe conditions of moisture and heat.

The manufacture of pharmacopeial plasters entails the making of the mass and the spreading of the same. The making of the mass offers little difficulty, for the formulas are intended to be of such nature that the pharmacist can prepare the mass in his own laboratory by fusing the various constituents, or in some cases softening them by gentle heat. Usually, they are made with the official lead plaster or adhesive plaster base. This mass is then rolled into appropriate sticks or left in the vessels in which they were prepared, until a spread plaster is called for.

The spreading of the plaster mass requires a high degree of skill, which can be achieved only by practice. The melted plaster mass is poured on a plaster skin, or cloth, and spread by means of a hot clean spatula or other flat utensil. Heat is necessary in the preparation of plasters; therefore, any volatile substances to be incorporated in plasters should be added last to prevent volatilization.

Plasters are cut or shaped to fit the various areas to which they are applied (Fig. 154).

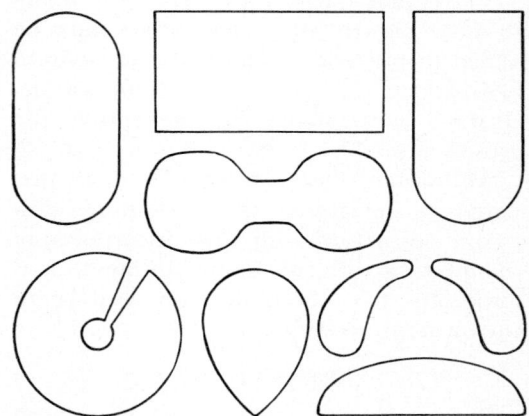

Fig. 154. Plasters for application to various areas of the body.

TABLE 27. PLASTERS OF THE U.S.P. AND THE N.F.

EMPLASTRUM	ENGLISH TITLE	COMPOSITION
Adhesive, U.S.P.	Adhesive Plaster	Rubber, resins, with a filler of an absorbent powder such as zinc oxide, orris root or talc
Belladonna, N.F.	Belladonna Plaster	Adhesive plaster and an extract of belladonna root
Mustard, N.F.	Mustard Plaster	Powdered black mustard seed in a base of pure rubber, dissolved in benzene and carbon disulfide
Salicylic Acid, U.S.P.	Salicylic Acid Plaster	Desired percentage salicylic acid in suitable base

Plasters are prepared also as porous plasters. The porosity is considered a mechanical advantage, in that it prevents the plaster's sliding from the point of application, each opening serving as a stop. It is also stated to be an advantage in the case of discharging surfaces, whereby the pores permit the outward flow of secretions, and this allows for greater cleanliness and prevents the reabsorption of possibly dangerous fluids which, of necessity, would accumulate under a nonporous covering.

COMMENTS

Mustard Plaster, N.F., is also known as Charta Sinapis, U.S.P. VIII, or mustard paper, because *U.S.P. VIII* directs the use of paper as the backing material for this preparation. *U.S.P. IX* gave permission to spread the material on cloth as well as paper, and the title was then changed to Emplastrum Sinapis.

Mustard Plaster is prepared by mixing powdered black mustard seed (deprived of its fixed oil by percolation with petroleum benzin) with a solution of pure rubber in benzene and carbon disulfide. The inert fixed oil is removed from the seed, for, if allowed to remain in the mustard paper, it would become greasy and disagreeable to handle.

This plaster serves as a rubefacient, a stimulant and a counterirritant. The major portion of this activity is due to the presence of the volatile allyl isothiocyanate. The latter is formed by hydrolysis of the glycoside sinigrin in the presence of the enzyme myrosin.

The action of the enzyme is initiated by thoroughly moistening the plaster in tepid water before applying it. The water should not be hot as this would inactivate the enzyme and prevent hydrolysis and subsequent liberation of the active allyl isothiocyanate.

CATAPLASMS

Cataplasms (Latin, *cataplasma*) or poultices are defined as wet masses of solid matter applied to the skin in order to reduce inflammation; or in some cases to act as counterirritants (mustard poultices). The solid matter used as the base is chosen with a view to its capacity to absorb and retain water, e.g., colloidal clay (kaolin), flaxseed and other mucilaginous drugs.

Cataplasms, like plasters, are one of our oldest forms of medication. They are listed in *De Medicina* by Celsus under the heading *"Malagma"* (poultice), and are classified as being "generally heating," but cooling poultices were applied to some areas. Usually they were applied to disperse diseased matter or to draw it out (*digerere, extrahere*); the latter were known as "epispastica," but also were used to relieve pain. They were often called after their inventor (Lysias, Andreas, etc.) as a recognition of his work.

Cataplasma Kaolini was official in *U.S.P. IX* but was dropped by the Tenth Decennial Revision and admitted to *N.F. V,* where it continued to be official as Kaolin Cataplasm until *N.F. X*. It consisted of kaolin, boric acid, thymol, methyl salicylate, peppermint oil and glycerin.

REFERENCES

1. Sauerland, F.: Biochem. Ztschr. **40**:65, 1912.
2. Sollman, T. H.: A Manual of Pharmacology, ed. 3, p. 76, 1926.
3. Bliss, A. R., Jr.: Drug and Cosmetic Ind. **35**:247, 1934.
4. Brown, M. W., and Scott, W. O.: J. Pharmacol. **50–51**:373, 1934

5. Fuller, A. T., Hawking, F., and Partridge, M. W.: Quart. J. Pharm. & Pharmacol. **15**:127, 1942.
6. Emmens, C. W.: J. Endocrinol. **2**:368, 1940–41.
7. Macht, D. I.: J.A.M.A. **110**:409, 1938.
8. Polano, M. K.: Skin Therapeutics, pp. 171–172, New York, Elsevier, 1952.
9. Michelfelder, T. J., and Peck, S. M.: J. Invest. Dermat. **19**:237, 1952.
10. Plein, E. M., and Plein, J. B.: J. Am. Pharm. A. (Sci. Ed.) **46**:705, 1957.
11. Beeler, E. C.: J. Am. Pharm. A. (Pract. Ed.) **3**:231, 1942.
12. Jones, E. R., and Lewicki, B.: J. Am. Pharm. A. (Sci. Ed.) **40**:509, 1951.
13. Johnston, G. W., and Lee, C. O.: J. Am. Pharm. A. (Sci. Ed.) **32**:25, 1943.
14. Elvin, N. C.: Arch. Ophthalmol. **27**:2, 373–374.
15. Harry, R. G.: Brit. J. Dermat. & Syph. **54**:1, 1942.
16. Husa, W. J., and Riley, D. E.: J. Am. Pharm. A. **23**:544, 1934.
17. Fiero, G. W.: J. Am. Pharm. A. **30**: 145, 1941.
18. Chakrauarty, D., Lach, J. L., and Blaug, S. M.: Drug Standards **25**:137, 1957.
19. Darlington, R. C., and Guth, E. P.: J. Am. Pharm. A. (Pract. Ed.) **11**:82 1950.
20. Barr, M., and Guth, E. P.: J. Am. Pharm. A. (Sci. Ed.) **40**:13, 1951.
21. Peronnet and Genet: J. Pharm. Chim. **26**:490, 1937.
22. Prout, W. A., Eddleman, M. S., and Harris, R. G.: J. Am. Pharm. A. (Sci. Ed.) **29**:372, 1940.
23. Prout, W. A., and Harris, R. G.: J. Am. Pharm. A. (Pract. Ed.) **2**:432, 1941.
24. Lesser, M. A.: Drug and Cosmetic Ind. **72**:616, 1953.
25. Rochow, E. G.: Chemistry of the Silicones, ed. 2, New York, Wiley, 1951.
26. Plein, J. B., and Plein, E. M.: J. Am. Pharm. A. (Sci. Ed.) **42**:79, 1953.
27. Casparis, P., and Meyer, E. W.: Pharm. acta Helv. **10**:101, 163, 1935.
28. Halpern, A., and Zopf, L. C.: J. Am. Pharm. A. (Sci. Ed.) **36**:101, 1947.
29. McClelland, C. P., and Bateman, R. L.: Chem. Eng. News **23**:247, 1945.
30. Smyth, H. F., Carpenter, C. P., and Weil, C. S.: J. Am. Pharm. A. (Sci. Ed.) **39**:349, 1950.
31. Rosenthaler, L.: Pharm. acta Helv. **18**: 262, 1943.
32. DeKay, H. G., and Kessler, N. A.: J. Am. Pharm. A. **33**:118, 1944.
33. Fantus, B.: Technic of Medication, p. 68, American Medical Assoc., Chicago, Ill., 1938.
34. Fantus, B., and Dyniewicz, H.: J. Am. Pharm. A. **28**:299, 548, 1939.

BIBLIOGRAPHY

Busse, L.: J. Am. Pharm. A. (Pract. Ed.) **4**:314, 1943.

Clark, W. C.: Am. J. Pharm. **111**:228, 1939.

Fantus, B.: Technic of Medication, p. 68, American Medical Assoc., Chicago, Ill., 1938.

Fantus, B., and Dyniewicz, H.: J. Am. Pharm. A. **28**:299, 548, 1939.

Fiero, G.: J. Am. Pharm. A. (Sci. Ed.) **29**: 18, 187, 458, 502, 1940; **30**:145, 1941.

Fuller, A. T., Hawking, F., and Partridge, M. W.: Quart. J. Pharm. & Pharmacol. **15**:127, 136, 1942.

Goodman, H.: Cosmetic Dermatology, McGraw-Hill Book Co., Inc., N. Y., 1936.

Johnston, G., and Lee, C. O.: J. Am. Pharm. A. (Sci. Ed.) **32**:25, 1943.

Langenham, H. A., and Noel, G. J.: N.F. Petroxolins and Parallel Preparations, Circular 5, Pharmaceutical Experiment Station, University of Wisconsin, Nov., 1918.

Martin, E. W., Husa's Pharmaceutical Dispensing, Fifth Ed., Mack Publishing Co., Easton, Pa., 1959.

Poucher, W. A.: Perfume Cosmetics and Soaps, 4th ed., vol. II, 1932.

Powers, J., and Crossen, G.: The Art of Compounding, The Blakiston Co., Phila., Pa., 1943.

Rosenthaler, L.: Pharm. acta Helv. **18**:262, 1943.

Sollman, T.: A Manual of Pharmacology, ed. 7 Saunders, Phila., 1948.

Unna, Eugen: J. Am. Pharm. A. **1**:673, 1912.

Urdang, G.: The Story of Ointments, What's New, Abbott Laboratories, North Chicago, Ill., 1942.

SIDNEY RIEGELMAN, Ph.D.
Associate Professor of Pharmacy and Pharmaceutical Chemistry
University of California

19

Suppositories

DEFINITION AND GENERAL CONSIDERATIONS
HISTORY
FACTORS AFFECTING DRUG ACTION VIA RECTAL ADMINISTRATION

SUPPOSITORY BASES
MANUFACTURE OF SUPPOSITORIES

DEFINITION AND GENERAL CONSIDERATIONS

Suppositories are a form of single dosage medication, usually conical or ovoid in shape, intended for insertion into the vaginal or rectal cavity for local or systemic action. Suppositories are most frequently prepared of semisolid bases which either melt when warmed to body temperature or dissolve or disperse when in contact with the body fluids. Modern commercial vaginal suppositories are usually prepared as a tablet compression in the shape of a flattened ovoid of lactose or of some other water soluble base. They are intended for local action by slowly dissolving in the vaginal fluids, thereby releasing their medication. Historically, suppositories also were prescribed for use in the urethra, in the nose or in the ear. These forms of suppositories are no longer administered. In their stead, tampons (cotton plugs soaked in the medicinal solution) are occasionally inserted in the ear or the nose, or the medication is administered by other traditional methods. Modern treatment of urethral infections utilizes parenteral drug administration.

Occasionally rectal medication is given as a single dosage rectal enema prepared from water or oil solution. They may be viewed as an extension of suppositories to liquid dosage forms. These retention enemas are available in plastic containers which may be used to propel the liquid from the container.

Drugs administered in the form of a suppository may have an effect that is either local or systemic, depending on the drug, its concentration and its rate of absorption. Frequently, a local response is desired from drug medication in suppository form in the treatment of vaginal and rectal conditions. Among the drugs so administered are emollients, astringents, local anesthetics, analgesics, estrogens and antibacterial agents. A drug which is not absorbed produces its action solely within the cavity in which it is confined. Even those drugs which are absorbed systemically may produce a local response. A drug applied in a concentration too low for systemic response may be entirely adequate for a transient local action. Estrogens are used locally in the vagina (to stimulate the generation of epithelial cells) in concentrations which are systemically relatively innocuous.

In the event that the drug is absorbed into the blood stream via the mucous surface, a systemic effect will be observed just as if the drug had been given orally. In contemporary medicine, when a systemic effect is desired, the use of rectal suppositories probably would be the overwhelming choice of physicians over vaginal and other suppository types.

HISTORY

Recorded history indicates that physicians of ancient Egypt and India used suppositories for local and systemic effect. In the writings of Hippocrates (400-370 B.C.) the special indications for suppositories and enemas were delineated for the first time. Dioscorides advocated the use of suppositories of hellebore to produce vomiting and those of poppy seed and mandrake to provide deep sleep. However, two centuries later, Galen reported that suppositories were used only to empty the intestines. He described the first soap suppository. Thus, suppositories had their brief period of popularity during Egyptian, Indian, Greek and Roman eras, only to fall into lesser use. It may have been the lack of a practical base for the suppository that discouraged their development.

In the late 18th century Antoine Baumé (1728-1809) discovered and developed cocoa butter as a suppository base. This introduced a new era in suppository medication. Following the work of A. B. Taylor and others, in the middle of the 19th century, attention was given to this form of medication, and much progress was made in methods of manufacture. Suppositories, with a base of cocoa butter, first became official in this country in *U.S.P. V.*

Suppositories were manufactured by manual manipulations until 1880 when metal molds were first manufactured. During the greater part of the 19th century suppositories were prescribed mainly for local action. When the fundamental anatomy and physiology of the rectum was understood more clearly, it became apparent that drugs can be absorbed from the lower regions of the rectum and can enter the general circulation. The rectal administration of digitalis in suppository form was tried and proved to be successful, particularly in children.

FACTORS AFFECTING DRUG ACTION VIA RECTAL ADMINISTRATION

The rectal use of a suppository may produce a systemic effect more rapidly than oral administration. Most of the drugs administered orally must pass through the stomach into the intestines before they are able to be absorbed. The time for passage of substances through the stomach depends on whether the drug was administered with, before or after meals, on the type of ingested food, on the amount of fluid taken with the medicine and on other factors. Since rectal absorption starts immediately after insertion, a more rapid response can be expected from rectal or vaginal administration of a drug than from oral administration.

A comparison of the routes of absorption of medication administered by oral, vaginal or rectal means will indicate another potential physiologic advantage for the rectal and the vaginal routes. Most of the drugs administered orally will pass into the hepatic-portal vein and, thereby, to the liver. Some of these compounds are modified biochemically by the liver, which reduces their potential systemic effectiveness. In addition to a lymphatic circulation, the compound is absorbed from the rectum by 3 different hemorrhoidal veins. The uppermost hemorrhoidal vein ultimately connects with the portal vein and leads to the liver. The lower and the middle hemorrhoidal veins connect with the general blood supply, circumventing the liver. The exact placement of the suppository within the rectal canal and the relative blood flow of the 3 veins influence the amount of the drug that will escape the liver. The studies of Bucher and others indicate that 50 to 75 per cent of a rectally administered drug will reach the general circulatory system without passage through the hepatic portal vein. However, lymphatic absorption must contribute to these results since the research of Fabre and his colleagues indicates that the blood and the lymphatic circulatory systems are nearly equal competitors as sites for the absorption of the rectally administered drugs. The entire blood supply of the vagina connects with the general circulation. Theoretically, not only will absorption begin more rapidly but also a larger portion of the intact active compound will enter the general circulation.

Symptoms of nausea and vomiting from local mucosal irritation occasionally are produced after oral administration of drugs. This difficulty is not experienced so frequently in rectal administration. Groedel has confirmed the lack of irritation and the relatively rapid absorption of digitalis and aminophylline after rectal administration. He concluded that rectal administration is comparable in its effect with intravenous injection and can be done without the physician's attendance.

While a number of experimenters have studied comparative rates of absorption via oral and rectal means, the results obtained are somewhat contradictory. Enesco and coworkers, in 1939, studied the absorption of aqueous solution of 6 drugs, both orally and rectally, on 63 normal individuals. Utilizing blood, urine and pharmacologic endpoints, they found that 5 of the 6 drugs were absorbed more quickly and in sufficient quantity rectally than on oral administration. These included sodium salicylate, chloral hydrate, methylene blue, atropine and morphine. Sodium iodide appeared to be absorbed more slowly from the rectum than by oral administration; however, the results varied considerably with the individual.

In the studies of Truitt and of Rudolfo and their co-workers the absorption of aminophylline was compared from the oral and the rectal sites of administration. Figure 155 gives the data obtained by Truitt et al. The administration of the dose of aminophylline from a solution results in a blood level nearly commensurate with intravenous administration. In contrast, oral

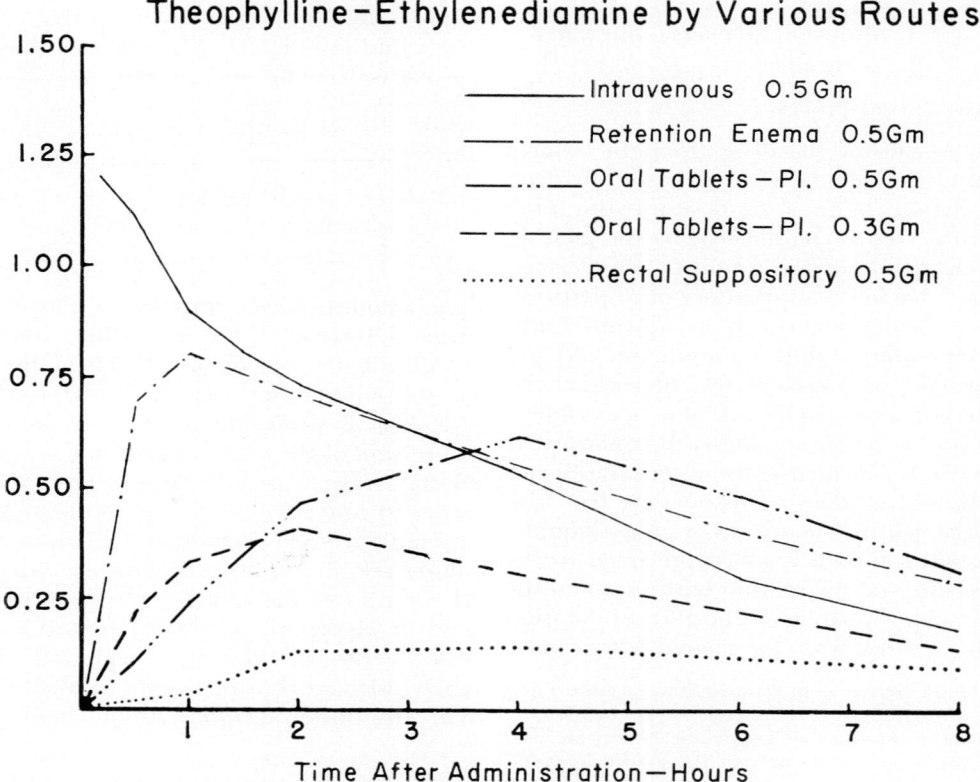

FIG. 155. Blood levels in mg./per cent vs. time for aminophylline administered by various routes. (Truitt *et al.*: J. Pharmacol. & Exper. Therap. **100**:309, 1950)

tablets appear to reach their maximum effect* only after a delay of 2 to 4 hours. Unfortunately, the suppository form utilized in this study and in most commercial bases consists of polyethylene-glycols which must dissolve prior to drug release.

Barach reports that rectal administration of aminophylline aqueous solutions results in relief of asthmatic attacks in 10 to 20 minutes. The studies of Cemeli on sodium salicylate indicate that significant blood levels are reached in 10 minutes from cocoa butter and selected substitutes. Contradictory results such as are found with aminophylline suppositories are probably related to the slow release of the drug from the suppository base to the absorption site.

In order for a drug to be absorbed systemically it must pass through the following stages:

Drug in Vehicle
↓ (may be rate-limiting step)

Drug in Solution
↓ (diffusion, pH effect, oil/water partition effect)

Absorption Process

The release of the drug from the vehicle to the body fluids is the first step in drug absorption. With a suppository, this rate-limiting step is complicated by the melting characteristics of the product. Drugs which are soluble in the suppository must partition out of the oily phase into the aqueous fluids. When water-soluble, oil-insoluble salts are used, they must pass to the interface of the water-oil and dissolve in the body fluids. Data to be presented later will confirm that it is far better to select a water-soluble, oil-insoluble salt than to dissolve the free base or free acid in the oil phase. For example, ephedrine sulfate is to be preferred to the free base, and the sodium barbiturate to the free acid. Apparently, the rate of solution in body fluids from the melted base is more rapid than the rate of partition of the dissolved drug.

The pH of the rectal mucosa is more acid than was previously believed. Schanker has found the colon and rectal area to be approximately 6.8. If a drug solution is more or less acid than this pH, the secretions will partially adjust the pH toward neutrality. However, it appears that the rectal fluids have little buffer capacity, and the dissolving drugs probably will determine the existing pH in accordance with their own acidity or basicity.

Schanker at the National Institutes of Health made a definitive study of the absorption characteristics of acidic and basic drugs in the colon and the rectum of anesthetized rats. The degree of ionization and the lipid solubility of the compounds are the most important factors determining their rates of absorption.

The student will recall that acid dissociation can be represented thus:

$$\text{HA} \rightleftharpoons \text{A}^- + \text{H}^+$$
(Lipid soluble undissociated) (Water soluble ionic salt)

while salts of bases may be looked upon as follows:

$$R_2NH^+ + Cl^- \rightleftharpoons R_3N + H^+ + Cl^-$$
(water soluble ionic salt) (lipid soluble free base)

The amount of each form of the particular drug is related to the ionization constant (pKa) of the acid or base.* When the pH of the environment is equal to the pKa, the drug is proportioned so that the concentration of the drug on each side is equal. Weak acids require a relatively high pH in order to convert them to the poorly absorbing anion. Acids whose dissociation constants are above 4.0 are absorbed rapidly. If the pKa of the acid is between 3 and 4, rate of absorption is slower, but still possible; below 3.0 the rate is negligible. Similarly, with weak bases whose pKa is below 8.5, absorption is quite rapid; those less

---

* Other independent data indicate a more rapid rate of oral absorption, but not as rapid as via the oral route. Further, aminophylline tablets are usually enteric coated to prevent the gastric irritation often experienced when the uncoated tablets are used; this delays the start of their absorption by more than an hour.

* The pKa of a base = $14 - pK_b$. This, in effect, is considering the salt as the conjugate acid of the base, just as the anion of the acid is the conjugate base of the free acid.

than 10 are slower, but still possible; but strong bases, such as quaternary ammonium salts, are insignificantly absorbed.

In each case, the uncharged drug molecule is selectively absorbed while the ionic form is poorly or negligibly absorbed. If buffer solutions are used to convert the pH of the rectum to a condition increasing the concentration of the uncharged form, the amount of the drug absorbed per unit time will increase. Schanker studied further a group of barbiturates. He found that the relative rate of absorption was dependent on their lipid solubility, the more lipid-soluble, the more readily absorbed from solution.

Even though the lipid-soluble form is the absorbing species, it is advisable to incorporate the salt form of the drug into the suppository so that the rate of solution in body fluids is enhanced. If the conditions are proper, the drug may be converted into the lipid-absorbing form by the neutralizing action of the environment or through the use of buffers.

Riegelman and Crowell utilized radioiodine-tagged drugs and followed absorption from the intact animal. They found that diffusion of the drug to the absorbing surface is one of the rate-limiting steps. Further, the mucous fluid secreted over the surface was a continuing barrier to the rapid absorption of some drugs. Other factors, such as particle size of the suspended drugs, were shown to be important in the rate of solution of the drug.

Dose. There is no uniformity of opinion as to the relation of the dose of a drug when given by mouth to the dose when given by suppository. In practice, the rectal dose is from ½ to 2 or more times the oral dose.

When a drug is administered in solution, such as in a retention enema, frequently it has been found to reach blood levels commensurate with intravenous injection and to exceed vastly the rate of absorption from oral adminstration. The aminophylline data given earlier is representative of such an effect.

The availability of the drug from a suppository vehicle is critically dependent on the physical characteristics of the base. Lack of appreciation of this fact is a cause of many of the discrepancies concerning dosage and much of the uncertainty over the usefulness of suppositories. The onset and the intensity of drug action are related directly to the blood and tissue concentration and the time required to reach the threshold concentration. Suppository bases modify drug action in proportion to the degree they modify the rate of drug absorption. When a drug is completely dissolved in a base, the initial rate of absorption is influenced by the percentage of saturation of the base. A 0.5-mg. dose of Diethylstilbestrol, U.S.P., in a 2-Gm. cocoa butter suppository (equivalent to a 1:4,000 solution) would be presumed to be less available than the same amount of drug dissolved in a glycerogelatin base. Such a conclusion is logical from the far greater solubility of the drug in the oil base. A very soluble drug present in a base in a low concentration will show a low escaping tendency. A more detailed discussion of the effect of percentage of saturation on drug release has been presented by Allawala and Riegelman.

SUPPOSITORY BASES

Theobroma Oil (Cocoa Butter). Prior to the introduction of cocoa butter in 1852, pharmacists used mixtures of lard and wax, as well as gums, honey, soap, resins and other fats, in suppository bases. Then, as until recently, the objective sought was a suppository base of a consistency that facilitated the introduction of the drug into the rectum and other orifices. Little consideration was given to the fate of a drug once the suppository was in position. The suppository was considered adequate if the finished product was solid at room temperature and liquid at body temperature. Cocoa butter answered these requirements admirably and was adopted widely.

Cocoa butter is a nonirritating, yellowish white triglyceride having a slight odor. When warmed to around 30° C., it begins to liquefy and usually melts at 34° to 35° C. However, even at temperatures below 30° C., it is a semisolid and consists of many

Table 28. Triglyceride Composition of Cocoa Butter

Tri-saturated glycerides	2-3	
Di-saturated glycerides	80-82	
P-O-S*		52-57
S-O-S		19-22
P-O-P		4-6
Monosaturated glycerides	13-18	
P-O-O		7-8
S-O-O		6-12
Unsaturated triglycerides	1-2	
O-O-O (Some linoleic)		1-2

* P = Palmitic acid, S = stearic acid, O = Oleic acid (includes approximately 2% linoleic acid)

Composite data from Hilditch and Slainsby: J. Soc. Chem. Ind. **35**, 957, 1936; Meara: J. Chem. Soc. 2154 1949; Chapman, D., Crossly A., and Davies, A. C.: J. Chem. Soc. 1502, 1957; Lutton, E. S.: J. Am. Oil Chem. Soc. **34**:5, 1957. See also Scholfield, C. R. and Dullon, H. J.: J. Am. Oil Chem. Soc. **36**:325, 1959.

crystals of solid triglyceride enmeshing a considerable portion of liquid. The liquid is held in place by surface-tension forces.

The data listed in Table 28 has been elucidated by different physical methods of analysis. It should be noted that cocoa butter contains predominantly symmetrical disaturated glycerides with the 2-oleo palmitostearin being the major component.

Most triglycerides are more diverse in their distribution of saturated and unsaturated fatty acids. For example, lard contains no more than 40 per cent of any one constituent. Probably as a consequence of this predominance of the disaturated triglycerides, cocoa butter exhibits marked polymorphism (the property of existing in different crystalline forms).

The rate of absorption of a drug suspended in a suppository vehicle is critically dependent on the melting characteristic of the base. Figure 156 illustrates the *in vitro* release of procaine hydrochloride and aminopyrine from cocoa butter suppositories as reported by Eckert. Procaine hydrochloride is suspended in the base while aminophylline is dissolved therein. The curves represent the per cent of the incorporated dose which is released to the water phase in 90 minutes relative to the immersion temperature of complete melting, the procaine hydrochloride crystals are able to transfer to the oil/water interface and to dissolve in the surrounding fluid. The rate of release of the dissolved aminopyrine is not so markedly affected by the melting process. When melting cocoa butter, the pharmacist frequently pays insufficient attention to the conditions of heating. Unfortunately, this careless practice results in a modification of the physical characteristics of the cocoa butter. When overheated, cocoa butter becomes completely liquid and loses all of the stable crystal nuclei with which to pattern its crystal form. It now must be supercooled, usually to below 15° C., and then it crystallizes into a meta stable crystalline form.

In order to explain these modifications fully, let us fill a thin-walled glass capillary tube with grated cocoa butter. We will heat it to 40° C., briefly supercool the melt to below 0° C. *just* until it solidifies and then immediately warm it to 15° C. The material appears translucent but is a solid. It is known as the gamma crystalline form.

As depicted in the center column of Figure 157, starting at the bottom at 15° C., we warm the capillary tube to 18° C., and the gamma form melts and resolidifies into

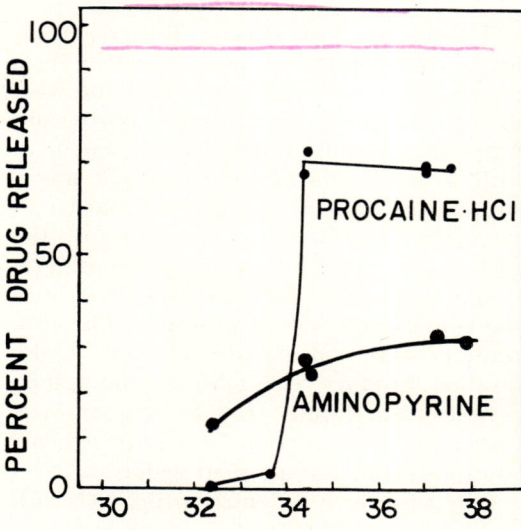

Fig. 156. The relative per cent of drug released in 90 minutes from cocoa butter suppositories exposed to various temperatures. (Echert: Ph.D. Dissertation, University of Basel, Switzerland)

another crystal form—the alpha form. The alpha form will melt at 22° C. and resolidify into the beta prime form. The beta prime form has a melting point of 28° C. and resolidifies into the stable beta form with a final melting point of 34.5° C. However, the melting and the cooling of a large mass of cocoa butter are not the same as in the above capillary experiment. Such factors as the rate and the time of cooling, the size and the shape of the suppository and the heat capacity of the mold influence the outcome. When overheated to above 36° C. and then quickly cooled in a chilled suppository mold, this larger mass of cocoa butter solidifies as a mixture of the unstable gamma, alpha and beta prime forms. When the mass is removed from the mold, we have a suppository that will melt if immediately allowed to warm to about 23° to 24° C. This procedure is indicated in the left-hand portion of Figure 157.

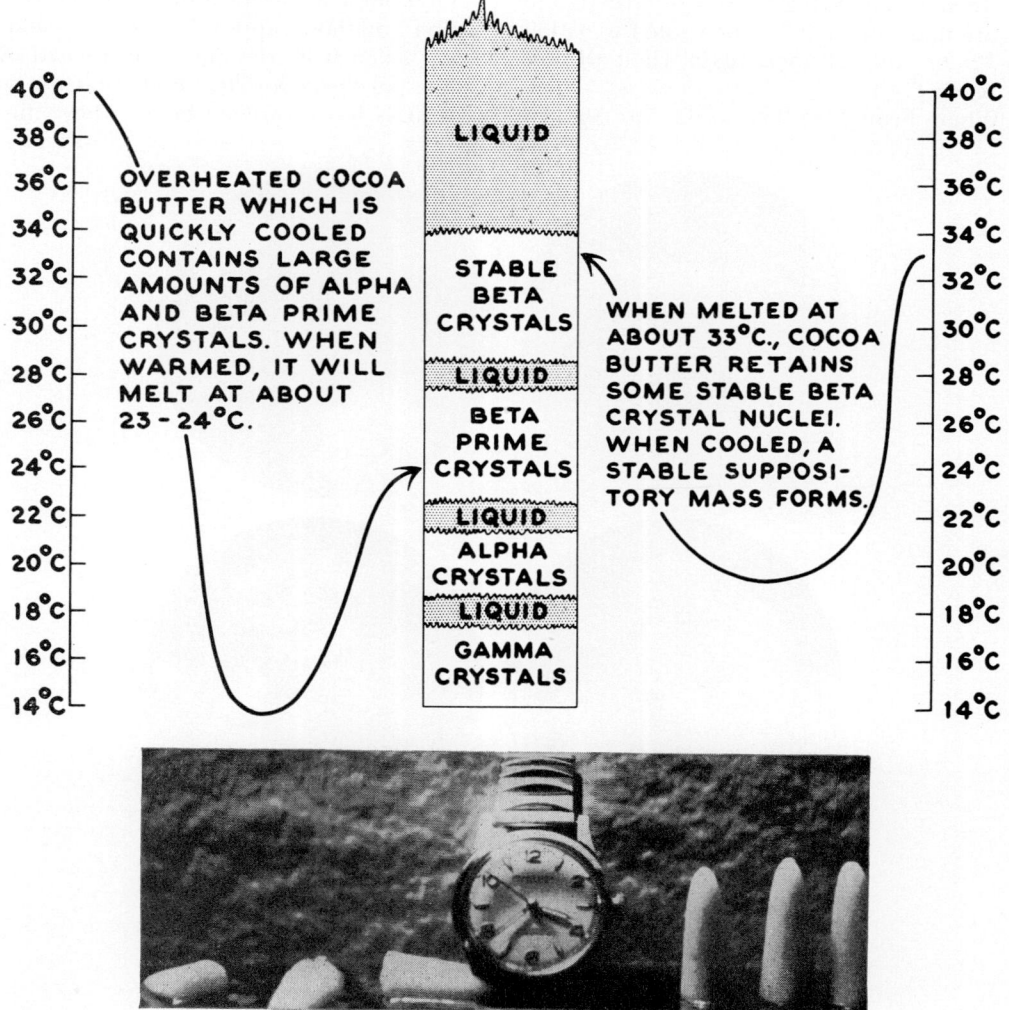

Fig. 157. (*Top*) The center diagram depicts the melting characteristics of the meta stable crystalline forms of cocoa butter. The left and the right inserts describe the results obtained when a large mass is melted.

(*Bottom*) Overheated and properly heated suppositories 7 minutes after removing from mold. (Air temperature, 35° C.)

354 Suppositories

The exact response of the melted cocoa butter mass depends, among other factors, on the speed of cooling and the difference between the temperature of the mass and the cooling environment. If cooled slowly with a small difference in temperature, the gamma form commences to form (at approximately 17.5° C.) and is transformed immediately into the alpha and then into the beta prime form. In contrast, if the melted cocoa butter is poured into an ice-cold mold the conversion from the gamma to the higher melting forms is retarded. The entire mass may have to be cooled to as low as 12° C. and will melt again when allowed to reach 15° C.

When heated to below 33° to 36° C., cocoa butter is sufficiently liquefied to be pourable, yet it will still retain crystal nuclei of the stable beta form. These crystal nuclei assist in the production of the beta crystals directly. A suppository made by this procedure will be composed essentially of the stable melting crystalline forms. The latter procedure is indicated in the right-hand portion of Figure 157. These summarized facts have been elucidated largely by the extensive researches of S. V. Vaeck in Belgium.

Occasionally, suppositories made by the fusion method appear perfectly shaped when taken from the mold and turned over to the patient, who later finds that the suppositories have softened before they can be

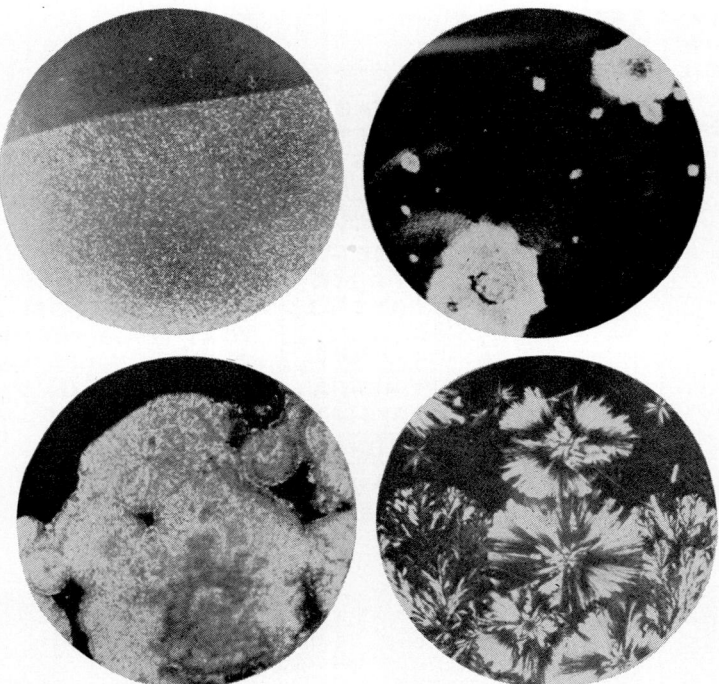

Fig. 158. Photomicrographs of cocoa butter. (*Top, left*) Freshly crystallized cocoa butter, alpha form.

(*Top, right*) After several days at room temperature, intermediate crystal forms occur. The large masses contain crystals of the stable beta form surrounded by mixtures of alpha and beta prime crystals.

(*Bottom, left*) About 2 weeks later, complete transition to the stable beta form has occurred.

(*Bottom, right*) Another photomicrograph of pure beta form grown under special laboratory conditions.

(From Dr. S. V. Vaeck and *International Chocolate Review*)

TABLE 29. SUMMARY OF POLYMORPHIC CHARACTERISTICS

Property	Gamma	Alpha	Beta
Relative stability....	Least	Intermediate	Most
Melting point......	Lowest	Intermediate	Highest
Gross appearance...	Glassy, partly transparent	Intermediate	Powdery, opaque
Obtained from liquid by other solid.	Rapid cooling not possible	Slow cooling from gamma form	Very slow cooling from alpha form*
Where found.......	Only in triglycerides	Triglycerides, monoglycerides and diglycerides, paraffins, esters	In all long-chain compounds

*An intermediate beta prime form found in mixed triglycerides.

used. The conversion of a low-melting suppository to one of the more stable melting forms take place spontaneously. Figure 158 shows 4 photomicrographs taken at 4 different times and indicates some of the transitional crystalline stages of cocoa butter. Fortunately, the conversion takes place more rapidly than is indicated in the photomicrographs. The time the suppository is kept frozen makes the difference. After a period of time, the frozen mass containing a mixture of other crystal forms slowly generates crystal nuclei of the stable beta form. When warmed, the meta stable crystals may all melt, leaving only the stable beta nuclei. These beta nuclei will seed the liquid for crystallizing into the stable form without going through all of the intermediate stages. But, will there be a sufficient network of beta crystals to hold the large volume of liquid and thereby retain the suppository shape? We all must agree that it is far easier to make the suppository correctly the first time than to trust to luck.

Meta stable crystalline forms, usually called polymorphic forms, are not uniquely a property of cocoa butter but are found in many organic compounds, particularly in long-chain compounds. Table 29 presents a summary of some of the general properties of these compounds and some of the conditions for their formation. Their existence in nearly all cases has been verified experimentally by x-ray diffraction analysis of the crystals and shows that the individual differences between each type of crystal are due to the relative closeness of packing of the molecules in the crystal. When tilted, the molecules can pack more closely; the result is a higher melting crystal. Table 29 includes a summary of the different types of long-chain compounds which are known to possess polymorphic crystal forms. If these substances are overheated and cooled quickly, they, too, might crystallize in meta stable forms. Experimental verification is not available at present.

As mentioned above, cocoa butter is composed of approximately 80 per cent of 2-oleo disaturated triglycerides, and it is this regularity in structure that results in the polymorphism. Most cocoa butter substitutes do not show significant polymorphism due to their heterogeneity of structure.

A further complication results with cocoa butter in contrast with the substitute triglycerides. The student will recall that the freezing point of a solution is lower than the pure solvent. The solute added to cocoa butter depresses the freezing point in proportion to its concentration in solution, usually expressed in terms of mole fractions. The proportionality constant is the molal freezing-point depression.[1]

Table 30 contains a list of the solubility data of various drugs in cocoa butter as obtained by Büchi and Oesch. Figure 159 illustrates the cooling curves for 20 per cent chloral hydrate suppositories as well as the pure bases.

Pure cocoa butter when melted at 35° C., solidifies at 22° C., as is noted in Figure 159.

---

[1] The molal freezing-point depression for cocoa butter might be estimated to be approximately 6°.

TABLE 30. SOLUBILITY OF CERTAIN DRUGS IN COCOA BUTTER

Ethyl aminobenzoate	0.5– 1.0*
Barbital	Less than 0.1
Camphor	8.0–10.0
Chloral hydrate	8.0–10.0
Menthol	10 –15
Phenobarbital	0.1– 0.5
Phenol	3.0– 4.0

* The figures represent a range of concentration. The upper figure indicates a concentration where soluble crystals were noted and the lower figure the next concentration tested which showed no solute crystals.

However, when chloral hydrate is added to the base it depresses and prolongs the cooling time. The suppository requires a temperature of approximately 8° C.* before it solidifies. Such a product will melt again at well below room temperature. A substitute triglyceride base of commerce, Imhausen H (see Table 31), is also shown in Figure 159. The pure Imhausen H solidifies at 25° C., and the addition of chloral hydrate only depresses the solidification point to 21° C.

Many new substitutes for cocoa butter have been developed in recent years, particularly in Europe. Many of these bases possess melting characteristics far superior to cocoa butter and have obtained much acceptance in Europe and in manufactured suppositories in this country. Table 31 includes a list of most of the commercial types available at present, including both American and European products. The fusion temperature as listed is temperature at which the product is completely fluid. The solidification point is also listed. These two temperatures are important in assisting the pharmacist in meeting his immediate need for a base which releases a drug quickly or one which can slow down the release (fusion point 38° to 41°). The information on solidification point will help the pharmacist to decide on a base to use with a drug that depresses the melting point of cocoa butter. Table 31 includes a classification of the commercial bases in physical and chemical groups. Some of these will be discussed later in this chapter.

When the melting point is lowered below the environmental temperature, it is necessary to raise the melting point through the addition of some fat-soluble, waxlike substance having a relatively high melting point. Although a variety of substances have been recommended, white wax and spermaceti are used most frequently. The addition of less than 3 per cent of white wax yields mixtures, after proper aging, having melting points lower than that of cocoa butter. The addition of more than 6 per cent gives rise to mixtures with melting point greater than 37° C. When wax is

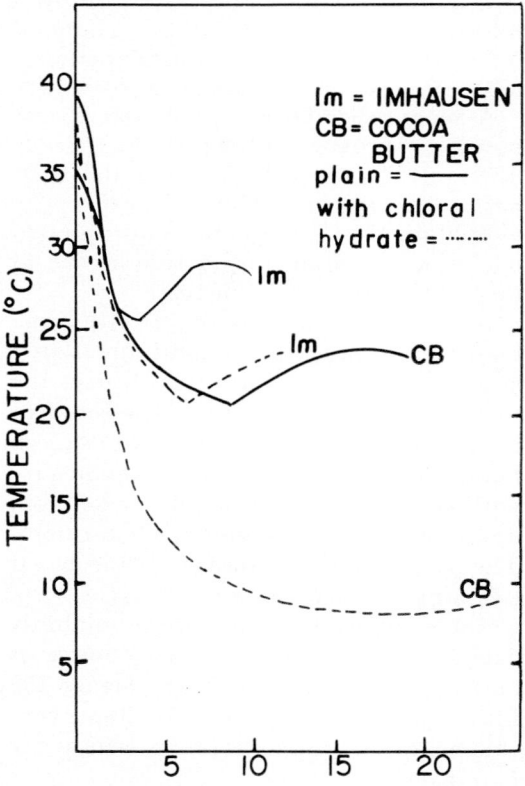

FIG. 159. Cooling curves for the melted cocoa butter and a triglyceride substitute (Imhausen H) in the presence and the absence of 20 per cent chloral hydrate. (Adapted from data by Pozo, A. D., Cemeli, J., and Galenia: Acta 7:144, 1954)

* Since this suppository is approximately 1.2 molal in respect to chloral hydrate, and the solidifying point is depressed 14° C., the molal freezing point depression of cocoa butter may be estimated at 12° C. per mole.

Table 31. Commercial Suppository Base Ingredients*

Trade Name		Property			Composition or Accessory Components	Manufacturer
		Fusion Pt.†	Solidification Pt.‡	Approximate Water No.		

I. Higher Melting Triglyceride Fraction of Vegetable Oils

Trade Name		Fusion Pt.	Solidification Pt.	Approx. Water No.	Composition	Manufacturer
Weecobee	W	35.5	33		Higher melting fraction of coconut oil prepared by fractional distillation. (All contain 0.25% lecithin.)	E. Drew Co., New York 10, N. Y.
	R	39	35	30–40		
	Cl	40	34			
	Bc	43	35			
Hard Butter S-70-XX					Transesterification of coconut oil type. (May be procured with or without 0.25% lecithin.)	Best Foods, Inc., Bayonne, N. J.
	Special low	36.5	32			
	Low	39	35			
	Medium	42	36.5			
	Hard	45	40			
Cebes		32	34	27.5	60	Modified coconut oil	Aarhus Oliefabrik, Aarhus, Denmark
		37	52	30			
Estarinum	A	34	32		Modified coconut oil, plus added monoglycerides	Edelfettwerke G.m. b.H., Hamburg-Eidelstedt, Germany
	B	35	30			
	C	38	30	30		
	D	42	40			

II. Hydrogenated or Modified Triglycerides

Trade Name		Fusion Pt.	Solidification Pt.	Approx. Water No.	Composition	Manufacturer
Cotomar		39			Partially hydrogenated cottonseed	Procter & Gamble Co., Cincinnati, Ohio
Coto Flakes		62			Hydrogenated cottonseed oil	
Oleum Arachis Hydrogenation		33	26		Hydrogenated peanut oil	Astra-Fett und Öl Werke, A. G., Steffesburg, Switzerland
Suppositol	S	37			Modified triglyceride	Fritz-Wetz, Hamburg-Wilhelmsburg, Germany
	T	37				
	R	385	31.5	45		
Supane		36	36	32	Hydrogenated triglyceride	Etablissement Nyco, Aubervilliers, Seine, France
	EM	36				
		39	39			

III. Triglycerides with Added W/O Emulsifiers

Trade Name		Fusion Pt.	Solidification Pt.	Approx. Water No.	Composition	Manufacturer
Massupol		36	32	50–100	Lauric acid triglyceride, plus monoglycerides	Crok & Laan, Wormeveer, Holland
		35	32.5	90		
Suppostal	N	39	37.5	50	Hydrogenated triglyceride, plus unsaturated fatty lanosterol or fatty alcohols (W/O emulsifiers)	Medifarma, S. A., Milan, Italy
	O	58		50		
	Eo	35.5	38	50		
Neo Suppostal		39	37	100	Hydrogenated triglycerides, plus polyethylene glycol fatty acid esters	Medifarma, S. A., Milan, Italy
		40.2	39	100		
		40	40	100		
Imhausen	H	36	32.5	100	Hydrogenated triglycerides of lauric acids, plus monoglycerides	Imhausen Co. G.m.b.H. Witten, Ruhr, Germany
	E	37	33	45		
	V	35	28	100		
DHW	I	36	33	100	Hydrogenated triglycerides	Deutsches Hydrierwerke, Düsseldorf, Germany
	II	39.5	37	100		

TABLE 31. COMMERCIAL SUPPOSITORY BASE INGREDIENTS*—(Continued)

TRADE NAME	PROPERTY			COMPOSITION OR ACCESSORY COMPONENTS	MANUFACTURER
	FUSION PT.†	SOLIDI- FICA- TION PT.‡	AP- PROXI- MATE WATER NO.		
IV. MISCELLANEOUS OLEAGINOUS COMPOUNDS					
Butyrum Tego G	34.5	32	100	Propylene glycol mono- and distearates	Atlas Goldschmidt, Essen, Germany
Monolene Aldo 25	46				Glyco Products Co., Brooklyn, N. Y. Kessler Chem. Co., Philadelphia 35, Pa.
Hexadienol	35			Hexa-2, 4-diene, -1-ol	Hexene-ol Laboratories Inc., Cleveland, Ohio
Hexene-ol	38			Hexadienol, plus hydrous lanolin, triethanolame glyceryl monostearate	
DHW III	37.5	33.5	100	Condensate of higher molecular saturated fatty alcohols	Deutsches Hydrierwerke, Düsseldorf, Germany
Adol 42§	35.5	34.4		Higher fatty alcohols (approximately 50% unsaturated)	Archer, Daniels & Midland Co., Chem. Product Div., Cleveland, Ohio
V. WATER DISPERSIBLE (POLYETHYLENE GLYCOLS OR THEIR ESTERS)					
Carbowax (UC) Polyglycol (D)				Polyethylene glycol (linear polymers of ethylene oxide)	Union Carbide & Carbon Co., New York, N. Y.
1000	41	38	Sol		
1540	47	42			
4000	48	40			Dow Chemical Co., Midland, Mich.
6000	49				
Postonal Scurol Supponal			Sol	European Trade Names for polyethylene glycol	
DN Suppopharm Polyethylene glycol (PEG) Monostearates (MS) PEG400 MS	25		Sol		Union Carbide & Carbon Co., New York, N. Y. (Kessler, Glyco—see above)
1000	41	37			
Myrj 51 (G2151)	425	39	Sol	Polyethylene glycol monostearates	Atlas Powder Co., Wilmington, Del.
Myrj 52 (G2152)	46	39	Sol		
Tween 61	39		Sol	Polyethylene glycol Sorbitan monostearate	Atlas Powder Co., Wilmington, Del.

* A portion of the data included in this table originally appeared in the Schweizerische Apotheker Zeitung **96**:205-220, 1958. It has been modified to include additional data of American source material and has been reorganized.

† The fusion temperatures are listed as the temperature for complete melting. The compounds usually melt over a range of 3 or more degrees.

‡ The solidification temperature is listed as **single** temperature although a small range is usually found.

§ Recent samples do not meet these melting point standards.

used to raise the melting point of cocoa butter, 3 to 6 per cent should be employed. The amount of spermaceti added to raise the melting point of cocoa butter suppositories is indefinite. A range of 20 to 28 per cent has been suggested.

Substances dissolved in cocoa butter may be referred to as "impurities" which create disorder within the normal molecular arrangement. Less energy is required to separate the molecules in this disordered arrangement resulting in a lowered melting point. The high-melting-point additives can cause disorder in certain ratios and lower the melting point.

When the suppository base is prepared, the high-melting-point additive is mixed with the cocoa butter, and the mixture is heated well above 36° C. This procedure destroys all of the stable crystal nuclei of the cocoa butter, and the mixture will crystallize in a meta stable crystalline form. Unless the suppository is allowed to age, the mixture may melt above body temperature, markedly restricting the release of the drug. When both a soluble drug and a high-melting-point additive are incorporated in the cocoa butter, the system is more complex. The suppository may have a lower melting point than the drug or the spermaceti by themselves. At present, no empirical rules are available to guide one to a choice of the proper ratio of drug and additive for any given formula. A practical solution to the problem of lowered melting point of cocoa butter in the presence of dissolved drugs (chloral hydrate, for example) would be to suggest to the physician that he select a vehicle which obviates this difficulty.

Substitutes for Cocoa Butter. Of the many fatlike mixtures that have been suggested as substitutes for cocoa butter, 2 will be mentioned. Martindale recommended a mixture of equal parts of stearic and oleic acids. After fusion, the cooled mixture melts rapidly at body temperature. A definite advantage of the stearic-oleic acid base over cocoa butter is that the melting point is adjusted easily by altering the ratio of the 2 acids. This base serves as a solvent for alkaloids, forming salts with them. Oleic acid is absorbed, in contrast with cocoa butter which is not absorbed; however, no data are available on the release of alkaloids or other drugs from the base. Another substitute for cocoa butter is a mixture of cetyl alcohol 17 per cent and almond oil 83 per cent. Other vegetable oils may be used with equal success.

Using one of these substitutes, a suppository can be prepared, avoiding the hazards of a lowered melting point of cocoa butter. For example, chloral hydrate or paraldehyde present a nearly insurmountable melting problem if cocoa butter is used for the base. An increase in the amount of the higher melting component assures the easy preparation of a properly melting finished suppository. Little or no adjustment of the formula is required when chloral hydrate is added to the stearic-oleic acid base. An excellent suppository results with the original formula. The chloral hydrate must be protected from evaporation by wrapping each suppository.

Glycerinated Gelatin.* Mixtures of glycerin and gelatin have been used widely as vehicles in the manufacture of suppositories since about 1870. Many formulas have been recommended, differing in the proportions of glycerin, water and gelatin. According to *U.S.P. XIV* formulation, one half of the weight of the suppository should consist of glycerinated gelatin, another material. Prepared glycerinated gelatin has been difficult to obtain in the commercial market, probably because there was small demand for it.

The formerly official method for making glycerinated gelatin is a tedious and time-consuming procedure. Water is mixed with the gelatin to initiate the solvation procedure, glycerin is added, and the mixture is heated until all of the water is driven off. This procedure dates from the time when gelatin was available only in sheet form and not in a finely powdered, purified form.

Tice and Abrams have proposed a direct method of preparing the finished glycerinated gelatin suppositories without requiring the prior preparation of the gel. The *U.S.P. XV* formula for glycerinated

---

* A more logical name for this mass would be gelled glycerin.

gelatin suppositories is based on their results,

The medicinal substance, the prescribed quantity
Purified water, a sufficient quantity to make .... 10 Gm.
Gelatin, granular .... 20 Gm.
Glycerin .... 70 Gm.

However, it differs slightly from the recommendations of Tice for the suppositories. The above formula was found to be adequate for vaginal suppositories but to be too hygroscopic and to lack adequate consistency for the common rectal suppository size. For the latter, Tice recommended that 25 per cent gelatin be used. The official directions for preparing the suppositories suggest the use of a steam bath to prepare the suppositories, but Tice found that the slightly higher heat source of a salt-water bath would accelerate rapid solvation of the gelatin particles since a higher temperature is produced than with tap water. This method of preparing glycerinated gelatin suppositories has the disadvantage of requiring the application of considerable heat. A heat-labile drug should be added at the end of the solvation period after the base has cooled to a temperature just above its solidification point.

Glycerin is not an ideal ingredient for the base. It is hypertonic; also, it is a poor solvent relative to propylene glycol or polyethylene glycols. The following has been studied in Switzerland as a substitute for the formula listed above:

Gelatin 25%
Water 37%
Polyethylene glycol 18%
Glycerin 20%

Propylene glycol can also be substituted for the glycerin. The advantage of the modification is that the suppository base can dissolve more of the water-insoluble compounds and make them more rapidly available for absorption.

Suppositories made of glycerinated gelatin do not melt at body temperature; instead, they slowly dissolve in the secretions or the contents of the body cavity into which they are inserted. The solution time varies according to a number of factors: the gelatin/glycerin/water ratio used, the gel strength of the gelatin and the presence of certain peptizing drugs or chemicals.

An important advantage to the use of type A or B gelatin in the preparation of glycerinated gelatin suppositories was pointed out by Tice and Abrams. By selecting either the cationic gelatin (type A) or the anionic gelatin (type B), it is possible to avoid most of the incompatibilities usually encountered in preparing suppositories from this vehicle.

U.S.P. XVI recognizes glycerin suppositories. This formula is a glycerin-sodium stearate gel. The suppository is official because of the laxative action resulting from the irritating effect of the soap and the osmotic effect of the glycerin. The suppositories rarely are prepared by pharmacists, since excellent commercial suppositories generally are available. Since it is not considered a basic suppository vehicle, drugs are not administered in this product. A slight modification in the relative ratio of glycerin to sodium stearate was made in the *U.S.P. XVI* formula in respect to the older formula.

U.S.P. XVI includes monographs for Aminophylline Suppositories and Carbarsone Suppositories. No base or dose is specified in either case; however, an excellent assay procedure is available for the standardization of each product.

Emulsifying Bases. Cocoa butter can be modified into o/w or w/o emulsions by the incorporation of suitable emulsifying agents. The addition of 2 per cent cholesterol or 5 to 10 per cent wool fat will assist in the formation of w/o emulsions. Approximately 10 to 20 per cent water or aqueous solutions may be added to such suppository vehicles. By the incorporation of a more hydrophilic surface-active agent such as sodium lauryl sulfate, aerosol OT, sodium stearate (all anionic agents), or 1 per cent lecithin (cationic), o/w emulsions are formed which allow the addition of up to 25 per cent water yet retain suppository characteristics. The suppositories are difficult to form, since more than 25 per cent water usually is necessary in order to obtain water as the external phase. Suppositories which form o/w emulsions are not stable for a long period of time, since the external aqueous phase rapidly evaporates.

Table 31 contains a list of triglycerides with added w/o emulsifiers (Section III), and miscellaneous oleaginous compounds which absorb water (Section IV). The *in vitro* data of Mühleman indicates that drugs dissolved in the aqueous internal phase of w/o bases are not as rapidly available as the same drug suspended in the vehicle. Even though the vehicles melt and allow the droplets of aqueous phase to move to the interface, additional force is required to cause the water droplet to cross the interface.

There is insufficient *in vivo* data available, comparing emulsified and anhydrous bases, to delineate their usefulness. The data of Eschenbrenner and of Büchi and Oesch seem to indicate that both water-insoluble and water-soluble compounds are released rapidly by the cocoa butter/water/lecithin base.

In 1936, Bird proposed propylene glycol monostearate, containing ½ to 1 per cent of sodium or ethanolamine stearate (as an emulsifying agent), as a useful suppository base. This raw material slowly, but spontaneously, forms a finely dispersed emulsion of the insoluble monostearate in body fluid, thus releasing the incorporated medication. The original material tested by Bird was reported to have a melting point of 37° C. However, commercially available samples of the compound appear to melt at around 42° C. The product has been proved to be nontoxic and safe for internal administration. When the product is placed in a beaker of water, it slowly swells to a soft jelly. When inserted into the rectum, analogous swelling will require osmotic transfer of considerable fluid into the rectal cavity for dispersion of the base. The author has found that the incorporation of 20 to 40 per cent of polyethylene glycol 400 monostearate (m.p. 23° to 25°) to propylene glycol monostearate produces a suppository base that will soften readily at body temperature.

Water-Soluble Bases. An important change of the postwar period in suppository medication has been the development of water-soluble suppository bases. Polyethylene glycols of high molecular weights are solids at room temperature and are very soluble in water. The *U.S.P. XV* mentions them as potential suppository bases for the official suppositories. The suppository uses of these substances were developed first in Germany and other European countries during World War II. (See Section V, Table 31.) Polyethylene glycol mixtures have melting points in the range of 45° to 50° C., and they, too, require the osmotic transfer of water into the rectal cavity for solution and release of the medication. The osmotic movement of water into the rectal cavity is not a uniform response and apparently varies from individual to individual and from one administration to another. Unless inserted well beyond the anal sphincter, the suppository will cause marked discomfort from the hard, slow-dissolving characteristics of the solid polyethylene glycol.

Many different formulas have been proposed for the polyethylene glycol suppositories. Hassler and Sperandio have proposed 2 interesting formulas in which 20 per cent water could be incorporated.

Formula No. 1
Polyethylene glycol 4,000.............. 33%
Polyethylene glycol 6,000.............. 47%
Water 20%

Formula No. 2
Polyethylene glycol 1,540.............. 33%
Polyethylene glycol 6,000.............. 47%
Water 20%

Polyethylene glycol suppositories must be prepared by the fusion process. They appear smooth and professionally acceptable when first prepared but frequently develop fractures on standing. The problem is even more pronounced with suppositories containing water in the formula. Since solid polyethylene glycols are soluble in water to the extent of about 60 per cent, the inclusion of 20 per cent water will produce a supersaturated system during the fusion process. On standing, the system undergoes slow crystallization or granulation which causes fractures in the suppository.

The systemic action of drugs included in polyethylene glycol suppository bases is markedly modified. Hassler and Sperandio utilized rats to evaluate the uptake of various water-soluble barbiturate salts from cocoa butter and from a water-soluble polyethylene glycol base. The absorption was judged by the onset of action (the time when the animal lost its righting reflex) and by the duration of action (the time when the animal regained its righting reflex). With the water-soluble barbiturates, the onset of action was consistently more rapid from the cocoa butter base than from the water-soluble base. But the water-soluble polyethylene glycol suppositories gave a longer duration of action than did the cocoa butter suppositories.

Charonat, Chevillard and Giono introduced methyl nicotinate into guinea pigs in the form of a rectal suppository. A thermocouple attached to each animal's ear measured the temperature rise produced by the compound. These authors found it extremely difficult to keep the solid polyethylene glycol suppository in place, since invariably the animals attempted to expel it. The polyethylene glycol suppository resulted in a slower onset but a longer duration of action than did the cocoa butter suppository. The slower release of drugs from the water-soluble base is expected as the base must dissolve in the body fluids to release the drug, while the cocoa butter quickly melts and permits more rapid absorption.

However, one cannot be too cautious in drawing generalities on the rate of release of medication from solid polyethylene glycol suppositories. Inadequate data are available for such conclusions, and much further research is required. Many drugs appear to complex with polyethylene glycols. These include any drug containing a phenolic group and probably with many other hydrogen-bonding groups. Such complexed molecules are available only slowly, if at all. It is apparent that many of these factors might be contributory to the fragmentary results we now possess. However, one cannot deny that many of the modern proprietary suppository formulations have selected solid polyethylene glycol as the basic vehicle.

Several other water-miscible formulations have been developed. Most of these include nonionic surface-active derivatives of polyethylene glycol. Examples of these are polyethylene glycol sorbitan monopalmitate (Tween 61) and polyethylene glycol monostearate (Myrj 51). The use of the latter compound has been proposed by Gross and Becker.

The release of the drugs from surface-active systems was discussed by Allawala and Riegelman, who concluded that surface-active agents can markedly modify the release of the drugs from these systems. In certain instances, the rate of uptake may be accelerated and in other formulations the opposite effect may result. This apparent anomaly is explainable in terms of the type of physical interaction of the drugs with the surface-active agents. It is theoretically possible for the drug to show systemic (and possibly toxic) action when formulated in suppositories containing surface-active agents while the drug normally would possess only local action from other suppository formulas.

Although analogous tests have not been attempted with solid polyethylene glycols in suppository form, the use of these agents in ointments has led to some significant modifications of therapeutic activity. Polano et al., found that a 25 per cent dispersion of salicylic acid in a polyethylene glycol ointment showed little or no peeling action (keratolytic activity), while 3 per cent or less of salicylic acid in petrolatum is a well-known keratolytic agent. Peck also found that polyethylene glycol ointments markedly retarded the transcutaneous absorption of tripelennamine free base (water insoluble) or Tripelennamine Hydrochloride, U.S.P. (water soluble). Although these water-miscible suppository bases have been used for over 10 years, too often their acceptance may have been based on physical appearance and ease of handling at environmental temperatures and too seldom on evidence which points to their pharmacologic superiority.

Comparative Evaluation of Different Suppository Bases. Rapp, Charonnot, Christian, Cemeli, Hassler, Riegelman and their co-workers each have conducted studies on the comparative absorption rate of drugs from different suppository bases. The recent studies of Pennati and Steiger-Trippi are particularly informative. They studied the absorption of a sulfonamide, that is sulfisomidine (Elkosin-Ciba) and its sodium salt in rabbits. They determined the blood levels obtained from a 150-mg. dose administered in a modified glycerinated gelatin (see p. 360) in cocoa butter, in a substitute triglyceride which melted at body temperature (Massupol), and in a polyethylene glycol suppository. Their results are given in Figure 160. In each instance the water-soluble sodium sulfonamide (NaS) was absorbed more rapidly than the poorly soluble free acid (HS). Furthermore, comparison of the rates of absorption of the sodium salt sulfonamide from the various vehicles indicates that the cocoa butter produces a more rapid onset followed by the substitute triglyceride and the gelatin bases. The blood concentration reached a 10 mg./per cent level in less than 1 hour with cocoa butter and at least 2 hours for any of the alternatives. The data of Figure 160 further indicates that the melting or dissolution of the vehicle and the subsequent solution of the drug in the body fluids is the rate-limiting step for drug absorption from the rectal medication.

MANUFACTURE OF SUPPOSITORIES

Suppositories are manufactured by 2 general methods. In the *hot* process, the drug is added to the melted base and the mixture allowed to cool after pouring into molds. In the *cold* process, the drug is incorporated with the unmelted base and the resulting mass shaped either by hand or by compression in a metallic press.

Size and Shape. According to the *U.S.P.*, rectal suppositories should weigh about 2 Gm. and should be tapered. Smaller sizes are used for infants. Generally, the suppository is tapered at one end so as to resemble a bullet. After giving consideration to the anatomy of the rectal canal, the late Sir Henry Wellcome designed a shape recommended as being retained more easily This suppository is tapered at both ends, the taper being greater at one end than at the other. Urethral suppositories (bougies) are pencil-shaped, pointed at one extremity, and either 7 cm. in length, weighing about 2 Gm. each, or 14 cm. in length, weighing about 4 Gm. each. The larger suppository is used for the male. Vaginal suppositories

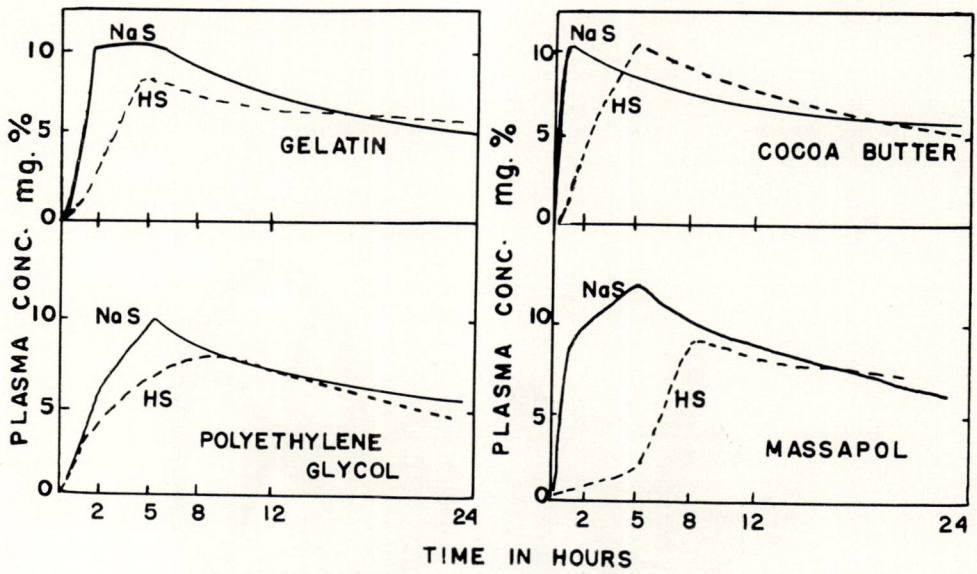

Fig. 160. Average blood levels in rabbits in mg. per cent vs. time of sulfisomidine, free acid (HS) and salt (NaS) administered in various suppository vehicles. (Data from Pennati, L., and Steiger Trippi, K.: Pharm. acta Helv. 33:663, 1958)

should be globular or oviform in shape and should weigh about 5 Gm.

Cold Process. Cocoa butter and other fat bases that do not require melting in order to secure mixing may be fashioned into suppositories by the cold process. This method is not suited to the use of glycerinated gelatin. The desired amount of grated cocoa butter is mixed with the medicament, or medicaments, and worked into a plastic mass with the aid of a mortar, pestle and spatula. A small quantity of fixed oil may be added to facilitate the preparation of a mass. Better distribution of the drug is obtained if it is first mixed with only a portion of the base. The remainder of the base can be worked in gradually. Powders should be triturated to a fine state of subdivision; solid extracts and powdered extracts often are incorporated more easily if they are first levigated with a small amount of dilute alcohol or glycerin. Small amounts of liquids may be taken up in an inert excipient (wool fat). The final mass must be kneaded until the drug is well dispersed. The mass then may be shaped by the use of either a metallic press or the fingers. Presses of various designs have appeared on the market; the type shown in Figure 161 is entirely suitable. When the metallic press is to be used, the well-kneaded mass should be thoroughly chilled and granulated. The prepared mass is then placed in a cylinder (chilled by ice or dry ice) fitted with a piston which forces the mass through an orifice into the attached mold. The molds are interchangeable and are obtainable in shapes suitable for the preparation of vaginal, rectal and urethral suppositories. Cold compression offers the advantages of ease of manufacture, uniformity of suppository and a superior looking product when

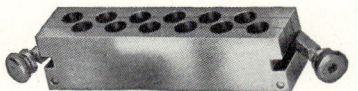

FIG. 162. Suppository mold opening longitudinally.

compared with the hand-molded suppository.

In the absence of a compression machine, the suppository may be molded by hand. The mass is rolled into a cylinder, as in the preparation of pills, the cylinder divided on a graduated pill tile, and the suppositories shaped by the use of the fingers and a spatula. The necessary skill is not too difficult to acquire. Since an individual's skin temperature may exceed the melting point of cocoa, it may be necessary to keep the hands cool by dipping in ice water. The use of starch as a dusting powder is an important aid to good technic. Lycopodium is contraindicated as it has allergic potentialities, and talc is to be discouraged since it is known to be the cause of surgical adhesions. The necessity of well-scrubbed hands is obvious.

Fusion Process. The preparation of cocoa butter suppositories by the fusion method requires careful attention to cer-

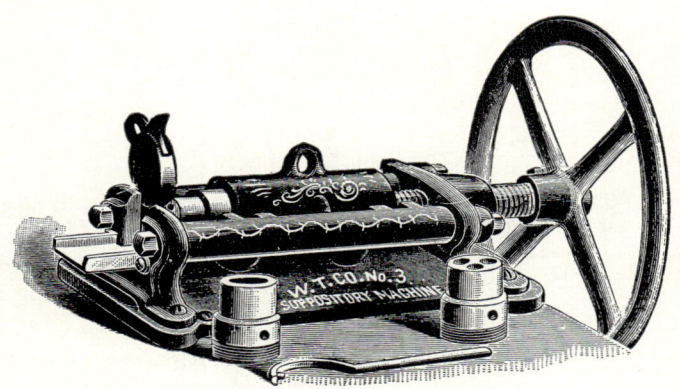

FIG. 161. Metallic press for shaping suppositories.

tain details. The fusion temperature as well as the temperature of the mold must be controlled carefully. The following procedure has been shown to be economical of time and to produce excellent suppositories:

1. Grate the cocoa butter carefully avoiding large particles.
2. Weigh the prescription ingredients and mix lightly with a stirring rod. The use of a stirring rod avoids the pressure usually encountered with the use of a pestle. Place the mixture in a small glass beaker.
3. Heat a slightly larger beaker about half full of water to around 50° C. Time may be saved by using hot water from the tap.
4. Place the beaker full of the prescription ingredients within the beaker of hot water. Glass beakers permit one to observe the mixture better than do other types of containers and the thin walls reduce the chance of overheating. Stir the mixture with a thermometer. The mass usually will soften at 31° C. and must be kept at or below 33° C.
5. When the mixture reaches 33° C., separate the beakers. Stir until the large cocoa butter particles melt and until the mixture appears uniform.
6. Pour the thick mixture into a metal mold at *room temperature*. After a minute or two, the suppositories will become somewhat firm; place the mold in a freezer for about 2 minutes. After this brief period in the freezer, open the lock nuts of the mold and apply pressure to the top of the suppositories. They will easily snap free from the mold.

Whether this procedure or another one is adopted, it is advisable to melt the mixture at a minimum temperature and to use a room-temperature mold. The use of a room-temperature mold will increase the over-all time of preparation no more than 2 or 3 minutes, while the use of a previously frozen mold may cause some supercooling and crystallization into the lower melting forms.

Very adequate aluminum alloy molds are available at moderate cost in 6-, 12- and larger-cavity capacities. A plastic mold is available; however, the slow rate of heat transfer makes this type of mold inferior to a metal mold in preparing not only cocoa butter suppositories but also many wax and water-miscible types. The plastic mold is adequate for preparing glycerinated gelatin suppositories.

The amount of base needed for each suppository depends on the size of the mold and the displacement value of the drug. Suppository molds differ in the amount of base accommodated. The pharmacist can ascertain the capacity of his mold by measuring the volume of water required to fill it. There are available several tables giving the amount of cocoa butter displaced by a given amount of drug. If necessary, the pharmacist may determine the displacement value for the particular formula as follows:

To the desired amount of medication, an amount of base known to be insufficient is added. The mixture is poured into the molds, and sufficient base is added to fill the molds completely. The suppositories are remelted, mixed and poured. Observation of the weight of the substances plus a simple calculation gives a displacement value that may be filed for future use.

When preparing suppositories in larger quantities with insufficient number of molds in which to pour the entire mass, one usually will find that the fused mass will solidify and require reheating. Szekely proposed that the fused mass be placed in a Dewar vacuum flask and one of the common commercial plastic siphon tubes be placed through a stopper in the top of the Dewar. The fused mass may be transferred from the Dewar by depressing the plunger on the top of the siphon.

BIBLIOGRAPHY

Allawala, N. A., and Riegelman, S.: J. Am. Pharm. A. **42**:267, 1954.
Andrews, M. J.: J. Am. Pharm. A. **23**:1002, 1934.
Barach, J.: J.A.M.A. **128**:589, 1945.
Bird, J. C.: J. Am. Pharm. A. **26**:475, 1937.
Bucher, K.: Helv. physiol. acta **6**:821, 1937.
Büchi, J., and Oesch, P.: Pharm. acta helv. **20**:129, 1945.

Caldwell, A. F.: J. Pharm. & Pharmacol. **12:** 680, 1939.

Cemeli, J., and Del Pozo, A.: Galenica acta **7:**249, 1954.

Charannat, R., Chevillard, L., and Giono, L.: Ann. pharm. franc. **7:**627, 1949.

Czetsch-Lindenwald, H. V.: *in* Suppositorien, Cantor (Ed.), Aulendorf, Württ, 1958.

Del Pozo, A., and Cemeli, J.: Galenica acta **7:**137, 1954.

Diepgen, P.: Das Analzapfchen in der Geschichte der Therapie, Stuttgart, Thieme, 1953.

Eckert, V., and Muhlemann, H.: Pharm. acta helv. **33:**649, 1958.

Eckert, V.: Die Abgabe von Arzneistoffen aus Fettartigen Suppositorien-Grundmassen, Dissertation for Pharmacy Doctorate, University Bern, Switzerland, Basel, Ameba, 1959.

Enesco, J., Branisteanu, D., and Dangeaunu, J.: Bull. acad. méd. roumanie 4:1, 1939.

Fabre, M. R., and Regnier, M.: Ann. Pharm. fran. **9:**318, 1951.

Gross, H. M., and Becker, S. H.: J. Am. Pharm. A. 42:90, 1953.

Hassler, W. H., and Sperandio, G. J.: J. Am. Pharm. A. (Pract. Ed.) **14:**26, 1953.

Michelfelder, T. J., and Peck, S M.: J. Invest. Dermat. **19:**237, 1952.

Miller, M., and Groedel, F. M. Am. J. Digest. Dis. **17:** 157, 1950.

Muhleman, H., and Neuenschwander, R.: Pharm. acta helv. **31:**305, 1956.

Pennati, L., and Steiger-Trippi, K.: Pharm. acta helv. **33:**663, 1958.

Peterson, C., Lee, C. O., and Christian, J. E.: J. Am. Pharm. A. (Sci. Ed.) **42:**731, 1953.

Polano, M. K., Bonsel, and VanderMeer: Dermatologica **101:**69, 1950.

Prout, W. A.: J. Am. Pharm. A. **25:**1123, 1936.

Rapp, R.: Pharm. Vtg. **72:**312, 1927.

Riegelman, S., and Crowell, W. J.: J. Am. Pharm. A. (Sci. Ed.) **47:**115; 123; 127, 1959.

Robinson, G. D.: J. Pharmacol. & Exper. Therap. **32:**81, 1927.

Rudolfo, A. S., *et al.*: Am. J. Med. Sc. **237:** 585, 1959.

Schanker, L. S.: J. Pharmacol. & Exper. Therap. **126:**283, 1959.

Szekely, I. J., and Lange, A. G.: J. Am. Pharm. A. (Pract. Ed.) **14:**385, 1954.

Tice, L. F., and Abrams, R. E.: Am. Prof. Pharm. **18:**327, 1952; J. Am. Pharm. A. (Pract. Ed.) **14:**24, 1953.

Truitt, E. B., McKusick, J. A., and Krantz, J. C., Jr.: J. Pharmacol. & Exper. Therap. **100:**309, 1950.

Vaeck, S. V.: Internat. Chocolate Rev. **6:**100, 1951.

Thomas Dudley Rowe, Ph.D.
Dean and Professor of Pharmacy, University of Michigan College of Pharmacy

20

Spirits and Elixirs

SPIRITS IN GENERAL
  HISTORY
OFFICIAL SPIRITS

ELIXIRS
  CLASSIFICATION OF ELIXIRS
  UNOFFICIAL ELIXIRS

SPIRITS IN GENERAL

Spirits may be defined as solutions of volatile substances in alcohol. The volatile substances in the majority of cases are volatile oils. The amount of volatile material in spirits varies greatly, and no fixed percentage can be given. In past editions, the N.F. contained a monograph, "Spirits of Volatile Oils," which specified that 6.5 per cent of volatile oil was to be used. This monograph is no longer official, presumably because the amount of oil indicated was considerably lower than that used in the majority of spirits and also because there was little demand for a general formula. In all cases, the volatile oil content of the official spirits is much greater than that of the corresponding aromatic waters.

Likewise, the alcohol content varies. The lowest percentage is in Compound Myrcia Spirit, N.F. XI, with a permissible range of 54 to 59 per cent. The highest is in Ethyl Nitrite Spirit, N.F. XI, with 85 to 93 per cent.

The term "essence" is often used in place of the word "spirit."

In preparing spirits, it must be kept in mind that the oils dissolved in alcohol are precipitated when the solutions are mixed with water. In order to avoid this precipitation, water, except as specified in the formula, should be avoided. Graduates and other equipment used should be thoroughly dry. Filter paper should be moistened with alcohol.

History

Although spirits are an older class of preparations than elixirs, their historical background and development is not established clearly. The introduction of spirits into pharmacy and medicine was brought about by the development of distillation procedures. By these means, volatile oils first were separated from the other constituents of the crude drugs in which they are found.

Brandy and whisky are the first spirits of which there is historical record. The exact date of their discovery is uncertain. However, the distillation of wine was carried out by the early Egyptians.[1] Brandy and whisky differ in many respects from the usual spirits of today inasmuch as they are not prepared by dissolving a volatile substance in alcohol. The first reference in European pharmacy to a spirit made from wine was by Arnaldus of Villanova, in the 13th century. He distilled herbs such as rosemary and sage with it, and highly recommended the medicinal virtues of these preparations.

Alcoholic solutions of volatile oils are probably an outgrowth of the perfume industry. As more and more volatile oils became known, it was only natural that they

367

368 Spirits and Elixirs

should be mixed and made into fragrant blends. This industry developed during the 15th and the 16th centuries, and in 1725 J. Maria Farina of Cologne introduced eau de cologne.[1] The perfumed spirit of *N.F. VIII* is similar to one introduced by Farina.

By the beginning of the 19th century, many volatile oils were known and some of their chemistry had been worked out. However, the term "spirit" for alcoholic solutions of these oils came into common use only very gradually. The first *U.S.P.* classified many of the earlier spirits as tinctures, primarily because the liquids were prepared by extracting the volatile oils from the crude drugs by maceration or percolation with alcohol. Either volatile oils were not obtainable easily at that time, or else it was thought that extraction from the crude drug gave a more suitable product. Through *U.S.P. III*, many of the spirits were still classified as tinctures. There were some official spirits but they usually consisted of both the crude drug extractive and a volatile oil. It was not until the 4th revision that the crude drugs were deleted as sources of volatile oils in the spirits. Prior to that time, some spirits were made from the crude drugs and some from the volatile oils.

The first *U.S.P.* (1820) had 3 spirits all made by distillation after maceration. There are now 3 in *U.S.P. XVI* and 6 in *N.F. XI*. There were 7 spirits official in *N.F. X*.

OFFICIAL SPIRITS

Even though the total number of official spirits is small, it is not possible to classify them to any extent into the therapeutic or pharmaceutical groupings. This situation exists because there is a different and separate medicinal action for nearly every one of the official spirits. Consequently, they are discussed for the most part individually rather than in groups.

Those used as carminatives and flavors are **Compound Cardamom Spirit (N.F. XI)** and **Peppermint Spirit (U.S.P. XVI).** Given orally in small doses, usually 1 ml., each of these spirits is effective as a carminative. **Peppermint spirit** is used extensively for that purpose.

Mixed with other drugs or preparations, they may be used also as flavors. Thus, each of them may be used alone or in mixtures. Both are prepared from volatile oils.

Peppermint spirit is more than a mere solution of the volatile oil in that a small amount of crude drug is used in its preparation as follows. First the leaves are macerated in water to remove tannins, xanthophyll and other principles soluble in water. The aqueous extract is discarded, the leaves expressed and then macerated in alcohol. The alcohol dissolves the chlorophyll so that the final product has a bright green color. To this alcoholic solution containing the chlorophyll, 10 per cent volatile oil is added. The leaves used do not impart any medicinal action to the preparation. This action comes from the volatile oil added to the alcohol.

Many of the commercial products of this spirit are colorless. Thus, they do not conform to the *U.S.P.* specification requiring green color but they do have the same therapeutic value.

Compound Orange Spirit (U.S.P.) is used almost entirely as a flavoring agent. It is a blend of several oils. It is prepared by simple solution and can be made up readily. It is an important ingredient of aromatic elixir.

Aromatic Ammonia Spirit (U.S.P.), frequently referred to (improperly) as "ammonia," is one of the best-known spirits. It will be found in a handy location in practically every drugstore. It acts as a carminative due to the volatile oils present, as an antacid and as a mild reflex circulatory stimulant. This latter effect is produced by the liberation of NH_3 from the ammonium carbonate which the spirit contains. This preparation occasionally is asked for by the dose and is used in cases of fainting. Because of the oils present, it makes a milky preparation when mixed with water. This precipitation does not affect its medicinal action and is a typical behavior of all spirits which contain volatile oils.

In making Aromatic Ammonia Spirit, the *U.S.P.* specifies the use of translucent pieces of ammonia carbonate. This specification is included because of the peculiar chemical nature of this compound. The official ammonium carbonate is a mixture of ammonium bicarbonate and ammonium carbamate. Its chemical formula is $NH_4HCO_3 \cdot NH_4NH_2CO_2$. The bicarbonate portion is insoluble in alcohol while the carbamate portion is alcohol-soluble. On exposure to air, more of the insoluble bicarbonate is formed by the loss of CO_2 and NH_3. The entire compound eventually becomes opaque. The opaque form is composed primarily of the alcohol-insoluble bicarbonate and is unsuitable for use in this preparation.

Diluted ammonia solution (10% NH_4OH) is used to dissolve the translucent ammonium carbonate. It converts all of the official ammonium carbonate to $(NH_4)_2CO_3$, which readily is soluble in alcohol.

Unless the original material is translucent, the conversion to the alcohol-soluble form is not complete due to the presence of excess NH_4HCO_3 in the opaque form. Therefore, the use of this form would produce a spirit below the required strength.

It takes several days to make this preparation. At the end of that time, it is usually colorless. On standing, it is apt to assume a pale amber color unless preserved according to U.S.P. directions. The color change is due to the oxidation of the oils. Apparently, the color change does not alter the medicinal action of the preparation.

Camphor Spirit, N.F., like aromatic ammonia spirit, is well known to the lay public. It is referred to as Tincture of Camphor and also as Camphor. This preparation is a simple solution of 10 per cent camphor in alcohol. It rarely is used internally, but its external use is very common. Usually it is applied to "cold sores" and similar ailments.

Ethyl Nitrite Spirit, N.F., usually is sold under its synonym of Sweet Spirit of Nitre or Spirit of Nitrous Ether. It is a well-known household remedy, widely used as a diaphoretic.

The ethyl nitrite decomposes readily when exposed to light and air, or when mixed with other drugs. Due to its unstable nature, the N.F. specifications for preservation should be followed closely.

This spirit often is prescribed with other liquids. In most cases, particularly if the second liquid is acid in reaction, the spirit decomposes within a very short time. For this reason, it is best if the spirit is not prescribed with other drugs.

The N.F. gives no method of manufacture for this preparation. A method formerly was given but it was too complex and dangerous to be carried out in the average pharmacy. When prepared in stores today, a concentrate of ethyl nitrite is used. This liquid comes in a sealed tube like a large ampul. The tube is kept refrigerated. When opened, the contents are dissolved in alcohol. The spirit prepared in this manner meets N.F. specifications.

Two spirits previously mentioned, **whisky** and **brandy**, are official in the N.F. The question of their therapeutic value is debated by physicians; however, many authorities[2-4] claim that both of these preparations have definite therapeutic value. They are used in the treatment of certain diseases of the vascular system, and in various discomforts associated with senescence. The therapeutic effect depends largely on their depressant action on the central nervous system. Both of them are made by distillation; whisky from the fermented mash of wholly or partially germinated malted cereal grains (barley, wheat, corn, rye) and brandy from "fermented juice of sound ripe grapes." The N.F. gives detailed specifications that apply to both preparations.

Compound Myrcia Spirit, N.F., is similar to bay rum which is sold so widely as a hair dressing and a shaving lotion. It is a blend of several oils in alcohol and water which together produce the pleasing odor commonly associated with bay rum.

ELIXIRS

Of the official liquid preparations for oral administration, elixirs probably are used the most widely. Their popularity is due to their pleasant flavor, their relative stability and the ease with which most of them are prepared.

Elixirs originally were defined as sweetened hydroalcoholic solutions containing flavoring materials, and usually medicinal substances. Their primary solvents were alcohol and water. This definition has limitations because of the many exceptions now on the market. Originally, however, elixirs were distinguished from other classes of preparations by the presence of sugar and alcohol in the finished product. Several of the official elixirs—compound pepsin elixir for example—do not contain sugar or any other sweetening agent. Furthermore, some commercial elixirs do not contain alcohol. Consequently, while the definition as presented covers many elixirs, it should be kept in mind that many commercial products and a few official ones do not meet the specifications of the definition given. In the official elixirs, the alcohol content varies from 4 to 40 per cent. Generally, there is just enough alcohol to keep volatile oils or the medicinal substances in solution.

Glycerin is also present in most elixirs. During World War II, the shortage of glycerin necessitated that it be replaced by some other liquid. Propylene glycol was found to be satisfactory, and the Bulletin of the *N.F.* published the formulas in which propylene glycol could be used to replace glycerin.[5] In most cases today, glycerin has been reincorporated as part of the formulas.

Although most elixirs can be prepared by simple procedures, their small-scale manufacture is often time-consuming and wasteful. These difficulties are encountered because of the need of filtering the liquids with talc. Under aromatic elixir, a more complete discussion of this problem is presented (p. 371).

Elixirs generally owe their pleasant flavor to the presence of sugar and the volatile flavoring agents. Their sugar content is lower than that of syrups.

History

Elixirs as we know them today are a comparatively new class of preparations. According to Lloyd,[6] the first published formula of an elixir containing sugar as a sweetening agent appeared in 1859. For centuries before that time, many substances were called elixirs, but the word was used to designate "the magical transformation powder, so much sought after, a pinch of which would convert a whole mass of base metal into gold."[6] Later, the word was used "to denote various preparations more or less alchemistic."[6] In the 18th century, the term was applied to liquid medicinal preparations. However, these preparations were more like our present-day tinctures and not comparable with modern elixirs.

Lloyd probably is responsible for the accepted pharmaceutical conception of elixirs. His book of elixirs,[6] published in 1883, clarified the confusion regarding these liquids and put them into a definite category. This book contained 283 formulas of these preparations. According to the *History of the National Formulary*,[7] it was this book and the *New York and Brooklyn Formulary*, also published in 1883, which stimulated the American Pharmaceutical Association to consider the publication of a national formulary.

Although elixirs are still popular today, they reached the height of their demand during the latter part of the 19th century. The first *N.F.*, which contained a total of 435 preparations, included 86 elixirs. Today, there are 17 official elixirs in *N.F. XI* of a total of more than 700 preparations included therein. *U.S.P. XVI* recognizes only 6 elixirs. Probably the main reason for the *U.S.P.* including so few and the *N.F.* so many is the difference in policy on admissions. As with many items, the chemicals are official in the *U.S.P.* on the basis of medical necessity and therapeutic value. The preparations containing these chemicals are official in the *N.F.* on the basis of physician demand or extent of use.

Classification of Elixirs

Elixirs divide naturally into 2 classes—*medicated* and *nonmedicated*. In many instances, it is difficult to decide into which group the elixir falls. As in many classifications, the grouping presented is an arbitrary one.

Nonmedicated Elixirs

Aromatic Elixir, U.S.P.
Red Aromatic Elixir, N.F.
Compound Benzaldehyde Elixir, N.F.
Glycyrrhiza Elixir, N.F.
Iso-Alcoholic Elixir, N.F.

All other elixirs are classified as medicated. Such elixirs as Compound Pepsin Elixir might easily be classed as nonmedicated, for their medical action is very slight. They frequently are used as vehicles.

While those of the nonmedicated group are chiefly vehicles, it should be emphasized that classification as a medicated elixir does not preclude its use for solvent purposes. Thus, phenobarbital elixir has a decided therapeutic action, yet it frequently is prescribed as the vehicle for other drugs.

The primary purpose of either type is to make it possible for medicines to be dispensed in a palatable form.

Aromatic Elixir. Of the elixirs in this group, aromatic elixir is by far the most widely used. It is used as the main solvent in 3 official elixirs. Of these 3, some are used to make other elixirs and in preparing other official preparations. It also is used extensively in extemporaneous prescriptions. Because of its importance, it is desirable to discuss it in detail.

By consulting the formula in the U.S.P., it will be seen that aromatic elixir is a rather simple preparation. Yet it is a difficult elixir to make properly. This difficulty arises because of the slowness with which it filters and the necessity for refiltration before the preparation becomes clear. Clearness is one requisite of all elixirs. On a small scale, it is not unusual for 10 to 20 per cent of the entire volume to be lost during filtration, due to the number of times that the liquid is passed through the filter. The loss of liquid is costly, and a long time is required. Consequently, many druggists do not attempt to prepare their own aromatic elixir but buy it from manufacturing houses.

Considerable research has been done to improve the method of making the preparation, but none of the results has been entirely satisfactory. Fantus,[8] Lee[9] and Burlage[10] have all suggested new methods for making this solution. None of their suggestions has been accepted by the U.S.P., with the result that the preparation today is much the same as it was many years ago.

The slowness in filtration results from the syrup's being added before the preparation is filtered. This ingredient, plus the talc, makes it nearly impossible to get a good rate of filtration. It is necessary to use talc as a filtering agent to help absorb the excess oils present. Fantus suggested dissolving the sugar in the filtrate to increase the rate.

The cloudiness is due to the insolubility in water of the oils present in compound orange spirit, which is one of the basic ingredients of this elixir. Burlage suggested the use of terpeneless oils (water-soluble) to avoid this difficulty. Both of these suggestions make it possible for the elixir to be made more rapidly. It is hoped that in future editions the U.S.P. will accept something along these lines to improve the preparation.

The sugar content of the finished product is about 31 per cent, or less than half that of syrup. The alcohol content is from 21 to 23 per cent by volume. It should be noted that this elixir may be diluted with water without becoming turbid. Consequently, it can be used with aqueous preparations without producing a milky liquid.

Red Aromatic Elixir, N.F., is aromatic elixir to which has been added amaranth solution to make it red in color. It can be used in most cases when a red-colored vehicle is desired.

Both of these preparations are stable under ordinary conditions.

Iso-Alcoholic Elixir is a comparatively new type, having first appeared in N.F. VI. It is composed of 2 separate parts: low alcoholic elixir with an alcohol content of from 8 to 10 per cent, and high alcoholic elixir with an alcohol content of from 73 to 78 per cent. By mixing these 2 solutions according to the directions given in N.F. XI, a final product may be obtained which has an alcohol content within the ranges given above. There is considerable need for this type of elixir. Doctors frequently prescribe aromatic elixir or some other liquid as a vehicle for drugs soluble only in high percentage alcohol. In such cases, the prescription must be dispensed as a shake mixture. If iso-alcoholic elixir were prescribed, the drug could be dispensed in solution by using the right proportion of the low and the high alcoholic elixirs. Unfortunately, this elixir has not become widely used. It is the type of preparation which pharmacists should call to the attention of physicians. It is easy to prepare, and both forms are stable. The product is similar in flavor and odor to aromatic elixir.

Other Nonmedicated Elixirs. These require little discussion. They are used when a flavor corresponding to their main ingredients is desired. Both **glycyrrhiza** and **benzaldehyde elixirs** are prepared by simple solution.

Medicated Elixirs

This group can be described best by further classifying them according to their therapeutic activity.

Sedatives and Hypnotics

This is the largest group of elixirs having a definite therapeutic action. In all, there are 8 elixirs in this division. They are:

Sodium Bromide Elixir, N.F.
Three Bromides Elixir, N.F.
Amobarbital Elixir, N.F.
Butabarbital Sodium Elixir, N.F.
Pentobarbital Elixir, U.S.P.
Phenobarbital Elixir, U.S.P.
Secobarbital Elixir, U.S.P.
Methyprylon Elixir, N.F.

Each of these preparations illustrates the primary function of an elixir—to present a drug in a palatable form. This function is particularly true of the elixirs containing bromides. These chemicals have a disagreeable saltlike flavor which is difficult to mask. Even in the elixirs, the saline flavor is still noticeable but is not so pronounced.

Elixirs Containing Bromides. The 2 elixirs containing bromides are old favorites and are in widespread use today. Of the 2, three bromides elixir probably is prescribed most. The dose (5 ml.) contains 0.4 Gm. of each of the bromides or a total of 1.2 Gm. per teaspoonful. The preparation is red in color, due to the presence of amaranth solution. It has a tendency to precipitate on standing.

Sodium bromide elixir contains .875 Gm. per 5-ml. dose

Both of the bromide elixirs are low in alcohol content, containing 3 to 7 per cent by volume. The low alcohol content is necessitated by the relatively slight solubility of the bromides in alcohol in comparison with their solubility in water. For example, 1 Gm. of sodium bromide will dissolve in 1.2 ml. of water, whereas about 16 ml. of alcohol is needed to dissolve 1 Gm. of this salt. With a fairly high concentration of bromide in each of the elixirs, it is obvious that low alcohol concentration is required in order to have the bromides remain in solution.

Elixirs Containing Barbiturates. There are 5 official elixirs in this category: Amobarbital Elixir and Butabarbital Sodium Elixir, both in the *N.F.*; and Pentobarbital Elixir, Phenobarbital Elixir and Secobarbital Elixir, all in the *U.S.P.*

Phenobarbital is used for long-acting sedation; amobarbital and butabarbital for intermediate duration; and pentobarbital and secobarbital are commonly used short-acting barbiturates.[11]

Each of these contains approximately 0.020 Gm. (⅓ gr.) of active ingredient per dose (5 ml.). When that amount of the drugs is taken, they act as mild sedatives. All 5 of the preparations often are used in combination with other drugs.

The method of dissolving the barbiturate differs in each case. In phenobarbital elixir, the active ingredient first is dissolved in alcohol before adding the other liquids. While phenobarbital dissolves readily in alcohol and will remain in solution when the alcohol content is lowered, it will dissolve with difficulty in the alcohol, water and glycerin mixture of the final product.

Actually, the amount of alcohol in the final product (12 to 15%) would not keep the phenobarbital in solution. The presence of the glycerin prevents the phenobarbital from precipitating. According to Krause and Cross,[13] "glycerin and glycerin water solutions are poor solvents for phenobarbital," but "the solubility of phenobarbital in alcohol is enhanced by the addition of glycerin." This point is illustrated further by one of their tables, which shows that 10 per cent alcohol will dissolve 0.19 per cent phenobarbital while 10 per cent alcohol to which is added 40 per cent glycerin will dissolve 0.5 per cent phenobarbital.

In amobarbital elixir, methenamine is used to increase the solubility of the amobarbital. In pentobarbital elixir, the sodium salt which is readily water-soluble is used. This compound, after being dissolved, later is converted to pentobarbital by adding diluted hydrochloric acid. The conversion is necessary because pentobarbital sodium is not stable in solution but decomposes on standing. By starting out with the sodium salt, the solution is prepared more readily.

The Durham-Humphrey law, a federal regulation, requires that preparations in which a barbiturate is one of the main ingredients must have a prescription, either oral or written, before they can be dispensed. This regulation applies to these 5 elixirs. Some state laws concerning the sale of barbiturate preparations are even more restrictive than the Durham-Humphrey law. In such cases, the state regulations must be followed.

Methyprylon Elixir, N.F. The chemical used in this elixir is a relatively new nonbarbiturate sedative and hypnotic. Drill[12] states, "The depressant effects of methyprylon on the central nervous system resemble those of the intermediate to short-acting barbiturates, pentobarbital and secobarbital."

He also states, "Methyprylon may be employed to advantage when the latter drugs (barbiturates) are contraindicated."

This elixir is official for the first time in N.F. XI.

Stomachics (Bitters)

There are 3 members of this, the second largest group of medicated elixirs. They are:

Iron, Quinine and Strychnine Elixir, N.F.
Iron, Quinine and Strychnine Phosphates Elixir, N.F.
Glycerinated Gentian Elixir, N.F.

Of those listed above, the two best known are: iron, quinine and strychnine elixir and iron, quinine and strychnine phosphates elixir.

Iron, quinine and strychnine elixir is used for its iron content as well as its stomachic properties and is well known to the laity. It is doubtful if it has enough iron present in the official 5-ml. dose to be of much value as a hematinic. It is bright green in color, due to the ferric citrochloride tincture used in this preparation.

Iron, quinine and strychnine phosphates elixir was introduced because it was thought at one time that the phosphates of the drugs involved were more effective than the other forms. This belief has never been substantiated, yet the preparation is preferred by some physicians over iron, quinine and strychnine elixir. Like the latter, this preparation has little action other than as a bitter. This elixir has a greenish-brown color which makes it easily distinguishable from the bright-green iron, quinine and strychnine elixir. Neither of these elixirs contains sugar.

Both of them owe their so-called "tonic" effect to the fact that they increase appetite.

Beef, Iron and Wine (N.F. XI) is not now classified as an elixir but in former *National Formularies* it was entitled Elixir of Beef and Iron. This preparation is well known to the laity and has been in use for many years in the same manner as the 2 elixirs mentioned above. It is less bitter than either of them.

The other elixir in this group presents no special problems. For the most part it is not used extensively.

Digestants

Compound Pepsin Elixir, N.F.

Although only one elixir is now official in this group, it is so widely used that it is placed in a separate classification. There are 2 commonly used synonyms for it—Compound Digestive Elixir and Lactated Pepsin Elixir. Usually it is prescribed under the latter name.

Pepsin is a proteolytic enzyme which aids in the digestion of proteins. It is generally agreed that pepsin as administered in this elixir, or other pepsin-containing elixirs, is of little therapeutic value. However, the lactated pepsin elixir is one of the most popular of all vehicles. It probably is used more generally as a vehicle in extemporaneous prescriptions than any other official elixir. It has a pleasant flavor, although no sugar is used in it, it is red in color, and it keeps better than some of the other elixirs. These properties are partly responsible for

Expectorants

The 2 elixirs included under this heading have an extensive use. They are: **Terpin Hydrate Elixir, N.F.,** and **Terpin Hydrate and Codeine Elixir, N.F.** Codeine is dissolved in the former to prepare the latter.

Neither of these elixirs can be diluted with much water or the slightly water-soluble terpin hydrate will precipitate. In this inability to mix with water, they differ from most of the other elixirs, to which water may be added in any quantity.

These elixirs contain the highest percentage of alcohol (39 to 44%) of all elixirs in order to keep the terpin hydrate in solution. The terpin hydrate and codeine elixir contains $9/10$ gr. of codeine per fluidounce and is, therefore, an exempt narcotic. If sold without a doctor's prescription, it must be recorded according to the directions given under the Harrison Narcotic Law.

Because of the high percentage of alcohol and glycerin in these 2 preparations, there are numerous nonofficial formulas in use. Most of these conform to the official preparations as far as the active constituents are concerned, but they are usually less viscous and less palatable.

They are probably the most efficacious cough remedies of all the official preparations.

Antihistaminics

Diphenhydramine Hydrochloride Elixir, U.S.P.

Tripelennamine Citrate Elixir, U.S.P.
Diphenhydramine Hydrochloride was introduced originally under the trade name Benadryl. Tripelennamine Citrate is the citrate form rather than the hydrochloride of tripelennamine which in the hydrochloride form was introduced as Pyribenzamine.

These two chemicals were among the first antihistamines to be used medicinally. They represent 2 different chemical classes of antihistamines, but both have the same general therapeutic action.

Diphenhydramine Hydrochloride Elixir was first official in *U.S.P. XV*. It was the first new elixir to appear in any *U.S.P.* since the 12th revision published in 1942. Tripelennamine Citrate Elixir is official for the first time in *U.S.P. XVI*.

There are many commercial elixirs on the market containing one form or another of the various antihistaminics. They are used extensively, and those official in the *U.S.P.* represent 2 types whose therapeutic merit have been well established over a period of years.

Miscellaneous Elixirs

Aminoacetic Acid Elixir, N.F., is a simple solution of the active ingredient in a palatable vehicle. The elixir is used in the treatment of achlorhydria.

Benzestrol Elixir, N.F., is official for the first time in *N.F. XI*. It presents an estrogen in a liquid dosage form suitable for oral use. The usual dose of 5 ml. contains about 2 mg. of Benzestrol.

UNOFFICIAL ELIXIRS

There are on the market many elixirs not or not yet recognized by the *U.S.P.* or the *N.F.* It would be impractical to attempt to include all of them in this chapter. However, there are some that are used so widely it is necessary that they be mentioned.

The 4 best-known types probably are:

Thiamine Hydrochloride Elixir
Ferrous Sulfate Elixir
Ferrous Sulfate and Thiamine Hydrochloride Elixir
Vitamin B Complex Elixir

Ferrous sulfate elixir is mentioned as a type of iron-containing elixir. Many preparations contain other ferrous salts in place of the sulfate. The end-results are the same in that an elixir is available which is of value in cases of mild iron deficiency. The amount of iron salt present is usually from 4 to 5 per cent.

Ferrous sulfate syrup was introduced in *N.F. VIII*. It is possible that this syrup was included to fill the demand for a liquid ferrous sulfate preparation. It was deleted from *N.F. IX;* it was official in *U.S.P. XV.* and now is in *N.F. XI*.

An elixir of ferrous sulfate with thiamine hydrochloride combines the advantages of both of these drugs. The elixir is particularly effective in cases of poor appetite. The quantity of ferrous sulfate is the same as in the plain elixir, and the thiamine hydrochloride is usually present to the extent of 5 to 10 mg. (1,665 to 3,330 units) per fluidounce.

The vitamin B complex elixir is similar to plain thiamine hydrochloride elixir. Here the entire B complex is present. There are also some B complex elixirs with ferrous salts.

All of these preparations appear under various trade names.

REFERENCES

1. Gildemeister, E., and Hoffman, F.: The Volatile Oils, ed. 2, Vol. I, translated by Edward Kremers, New York, Wiley, 1913.
2. Goodman, L., and Gilman, A.: The Pharmacological Basis of Therapeutics, New York, Macmillan, 1955.
3. Cushny, A. R.: Pharmacology and Therapeutics, ed. 13, revised by C. W. Edmunds and J. A. Gunn, Philadelphia, Lea & Febiger, 1947.
4. Sollman, T.: A Manual of Pharmacology, ed. 7, Philadelphia, Saunders, 1948.
5. Bull. National Formulary Comm. 11: 201, 1943.
6. Lloyd, J. U.: Elixirs, Cincinnati, Clarke, 1883.
7. National Formulary, ed. 10, Washington, D. C., American Pharmaceutical Association, 1955.
8. Fantus, B., Dyniewicz, H. A., and Dyniewicz, J. M.: J. Am. Pharm. 22:655, 1933.
9. Lee, C. O., and Close, M.: J. Am. Pharm. A. 23:236, 1934.
10. Smith, W. J., and Burlage, H. M.: J. Am. Pharm. A. 25:123, 1936.
11. Modell W. (Ed.): Drugs of Choice 1958-59, St. Louis, Mosby, 1958.
12. Drill, V. A. (ed.): Pharmacology in Medicine, New York, McGraw-Hill, 1958.
13. Krause, G. M., and Cross, J. M.: J. Am. Pharm. A. 40:137, 1951.
14. Salter, W. T.: A Textbook of Pharmacology, Philadelphia, Saunders, 1952.

WILLIAM ARTHUR PURDUM, Ph.D.

Vice President in Charge of Production and Development, Burrough Brothers Manufacturing Co., and Professor of Hospital Pharmacy, University of Maryland

21

Vinegars, Tinctures, Fluidextracts, Fluidglycerates and Extracts

VINEGARS
TINCTURES
    TINCTURES OF THE U.S.P.
    TINCTURES OF THE N.F.
    NONOFFICIAL TINCTURES
FLUIDEXTRACTS
    FLUIDEXTRACTS OF THE U.S.P.
FLUIDEXTRACTS OF THE N.F.
NONOFFICIAL FLUIDEXTRACTS
FLUIDGLYCERATES
EXTRACTS
    EXTRACT OF THE U.S.P.
    EXTRACTS OF THE N.F.
    NONOFFICIAL EXTRACTS

VINEGARS (ACETA)

GENERAL CONSIDERATIONS

Medicated vinegars are liquid preparations made by extracting drugs with diluted acetic acid. Originally, they were made by using vinegar as the menstruum, but this practice was discontinued because of the lack of uniformity of different lots of vinegar, these varying in both acetic acid content and color. Diluted acetic acid contains from 5.7 to 6.3 Gm. of $C_2H_4O_2$ in each 100 ml. and is the weakest of the 3 strengths of this acid which are recognized officially.

HISTORY

Medicinal vinegars represent one of the oldest classes of galenic preparations. The ancients recognized the superior solvent powers of vinegar over water and also realized that products made with vinegar kept for a longer period of time than did the infusions and the decoctions prepared with water. This, of course, was centuries before distilled spirit (alcohol) was known.

Vinegars are little used today, and none is official. Tinctures and fluidextracts largely have taken the place of the vinegars of former years.

SQUILL VINEGAR, N.F. X
Acetum Scillæ

Squill Vinegar is a very old preparation—in fact, it is believed that the original formula was devised by **Galen** during the 2nd century.

It is prepared by maceration of coarsely powdered squill in diluted acetic acid for 7 days. Then, the mixture is strained to remove the marc, the strained liquid is brought to a boil to coagulate albuminous material and then filtered while hot. The boiling must not be prolonged because acetic acid is volatile.

The product is not permanent, usually depositing solid matter after some weeks of standing, and should be prepared in reasonably small quantities. It is used in the manufacture of squill syrup.

TINCTURES

Tinctures are alcoholic or hydroalcoholic solutions of chemicals or of the soluble constituents of vegetable or animal drugs. The great majority of tinctures are prepared from drugs of vegetable origin; however, a few are derived from the other sources.

History

Preparations which can be considered as tinctures in the modern meaning of the term and actually called Tincturae were introduced into therapy as a special group by Paracelsus (1493–1541). The name "tincture" is derived from their being tinged by the extractives dissolved in the alcoholic menstrua which are employed in their manufacture. Official therapy recognized them very hesitantly. For instance, it was not until 1666 that the *Dispensatorium Valerii Cordi* listed Tincturae, among them a Tinctura Aurantiorum Corticis (Tincture of Orange Peel).

Several tinctures have replaced the medicated wines of former editions of the *U.S.P.* and the *N.F.* These wines, one of the older classes of galenic preparations, were hydroalcoholic solutions made from various drugs and employing white (sherry) or red (port) wine as the principal solvent or menstruum. *U.S.P. VIII* recognized red wine, white wine and 8 medicated wines. *N.F. IV* included formulas for 15 wines, all of which were made with sherry, but none has been official in later editions. The absence of uniformity in commercial wines, the adequacy of other preparations such as tinctures and fluidextracts, and the legal restrictions affecting the use of wines during the period of national prohibition, account for the decline in popularity of medicinal wines and their eventual deletion from official compendia. Detannated wine is now used rather extensively as the vehicle for a number of proprietary elixirs, notably those of thiamine hydrochloride.

Preparation of Tinctures

Unlike fluidextracts, all of which bear a uniform potency relationship to the drug or drugs from which they are prepared, tinctures vary markedly in strength. However, most of these preparations fall into 2 categories: (1) potent and (2) nonpotent. Tinctures prepared from potent drugs are of such strength that 100 ml. represents the activity of 10 Gm. of drug. This is in conformity with the recommendation of the Brussels Conference (International Conference for the Unification of Potent Remedies). These preparations frequently are referred to as 10 per cent tinctures. Before completion, some of these products must be subjected to an assay, either chemical or biologic, and, according to the result of this determination, carefully adjusted to a definite prescribed standard of potency. Nonpotent tinctures usually represent 20 Gm. of drug per 100 ml. of product and, accordingly, are called 20 per cent tinctures. Formulas for several compound tinctures are given official recognition, but no generalizations regarding their strength can be drawn. Two tinctures in the *U.S.P.* are prepared from drugs in the fresh condition, and, in these, 50 Gm. of drug is represented in 100 ml. of liquid. In addition to these, the *N.F.* formerly provided a general formula for the manufacture of tinctures from fresh drugs which are not recognized officially. Years ago, products called "Ethereal Tinctures" were used. While none of these is official at the present time, *N.F. VII* gave a formula for the preparation of any ethereal tincture that may be ordered.

Tinctures are prepared chiefly by percolation and by maceration, although several are made by simple solution of the medicinal agents in suitable solvents.

Percolation is the procedure of choice, where applicable. Crude drugs which are cellular in structure are well-adapted to the process of percolation, whereas a number of plant exudates (such as gum resins and balsams) are very liable to become impacted in the percolator and, thereby, retard or stop the flow of percolate. In these cases, maceration must be employed.

In the preparation of tinctures by percolation, experience has demonstrated that moderately coarse powders of vegetable drugs usually are preferable to powders of other degrees of comminution. Coarse powders are penetrated by menstrua more slowly than are the moderately coarse, and fine powders tend to pack tightly in the percolator and obstruct the passage of percolate. In several instances, fine powders are specified because of the difficulty encountered in completely extracting coarser grades.

The usual menstrua employed are alcohol or mixtures of various proportions of alcohol and water. In some cases, small amounts of either an acid or glycerin are added to the alcohol-water mixtures. The choice of menstruum by the *U.S.P.* or the *N.F.* for the extraction of a particular drug was dependent on a number of considerations, and the selection was made only after much study and experimental investigation. Knowledge of the crude drug's constituents, active and inert, is essential, as is a knowledge of the solubility of these constituents in the commonly employed solvents with a view toward the complete removal of desired principles and the exclusion of as much extraneous matter as practicable. Frequently, it is not possible to prevent the extraction of inert matter, and, if this material is not objectionable, it is permitted to remain in the tincture. In those cases in which the dissolved inactive matter is undesirable and could be responsible for the production of a malodorous preparation or one subject to deterioration, the tincture is given special treatment to ensure removal of the offending substance. For a more detailed discussion of menstrua, the reader is referred to Chapter 8.

Both the *U.S.P.* and the *N.F.* carry a general chapter on tinctures which give 2 procedures for the manufacture of these products. One of these methods involves percolation; the other, maceration. They are designated as Process P and Process M, respectively. When these processes are applicable, the individual tincture monographs direct the use of the one better suited for the particular drug or drugs to be extracted. In addition to referring to the procedure to be followed, the monographs also state the quantities of the drugs to be used, their degree of comminution and the menstrua to be employed.

Process P is as follows:

Carefully mix the ground drug or mixture of drugs with a sufficient quantity of the prescribed menstruum to render it evenly and distinctly damp, allow it to stand for 15 minutes, transfer it to a suitable percolator and pack the drug firmly. Pour on enough of the prescribed menstruum to saturate the drug, cover the top of the percolator, and when the liquid is about to drip from the percolator, close the lower orifice and allow the drug to macerate for 24 hours or for the time specified in the monograph. If no assay is directed, allow the percolation to proceed slowly, or at the specified rate, gradually adding sufficient menstruum to produce 1,000 ml. of tincture, and mix. If an assay is directed, collect only 950 ml. of percolate, mix this and assay a portion of it as directed. Dilute the remainder with such quantity of the prescribed menstruum as calculation from the assay indicates is necessary to produce a tincture that conforms to the prescribed standard, and mix.

The drug is dampened and allowed to stand for a short period of time prior to packing in the percolator to permit expansion to occur as menstruum is absorbed by the drug. If the drug were placed in a cylindrical percolator in the dry state and then moistened, the ensuing swelling would cause the drug to become packed so tightly that percolation could not proceed properly. The lower orifice of the percolator is kept open while saturating the drug with menstruum so that air which is occluded between the particles of drug can escape during the descent of menstruum. Maceration for the prescribed period of time before percolation permits saturation or near-saturation of the menstruum in contact with the drug, thereby assuring a more nearly complete exhaustion of the drug than if percolation were begun immediately after packing of the drug.

The rates of percolation as defined by official compendia refer to the extraction of 1,000 Gm. of drug. The expression *"percolate slowly"* means a rate not exceeding 1 ml. per minute; *"percolate at a moderate rate"* means the collection of from 1 to 3 ml. per minute; *"percolate rapidly"* means a rate of from 3 to 5 ml. per minute. The extraction of quantities larger or smaller than 1,000 Gm. necessitates a proportionate increase or decrease in the speed of percolation.

In preparing those tinctures which must be assayed, only 950 ml. of percolate is collected as a precautionary measure. Should a substandard drug be used or incomplete extraction effected, calculation from the result of the assay will indicate that the tincture should be diluted with menstruum to a volume of somewhat less than 1,000 ml. in order to meet official standards. If, on the other hand, 1,000 ml. of percolate is collected, a tincture falling below official requirements may result.

Process M. The pharmacopeial directions for preparing tinctures by Process M are as follows:

Macerate the drug with 750 ml. of the prescribed menstruum, in a container that can be closed, and put in a warm place. Agitate it frequently for 3 days or until the soluble matter is dissolved. Transfer the mixture to a filter, and when most of the liquid has drained away, wash the residue on the filter with a sufficient quantity of the prescribed menstruum, combining the filtrates, to produce 1,000 ml. of tincture, and mix.

The use of a closed vessel is directed to prevent loss of volatile drug constituents or of menstruum through evaporation. Since heat increases the solubility and the rate of solution of most substances, the maceration should be conducted in a moderately warm place. Menstruum in contact with the drug at the bottom of the container soon becomes saturated and, therefore, incapable of further exerting its solvent action on the drug. Frequent agitation during the period of maceration dilutes this strong layer with the weaker stratum above, and the process of solution continues. The initial quantity of menstruum used, equal to three fourths of the volume of tincture being prepared, is sufficiently small to permit ample washing of the undissolved residue with fresh portions of menstruum after removal of the first portion by filtration. This washing is necessary because an appreciable amount of liquid containing dissolved constituents is retained by the marc and must be displaced by other menstruum.

Circulatory maceration is a convenient and efficient modification of Process M. In this modified process, the drug is placed in a cloth bag and suspended in the menstruum at a point just below the top surface of the liquid. The solvent in contact with the drug dissolves soluble material and thereby becomes more dense than the surrounding liquid. Because of this increase in density, the solution falls to the bottom of the container, and fresh menstruum passes into the bag. This circulation of liquid continues until the drug is exhausted or until the menstruum is saturated. The chief advantage of this procedure over ordinary maceration lies in the fact that agitation is unnecessary. For small-scale operations, the infusion pot is useful if the spout is stoppered to prevent evaporation.

As a general rule, tinctures should not be prepared by diluting fluidextracts or other more concentrated preparations. However, *N.F. VI* and *N.F. VII*, permitted the manufacture of a tincture by diluting an official fluidextract with the official menstruum of the fluidextract. The tincture so prepared had to meet official requirements as to drug strength, alcohol content and content of other menstruum ingredients. Because the alcohol content of a tincture frequently differs from that of the fluidextract made from the same drug, the number of tinctures which may have been prepared by dilution was actually quite limited.

With few exceptions, tinctures are stable products when kept under optimum storage conditions. However, it is not uncommon for precipitation to occur after a period of standing. Fortunately, the precipitate is usually inactive and may be separated from the liquid without detracting from the potencies of the tincture. Tightly stoppered bottles are required to prevent evaporation of volatile components. Light-resistant containers such as amber bottles must be employed to avoid deterioration caused by photochemical change. For this same reason, the preparations must be protected from exposure to direct sunlight. High temperatures exert a deleterious effect on many substances, organic and inorganic; therefore, contact with excessive heat must not be permitted. The pharmacopeial terms "tight container," "light-resistant container" and "excessive heat" are defined in the General Notices of the *U.S.P.*

TINCTURES OF THE U.S.P.

BELLADONNA TINCTURE
Belladonna Leaf Tincture

Because Belladonna Tincture has much in common with the tinctures of hyoscyamus and stramonium, all 3 preparations will be discussed at this time. They are prepared by Process P, as modified for assayed tinctures, the menstruum consisting of 3 volumes of alcohol and 1 volume of water. This menstruum was first prescribed by *U.S.P. XI*, earlier revisions having called for the use of diluted alcohol. Both menstrua have advantages and disadvantages. The change to a menstruum of higher alcohol content was made because the tinctures prepared with diluted alcohol had a displeasing brownish-green color. The present menstruum extracts more of the alcohol-soluble chlorophyll to the partial exclusion of the water-soluble brown coloring matter, thereby producing green tinctures which are esthetically superior to the older products. From the standpoint of compatibility, the present official tinctures, when mixed with aqueous preparations or preparations having a low alcohol content, are objectionable because of the precipitation of resinous matter and the separation of oily globules.

The tinctures are assayed chemically for their content of total alkaloids, the same procedure being employed for all three. However, it should be noted that hyoscyamus contains a much smaller proportion of alkaloids than do the other two. The important alkaloids present are atropine, hyoscyamine and scopolamine (hyoscine).

The above-named constituents comprise an important group of parasympathetic depressants, and the tinctures are used in the treatment of a number of ailments. While certain preparations of the crude drugs are applied externally, nearly always the tinctures are administered by mouth. When so given, they exert sedative, narcotic and antispasmodic activity. They check excessive body secretions and, because of this property, frequently are employed in the treatment of coryza. The griping action of cathartics may be overcome, partially at least, by use of these tinctures.

COMPOUND BENZOIN TINCTURE

This preparation represents a modification of formulas, some proprietary, in use during the past 2½ centuries and probably longer. Among the more prominent of numerous names under which similar preparations have been sold may be mentioned Friar's Balsam, Jesuit's Drops and Turlington's Drops. The *Pharmacopœia Londinensis* of 1746 called it Traumatic Balsam.

Compound Benzoin Tincture contains the alcohol-soluble principles of the drugs aloe, benzoin, storax and tolu balsam. These drugs are not suited for percolation, and Process M is employed for its manufacture. Benzoin Tincture, N.F. (q.v.), also is prepared by Process M for the same reason.

Inasmuch as the complete transfer of a weighed quantity of storax, a sticky, viscous liquid, from one vessel to another is troublesome, it is suggested that the container in which the tincture is to be prepared be tared and the storax be weighed directly in it. Refer to the remarks on tolu balsam tincture (p. 386) for the procedure recommended for the handling of tolu balsam.

Compound Benzoin Tincture is infrequently administered internally in doses of from 1 to 4 ml. as a stimulating expectorant. More often, it is employed as an inhalant in the treatment of respiratory affections such as acute bronchitis and laryngitis by placing a teaspoonful of it in a pint of boiling water and inhaling the vapors. It is also used in external demulcent and cosmetic preparations as a protective.

IODINE TINCTURE

Iodine Tincture is one of two official tinctures which contain iodine. The other is Strong Iodine Tincture, N.F. Iodine Tincture contains 2 per cent (w/v) of iodine whereas strong iodine tincture contains 7 per cent (w/v) of iodine. *U.S.P. XII* recognized these preparations under the titles Mild Tincture of Iodine and Tincture of Iodine, respectively. At the same time, *N.F. VII* gave official recognition to Stronger Tincture of Iodine, also known as Churchill's Tincture of Iodine, which contained 16.5 per cent (w/v) of iodine. These changes in nomenclature and the deletion of the 16.5 per cent preparation undoubtedly have caused confusion, especially among lay people. Therefore, pharmacists must exercise care in the dispensing of these tinctures, making sure that they are giving the desired products regardless of the names used in ordering.

Years ago, Iodine Tincture was prepared simply by dissolving iodine in alcohol. This preparation lost strength rapidly because of a chemical reaction resulting in the formation of ethyl iodide. To prevent this reduction in strength, sodium iodide is included and reacts with the iodine to form sodium triiodide

$$I_2 + NaI \rightleftharpoons NaI_3$$

Potassium iodide, rather than the sodium salt, is used in preparing the strong or 7 per cent tincture, although it is believed that sodium iodide is less irritating to body tissues. In preparing the strong tincture, time can be saved by closely following the official directions that the iodine be dissolved completely in the aqueous solution of potassium iodide before adding the alcohol, because iodine dissolves more quickly in strong aqueous solutions of iodides than it does in alcohol.

It is imperative that these preparations be kept stoppered tightly. If not so stored, the alcohol present evaporates more rapidly than the iodine sublimes, thereby resulting in an increase in the proportion of iodine and a consequent increase in irritating properties. Cork and metallic stoppers are wholly unsuited, as they are attacked by the iodine. Glass closures are satisfactory; rubber stoppers are satisfactory for a limited time only.

Because of the high tax on alcohol, these tinctures seldom are prepared in the drugstore. By complying with certain government regulations, pharmaceutical manufacturers may obtain, tax-free, specially denatured alcohol suitable for use in these tinctures. The denaturants are iodine and either potassium or sodium iodide, which are added under government supervision before the alcohol is released from bond.

Iodine Tincture is rapidly replacing Strong Iodine Tincture as an external antiseptic for general first-aid and household purposes, the 7 per cent preparation being too irritating. However, Strong Iodine Tincture is useful as a counterirritant and as a preoperative sterilizing agent for the skin. The formerly official stronger tincture containing 16.5 per cent of iodine is employed occasionally as an escharotic.

LEMON TINCTURE

Lemon Peel Tincture

Lemon Tincture is made from the *outer yellow* rind of the *fresh* lemon by a procedure identical with that for sweet orange peel tincture.

It has been suggested that, in order to produce the tincture more economically and to make it more uniform in flavor, it be prepared by dissolving 5 per cent of lemon oil in alcohol and coloring the product with tartrazine. However, up to the present time, this proposal has not met with official acceptance.

The preparation is used as a flavoring agent and serves as the flavoring constituent of the widely used citric acid syrup.

OPIUM TINCTURE

Laudanum, Deodorized Opium Tincture

The name "laudanum," a popular synonym for Opium Tincture, was originated, in all probability, by Paracelsus and was used by him as a name for a number of his concoctions. One of the earliest, if not the very first, of the liquid preparations of opium was formulated by Thomas Sydenham, a physician of the 17th century. It contained opium, saffron, cinnamon and clove. Sydenham's laudanum was recognized by *N.F. V* under the title Tincture of Opium with Saffron. The synonym Deodorized Opium Tincture originally was used to distinguish the present Opium Tincture from the one-time official tincture which was not treated (as explained below) to remove the malodorous and nauseating constituents.

While containing about 25 alkaloids, Opium Tincture is standardized only for anhydrous morphine. The alkaloids occur chiefly as the salts (meconates and sulfates) which are soluble in water. U.S.P. X directed that the aqueous extraction of the opium be concentrated by evaporation on a water bath, but tinctures thus prepared form a large quantity of light, muddy, albuminous sediment on standing. This objectionable precipitation can be prevented by boiling the aqueous solution for at least 15 minutes, as required by U.S.P. XVI. Treatment with melted paraffin effects removal of the undesirable substances of a fatty or waxy nature which are responsible for the characteristic sickening odor of opium. This operation is an application of the principle of extraction with immiscible solvents, which is described in detail on p. 171.

This preparation is a narcotic and is subject to the restrictions of the Federal narcotic regulations. It is a valuable analgesic and somnifacient, but its continued use is accompanied by the danger of addiction. Opium Tincture is employed frequently in the treatment of diarrhea because of its property of reducing excessive intestinal peristalsis. It also is used in the manufacture of Ipecac and Opium Tincture, N.F. VIII, and may be employed in the preparation of camphorated opium tincture.

Camphorated Opium Tincture
Paregoric

Camphorated Opium Tincture, popularly called paregoric, originally was introduced by Le Mort, of the University of Leyden, in the early years of the 18th century. Since that time, the original formula and its modifications have been known variously as Elixir Paregoricum, Elixir Asthmaticum, Tinctura Camphora Composita and Tinctura Opii Benzoica.

In order to simplify its manufacture by the pharmacist, U.S.P. XI directed that the tincture be made from opium tincture by a simple process of solution, whereas formerly the formula called for powdered opium and involved the use of Process M. While convenient, the preparation of the camphorated tincture from the plain tincture is more costly than its preparation from powdered opium, and this expense gave rise to numerous complaints from large manufacturers. Consequently, a supplemental monograph was issued which included an alternate formula, again calling for powdered opium. Both formulas are given in U.S.P. XVI.

According to Federal law, Camphorated Opium Tincture is an exempt narcotic and can be sold at retail in limited quantities without a prescription as long as sales are made in good faith and are recorded properly. This exemption had led to the widespread illicit use of the tincture by opium addicts, and a number of states have enacted legislation in recent years forbidding its sale except on bona fide prescriptions. The preparation is employed widely as a mild anodyne in cough mixtures; it is an ingredient in the popular household cough preparation, Brown Mixture. Huge quantities of paregoric have been administered by ignorant mothers to colicky babies—a practice which should be discouraged strongly because of the danger of addiction. The tincture also is used in the treatment of diarrhea and to relieve the abdominal pains often associated with diarrhea.

Sweet Orange Peel Tincture

Attention is called to the requirement that only the *outer* rind of the *ripe* fruit be employed in preparing Sweet Orange Peel Tincture. The inner, white portion of the rind is somewhat bitter and should be excluded. Owing to chemical treatment, artificially colored oranges must not be used. While alcohol alone is used as the menstruum, the alcohol content of the tincture is between 62 and 72 per cent (v/v) because of the moisture content of the fresh peel. The tincture is prepared by Process M and, in common with other tinctures of fresh drugs, it represents 50 per cent (w/v) of crude drug.

Having a very agreeable flavor, the tincture is the source of orange flavor in the popular orange syrup and in other official products.

TINCTURES OF THE N.F.
Arnica Tincture

To ensure complete extraction of the arnica flowers, a modification of Process P is employed. After collection of one half of the percolate, the partially extracted drug is again macerated before completing the percolation. A former process *(U.S.P. VIII)* required maceration and expression with 3 successive portions of menstruum. Later *(U.S.P. IX)*, it was prepared by percolation with a period of maceration between the collection of each fourth of the percolate.

At one time, Arnica Tincture was a popular household liniment, being employed as a mild counterirritant in the treatment of sprains and bruises. It seldom is used today.

Benzoin Tincture

The balsamic resin benzoin is unsuited for percolation; therefore, this tincture, as well as Compound Benzoin Tincture *(q.v.)*, is prepared by Process M.

Benzoin Tincture occasionally is taken internally for the relief of respiratory affections, but it finds its principal use as an ingredient in external preparations such as skin lotions.

Capsicum Tincture

Experiments have determined that 4 volumes of alcohol and 1 volume of water is the menstruum best suited for the extraction of capsicum. However, as the tincture sometimes is mixed with volatile oils in the manufacture of liniments, a higher alcohol content is necessary to dissolve the oils; hence, a menstruum of 9 volumes of alcohol and 1 volume of water is prescribed.

For this tincture, *N.F. VII* gave an organoleptic test for quality. In this test, a very dilute sweetened sample of the tincture must produce a sensation of pungency when swallowed by humans. Although interesting, the test is not reliable, and the Second Supplement to *N.F. VII* ordered its deletion.

Internally, the tincture is an aromatic stomachic and sometimes is used in the treatment of chronic alcoholism to furnish a substitute for the local irritant action of alcohol in the stomach. The preparation also is used externally for counterirritation.

Compound Cardamom Tincture

The name of each of the 4 drugs (cardamom, cinnamon, caraway, cochineal) represented in this tincture bears the initial letter C, and for this reason the preparation sometimes is called Tincture of Four C's. This combination of crude drugs is satisfactory for extraction by percolation, but, inasmuch as the total quantity of drugs is small in comparison with the volume of tincture to be prepared, the tincture can be made satisfactorily and conveniently by Process M.

Compound Cardamom Tincture possesses mild carminative properties as well as a pleasing flavor and a rich red color. These properties account for its extensive use as a pharmaceutical vehicle.

Digitalis Tincture

Digitalis leaf contains inert fatty material which, at one time, was required to be removed in the manufacture of the tincture. This was accomplished by percolation of the finely powdered digitalis with solvent hexane prior to extraction of the active glycosides. Today, however, the fat is not considered to be objectionable, and the tincture is prepared simply by Process P, as modified for assayed tinctures, employing a hydroalcoholic menstruum.

No satisfactory method for the estimation of the potency of digitalis by chemical procedures has been devised as yet, and the *N.F.* requires that the tincture be standardized biologically. For several decades, the bio-assay has been the topic of considerable research and controversy, and numerous procedures employing various test animals have been proposed. The present method of assay calls for the use of pigeons, whereas early revisions of the *U.S.P.* prescribed the employment of frogs, and more recently cats have served as the test animals. By any of these procedures, the activity of the unstandardized product is compared with the activity of a reference standard.

The tincture is the most popular of the several liquid preparations of digitalis, none of which is satisfactory from the standpoint of keeping quality. All are subject to deterioration, resulting in a diminution of physiologic activity. On the other hand, the properly dried and powdered leaf retains its potency over a longer period of time than does the tincture. Consequently, although use of the tincture is somewhat on the decline, the use of tablets and capsules made from the powdered leaf remains popular.

Digitalis Tincture was an important medicinal preparation. It has prolonged the lives of millions of victims of heart disease through its direct stimulating action on heart muscle. This action increases the efficiency of the heart and improves the circulation by slowing the heart rate and strengthening the beat. Digitalis also exerts an indirect stimulating action on the kidneys, bringing about diuresis. Because of this property, digitalis is of value in the relief of dropsical conditions.

Ferric Chloride Tincture

Iron Tincture

On standing, Ferric Chloride Tincture develops an aromatic odor as the result of the formation of a small amount of ethyl chloride by the interaction of the alcohol with the hydrochloric acid in the ferric chloride solution. Furthermore, the oxidation of part of the alcohol to acetic acid, which in turn combines with alcohol, results in the production of a trace of ethyl acetate. Since these reactions are very slow, former pharmacopeial directions required that the tincture be aged for 3 months before dispensing. Because of the acidity of the preparation, it should be stored in glass-stoppered bottles.

Some years ago, the tincture was valued as a hematinic, but today, because of its astringent and irritating properties, other iron compounds, notably ferrous, have come into favor. When taken by mouth, the tincture should be diluted well and administered by means of a drinking tube to protect the teeth. It is a protein precipitant and is employed externally as a styptic for minor hemorrhages. Because of its astringent qualities, it is diluted and used as a throat application in the treatment of pharyngitis. It sometimes is applied locally in the prevention and the treatment of rhus poisoning.

In prescription compounding, the tincture is the source of numerous incompatibilities. Notable among these are the deep discolorations produced with tannins, the precipitation of ferric hydroxide in the presence of alkalis, the gelatinization of acacia solutions and, in the presence of soluble iodides or hydriodic acid, the reduction of the ferric ion to the ferrous with the liberation of iodine.

Ferric Citrochloride Tincture

Ferric chloride tincture and Ferric Citrochloride Tincture have the same iron content, but the latter is prepared by treating ferric chloride solution with sodium citrate. The exact composition of the compound formed is not known, but the characteristic reddish brown ferric color changes to green during the reaction. The following has been proposed to represent the formation of this complex salt:

$$Na_3C_6H_5O_7 + HCl \rightleftharpoons Na_2HC_6H_5O_7 + NaCl$$
$$Na_2HC_6H_5O_7 + FeCl_3 \rightleftharpoons (FeHC_6H_5O_7)Cl + 2NaCl$$

The saline matter which precipitates during several days of storage in a cold place after the addition of alcohol is sodium chloride. It has been shown that the iron in this compound ionizes very slightly and fails to exhibit the chemical properties of the ferric ion except on long standing. Therefore, the preparation is a very useful substitute for ferric chloride tincture in mixtures where ferric iron is a source of incompatibility. For example, no inky discoloration accompanies its admixture with tannin-bearing preparations. The tincture is practically devoid of astringent action and should not be employed where astringency is desired. On the other hand, this lack of astringency is a distinct advantage in many cases, inasmuch as the preparation is considerably more palatable than ferric chloride tincture. Ferric Citrochloride Tincture is an ingredient in the popular tonic iron, quinine and strychnine elixir.

Exposure to light causes a gradual darkening of the preparation, and storage in amber bottles is recommended.

Compound Gentian Tincture

Compound Gentian Tincture is prepared by Process P and represents 10 per cent (w/v) of gentian together with small quantities of bitter orange peel and cardamom seed. A mixture of glycerin, alcohol and water is used to extract the mixed drugs, the glycerin serving to retard the precipitation of tannin and other substances resembling tannin.

This tincture is probably the most popular of the several official galenic preparations of gentian. It is often prescribed as a bitter tonic to improve the appetite. Because of its content of tanninlike principles, it is incompatible with most preparations of iron. However, the tincture can be mixed with ferric citrochloride tincture in which the iron is bound in a complex ion due to the presence of sodium citrate.

Hyoscyamus Tincture
Henbane Tincture

See Belladonna Tincture (p. 380).

Strong Iodine Tincture

See Iodine Tincture (p. 380).

Myrrh Tincture

Myrrh Tincture is prepared by Process M, using alcohol as the menstruum. Myrrh is a gum resin and, therefore, not suited for percolation. It contains somewhat more than 30 per cent of alcohol-soluble extractive, chiefly volatile oil and resin, as well as a high proportion of gum, which is not soluble in alcohol.

The tincture is employed principally as a local stimulant to the mucosa of the mouth in stomatitis and other sore or ulcerated conditions.

Nitromersol Tincture

Nitromersol Tincture was recognized officially for the first time in *N.F. VIII*. The tincture, as well as other preparations of nitromersol, has been available for some years under the registered trade name of Metaphen.

Nitromersol is insoluble, or nearly so, in most of the common pharmaceutical solvents, including acetone, alcohol and water. However, it is soluble in weak solutions of alkalies, which explains the presence of 0.1 per cent of sodium hydroxide in the formula for the tincture.

This preparation is employed as a general antiseptic for disinfection of the intact skin and for open cuts and wounds. Unlike certain other organic mercurial antiseptics, it is relatively free from irritating qualities. The tincture possesses a distinct red to reddish-brown color but does not stain the skin. Where staining is desired, a nonofficial tinted tincture containing certified dye is commercially available.

Nux Vomica Tincture

Nux Vomica Tincture is prepared by Process P, as modified for assayed tinctures. The hydroalcoholic menstruum contains a small quantity of hydrochloric acid, which facilitates the extraction of the alkaloids present in the drug by converting them to the more soluble hydrochlorides. *U.S.P. X* employed acetic acid for this purpose, but the tinctures prepared in this manner frequently deposited solid matter on standing. Although containing several alkaloids, the tincture is standardized chemically only for its content of strychnine. After adjusting the product to its proper volume as determined by the assay, it is chilled to 5° C. for a half hour and filtered while cold in order to remove inert fatty material.

The tincture is employed principally as a bitter tonic and a stomachic. It seldom is used where the systemic stimulating action of strychnine is desired because of the small content of strychnine present.

Aromatic Rhubarb Tincture

This tincture contains 10 per cent (v/v) of glycerin to reduce precipitation of tannoid material during storage. This is also true of the formerly official (*N.F. IX*) Rhubarb Tincture and Sweet Rhubarb Tincture. However, the preparations are not entirely satisfactory, as some precipitation does occur on standing. Rhubarb Tincture formerly was called Compound Tincture of Rhubarb, as it represents, in addition to rhubarb, a small amount of cardamom seed. Rhubarb Tincture and Aromatic Rhubarb Tincture represent 20 per cent (w/v) of rhubarb whereas Sweet Rhubarb Tincture represents only one half as much of the drug—a fact which makes it especially suited for administration to children.

Rhubarb is one of the group of anthraquinone cathartics. The aromatic tincture is used primarily in the preparation of aromatic rhubarb syrup.

STRAMONIUM TINCTURE

See Belladonna Tincture (p. 380).

THIMEROSAL TINCTURE

Thimerosal Tincture, official for the first time in *N.F. X*, is much better known as Merthiolate Tincture.

Small amounts of ethylenediamine solution and monoethanolamine are included in the formula for the tincture for their stabilizing influence on the thimerosal. It is believed that this stabilizing effect results from their chelating action on traces of metallic impurities which may be present in the preparation. A number of metals, notably copper, cause decomposition of Thimerosal Tincture, a fact which explains the caution appearing in the monograph which reads: "*Manufacture and store Thimerosal Tincture in glass or suitably resistant metal containers.*" Years of experience in the manufacture and the handling of the tincture have shown that silver and certain grades of stainless steel are compatible with it. It is permissible to color the product with one or more of the certified coal-tar colors. The commercial Merthiolate Tincture has an orange-red tint with a greenish fluorescence and it leaves a red stain on the skin which is helpful in defining the area of application.

Thimerosal Tincture is employed as an antibacterial agent for topical use. It is used extensively as a household antiseptic for application to contaminated wounds, and it also is used for disinfection of the skin in the preparation of patients for surgery.

TOLU BALSAM TINCTURE

Tolu Tincture

At room temperature, tolu balsam is a tenacious, plastic mass and, for convenience in handling and weighing, it is recommended that the balsam be chilled to render it brittle and easily broken into fragments of suitable size for use in preparing the tincture.

Tolu balsam possesses a pleasant flavor, and the tincture is used to make tolu balsam syrup, which is employed widely as a vehicle for cough syrups.

VANILLA TINCTURE

The ordinary process of percolation usually does not effect complete extraction of the flavoring principles of vanilla and, for this reason, the *N.F.* directs the use of a procedure involving both maceration and percolation.

Vanilla Tincture often is referred to as **extract** or **essence** of vanilla. For many years, synthetic substitutes, usually sweetened and colored hydroalcoholic solutions of coumarin and vanillin, have been marketed legitimately as imitation vanilla extracts and all too frequently as the true tincture, to which they are far inferior in flavor. This deception has declined in extent in recent years because of improved Federal control over food and drug products. The Food and Drug Administration requires that each gallon of vanilla extract contain the soluble material from at least 13.35 oz. (avoir.) of vanilla beans with at least 35 per cent ethyl alcohol. The *N.F.* tincture satisfies these requirements.

Recent (1953) pharmacologic studies have shown that coumarin produces serious liver damage in experimental animals. While coumarin has been used as a constituent of flavors and foods for more than 80 years, and while there is no evidence of any injurious effects in man, the primary producers of this compound voluntarily withdrew it from sale to the food industry. Ethyl Vanillin is regarded as a satisfactory replacement for coumarin in food products.

The tincture is employed extensively as a flavoring for pharmaceutical preparations and foods.

NONOFFICIAL TINCTURES

ACONITE TINCTURE, N.F. X

This potent preparation is made by Process P, as modified for assayed tinctures, using a hydroalcoholic menstruum. However, before assaying the product, it is required that the pH of the percolate be adjusted to 3 ± 0.2 by the addition of hydrochloric acid. This is done to stabilize the tincture. Experiments have shown that, at higher pH values, it decreases in potency over a period of time due to hydrolysis of the active alkaloid, aconitine, and that careful control of the acidity reduces this deterioration to a minimum. After being assayed and diluted to the proper volume, readjustment of the pH is necessary.

Aconite Tincture is standardized biologically on guinea pigs by comparing its potency with that of a standard reference aconitine.

Aconite Tincture is infrequently administered internally as a cardiac sedative but, because of its toxicity, it must be used cautiously. Aconite also possesses local anesthetic properties, and occasionally the tincture is used in liniments and dental preparations.

Asafetida Tincture, N.F. X

The oleo-gum-resin, asafetida, being unsuited for percolation, is extracted by Process M in the preparation of the tincture.

Asafetida Tincture is medicinally unimportant and rapidly falling into disuse. It is employed as a sedative in hysteria, and its effect, largely psychological, generally is attributed to its extremely unpleasant odor.

Cantharides Tincture, N.F. X

The extraction of cantharides or Spanish flies has been the subject of considerable research. Former editions of the U.S.P. have directed that the tincture be prepared by ordinary percolation with alcohol at room temperature, and by digestion with alcohol at 50° to 55° for 24 hours, followed by percolation. The present menstruum is composed of a mixture of glacial acetic acid and alcohol, since it has been shown that the acid aids in the extraction of the active constituent, cantharidin, and retards its subsequent precipitation.

Cantharides is a powerful irritant, externally and internally, and the tincture must be used cautiously. It formerly was employed as a diuretic, but its internal use is inadvisable because of the danger of nephritis and other ill effects, such as damage to the alimentary tract. It is used as a local stimulant in scalp preparations. Occasionally, it is used as a vesicant, although Cantharides Cerate, N.F. VIII, is preferred for this purpose.

Colchicum Seed Tincture, N.F. X
Tinctura Colchici Seminis

This preparation has replaced the formerly official wine of colchicum (seed). Colchicum seed is difficult to extract, and the percolation should be conducted slowly. Following percolation, the tincture is assayed chemically and standardized for its content of the alkaloid colchicine.

Colchicine and colchicum preparations have long been employed empirically in the treatment of gout. While the action of colchicum is obscure, it is useful for relieving the pain and appears to shorten the duration of an acute attack. The tincture of the seed generally is preferred to that of the corm.

Larkspur Tincture, N.F. IX
Tinctura Delphinii

and

Acetic Larkspur Tincture, N.F. IX
Tinctura Delphinii Acetica

Acetic Larkspur Tincture is prepared by a combination of the processes of decoction and maceration. The drug is boiled with acetic acid, glycerin and water, the acid aiding in the extraction of alkaloids. The vessel should be covered loosely during the boiling to prevent undue loss of the volatile acetic acid.

Both the plain and the acetic tincture are used externally to kill head and pubic lice, but their use is considered dangerous because of the likelihood of systemic absorption. On calls for larkspur lotion, the acetic tincture should be dispensed.

Compound Lavender Tincture, N.F. X
Compound Lavender Spirit

Compound Lavender Tincture was recognized in the *London Pharmacopœia* of 1721. It was made with French brandy and 27 other ingredients, most of which were aromatic subtsances.

In the present formula, because the total quantity of combined drugs is relatively small, the tincture is prepared by Process M as a matter of convenience, even though the drugs are well suited for percolation.

The tincture is employed as a mild carminative in the treatment of flatulence and nausea. It is also used as a coloring and flavoring agent.

Lobelia Tincture, N.F. X

The small amount of acetic acid in the menstruum renders the alkaloids of lobelia more soluble.

Bitter Orange Peel Tincture, N.F. X
Tinctura Aurantii Corticis Amari

It should be observed that this tincture is prepared from bitter orange peel, the *dried* rind of the *unripe* fruit of the official species of orange in contrast with sweet orange peel, which is still recognized officially.

A flavoring agent with mild stomachic properties, this tincture frequently is combined with simple bitters. Its flavor is not so pleasant as that of Sweet Orange Peel Tincture.

Some nonofficial tinctures which still find occasional use are the following:

Aloe Tincture, N.F. IX
Antimony Tincture, N.F. VII
  (Tincture of Tartar Emetic)
Compound Cinchona Tincture, N.F. IX
Strong Colchicum Corm Tincture, N.F. IX
Gelsemium Tincture, N.F. IX
Ammoniated Guaiac Tincture, N.F. IX
Hydrastis Tincture, N.F. IX
Iodides Tincture, N.F. IX
Ipecac Tincture, N.F. IX
Rhubarb Tincture, N.F. IX
Sweet Rhubarb Tincture, N.F. IX
Veratrum Viride Tincture, N.F. IX

The following represent special types of tinctures which were used at an earlier time.

Ethereal Tinctures, N.F. VII
Tincturæ Æthereæ

Under the above title, *N.F. VII* presented a general formula and procedure for the manufacture of ethereal tinctures, since no specific preparations of this type are recognized in this country. They represent 10 per cent (w/v) of the crude drug and are prepared by Process P, employing a menstruum consisting of 1 volume of ether and 2 volumes of alcohol. To avoid loss of this highly volatile menstruum, a closed system having an air vent from the receiver to the top of the percolator should be used.

These preparations are called for very seldom.

Fresh Drug Tinctures, N.F. VII
Tincturæ Medicamentorum Recentium,
Tincturæ Herbarum Recentium

The formula and the procedure given for tinctures of fresh drugs is intended as a guide to the pharmacist on those infrequent occasions when nonofficial tinctures of this type are to be supplied. They represent 50 per cent (w/v) of the contused or cut drug and are made by Process M with alcohol as the menstruum. Instead of the customary 3-day period of maceration, 14 days are required.

FLUIDEXTRACTS

Fluidextracts are concentrated liquid preparations representing the therapeutically active principles of vegetable drugs. As a class, they have much in common and form one of the best-defined classes of galenics. All are prepared by some modification of the process of percolation. They are uniform in strength, being adjusted so that each milliliter of liquid represents the soluble components of 1 Gm. of the standard, dried drug. This relationship holds even for the several nonofficial compound fluidextracts in which a total of 1,000 Gm. of mixed drugs is used to prepare 1,000 ml. of fluidextract. Without exception, these products contain alcohol, the concentration of which varies, depending on the nature of the drugs to be extracted. In a few, the drugs are extracted by percolation with water, and the alcohol is added to the percolate as a preservative.

History

A survey of the general historical development of percolation has been given in Chapter 8, "Extraction." As to its admittance into the *U.S.P.*, it was in the edition of 1842 (2nd revision, 3rd edition) that the "method of displacement" (percolation) was introduced, although merely as a matter of choice. As a special class of official preparations, percolates were recognized for the first time in the *U.S.P.* of 1850, although from then until the time of *U.S.P. VIII* (1906), when the coined Latin word *fluidextractum* first made its appearance, the products were designated as *Extractum* [name of the drug] *Fluidum*. To this day, the *British Pharmacopœia* recognizes these preparations under the general title Liquid Extracts. Occasionally, American physicians of the older generation still prescribe fluidextracts by their former names.

About 60 years ago, a class of products called *fluidacetracts* was recommended to replace fluidextracts. These preparations were made with a menstruum consisting of acetic acid and water. The particular advantages claimed for them were stability, low cost and miscibility with water, but they never gained popularity.

Preparation of Fluidextracts

The menstrua employed in the manufacture of fluidextracts have been selected with a view toward the complete and economical extraction of desired constituents. At the same time, it is desirable that the menstrua, insofar as possible, eliminate inert matter which later may cause precipitation or other forms of deterioration.

A cylindrical percolator usually is preferred because a concentrated percolate is wanted. The passage of menstruum through a long column of drug yields a percolate richer in dissolved material than would be possible when using a squat or flared form of percolator. The use of a cylindrical percolator also effects a substantial saving in the quantity of menstruum needed to exhaust the drug and thereby reduces the cost of the preparation. If the drug is one which swells to a considerable degree on being moistened, a conical percolator may be used to advantage. If the drug be permitted to expand in a cylindrical percolator, it is quite likely to become packed so firmly as to slow down or stop completely the passage of percolate.

The period of maceration of the drug in the menstruum prior to percolation is varied for different drugs, depending on their ease of extraction. For example, only 2 hours of maceration are required for glycyrrhiza, whereas 72 hours are prescribed for ipecac; the large majority of drugs are required to macerate for 48 hours.

Three terms, namely, "percolate slowly," "percolate at a moderate rate" and "percolate rapidly," are used by the *U.S.P.* and the *N.F.* to designate the proper speeds for the collection of percolate. For the extraction of 1,000 Gm. of drug, these terms, respectively, mean a rate not exceeding 1 ml. per minute, a rate of from 1 to 3 ml. per minute and a rate of from 3 to 5 ml. per minute.

A few fluidextracts are manufactured by special procedures, but the great majority are made by 5 processes which are described in detail in the general chapter on fluidextracts in the *N.F.*

Process A, the first of these (see *N.F. XI*, p. 428, for details of the process), is prescribed much more often than the other four. It involves the usual method of percolation, and the menstrua employed are alcohol or mixtures of alcohol and water. The drug is moistened with menstruum and allowed to stand for about 15 minutes prior to packing in the percolator to permit its expansion through absorption of liquid. The lower orifice of the percolator is left open while saturating the packed drug with menstruum to allow for the escape of air trapped between the particles of drug. The first portion of percolate (850 ml.) is more concentrated than the percolate collected thereafter. For this reason, the strong percolate is set aside, and only the weaker second percolate is subjected to concentration by heating, which may affect certain dissolved principles adversely. Evaporation at the specified temperature is slow, and large manufacturers usually conduct the operation under reduced pressure in order to hasten the concentration. It should be noted that "a mixture of alcohol and water" is used to adjust the preparation to its final volume. This mixture will not necessarily contain the same proportion of alcohol as was used in the menstruum. Upon dissolving the soft extract, from which practically all alcohol has been evaporated, the alcohol content of the reserved percolate will be somewhat reduced. In order that the completed fluidextract will contain the prescribed amount of alcohol, the diluting mixture may contain more alcohol than was contained in the menstruum.

Process B (see *N.F. XI*, p. 428) differs from Process A only in that 2 menstrua are employed successively. The first menstruum contains a small quantity of either an acid or glycerin in addition to the alcohol or the mixture of alcohol and water prescribed; the second is alcohol or an alcohol-water mixture. Where an acid is called for as an ingredient of the first menstruum, it serves to ensure the complete extraction of alkaloids from the drug by conversion of these alkaloids to their respective salts, thereby increasing their solubility in the menstruum. The presence of glycerin in Menstruum I facilitates the extraction of tannins or other similar glycosidal substances and, to some extent, prevents the subsequent precipitation of these principles or the precipitation of products resulting from their hydrolysis.

Process C (see *N.F. XI*, p. 428) is known officially as *fractional* or *divided percolation* and is a modification of the process of repercolation introduced by Squibb. Process C is intended especially for the preparation of fluidextracts from drugs having constituents which are decomposed or volatilized by heat and, in addition, the process may be employed as an alternative for Processes A or B. It is important to note that the use of this elaborate procedure involves no heating or concentration of any of the numerous portions of percolate. The first or reserved percolate collected from the first portion of drug is either saturated or nearly saturated with dissolved material and is of no further value as a solvent. Portion No. 1 is weaker than the reserved percolate; portion No. 2, still weaker; and so on down to No. 5, which contains little or no dissolved substances. When using these 5 numbered portions as menstruum for the extraction of the second portion of drug, care should be taken to prevent, as far as possible, the admixture of these portions within the percolator. This can be accomplished by waiting until the upper level of each successive portion reaches the top surface of the drug before pouring in the next. If this precaution is not observed, and the various fractions are poured into the percolator in rapid succession, thereby becoming mixed more or less uniformly, the effort expended in the separate collection of these portions will have been wasted and an incomplete extraction effected because of retention by the marc of liquid containing dissolved material. This precautionary measure also applies with equal force to the extraction of the third portion of drug.

Process D (see *N.F. XI*, p. 429) is applicable to the extraction of drugs the desired principles of which are soluble in water. Boiling water is employed as the menstruum, and, after concentration of the aqueous percolate, alcohol is added to preserve the product. A metallic rather than a glass percolator should be used because of the danger of cracking the glass upon addition of the boiling water. The lining of the percolator should be of material which does not react chemically with plant principles. For this purpose, tin is preferred. The period of standing after addition of alcohol to the concentrated percolate permits the precipitation of alcohol-insoluble constituents. While the *N.F.* specifies "several days" of standing, an even longer period is desirable because the deposition of insoluble material may continue for several weeks.

Process E (see *N.F. XI*, p. 429) was recognized officially for the first time in *N.F. VII*. It is a process of pressure percolation and in many respects is similar to the process of diacolation described on page 170. At the present time, the process is recommended specifically for the preparation of only one fluidextract, although it is suggested as an alternative for Processes A, B or C. The employment of Process E is advantageous over Processes A and B in that the former effects a substantial saving of menstruum and eliminates the necessity of concentrating weak percolate by vacuum distillation. Over Process C, Process E possesses the advantages of obviating the division of the crude drug into 3 weighed portions and the collection of 13 separate measured fractions of percolate. The percolator or series of percolators used need not be a single vertical tube or series of tubes mounted one upon the other. On the large scale, such an arrangement may mean the extension of the equipment through several floors of the manufacturing plant. Obviously, this set-up would be expensive to install, inconvenient to pack and difficult to clean. Experiments have shown that an up-to-standard fluidextract can be prepared by extracting the drug in an apparatus consisting of a number of parallel vertical tubes joined together with U-shaped tubes. The previously moistened drug is packed into each straight tube and U-tube; a U-tube is then attached to the bottoms of the first and the second straight tubes, a second U-tube to the tops of the second and the third straight tubes, and so on until the assembly is complete. Then a suitable reservoir for menstruum is joined to the top of the first tube, and means are provided for forcing menstruum through the system under pressure.

Soon after their completion, most fluidextracts begin to precipitate solid matter. The period of time over which this deposition continues is variable with different products, and at times may be as long as several months. The sediment formed is nearly always inert, but occasionally it may contain active material. The official compendia allow the removal of this sediment "provided the resulting clear liquid conforms to the official standards." Therefore, manufacturers age their fluidextracts for the length of time necessary to ensure complete precipitation, and then clarify them by filtration or by means of a continuous type of centrifuge. Time can be saved by decanting the clear supernatant portions of the products and clarifying only the cloudy parts. As in the case of tinctures, fluidextracts should be stored in well-stoppered, light-resistant containers, and their exposure to direct sunlight or to excessive heat should be avoided. The reasons for these requirements have been given previously.

Fluidextracts seldom are prescribed alone for direct consumption by the patient, particularly when a tincture of the same drug is available. The dose of a fluidextract, when compared with that of a tincture, is small, and the accurate measurement of a small volume of liquid by the layman with ordinary household measuring devices is not possible. For example, the usual dose of belladonna leaf fluidextract is 0.06 ml. (1♏) and its measurement by the patient would be impracticable, whereas a 0.6 ml. (10♏) usual dose of the tincture can be obtained with reasonable accuracy. Relatively few of the fluidextracts are prescribed today in extemporaneous prescription formulas since physicians prefer more palatable preparations for their patients. However, the fluidextracts are useful for manufacturing purposes and often appear in the formulas for official syrups and elixirs which are much more agreeable to the taste than are the fluidextracts.

FLUIDEXTRACTS OF THE *U.S.P.*

Aromatic Cascara Sagrada Fluidextract

Magnesium oxide is mixed with the cascara sagrada before percolation to neutralize and thereby partially to prevent the extraction of the bitter cathartic constituents. After concentration of the percolate, pure glycyrrhiza extract is added to sweeten and flavor. In addition to the extract, saccharin further sweetens the product, and the oils of anise, coriander and wintergreen (methyl salicylate) impart their characteristic flavors.

Aromatic Cascara Sagrada Fluidextract is a popular preparation for the relief of habitual constipation. Small repeated doses which gradually may be reduced seem to be more effective than single large doses. While not entirely bitterless, this preparation is considerably more palatable than the plain fluidextract, but, since the magnesium oxide prevents the complete extraction of the drug, it is less active physiologically, and a proportionately larger dose must be taken to secure the desired effects.

Glycyrrhiza Fluidextract
Licorice Root Fluidextract

A slight excess of diluted ammonia solution is added to the aqueous percolate to convert the extracted glycyrrhizin to its ammoniated form, which is more soluble and sweeter than glycyrrhizin itself. This percolate is particularly susceptible to fermentation and should be evaporated promptly to prevent spoiling. Active boiling under normal atmospheric pressure causes coagulation of albuminous material which, if allowed to remain in solution, would precipitate later and produce an unsightly product. The percolate is filtered after partial concentration because, at this stage, it is still sufficiently fluid to pass through the filter readily: if the evaporation is completed before clarifying, the resulting liquid is too viscous.

This fluidextract is highly esteemed as an agent for masking the disagreeable taste of bitter and saline drugs. It is an ingredient in glycyrrhiza syrup and in several other official preparations. Recent laboratory and clinical findings indicate that glycyrrhiza has an adrenocortical-hormonelike effect in experimental animals and in patients suffering from Addison's disease. This effect is attributed to the constituent glycyrrhetinic acid. In some of this work, Glycyrrhiza Fluidextract has been employed as the source of glycyrrhetinic acid.

Ipecac Fluidextract

Ipecac is not adapted to extraction by any of the usual procedures for the manufacture of fluidextracts; therefore, it must be given special treatment. After percolation, the liquid is concentrated to remove most of the alcohol, and to the remaining liquid is added a large volume of water which causes the precipitation of resin. The fluidextract is used almost exclusively for the manufacture of ipecac syrup, and the removal of resinous material from the fluidextract is necessary for the production of a clear syrup. Hydrochloric acid is added to stabilize the product by converting the alkaloids to their hydrochlorides. The important alkaloids of ipecac are emetine and cephaëline.

FLUIDEXTRACTS OF THE N.F.
Belladonna Leaf Fluidextract

Belladonna Leaf Fluidextract may be prepared either by Process A, as modified for assayed fluidextracts, or by Process E. This is the only official fluidextract for the preparation of which Process E is specifically recommended. It should be observed that, when Process E is used, a lower concentration of alcohol is employed as the menstruum than when Process A is used.

Hyoscyamus and stramonium fluidextracts (N.F. IX) also were prepared by Process A, as modified for assayed fluidextracts, using a menstruum consisting of 3 volumes of alcohol and 1 volume of water, the same as that prescribed for Belladonna Leaf Fluidextract when prepared by this process. For all 3, the period of maceration (48 hours) and the rate of percolation (moderate) are identical. Furthermore, the 3 preparations are assayed chemically by identical procedures.

Belladonna Root Fluidextract

Since Belladonna Root Fluidextract is 50 per cent stronger in alkaloids than the fluidextract prepared from the leaf, the 2 products must not be used interchangeably.

Cascara Sagrada Fluidextract
Rhamnus Purshiana Fluidextract

The cathartic principles of cascara sagrada are soluble in water, hence the employment of Process D. Because this preparation is intensely bitter, it is not used as extensively as the aromatic fluidextract prepared from the same drug.

Ergot Fluidextract

Because the active constituents of ergot are destroyed by heat, Ergot Fluidextract is prepared by Process C. Hydrochloric acid is combined with the other menstruum ingredients to facilitate the extraction of the active alkaloids and amines by converting them to their respective hydrochlorides. Ergot contains an appreciable quantity of inert fatty material which would be objectionable in the final product. Two procedures are given for the removal of this fat.

In one, the crude drug, prior to the removal of desired principles, is subjected to percolation with solvent hexane. The alternative procedure calls for chilling the combined reserve percolates to a temperature of −14° C. and filtering off the congealed fat while maintaining this temperature.

Former revisions of the *U.S.P.* required that the fluidextract be standardized by biologic means, but more recent revisions have eliminated this requirement. However, the crude drug from which the fluidextract is prepared must be of standard quality.

The keeping quality of Ergot Fluidextract is extremely poor. Certain manufacturers even place an expiration date on the label of their product. Dated or undated, the preparation should be preserved in small, well-filled bottles in a cool, dark place.

For a long time, the preparation has been used as an ecbolic in childbirth and in the prevention of postpartum hemorrhage. In modern therapeutics, the fluidextract is being supplanted largely by the alkaloids, ergonovine and ergotamine.

Eriodictyon Fluidextract
Yerba Santa Fluidextract

Eriodictyon Fluidextract is valued for its content of resinous matter, the extraction of which requires a rather highly alcoholic menstruum. The fluidextract and the aromatic syrup which is prepared from the fluidextract are used to disguise the unpleasant flavor of numerous drugs, particularly bitter substances. Occasionally, eriodictyon preparations are employed as tonics and expectorants.

Gentian Fluidextract

This fluidextract is prepared by Process A by percolation with diluted alcohol.

It is used principally in the manufacture of glycerinated gentian elixir.

Nux Vomica Fluidextract

Nux Vomica Fluidextract owes its activity to its content of strychnine and, to a lesser degree, brucine. Acetic acid, which is a part of the first menstruum, assists in the extraction of these alkaloids by converting them to acetates which are more easily dissolved than the free bases. Inert fatty material should be removed from the preparation by chilling the percolate, a process which causes solidification of the fat, and filtering while cold.

Rhubarb Fluidextract

Rhubarb Fluidextract, prepared by Process A, is used principally in the manufacture of rhubarb and soda mixture.

Sarsaparilla Fluidextract

This preparation, now generally recognized as devoid of therapeutic activity, is used principally as an ingredient in the official compound sarsaparilla syrup which, in turn, is employed chiefly as a vehicle for the administration of saline drugs.

Senna Fluidextract

This fluidextract is prepared by Process A and is employed in the manufacture of senna syrup.

Taraxacum Fluidextract
Dandelion Root Fluidextract

This fluidextract, seldom prescribed today, continues to warrant official recognition because it is an ingredient in glycerinated gentian elixir.

NONOFFICIAL FLUIDEXTRACTS

Buchu Fluidextract, N.F. X

To prevent loss of volatile oil during the manufacture of Buchu Fluidextract, Process C is now prescribed instead of Process A, which formerly was employed.

Colchicum Seed Fluidextract, N.F. X
Fluidextractum Colchici Seminis

Colchicum seed contains a considerable amount of inactive fatty material which should be removed by percolation with solvent hexane prior to extraction of the useful constituents. Attention is called to the requirement that Colchicum Seed Fluidextract contain a somewhat greater amount of colchicine than the fluidextract prepared from colchicum corm.

Ginger Fluidextract, N.F. X
Fluidextractum Zingiberis

Ginger Fluidextract is prepared by Process A with a menstruum containing 9 volumes of alcohol and 1 volume of water. A highly alcoholic menstruum is needed for effective extraction of the volatile oil and resin in the drug.

The product finds its chief use in the manufacture of ginger syrup.

Grindelia Fluidextract, N.F. X

Grindelia Fluidextract contains resinous material which is precipitated upon admixture of the fluidextract with aqueous liquids. Certain manufacturers of pharmaceuticals offer preparations for sale under the names of Fluid Grindelia Soluble or Fluid Grindelia Miscible. These products are unlike the formerly official fluidextract in that they contain little or no resin and form clear solutions with water. Therefore, they should not be employed when the fluidextract is called for.

Hydrastis Fluidextract, N.F. X
Goldenseal Fluidextract

This fluidextract, prepared by Process A, as modified for assayed fluidextracts, is standardized for its content of ether-soluble alkaloids.

Senega Fluidextract, N.F. X
Fluidextract of Seneca Snakeroot

After Senega Fluidextract has been prepared by Process A, and before it has been diluted to its final volume, it should be rendered feebly alkaline by the careful addition of diluted ammonia solution. By this procedure, acidic pectinous bodies present in the preparation are converted to soluble ammonium salts, and subsequent gelatinization of the fluidextract is averted.

Squill Fluidextract, N.F. X
Fluidextractum Scillæ

Squill Fluidextract cannot be prepared satisfactorily by any of the usual procedures for the manufacture of fluidextracts, special manipulation being necessary to eliminate certain inert material from the final product. Damage to the active glycosides from heat is held to a minimum by evaporating the percolate at a temperature not exceeding 45° C. The large volume of alcohol that is added to the concentrated percolate causes precipitation of albuminous and pectinous matter which later may result in precipitation, or even gelatinization of the fluidextract. N.F. VI required that the preparation be assayed biologically and adjusted to a prescribed standard of strength.

Wild Cherry Fluidextract, N.F. X
Fluidextractum Pruni Virginianæ

Wild cherry bark contains the glucoside amygdalin. When the bark is moistened with the initial menstruum, an enzyme present, emulsin, promotes hydrolysis of the amygdalin, resulting in the formation of hydrocyanic acid, benzaldehyde and glucose as follows:

$$C_{20}H_{27}O_{11}N + 2H_2O \xrightarrow{emulsin} HCN + C_6H_5CHO + 2C_6H_{12}O_6$$

The advisability of preparing the fluidextract by Process B is to be questioned since the desired constituents, benzaldehyde and hydrocyanic acid, are volatile, and since the process involves the concentration of weak percolate by heating.

The bark also contains tannin, which in the fluidextract is objectionable and may be the cause of incompatibility when the fluidextract is mixed with other substances. In order to facilitate partial exclusion of the tannin from the completed preparation, it is directed that the period of maceration be relatively brief and that the percolation be conducted at a rapid rate. As it is not possible to prevent the extraction of tannin entirely, glycerin is employed as a preservative.

FLUIDGLYCERATES

Fluidglycerates are liquids made by extracting vegetable drugs with a menstruum containing glycerin and water. They represent the same weight of crude drug per unit of volume as do fluidextracts; that is, each milliliter of preparation contains the useful constituents from 1 Gm. of drug. They contain about 50 per cent, by volume, of glycerin and no alcohol.

These products are intended as substitutes for fluidextracts where the administration of alcohol is therapeutically contraindicated. Furthermore, they are prepared more economically than fluidextracts, and it is claimed that they fill the need for stable concentrated infusions. On the other hand, their preparation is restricted to those drugs whose active principles are extracted by the solvents named.

History

Fluidglycerates were proposed first in 1907. They have never been adopted by the *U.S.P.*, but *N.F. IV* and *N.F. V* recognized a general chapter and also specific monographs on the fluidglycerates of cascara sagrada, aromatic cascara sagrada, glycyrrhiza, krameria and rhubarb. Because they failed to gain the favor of medical practitioners, only the general monograph was retained by *N.F. VI* and *N.F. VII*. Not even this general monograph appears today.

Preparation of Fluidglycerates

N.F. VII states that fluidglycerates made from drugs that do not require either an acid or an alkaline menstruum may be prepared by the following general process:

The Drug, in coarse powder....	1,000 Gm.
Glycerin	500 cc.
Water	1,500 cc.
Chloroform Water, a sufficient quantity,	
To make	1,000 cc.

Mix the glycerin and the water; moisten the drug thoroughly with a portion of the mixture; then pack it very lightly in a cylindrical percolator and add enough of the menstruum to saturate the powder and leave a stratum above it. When the liquid begins to drop from the percolator, close the lower orifice, cover the percolator and macerate 48 hours. Then allow the percolation to proceed slowly until the drug is practically exhausted, using first the remainder of the menstruum and then chloroform water.

Reserve the first 500 cc. of the percolate and evaporate the remainder on a water bath, the weaker portion first, then the stronger, until reduced to 600 cc.; then add the reserved portion and continue evaporation until the product measures 1,000 cc. Allow the preparation to stand for a few days, then decant the clear portion, strain the remainder and mix well.

Whereas moderately coarse (No. 40) powders of vegetable drugs generally are satisfactory for the manufacture of fluidextracts, they have a tendency to become too firmly packed in the percolator in the presence of a glycero-aqueous menstruum, thereby obstructing the descent of the percolate. This explains the requirement above, that the drug be in the form of a coarse (No. 20) powder. Chloroform water, rather than plain water, is used as the second menstruum to prevent deterioration from the growth of micro-organisms. If plain water were used, fermentation and mold growth would soon occur after the glycerin was washed from the percolator. However, the chloroform does not enter the final product because it is dissipated completely during the concentration of the weak percolate by evaporation. To minimize the possible injury to active material by prolonged heating, the several portions of percolate are evaporated by starting with the weaker and successively adding the stronger.

EXTRACTS

Extracts are concentrated solid, semisolid or viscous liquid products made from vegetable or animal drugs. The drugs are extracted by percolation or other extraction procedures, the resulting liquids evaporated to, or nearly to, dryness, and the residues adjusted to prescribed standards of strength or consistency.

History

Although extracts are a very old class of pharmaceutical preparations and some, for example, opium extract and an aqueous extract of rhubarb, are known to have been in use for at least 2000 years, not until the late 16th century were they given special emphasis by the followers of Paracelsus, who called them quintessences and recommended them highly. The ancient and fallacious belief that nature was composed of the 4 elements—earth, air, fire and water—may be responsible for the term "quintessence," which refers to the 5th or uppermost essence in a natural substance. Another more realistic explanation of the term is that, in the opinion of Paracelsus, the "quinta essentia," although representing only 5 from 100 of the raw materials concerned, contained all the efficacious constituents, hence was 20 times stronger than the same amount of the drug from which it was prepared.

PREPARATION OF EXTRACTS

Extracts present the useful or active constituents of drugs in a concentrated condition convenient for use in many solid or semisolid forms of medication, and, occasionally, in liquid preparations. One official extract is a viscous liquid. All of the others are either dry powders, known as powdered extracts, or semisolid plastic masses, known as pilular or solid extracts. Neither the *U.S.P.* nor the *N.F.* defines *pilular*, but the accepted inference is that products so described are of such consistence that they can be rolled into pills which will retain their shape without the addition of drying excipients. Few, if any, of the commercial pilular extracts are nearly so viscid, softer preparations being more desirable pharmaceutically, since they may be mixed more easily with other substances. In 2 cases, both the powdered and the pilular forms of an extract of a particular drug are official and, although identical in medicinal activity, each type has distinct advantages over the other in certain compounding operations. For example, the pilular products are preferred where extracts are to be used in the manufacture of ointments, suppositories and pill masses, whereas powdered extracts are better adapted to incorporation into bulk or divided powders, capsules and cachets.

The *N.F.* contains a general chapter on extracts. However, it does not give general processes for making these products such as are given for tinctures and fluidextracts. Therefore, detailed directions for the preparation of most of the extracts officially recognized are given in the individual monographs. The great majority are prepared by percolation; a few by maceration, infusion, decoction and simple trituration of several powdered ingredients.

The menstrua employed are water, alcohol or mixtures of alcohol and water. The menstruum prescribed is sometimes more highly alcoholic than that used for the preparation of a tincture or a fluidextract of the same drug. This enables the production of a more concentrated extract by excluding, partially at least, inert water-soluble extractive. It is permissible to use specially denatured alcohol containing not more than 10 per cent by volume of methanol (wood alcohol) or acetone in place of official alcohol, the denatured products not being subject to the high Federal tax levied on pure alcohol. To effect this saving, manufacturers must obtain a special permit and must comply with numerous other regulations. The use of these denatured alcohols in no way affects the quality of the finished extracts, as all the solvent is removed by distillation.

Where percolation is directed as the method of extraction, it is important, for reasons of economy, that the prescribed rate of flow not be exceeded. These rates of flow are defined under Fluidextracts (p. 389). If the percolation is conducted too rapidly, more menstruum is needed to exhaust the drug, with a consequent increase in volume of percolate to be evaporated; whereas percolation at the proper rate produces a smaller volume of more concentrated liquid.

Evaporation under reduced pressure frequently is directed in order to speed up the concentration of percolates. The operation involves the use of expensive equipment, and for this reason extracts seldom are prepared by the retail druggist. In a number of cases, definite maximum temperatures for the evaporation, often 60° C., are given. The stated temperatures should not be exceeded if damage to active constituents is to be avoided.

Nearly all of the official extracts are adjusted to definite standards. In some instances, the adjustment is made following a determination of the amount of active material present by chemical assay; in others, where satisfactory assay methods are not available, the evaporated products are adjusted, by the addition of suitable diluents, to weigh a certain proportion of the weight of drug represented.

Starch, previously dried at 100° C., usually is directed as the diluent for powdered extracts, although any of the following substances may be used: sucrose, lactose, powdered glycyrrhiza, calcium phosphate or the finely powdered marc remaining after the extraction of the drug. In addition, magnesium carbonate and magnesium oxide may be employed except for the powdered extracts of belladonna, hyoscyamus and stramonium. Liquid glucose is directed as the diluent for official pilular extracts, but it is permissible to use malt extract or glycerin instead.

If substantial amounts of white powders such as starch or lactose are added to powdered extracts, the normal color of the extract will be lightened materially. No color standards are given in the official compendia, but they do permit the artificial coloring of the diluents to approximate the natural colors of the extracts. Caramel and chlorophyll are used to impart brown and green colors, respectively.

A number of the drugs from which extracts are prepared contain inert oily material which would interfere with obtaining satisfactory dry powdered extracts. This fat or oil should be removed by any one of several procedures. Removal may be accomplished by percolation of the crude drug with solvent hexane prior to extraction of the desired constituents or, as the N.F. recommends, by washing the extract with several portions of solvent hexane and then drying at a temperature not above 70° C. Another method suggested in the N.F. involves washing of the extract with 3 successive portions of hot acidulated water, skimming off fatty matter which has risen, combining the aqueous fluids and evaporating them at a temperature not exceeding 70° C. The residue then is combined with the undissolved extract and evaporated to dryness at the stated temperature. It is recommended that the acidulated water contain about 0.05 per cent of HCl or about 0.2 per cent of tartaric acid.

Extracts usually are marketed in small wide-mouthed amber jars or bottles with tight-fitting stoppers. They should be stored preferably at room temperature; higher temperatures may hasten decomposition of active constituents in some extracts and lower temperatures may increase the viscosity of pilular extracts to the point where they are difficult to handle. Proper preservation demands that extracts be kept tightly stoppered. If exposed to the air, powdered extracts absorb atmospheric moisture and eventually form a solid cake. Pilular extracts, on exposure in a dry atmosphere, slowly dry out and become hard, and thereby are rendered unfit for further use. This absorption or loss of moisture not only affects the physical state of the products, but also, even more important, their strength is decreased or increased proportionately. Some manufacturers put up pilular extracts in collapsible tin tubes because products so packaged keep considerably better than those in wide-mouthed jars. When jars are used, they should be light-resistant to prevent possible deterioration through photochemical action.

The U.S.P. of 1880 recognized a special class of extracts which were called *abstracts*. These products were standardized so that 1 part of abstract represented 2 parts of the drug.

Another class of preparations, closely allied to the extracts and used in some of the European countries, are *inspissated juices*. These products are made by contusing fresh plant parts, expressing the juice and drying the expressed liquid.

EXTRACT OF THE U.S.P.

PURE GLYCYRRHIZA EXTRACT

Pure Licorice Root Extract

Pure Glycyrrhiza Extract is prepared from glycyrrhiza, in granular powder. The term "granular powder" is not defined, but a No. 8, or very coarse, powder is suitable. Following exhaustion of the drug with boiling water, diluted ammonia solution is added to the percolate to convert the extracted glycyrrhizin to its ammoniated form. The liquid readily ferments and should be concentrated promptly by boiling under atmospheric pressure. This boiling coagulates albuminous extractive, which is removed by filtering before the liquid has increased sufficiently in viscosity to impede rapid filtration. The clear liquid then is evaporated to a pilular condition; no diluent is added. The yield and the quality of extract obtained are subject to variation and depend mainly on which of the several official varieties of glycyrrhiza is employed. Naturally, the degree to which the percolate is concentrated also affects the yield as well as the consistence.

The pure extract is used to mask the taste of cascara sagrada in the aromatic fluidextract of this drug. In the extemporaneous preparation of pills at the prescription desk, it is useful as an adhesive excipient.

EXTRACTS OF THE N.F.

Beef Extract

Extractum Carnis

The beef used for the preparation of the extract should be chopped or ground before cooking. The use of a pressure cooker is advantageous in that more of the odoriferous principles of the beef are retained than when the cooking is conducted in an open vessel. Although lean beef is prescribed, it is impracticable to exclude all fat from the raw meat; however, fat easily may be removed from the broth by chilling and filtering while cold.

Beef Extract, long used as a food for the sick, actually has little value as a nutrient, since fat is excluded and most of the protein is coagulated during the process of cooking. However, its agreeable flavor seems to have a stimulating effect on the appetite; therefore, it is much used in anorexia. It is also an ingredient in the popular hematinic beef, iron and wine.

Belladonna Extract

The extracts of belladonna, hyoscyamus and stramonium have much in common. For belladonna and hyoscyamus, both the pilular and the powdered forms are recognized for the convenience of the pharmacist. This is true also of Stramonium Extract, *N.F. IX*. For the powdered extracts, alcohol is employed as the menstruum, as this is evaporated to dryness more easily than a mixture of alcohol and water. On the other hand, in preparing the pilular extracts, a menstruum consisting of 3 volumes of alcohol and 1 volume of water is used because moisture is needed in the completed products to maintain a pilular consistence. The preparations are assayed chemically for their content of alkaloids and adjusted to specified standards of strength by the addition of diluents. These standards are approximately 4 times the minimum alkaloidal potency of the respective standard drugs. Attention is called to the fact that magnesium carbonate and magnesium oxide should not be used as diluents for the powdered products. In the presence of atmospheric moisture, the alkalinity of these diluents would cause the slow hydrolysis of the active alkaloids and, thereby, bring about a decrease in potency.

These extracts are employed widely for their anodyne and drying effects in pill, tablet and capsule formulas for relief of the common cold. Their tendency to relieve the griping of vegetable cathartics accounts for their presence in numerous proprietary and official laxative pill combinations. The extracts of belladonna and stramonium often are used in hemorrhoidal ointments and suppositories for their pain-relieving property.

Cascara Sagrada Extract

Powdered Cascara Sagrada Extract; Rhamnus Purshiana Extract

Cascara Sagrada Extract is prepared by percolation of the drug to exhaustion with boiling water, evaporation of the percolate to dryness and addition of sufficient dried starch to make the extract weigh one third of the weight of drug used.

The extract serves as a convenient means for the administration of cascara sagrada in the forms of tablets, pills or capsules.

Chondrus Extract

Irish Moss Extract

Official for the first time as an extract in *N.F. IX*, this product was recognized years ago in the first 2 editions of the *N.F.* under the title Irish Moss Gelatin. No procedure for its preparation is given, but it may be prepared by evaporating chondrus mucilage to dryness.

Large quantities of the extract are manufactured commercially, and, while consumed chiefly in the food industry in foods such as ice cream, chocolate milk, soups, cheese and canned meats, sizable quantities also are used in the manufacture of proprietary medicines. Chondrus mucilage (see p. 251) is an excellent suspending and emulsifying agent, but it has never been very popular at the prescription desk because it ferments readily, must be prepared freshly, and its preparation from chondrus is rather troublesome. The mucilage now may be prepared from the extract by a procedure somewhat simpler than that from chondrus itself, but it is doubtful that pharmacists will adopt it for the extemporaneous preparation of small quantities of suspensions and emulsions.

COLOCYNTH EXTRACT

Bitter Apple Extract

Colocynth Extract is prepared by percolation of the drug with a menstruum containing 4 volumes of alcohol and 1 volume of water, evaporation of the percolate to dryness, reduction of the residue to a fine powder and the addition of dry starch to the powder to make the extract weigh one fourth of the weight of the colocynth taken.

Occasionally called for in cathartic prescriptions, it is employed more often in preparing compound colocynth extract.

COMPOUND COLOCYNTH EXTRACT

This is prepared by simple admixture of colocynth extract with ipomea resin, aloe and cardamom seed, all powdered finely.

Compound Colocynth Extract is used in the manufacture of compound mild mercurous chloride pills.

GLYCYRRHIZA EXTRACT

Licorice Root Extract; Licorice

No procedure is given in the N.F. for the manufacture of Glycyrrhiza Extract, but its preparation is quite similar to that given for pure glycyrrhiza extract (q.v.). The extract usually is marketed in the form of large molded blocks and less often as cylindrical sticks or as a powder. Commercial samples often have been adulterated with starches and other insoluble substances. This unscrupulous practice accounts for the official requirements of a limit on the amount of insoluble matter present and a test for the detection of foreign starch.

While used in the manufacture of pharmaceuticals, principally in proprietary troches, much larger quantities are used in the tobacco and the confectionary industries.

HYOSCYAMUS EXTRACT

Henbane Extract

See Belladonna Extract (p. 398).

LIVER EXTRACT

Dry Liver Extract

Before being marketed, Liver Extract must meet the specifications for antianemia preparations presented on page 407 of N.F. XI and must be approved by the N.F. Antianemia Preparations Advisory Board. These requirements make it impracticable for the retail pharmacist to prepare the extract; therefore, no procedure for its manufacture is given. While a number of assays have been proposed, none is regarded as reliable, and the activity of commercial preparations must be determined by clinical trial. The products of various manufacturers differ in their process of manufacture and degree of concentration, and, for these reasons, the proper dosage must be stated on each package of the extract.

The extract may be prepared by extracting ground fresh mammalian livers with water. Protein is removed by adjusting the liquid to the iso-electric point, heating to cause coagulation and filtering. The clear solution is concentrated at a low temperature and alcohol added to precipitate the hematopoietic fraction, which is then dried and powdered.

Liver is invaluable in the treatment of pernicious (primary) anemia. The ingestion of large quantities of liver by patients suffering from pernicious anemia causes production of normal red blood cells, but liver therapy must be continued indefinitely or a relapse occurs. The fact that patients soon tire of eating one-half pound or more of fresh liver daily has stimulated the search for more concentrated preparations which are not offensive to take. The extract, which is taken by mouth, is one of 10 liver preparations now recognized by the N.F. It should be observed that some of these products are not intended for the treatment of pernicious anemia but are employed as vitamin supplements.

Liver with Stomach, official for the first time in *U.S.P. XIII,* more properly may be called liver extract with stomach, because actually it is prepared by combining a concentrated solution of liver principles with hog stomach tissue. This preparation also is employed in the treatment of pernicious anemia and produces effects clinically identical with those of Liver Extract.

Liver preparations no longer are recognized by the *Pharmacopeia,* having been supplanted by cyanocobalamin (vitamin B_{12}).

Liver, combined with iron preparations, frequently is employed in the treatment of secondary anemias, as there is clinical evidence that the two together are more beneficial than iron therapy alone.

Malt Extract

Malt Extract is prepared by infusing barley malt with water at 60° C., after which the separated liquid is evaporated under reduced pressure at a temperature not exceeding 60° C. to the consistence of a viscous liquid. It is customary afterward to add 10 per cent of glycerin as a preservative. In order to prevent destruction of the starch-digesting enzyme, diastase, the moderate temperature prescribed should not be exceeded. The preparation is assayed for diastatic power by a procedure involving the conversion of potato starch into water-soluble sugars.

The extract often is employed as a digestant and an easily assimilated nutrient. Pharmaceutically, it is used as a flavoring agent and a vehicle for distasteful drugs, as a nutrient, as a diluent for pilular extracts and as an emulsifying agent, notably for cod-liver oil.

Nux Vomica Extract
Powdered Nux Vomica Extract

After removing inert fatty matter from the drug by percolation with solvent hexane, Nux Vomica Extract is prepared by Process B for fluidextracts followed by evaporation of the percolate, assay and adjustment to the proper weight. The use of acetic acid in Menstruum I converts the alkaloids present to more soluble acetates, thereby facilitating their extraction. Formerly, the extract was assayed for total alkaloids, but now it is assayed only for the most active, strychnine.

Ox Bile Extract
Powdered Oxgall Extract

At present, no procedure is given for the preparation of Ox Bile Extract, but the *N.F.* requires that the extract contain "an amount of the sodium salts of ox bile acids equivalent to not less than 45 per cent of cholic acid ($C_{24}H_{40}O_5$)." The preparation is assayed colorimetrically.

U.S.P. XI directed that the extract be prepared as follows:

Evaporate 800 Gm. of ox bile to a volume of 200 cc. and slowly add 500 cc. of alcohol with constant stirring. Allow the mixture to stand for 24 hours, with occasional stirring, then decant the clear liquid. Mix the residue with 250 cc. of alcohol, filter, and wash the filter with 250 cc. of alcohol. Combine the alcoholic solutions, filter this liquid if necessary, and evaporate it to dryness at a temperature not exceeding 80° C. Powder the residue and mix it with sufficient starch, dried at 100° C., to make the product weigh 100 Gm.

The addition of alcohol to the concentrated bile effects precipitation of albuminous material but permits the desirable principles to remain in solution. Formerly, when no assay was directed, products made by this procedure varied considerably in strength and were inferior to the assayed preparation now official.

The extract, usually administered in the form of capsules or tablets, is employed to increase the efficiency of resinous hydragogue cathartics and also, at times, as a mild laxative itself. Bile is necessary to promote absorption in the intestine of fats and fat-soluble accessory foods such as carotene and vitamins D, E and K. The extract is indicated if a deficiency of bile causes nonabsorption of these substances.

NONOFFICIAL EXTRACTS

OPIUM EXTRACT, N.F. IX
Powdered Opium Extract

Opium contains a factor which is practically insoluble in water and frequently causes nausea and vomiting in many persons. However, the extract appears to produce these undesirable reactions less often. This observation has been explained by the fact that the extract is prepared by extracting opium with water.

RHUBARB EXTRACT, N.F. IX
Extractum Rhei; Powdered Rhubarb Extract

Rhubarb contains a high proportion of soluble material which prevents a high degree of concentration in the preparation of the extract. No assay is provided, but, after evaporation of the percolate to dryness, adjustment of strength is made by the addition of dried starch or other powdered diluents to make the extract weigh one half the weight of the drug used.

RICE POLISHINGS EXTRACT, U.S.P. XIV
Extractum Perpolitionum Oryzæ; Tikitiki Extract, Rice Bran Extract, Extracto de Salvado

Rice Polishings Extract, a viscous liquid, is valued for its content of thiamine (vitamin B_1) which amounts to not less than 0.06 mg. per ml. of extract. Other substances which have been reported as present are riboflavin, nicotinic acid, tocopherol, pyridoxine and an antianemia factor. Neutral or alkaline thiamine preparations are much reduced in potency at elevated temperatures, a fact which accounts for the moderate temperature prescribed for the concentration of the extract.

The extract seldom is employed in the United States, but it enjoys wide usage in the Philippine Islands in the treatment of beriberi and other diseases associated with a deficiency of thiamine. The other constituents, named above, are present in too small an amount to warrant the use of the extract where therapy with these substances is indicated.

STRAMONIUM EXTRACT, N.F. IX
See Belladonna Extract (p. 398).

BIBLIOGRAPHY

TINCTURES

Beal, G. D., Waters, K. L., and Block, P., Jr.: J. Am. Pharm. A. (Sci. Ed.) **36**:203, 1947.

Burlage, H. M., and Hawkins, D. B.: J. Am. Pharm. A. (Sci. Ed.) **35**:379, 1946.

Davy, E. D.: J. Am. Pharm. A. **8**:112, 1919.

Jackson, R. M., and Rowe, T. D.: J. Am. Pharm. A. (Sci. Ed.) **33**:188, 1944.

Scoville, W. L.: J. Am. Pharm. A. **4**:1472, 1915; **8**:799, 1919; **16**:1136, 1927.

FLUIDEXTRACTS

Arny, H. V., and Oxley, F. H.: Proc. Am. Pharm. A. **58**:1104, 1910.

Burlage, H. M., and Hawkins, D. B.: J. Am. Pharm. A. (Sci. Ed.) **35**:379, 1946.

Scoville, W. L.: Proc. Am. Pharm. A. **58**:874, 1910; J. Am. Pharm. A. **8**:799, 1919; **16**:1136, 1927.

Squibb, E. R.: Proc. Am. Pharm. A. **13**:201, 1865; **15**:391, 1867; **26**:708, 1878.

Thompson, W. B.: Am. J. Pharm. **71**:67, 1899.

FLUIDGLYCERATES

Beringer, G. M.: Proc. Am. Pharm. A. **56**:981, 1908.

EXTRACTS

Gillis, E., and Langehan, H. A.: J. Am. Pharm. A. **20**:746, 1931.

Hallberg, C. S.: Proc. Am. Pharm. A. **29**:424, 1881.

Squibb, E. R.: Proc. Am. Pharm. A. **13**:201, 1865.

GENERAL

Brochmann-Hanssen, E.: J. Am. Pharm. A. (Sci. Ed.) **43**:27, 1954.

Coblentz, V.: Proc. Am. Pharm. A. **33**:424, 1885.

Greco, S. J., and DuMez, A. G.: J. Am. Pharm. A. (Sci. Ed.) **39**:560, 1950.

NOEL E. FOSS, PH.D.
Dean, School of Pharmacy, University of Maryland

22

Resins and Oleoresins

RESINS
  HISTORY
  COMMENTS ON THE RESINS
  NATURAL RESINS
  SYNTHETIC RESINS

OLEORESINS
  HISTORY
  COMMENTS ON THE OLEORESINS

RESINS

The galenical resins are a class of preparations made by percolating the drug with an alcoholic menstruum, removing the volatile portion of the menstruum from the percolate by distillation and subsequently evaporating, and precipitating the resins by pouring the concentrated percolate into water or acidulated water. They differ from the so-called natural resins in that they are not exudates and in that they contain some extractive matter in addition to resins.

The natural resins are collected as exudates from plant products. They are liquid when first collected, but, on exposure to air, they become solid. Guaiac, mastic and rosin are examples of natural resins.

The galenical or prepared resins are obtained from the powdered crude drug. Although they are of indefinite composition, they are generally acidic in nature, and thus can be saponified by alkalies, which property is utilized in several official preparations. Resins are soluble in alcohol, chloroform and ether, and they are insoluble in water.

HISTORY

Resins first became official in the *U.S.P.*, as a class of galenicals, in 1860, at which time the resins of jalap, podophyllum and scammony were admitted. In the 1920 edition of the *U.S.P.*, the resin of scammony was replaced by the resin of ipomea. The resins of ipomea, jalap and podophyllum were admitted to the *N.F.* as soon as they were deleted from the *U.S.P.*, and all 3 were recognized officially by the *N.F.* from the 1940 edition until 1955, when podophyllum resin was again admitted to the *U.S.P.*, where it continues to be official. The resins of ipomea and jalap were retained in *N.F. X* and continue to be described in the current *N.F.*

To what extent, if any, the eclectic resinoids, made by a process similar to the one now prescribed officially for making the resins, influenced the introduction of resins into the *U.S.P.* cannot be stated definitely, but it is interesting to note that such preparations as resinoid of caulophyllum, resinoid of cimicifuga, resinoid of euonymus and resinoid of leptandra were being manufactured and advertised commercially as early as 1855.

For brief descriptions of the official methods of preparing the resins, see Table 32.

COMMENTS ON THE RESINS

Podophyllum Resin, U.S.P. Podophyllum Resin, official in the *U.S.P.* from the 1860 edition to the 1940 edition, and in the *N.F.*

TABLE 32. GALENICAL RESINS*

Resin	Drugs Used	Menstruum	Method of Preparation
U.S.P.: Podophyllum Resin...	Podophyllum in a fine powder	Alcohol	Percolation to exhaustion, concentration of the percolate and precipitation of the resin by pouring the concentrated percolate into 1,000 ml. of acidified water previously cooled to a temperature between 5° and 10° C.
N.F.: Ipomea Resin........	Ipomea in a moderately coarse powder	9 vols. of alcohol and 1 vol. of water	Percolation, concentration of percolate and precipitation of resin by pouring the concentrated percolate into 2 times its volume of hot water
Jalap Resin..........	Jalap in a fine powder	9 vols. of alcohol and 1 vol. of water	Percolation, concentration of percolate and precipitation of resin by pouring the concentrated percolate into 12 times its volume of hot water

* Synopsis of methods given in the present official compendia for the preparation of resins. For more detailed descriptions, the compendia should be consulted.

until the 1955 edition, continues to be official in the *U.S.P.* It is known to eclectic practitioners, who used it prior to its official recognition, under the name Podophyllin.

The resin is prepared by pouring the concentrated percolate into 1,000 ml. of water acidulated with hydrochloric acid and previously cooled to a temperature between 5° and 10° C. This procedure is followed because a greater yield of resin is obtained than when pure water is used. The yield is about 5.5 per cent with acidulated water and only 5 per cent with water alone. In the past, some manufacturers have precipitated the resin by pouring the concentrated percolate into a dilute solution of alum, even though the yield is only about 4.9 per cent, to obtain a greenish-yellow product. The product obtained by the official process is light brown in color. It should be handled with caution, since it is highly irritating to the eye and to mucous membranes in general.

The resin is employed as a caustic by virtue of its cytotoxic effect for certain papillomas or epithelial tumors. It is usually applied topically in the form of a 25 per cent dispersion in liquid petrolatum, preferably containing up to 20 per cent paraffin. In addition, the resin is considered to be among the most drastic of hydrogogue cathartics and is usually dispensed in combination with drugs in pills or capsules. The resin is an ingredient of an official pill as well as several nonofficial pills and capsules.

Ipomea Resin, N.F. Ipomea Resin, also known as Mexican scammony resin, was admitted to *U.S.P. X*, in which it replaced resin of scammony, which had been official up until that time. The change was made because the therapeutic properties of the two resins were similar, and genuine resin of scammony had disappeared almost completely from the market.

In the preparation of the resin, which is now in the *N.F.*, it is directed that the concentrated percolate be poured into twice its volume of hot water. Hot water is specified because cold water yields a precipitate of large aggregates from which it is difficult to remove impurities by washing. Constant stirring also aids in producing a fine precipitate. This also applies to the preparation of the other official resins.

Ipomea Resin is a hydrogogue cathartic and usually is dispensed in combination with other drugs in pills and capsules. It is an ingredient of Compound Colocynth Extract, N.F.

Jalap Resin, N.F. Resin of Jalap was official in the *U.S.P.* from the 1860 edition to the 1920 edition, inclusive. Then it was taken over by the *N.F.*, in which it is now official.

It is directed to be prepared by pouring the concentrated percolate into 12 times its volume of hot water. The use of a comparatively large volume of water is necessary to produce a fine precipitate free from impurities.

Sometimes the resin is adulterated with rosin, guaiac and other resins, also with aloe. Therefore, the N.F. prescribes tests for these adulterants.

Jalap Resin is used as a hydrogogue cathartic in combination with other drugs. It is an ingredient of an official and several nonofficial pills.

NATURAL RESINS

Mastic, N.F. Mastic is the concrete resinous exudation from *Pistacia lentiscus*. The resin yields not more than 3 per cent of ether-insoluble residue and not more than 20 per cent of alcohol-insoluble residue.

Mastic is used as an ingredient of compound mild mercurous chloride pills.

Rosin, N.F. Rosin, also known as Resina and Colophony, is the solid resin obtained after the distillation of turpentine. The volatile portion of turpentine is known as oil of turpentine. Turpentine is an oleo-gum resin obtained from *Pinus palustris* and from other species of *Pinus*.

Rosin is used as a component of many ointments and plasters and as an adhesive.

SYNTHETIC RESINS

In recent years a new class of chemical compounds has been introduced. These are polymers of high molecular weight which are closely related to the plastics. Because of their physical and chemical similarity to natural resins they have been classified as synthetic resins. The use of such compounds in pharmacy is based primarily upon their ability to remove positively or negatively charged ions from solution by a mechanism which is called ion-exchange. This is described under the preparation of Purified Water, page 176.

Both cation-exchange and anion-exchange resins have been used in therapeutics. The anion-exchange resins have been used to neutralize excess gastric acidity, while the cation-exchange type have been used in an attempt to remove excess sodium ions from the system by retaining such ions in the intestinal tract. One of the major difficulties encountered has been the comparatively large dosage required. The *U.S.P. XVI* has included one preparation of the synthetic resin type. Although its use is based upon the ion-exchange principle, it is intended as a diagnostic aid.

Azuresin, U.S.P., is also known as Azure A Carbacrylic Resin. It consists of a combination of a complex dye, known as Azure A dye, and a carbacrylic cation exchange resin. It contains in each Gm. not less than 50 mg. and not more than 70 mg. of the dye calculated on the dried basis. The *U.S.P.* suggests that this preparation be given in a dose of 2 Gm. with 500 mg. of Caffeine and Sodium Benzoate. The Caffeine and Sodium Benzoate stimulates gastric acid secretion. The hydrogen ions of the acids are then exchanged for the molecules of dye which have previously been complexed with the resin. The released dye is absorbed into the blood stream and excreted in the urine, producing a blue color. After a suitable period of time, the absence of color in the urine is presumptive evidence of hypochlorhydria or achlorhydria. Then further tests can be performed to determine the nature of the disease which is present. The preparation is commercially available as Diagnex Blue.

OLEORESINS

Oleoresins as a class of galenicals are extracts prepared, as a rule, by percolation of the drug with a highly selective solvent and the subsequent removal of the latter from the percolate by evaporation. Ether is the solvent most widely used for this purpose. It was replaced by acetone in *U.S.P. VIII*, but it was again the solvent directed to be used by *U.S.P. XIV* and *XV* for the preparation of aspidium oleoresin. The *U.S.P.* does not specify any solvents but merely states that the oleoresin is obtained from aspidium by suitable extraction. The *N.F.* permits a choice of ether or acetone in the preparation of ginger oleoresin.

The galenical oleoresins do not necessarily correspond in composition to the so-called natural oleoresins, such as turpentine, which consist almost wholly of volatile oil and resin. As a matter of fact, some of the galenical oleoresins contain little or no volatile oil and only a small amount of resin, as, for instance, the capsicum oleoresin.

History

The oleoresins were, at one time, a fairly popular form of medication, but their popularity has waned rapidly in the last 4 decades. They first appeared as a separate class of galenical preparations in the *U.S.P.* in 1860, which contained monographs for the preparation of no less than 5 oleoresins. Six were official in the 1910 edition. The present edition recognizes only the aspidium oleoresin. However, 2 of the oleoresins formerly official in the *U.S.P.*—capsicum and ginger—have been retained by the *N.F.*

The suggestion for the name oleoresin appears to have come from Buchner, though first applied as the name of a galenical by Peschier. In 1825, Peschier had prepared an ethereal extract of male fern which he designated *Huile de Fougere Mâle*. Buchner objected to this name, suggesting the title *Extractum resinosum*. However, in reporting Peschier's work, Buchner speaks of the constituents of the ethereal extract as the *œlharzige Bestandtheile* of male fern, and, later in his account, he refers to the finished preparation as the *œlharzige Extract*, i.e., an oleoresinous extract. Therefore, it would appear that when Peschier, in his second account (1828), speaks of *oléorésine*, our English oleoresin, he took his suggestion from Buchner's use of the German *œlharzig*.

Buchner's suggestion that these preparations be called *Extracta* appears to have met with general favor throughout Europe as indicated by the European pharmacopeias, in which they are classed with the extracts. In this country, a Latinized form of Peschier's title, *oléorésine,* was adopted, and these preparations are listed in our official compendia as *Oleoresinæ*.

For brief descriptions of the official methods of preparation of the *N.F.* oleoresins, see Table 33.

Comments on the Oleoresins

Aspidium Oleoresin, U.S.P. The Aspidium Oleoresin, also known as Male Fern Oleoresin, was introduced into the *U.S.P.* of 1870 and has been official in all subsequent editions.

Inasmuch as aspidium deteriorates rapidly when in the powdered form, the oleoresin is usually prepared from the freshly powdered drug. As a matter of fact, it is rarely, if ever, prepared by the pharmacist, because all of the drug must be imported from Europe, and most of it is in a deteriorated condition when it reaches this country. European manufacturers are aware of this, and practically the entire crop of the drug is made into oleoresin by these manufacturers immediately after the annual harvest. That which is not required for home consumption is offered for sale to importers in this and other countries.

Because of the comparatively high cost of production and the necessity of using fresh drug to obtain a good product, the oleoresin has been adulterated by dilution with castor oil to increase profits or by the addition of chlorophyll to mask the brown color imparted by the use of old deteriorated drug. The former can be detected by testing its solubility in 95 per cent alcohol

Table 33. *N.F.* Galenical Oleoresins*

Oleoresin	Drugs Used	Menstruum	Method of Preparation
Capsicum Oleoresin	Capsicum in a coarse powder	Acetone or ether	Percolation and subsequent distillation and evaporation of the solvent. Liquid portion separated from fatty matter by straining or decantation
Ginger Oleoresin	Ginger in a moderately coarse powder	Acetone, alcohol or ether	Percolation and subsequent distillation and evaporation of the solvent

* Synopsis of methods given in the present official compendia for the preparation of oleoresins. For more detailed descriptions, the compendia should be consulted.

and the latter by the official assay for filicic acid content.

Aspidium Oleoresin is used primarily as an anthelmintic for intestinal tapeworms, its effectiveness for this purpose depending largely on its state of preservation. The active constituents, known collectively as filicic acid and of which filmaron is the most important, break down on exposure to air and aging into compounds which are inactive. Therefore, the oleoresin should be stored in tightly stoppered containers in a cool place and should be used within a reasonable period of time—about 1 year.

The *U.S.P.* directs that the granular, crystalline precipitate usually found in the oleoresin after storage be mixed with the liquid portion before dispensing.

Aspidium Oleoresin is a toxic preparation and should be administered with care. The usual dose is now 5 Gm. with a range of from 3 to 5 Gm. Before the oleoresin is administered, it is recommended that the patient be placed on a fat-free diet for 24 hours preceding the ingestion of the oleoresin. After administering a saline cathartic, the Aspidium Oleoresin is taken, followed by a saline laxative in 3 hours. These precautions are recommended to ensure the elimination of the Aspidium Oleoresins. It is usually recommended that an oily cathartic should not be given, since the oleoresin is soluble in oils and there might be danger of absorption. Aspidium Oleoresin is a thick green liquid and usually is administered in capsule form and less frequently in the form of an emulsion.

Capsicum Oleoresin, N.F. The Capsicum Oleoresin was official in the *U.S.P.* from the 1860 edition to the 1920 edition, inclusive. Since then, it has been official in the *N.F.*

When prepared by percolating the drug with acetone or ether, the oleoresin contains a considerable amount of fats which are solids at ordinary room temperature. The *N.F.* directs that these fats be removed by decantation or by straining the mixture through a pledget of cotton. A more convenient method of accomplishing this is to chill the mixture in a refrigerator, then punch a hole in the layer of solid fat which has formed on the surface and pour off the liquid.

The chief therapeutic uses of the oleoresin are as a rubefacient and as a counterirritant. For these purposes, it usually is applied in the form of a plaster or ointment. It is also employed internally in dilute solution as a carminative. Its main use, from the standpoint of quantity consumed, is in the manufacture of carbonated ginger beverages, to which it is added to increase pungency. It is interesting to note that a compendium as recent as the *N.F. VII* included an organoleptic assay for Capsicum Oleoresin. This assay specified a characteristic pungent taste when the oleoresin had been diluted to an approximate concentration of 1 to 2,200 with a syrup containing 10 per cent of sucrose.

Ginger Oleoresin, N.F. The Ginger Oleoresin, which was official in the *U.S.P.* from the 1860 edition to the 1910 edition, was taken over by the *N.F.*, in which it is official at the present time.

Ether is the solvent which was directed by the *U.S.P.* to be used in making this oleoresin, except in the 1900 edition, when acetone was directed to be used. The present edition of the *N.F.* permits the use of acetone, alcohol or ether for this purpose, because there is little difference in the efficacy of these 3 solvents insofar as the extraction of the pungent principles of ginger is concerned.

The pungency of Ginger Oleoresin is attributed to a volatile ginger oil. It is used chiefly as a flavoring agent and in the manufacture of ginger beverages. Sometimes it is adulterated with Capsicum Oleoresin to increase its pungency.

BIBLIOGRAPHY

Resins

Beach and Little: Am. J. Pharm. **48**:385, 1876.

Husa and Fehder: J. Am. Pharm. A. **27**:121, 220, 319, 1246, 1937.

Husa and Lee: J. Am. Pharm. A. **28**:593, 1939.

Husa and Macek: J. Am. Pharm. A. (Sci. Ed.) **29**:455, 1940.

Husa and Magid: J. Am. Pharm. A. **23**:891, 1934.

Kaplan: New Orleans M. and S. J. **94**:388, 1942.

King and Sullivan: Science **104**:244, 1946.

Lloyd: Proc. Am. Pharm. A. **35**:65, 1887; Am. J. Pharm. **62**:242, 1890.

Ough: Chem. and Drug. **51**:524, 1897; **52**: 86, 548, 1898; **53**:183, 1898; **55**:299, 561, 1899; **56**:158, 735, 1900.

Parker: Pharm. J. **12**:41, 62, 1881.

Scoville: Proc. Am. Pharm. A. **57**:897, 1909.

Warren: J. Am. Pharm. A. **21**:217, 1932.

OLEORESINS

Beringer: Am. J. Pharm. **64**:145, 1892.

DuMez: The Galenical Oleoresins, pp. 1–288. Bull. Univ. of Wisconsin, Madison, 1917.

Maish: Proc. Am. Pharm. A. **48**:495, 1900.

Sherrad: Chem. and Drug. **40**:523, 1892.

PERRY ALBERT FOOTE, Ph.D.
Dean, College of Pharmacy, University of Florida

23

Powders, Capsules and Related Dosage Forms

POWDERS
    DISPENSING POWDERS
    SPECIAL PROBLEMS IN COMPOUNDING
      POWDERS
    U.S.P. POWDERS
    N.F. POWDERS
CAPSULES
    HARD CAPSULES
    DISPENSING CAPSULES

SPECIAL PROBLEMS WITH CAPSULES
ELASTIC CAPSULES
PEARLS AND GLOBULES
OFFICIAL CAPSULES
WAFERS, CACHETS, KONSEALS
OIL-SUGARS
CANDY MEDICATION
TRITURATIONS

Throughout history, pharmacists and physicians have sought new and better drugs to allay disease and suffering. Also, they have designed new methods and have improved on existing modes of administration to give the patient more efficient medication. The form of a drug may affect greatly its therapeutic action, appearance and palatability. The form of medication should be chosen also with such factors in mind as stability, ease of handling and dispensing, cost and convenience to the patient. Like other modes of administration, powders, capsules, cachets, oil-sugars and triturations have found their place among dosage forms. Their use in drug therapy gives the pharmacist a further opportunity to acquaint physicians with the desirable prescription service he can render.

POWDERS

Powders (Latin, *pulvis*; plural, *pulveres*) are mixtures of drugs and/or chemicals prepared in dry powder form. They are used internally, externally, as snuffs and as insufflations for body cavities. Occasionally, they are used to make solutions, such as douches. They are compounded in bulk and in divided doses (*chartulae*).

Powders were designed originally as a convenient mode of administration for such hard vegetable drugs as roots (rhubarb), barks (cinchona) and woods (charcoal). When chemical remedies were introduced, this mode was extended to them. In particular, this method was found convenient for dispensing insoluble compounds such as calomel, bismuth salts, mercury and chalk. Greater diffusion of drugs is obtained from powders than if the drugs are given in a compact form. When pills, tablets and capsules are difficult for children and others to swallow, the powder form often is desirable. Powders are economical and convenient. Because liquid vehicles are not present, many incompatibilities are avoided, as well as deterioration in some cases. (For example, acetylsalicylic acid is unstable in the presence of moisture.) On the other hand, this dosage form is not the best for administering bitter and corrosive drugs and those which readily change on exposure to the air, such as deliquescent and efflorescent bodies. Combinations which form eutectic or explosive mixtures should be avoided if possible; otherwise, they become special compounding problems.

Powders should be in a fine state of subdivision. The degree of fineness frequently has a bearing on their therapeutic action, such as bismuth compounds when given for coating the intestines. Fine powders are absorbed more readily, for example, calomel, arsenious oxide and dicalcium phosphate. Dusting powders, snuffs and insufflations might be irritating if coarse particles were present. They should be passed through a bolting cloth sieve of 120 to 150 mesh.

Administration of Powders. Powders are administered orally by being placed on the tongue followed by a drink of water or other liquid. An alternative method is to mix with water first, especially if the bulk is large. The mixing of powders with honey, syrup or jam will assist in masking an unpleasant taste. The bitterness of soluble salts may be overcome partially by dissolving in a sweet fruit juice. Dusting powders are applied conveniently from sifter-top cans. Snuffs are inhaled. Insufflations are blown into body cavities by a powder blower called an insufflator.

Mixing Powders. All processes for mixing powders are based on agitation produced by some method or device. Motion must be imparted to the particles to cause them to diffuse. Therefore, the spatula frequently is used to mix powders on a pill tile or paper, and the pestle is used to mix them in a mortar. The method of sifting or bolting produces motion for diffusion and also classifies the particles as to size. Some pharmacists mix powders on a sheet of paper, giving the paper a rolling motion while holding its ends. Because the efficiency of this procedure is questionable, it cannot be advocated when a potent drug is present. In large-scale production, power mixers are used, followed by sifting. Some

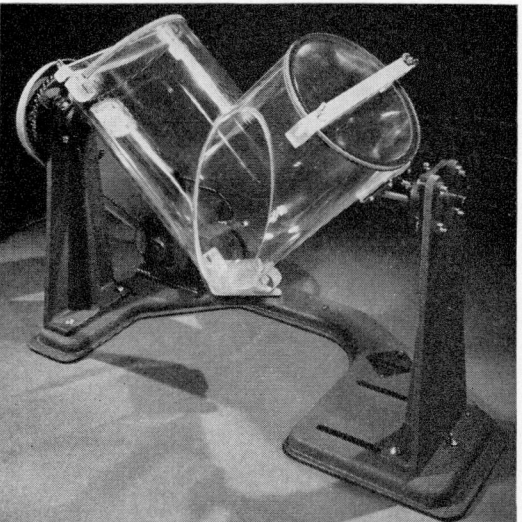

FIG. 163. Standard plastic laboratory twin shell blender. The dust-tight shell is made of heavy, transparent Lucite. (Patterson-Kelley Co., Inc., East Stroudsburg, Pa.)

pieces of equipment combine a mixer and a sifter.

During recent years, patented "twin shell" blenders (Fig. 163) have been introduced for laboratory size or larger quantities of powders. These are available in capacities of 4 quarts and larger. Transparent plastic shells and special shells of stainless steel and other metals can be obtained. These blenders are very efficient.

The general principle of mixing which should be observed in all cases is to start with the smallest (or most potent) ingredient and add an equal volume of diluent or other ingredient to it. Mix thoroughly. Then add another quantity of another ingredient equal to the bulk already mixed. Mix and repeat the process until all the ingredients are combined, resulting in a uniform distribution of each ingredient. The importance of uniformity is magnified in the case of potent drugs and large-scale manufacturing. In the latter case, the finished product should be assayed. Powders should be divided finely before mixing. If not, they should be triturated previously to the proper degree of fineness. The character and the quantity of the ingredients as well as the use of the finished product will largely determine the method.

MORTAR METHOD. The method used most frequently by American pharmacists is the mortar method. Its principal advantage is pulverization and diffusion in one operation. Therefore, it is better for crystalline salts. If all ingredients are in a fine state of subdivision, light trituration should be used unless it is desired to make them more compact. In the latter case, heavy trituration should be used. In most cases, the mortar method will give more compact powders than sifting. If possible, heavy trituration should be avoided, because the trituration is primarily for mixing. Heavy trituration might delay this process as it sometimes causes caking and sticking to the pestle and the sides of the mortar. Magnesium oxide is an example. Occasionally, the mortar and the pestle should be scraped with a spatula.

Composition mortars such as the Wedgwood and the porcelain types usually are preferred. A rough interior surface is desirable. Smooth mortars may be roughened by triturating in them some abrasive such as carborundum powder, coarse emery or sand. Glass mortars are too smooth; however, pharmacists find them advantageous for combining small amounts of powerful or costly drugs as there is less possibility of absorption and sticking to the mortar and the pestle. Glass mortars also are desirable for drugs that might stain the porcelain or the Wedgwood types; iodine is an example.

SPATULA METHOD. This method consists of stirring the ingredients on a pill tile or paper. In particular, it is used for small quantities and those cases where trituration would bring about a too compact powder, e.g., as with powders containing magnesia. Powders so mixed usually diffuse more readily in water.

SIFTING METHOD. This method usually is practiced at the prescription counter by using a kitchen-type flour sieve. Regular covered standard sieves also are available and are very desirable. In large-scale manufacturing, power-operated, dustproof mixers and sifters are almost necessary. To ensure enough mixing, powders should be put through sifters 2 or 3 times.

Coarse particles which do not pass through the sieve should be triturated to a finer state and mixed in by repeated sifting. The method of sifting is advantageous in producing a fine powder, well-mixed and free from foreign matter such as pieces of the glass or the paper container in which the ingredients were shipped. It is an excellent method for incorporating colors.

DISPENSING POWDERS

Powders are prescribed in bulk quantities and divided doses.

Bulk Powders. These usually are limited to: (1) those which are relatively nontoxic and can be measured safely in a spoon by the patient; (2) dusting powders. Douche powders frequently are dispensed in bulk with directions for measuring when used. The usual containers for bulk powders are round pasteboard boxes or wide-mouth screw-cap glass jars. The opening should be large enough to insert a spoon. If a cork-stoppered bottle is used, it is well to fit a piece of glazed paper between the cork and the neck of the bottle so that particles of the cork cannot get into the powder. Bottles should be used for volatile or hygroscopic substances. Sifter-top cans are preferred in the dispensing of dusting powders. Powders intended for external or local use always should be dispensed with *"external use"* or *"local use"* labels printed in red to distinguish them from powders used orally.

Divided Powders. These are prescribed to make certain that the patient gets the proper dosage. The ingredients having been mixed according to one of the above methods, the pharmacist must choose the best method for dividing the bulk into the required number of doses. Great accuracy is necessary for potent drugs. For less potent drugs, a great degree of accuracy is not so essential. The required accuracy and the comparative amount of time involved will assist the prescriptionist in choosing one of the following methods:

1. WEIGHING. Weighing each powder is the most accurate and is the only safe method for potent drugs. Because the pharmacist is skilled in weighing, this method may not consume much more time than other methods. Since powder papers have

been found to vary in weight, the same one or a watch crystal should be used for all weighings in each prescription. This will save time in balancing. Due to slight losses of material in compounding, the last powder weighed frequently will be too light. This difficulty may be overcome by compounding enough of the ingredients to make an additional powder which also would fall short of the required weight and should be discarded. However, if one of the ingredients is a narcotic drug, none may be discarded. In such a case, the pharmacist should be very particular to lose as little drug as possible. The loss should be divided equally among all the powders.

2. BLOCKING AND DIVIDING. Perhaps the most common method is blocking and dividing powders, although it is not so accurate as weighing. By this procedure, the mixed powder is placed on a pill tile and formed into a rectangle with a spatula, making reasonably certain that the powder is of uniform depth and packing. The rectangular block is then divided with the edge of a spatula into the required number of doses (little blocks). For example, if 12 powders are called for, 4 divisions may be made vertically and 3 horizontally. The scale on the pill tile should be used for the proper dividing. Some powders having a tendency to flow cannot be blocked uniformly and should be divided by weighing.

3. MEASURES IN SPECIAL FORMS sometimes are used for powders of comparatively large bulk. This method lends itself to large-scale packaging of nontoxic powders. A wooden cup for Seidlitz powders is an example, although such cups are seldom used at present. Packing must be uniform, and continued usage may wear down the edges of such a cup and thus lower its capacity.

4. MECHANICAL POWDER DIVIDERS. These have been invented, but they rarely are used at prescription counters today. Some are illustrated in older textbooks.

The practice of estimating with the eye the proper amount of powder in a dose is dangerous and should be condemned.

Packaging Divided Powders

Choosing the Paper. Divided doses are dispensed in so-called powder papers. Several different kinds of paper may be used for this purpose, but the most popular are a special paraffin (glassine) paper and vegetable parchment paper. These are best for hygroscopic substances, especially the former. Other types infrequently used are white unsized paper and light-weight bond paper. These are not moisture-proof and therefore should be wrapped again with a paraffin paper for hygroscopic drugs. Occasionally, a pharmacist will have his

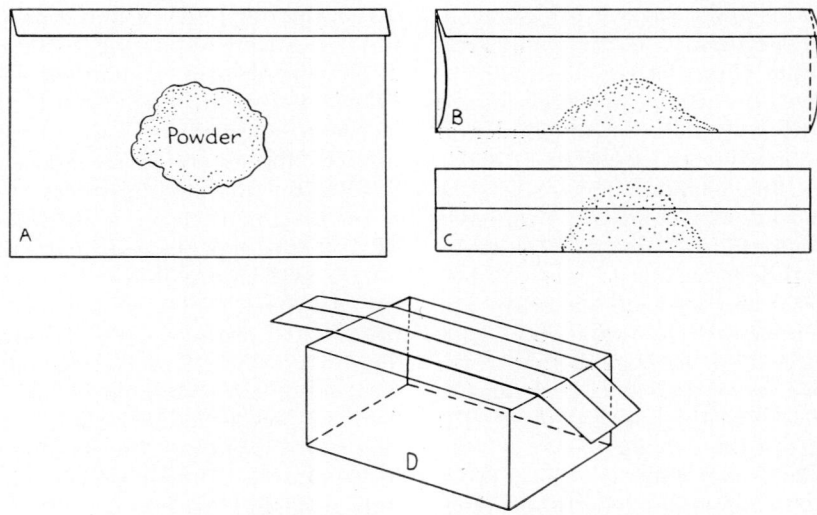

FIG. 164. Steps in folding powders in papers.

name printed on powder papers in such a position that it will appear at the top of the paper after folding.

Colored papers are used to distinguish powders. Thus, if a patient has to take 2 different powders, one may be dispensed in a white paper and one in a colored paper. An official illustration is Seidlitz powders.

It is not necessary for the pharmacist to cut powder papers, as they are available at low cost in different sizes. The correct size to choose will be governed by the amount of powder to be dispensed and the size of the powder box. The most popular size for adults is $3\frac{1}{2}'' \times 4\frac{1}{2}''$. Powders for babies and small children usually are wrapped in $2\frac{1}{2}'' \times 3\frac{1}{2}''$ papers.

Folding the Paper. With a little experience, this procedure can be done uniformly and neatly. The steps are as follows (Fig. 164):

1. Fold down a long edge approximately $\frac{1}{2}''$ for the average size paper. Several may be folded at once to save time. This fold will be the top of the finished powder paper (Fig. 164A).

2. Lay the papers on the prescription counter in a uniform manner so that the tops will be away from the compounder. For example, if 12 powders are prescribed, lay out 3 rows of 4 each.

3. Place the divided portions of the powder on the center of each paper (Fig. 164A).

4. Bring the lower edge of the paper to the creased line under the top fold. Press down the latter (Fig. 164B).

5. Now pull the top creased edge toward yourself until it divides the remainder of the paper approximately in half (Fig. 164C). Thus, a new top is made. The correct line for the last fold will depend on the style and the height of the powder box to be used. For slide-type boxes, the finished powder should be even with the edge. For hinged-top boxes, the powder should be slightly higher than the edge so that it can be picked out easily. It is usually better not to crease the top of the paper as this might unduly compact the powder.

6. Now fold the ends of the powder paper by pressing equal lengths of them down over the powder box while you gently press in the ends of the box (Fig. 164D). Sharply crease the end folds with a spatula. Instead of folding the powder papers over the box, a powder-paper folder may be used. This device has 2 edges; the distance between them may be adjusted to the desired length of the folded powder papers.

7. Then place the powders in the box according to one of the following plans: (A) all tops up and folds toward the operator; (B) all tops up, half the folds toward the operator and half away from him; (C) half the tops up and half down. Method A usually is used. Method C is advantageous where the powders are bulky.

Choosing the Box. The slide-type box is the most popular and the cheapest. The more expensive boxes have the name of the pharmacist or the store printed or engraved on the top of a removable lid. The latter may be hinged with the label placed on the under side so that lids and directions on 2 or more boxes cannot be interchanged by accident. When only 2 or 3 powders are prescribed, they usually are dispensed in an envelope.

SPECIAL PROBLEMS IN COMPOUNDING POWDERS

Small Quantities of Ingredients. These, which are impossible to weigh, must be diluted with an inert powder such as lactose and an equivalent amount used. Powdered sucrose plus 10 per cent cornstarch was a wartime substitute for lactose as a diluent. In diluting potent substances with lactose, it is well to put about 5 gr. of the lactose in a mortar, add the drug with trituration and finally the remainder of the lactose. By this method, there is little loss of the drug in adhering to the mortar. Volatile solvents may be used in certain cases to obtain an even distribution of a small quantity. An illustration of this is the incorporation of iodine in powders. Dissolve the iodine in powders. Dissolve the iodine in the volatile solvent contained in a glass mortar. Add the powder and triturate until the solvent has evaporated. A series of experiments incorporating iodine in powdered boric acid indicated that benzene gave better results than ether, chloroform or other solvents. Due to the volatility of the iodine, the finished product should be packaged immediately.

When sucrose is an ingredient, the powdered variety should be used. This is available on the market as confectioner's sugar.

Liquids. Liquids should not be incorporated into powders if it can be avoided. Small amounts of liquid may be added successfully to a portion of the powder while triturating, with addition of the remainder of the powder in divided parts. If alcoholic preparations such as fluidextracts and tinctures are prescribed in powder mixtures, the difficulty might be overcome conveniently by obtaining the consent of the physician to use an equivalent amount of the powdered extract of the same drug. If this cannot be done, the tincture or the fluidextract may be concentrated by heating on a water bath. After reduction to a small volume, some inert substance such as lactose should be added. When practically dry, powder the product and compound it into the powder mixture. Another method for incorporation of small amounts of tinctures and fluidextracts is as follows: warm a pill tile with an alcohol lamp, then drop the liquid ingredient on the pill tile, spacing the drops a few millimeters apart. Allow to evaporate, then scrape up the residue with a spatula and mix with the other ingredients.

Pilular Extracts. These are undesirable ingredients due to their semisolid nature. If the powdered extract cannot be used, the pilular extract should be converted to a dry form by the addition of an inert ingredient —e.g., lactose.

Essential Oils. If essential oils and other volatile drugs such as menthol and camphor are incorporated into powders, special care should be observed to prevent evaporation. Inert absorbent powders are helpful, as well as double powder papers or cellophane envelopes which are sealed by heat.

Liquefaction of Powders. This is caused by one or more of three conditions:

Eutectic Mixtures. Certain solid substances, when thoroughly mixed with each other, will form a liquid due to a lowering of the melting point. The proportions used will determine the melting point. These substances are found usually among aldehydes, ketones, phenols and alcohols. They include such commonly used drugs as chloral hydrate, camphor, phenol, menthol and thymol. Antipyrine, acetanilid and acetophenetidin are also in this category. When such cases occur, the difficulty usually is obviated by mixing the ingredients separately with an absorbing agent such as kaolin, dry starch, calcium phosphate, magnesium oxide or magnesium carbonate. The different lots then are compounded into the final powder mixture.

Water of Crystallization. Sometimes water of crystallization is liberated from such salts as sodium phosphate, sodium sulfate, alum and ferrous sulfate during or after trituration, particularly if they are triturated heavily during mixing. Pressure promotes liberation of water. Light mixing is necessary. The best method is to use the anhydrous forms of the salts. If these are not available, the hydrous forms may be dried before mixing. Absorbents can be used as described for eutectic mixtures.

Hygroscopic Drugs. These should not be dispensed in powders if it can be avoided. A solution of them is a better dosage form. If the powder form is required, the problem may be solved by the use of an absorbent, light mixing and double wrapping in moisture-proof powder papers or by the use of sealed cellophane envelopes.

Additional methods of solving the foregoing problems include the making of a mass to be dispensed in capsules and the dispensing of troublesome ingredients in separate powder papers. The pharmacist should obtain the physician's approval before resorting to any of these methods.

Explosive Mixtures. These usually consist of oxidizing agents and organic compounds; they include potassium chlorate and potassium permanganate as sources of oxygen and such organic compounds as starch, sugar, tannic acid and gums. Sulfur and sulfides also may be oxidized with explosive violence. Trituration of such mixtures must be avoided. Some authorities advise triturating the powders separately, then mixing lightly on a pill tile or paper, or dispensing in separate powder papers. The author of this chapter advocates the latter, with the belief that such mixtures should not be dispensed. Explosions of this nature may occur several hours after dispensing, as illustrated by the following case.

A pharmacist compounded a prescription consisting of sodium perborate and aspirin and dispensed it in a screw-cap bottle. After the patient had retired that night, the mixture exploded, making it necessary for the pharmacist to pay for damaged household effects.

Flavors. Small amounts of essential oils may be incorporated to flavor powders. Peppermint and cinnamon oils are used most frequently. The oil-sugars of *N.F. VII* are valuable for this purpose, as well as Aromatic Powder, N.F. IX.

Colors. Sometimes colors are added; these include certified food and drug dyes, solutions of carmine or cochineal, red saunders and charcoal.

U.S.P. Powders

U.S.P. XVI lists only 2 formulas for powders.

Absorbable Dusting Powder, U.S.P. (*Starch-derivative Dusting Powder*). This is a biologically absorbable powder prepared from cornstarch by etherification with epichlorohydrin. The starch derivative is mixed with magnesium oxide, 2 per cent, and small residual amounts of sodium sulfate and sodium chloride. It is used for lubrication of the hands in donning rubber gloves and as a substitute for talcum powder in hospital routines. It has the advantage of biologic absorbability and is nonirritating and nontoxic. The powder should be sterilized by autoclaving. Slight clumping which occurs after repeated autoclaving may be broken up readily with moderate pressure. Dry heat sterilization is not recommended for bacteriologic reasons, and also should be avoided because of the possible flammability of the powder. However, the powder will flash only to about the same degree as cotton, so that flammability is not a hazard to its use in surgery. This powder is available under the name of Powder Bio-Sorb (Ethicon Suture Labs.).

The powder should be preserved in sealed paper packets.

Compound Iodochlorhydroxyquin Powder, U.S.P. (*Pulvis Iodochlorhydroxyquini Compositus*). This powder was recognized officially for the first time in *U.S.P. XIV* and is designed for treating *Trichomonas* vaginitis by intravaginal insufflation. It consists of iodochlorhydroxyquin 25 per cent, boric acid 10 per cent, lactic acid 2.5 per cent, zinc stearate 20 per cent and lactose 42.5 per cent. The *U.S.P.* directs that the lactic acid be mixed with the lactose, then add the boric acid, the iodochlorhydroxyquin and the zinc stearate and mix thoroughly. This powder is available under the name of Vioform Insufflate (Ciba). It should not be confused with Iodochlorhydroxyquin, U.S.P. (Vioform—Ciba).

The powder should be preserved in tight, light-resistant containers.

N.F. Powders

Compound Effervescent Powders, N.F. (*Seidlitz Powders*). This well-known saline cathartic was named after the Seidlitz Spring in Germany, not because it duplicated the contents of that water but probably because the name of that famous spa aided its sale as a secret nostrum. The original product, sold more than a century ago, consisted of a combination of 2 powders. One was sodium bicarbonate wrapped in blue paper to distinguish it from the other, which was tartaric acid. A colorless paper was chosen for the acid since it might react with the dye from a colored paper, particularly if it had absorbed moisture.

The *N.F.* recognizes a better formula: 30 Gm. of dry sodium bicarbonate (60 mesh) is mixed thoroughly with 90 Gm. of dry potassium and sodium tartrate (40 mesh) and divided into 12 equal powders, each to be wrapped in a blue paper; 26 Gm. of dry tartaric acid (40 mesh) is divided into 12 equal parts and each wrapped in a white paper. The contents of the blue paper is called the "Seidlitz Mixture" and may be purchased in bulk.

The old method of measuring Seidlitz powders by wooden cups rarely is used in pharmacies today. Weighing is more accurate. Moreover, most pharmacists buy Seid-

TABLE 34. POWDERS OF N.F. XI

Official Title	Percentage of Ingredients	Usual Dose (Approximate Equivalent in Parentheses)
Effervescent, Compound (Seidlitz Powders)	See description of ingredients, p. 414	See description of ingredients, p. 414
Furazolidone and Nifuroxime	Furazolidone 0.1%, Nifuroxime 0.5%, Slightly Acidified Powder Base 99.4 %	No dose (external use)
Ipecac and Opium (Dover's Powder)	Ipecac 10%, Powdered Opium 10%, Lactose 80%	300 mg.
Senna, Compound (Compound Licorice Powder)	Senna 18%, Glycyrrhiza 23.6%, Precipitated Sulfur 8%, Fennel Oil 0.4%, Sucrose 50%	4.0 Gm.
Sodium Bicarbonate and Calcium Carbonate (Sippy Powder No. 1)	Precipitated Calcium Carbonate 23%, Sodium Bicarbonate 77%	2.6 Gm.
Sodium Bicarbonate and Magnesium Oxide (Sippy Powder No. 2)	Magnesium Oxide 50%, Sodium Bicarbonate 50%	1.3 Gm.
Zinc Sulfate, Compound	Salicylic Acid 0.5%, Phenol 0.1%, Eucalyptol 0.1%, Menthol 0.1%, Thymol 0.1%, Zinc Sulfate 12.5%, Boric Acid 86.6%	No dose (external use)

litz powders already packaged by manufacturers.

If the ingredients were mixed together, the product would simulate the chemical composition of an effervescent salt (Chapter 24). In such mixtures, a chemical reaction occurs in the presence of moisture. Since the tartaric acid in Seidlitz powders is in a separate paper, this reaction cannot occur. This is an important advantage, particularly in an atmosphere of high humidity.

This dosage form is based on the principle that carbonation renders solutions of salts more palatable. The average dose is the contents of a white and a blue paper, each dissolved in about 2 fluidounces of water, the solutions mixed and administered just after effervescence begins to subside. The reaction is as follows:

$$2NaHCO_3 + H_2C_4H_4O_6 \rightarrow Na_2C_4H_4O_6 + 2H_2O + 2CO_2$$

Furazolidone and Nifuroxime Powder, N.F. This preparation has been recognized for the first time in N.F. XI. The drug content and description corresponds with that of the patented preparation Tricofuran Vaginal Powder, Improved of Eaton Laboratories. The preparation has been recommended particularly for use in vaginitis due to *Trichomonas vaginalis* and *Candida albicans*. It is categorized as a local antibacterial and antiprotozoan. Since it is applied by insufflation, there is no statement of dose.

Ipecac and Opium Powder, N.F. This narcotic preparation is the well-known Dover's powder. The formula illustrates the use of lactose as a diluent. The N.F. specifies that this ingredient be coarsely powdered. During trituration to a fine powder, the coarse particles will assist in the subdivision of the ipecac and the opium. It is used primarily as a diaphoretic in incipient colds.

Compound Senna Powder, N.F. The fennel oil should be mixed thoroughly with about one half of the sucrose, then the remainder of the sucrose and the other ingredients should be added and mixed thoroughly. Finally, pass the powder through a No. 80 sieve, pulverize the residue; if any should be left on the sieve, add it to the sifted powder and mix thoroughly. The N.F. permits replacing 3 per cent of the sucrose with powdered starch. If it becomes hard or compact, it should not be dispensed.

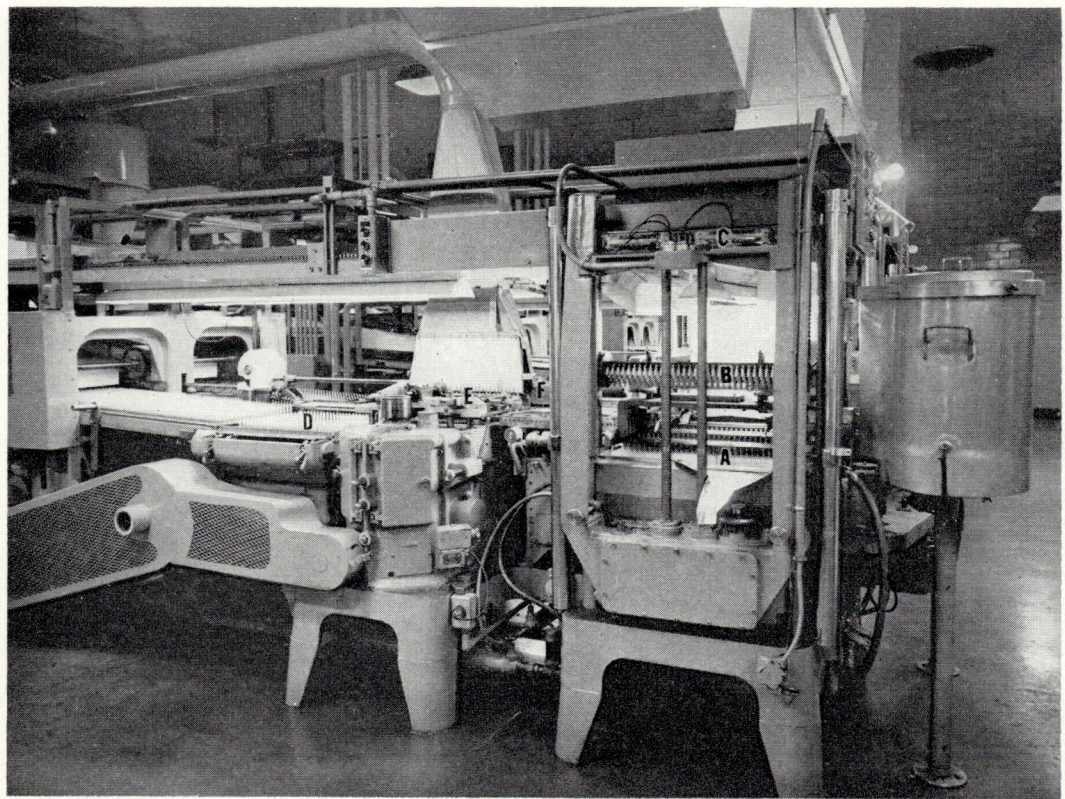

Fig. 165. Automatic capsule-making machine at Eli Lilly and Company. (A) Stainless-steel body molds are dipped in gelatin solution; molds for caps are treated similarly on the opposite side of the machine; (B) molds are rotated as they are raised to the top of the machine to ensure uniform distribution of gelatin; (C) molds are conveyed to the drying kiln; (D) molds are conveyed from the drying kiln; (E) dried gelatin is stripped from the molds and trimmed and bodies and caps joined; (F) finished capsules are delivered on other side.

Compound Zinc Sulfate Powder, N.F. The *N.F.* directs that the salicylic acid and the zinc sulfate be triturated to a fine powder. To this are added the phenol, the eucalyptol, the menthol and the thymol, previously liquefied by trituration. The boric acid is added with trituration until a uniform mixture is obtained. The powder is then passed through a very fine sieve. This preparation is used for making mild astringent washes and douches. It is criticized as being unnecessarily complex.

N.F. Tooth Powder. This is an official synonym for the **N.F. Dentifrice** (official title) and is classified by the *N.F.* as a dentifrice. For the formula and the method of compounding, see *N.F. XI*.

CAPSULES

Capsules (Latin, *capsulae*) are shells of gelatin used for the administration of solids, masses and liquids (Fig. 166). Efforts in the United States to produce satisfactory capsules of methyl cellulose have not been successful. Some use of them has been made in England. Historical records reveal that, in 1834, two French patents were granted to Mothes and Dublanc for the employment of soft gelatin capsules. The inventor was Mothes. Dublanc was an apothecary who improved the invention for pharmaceutical use. In 1848, Murdock patented the 2-piece hard gelatin capsule which is easier to fill and close. Soft capsules are composed principally of gelatin, glycerin and water. Gelatin hard capsules consist of such other ingredients as sugar, acacia and a very small amount of water.

Advantages. The popularity of capsules as a mode of administration is based not only on elegance and portability but also on other advantages, as follows:

1. To the Patient. Capsules mask the taste and the odor of drugs. The gelatin shell is soon dissolved in the stomach, and the contents are absorbed more readily because no excipients are present, as in the case of tablets and pills. Swallowing and disintegration are facilitated by a draught of water. For more rapid disintegration and absorption, the capsule may be pricked several times with a pin and swallowed with hot water. Capsules can be administered rectally, if necessary, preferably after moistening with water. A special rectal capsule has been manufactured, but is not presently on the market in the United States (Fig. 167).

A newly patented and unique method for bringing about continuous therapeutic effects from the contents of one capsule was introduced several years ago. The capsule contains hundreds of tiny pellets with varying disintegration times. Release of medication is extended over a period of 8 to 10 hours, with therapeutic effect lasting for approximately 10 to 12 hours.

2. To the Physician. He may prescribe different combinations of drugs and vary the proportion to suit the patient's needs.

3. To the Pharmacist. Convenience. Quick filling. They can be dispensed within

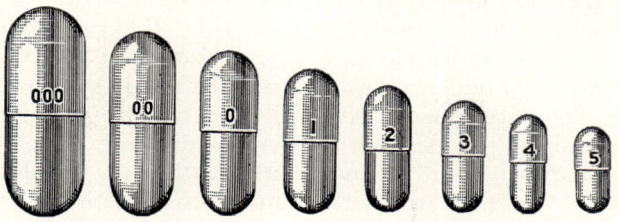

Fig. 166. Actual sizes of empty gelatin capsules.

5 per cent tolerance with confidence provided that the contents does not weigh less than 2 grains and that each filled capsule is weighed.

4. To Make Solutions. Solutions of a definite strength sometimes are made by adding the contents of a capsule to a given volume of water.

Capsules are undesirable as a dosage form for aqueous or hydroalcoholic liquids which would dissolve the gelatin and for very soluble salts. Such compounds, when released in the stomach, would make irritating concentrated solutions. Bromides, iodides and chloral hydrate fall in this group. Fantus warned that practically insoluble powders such as bismuth subnitrate should not be prescribed in capsule form because of the possible formation of enteroliths. He cautioned against the use of capsules, pills and tablets in ulcerative conditions of the alimentary tract.

Hard Capsules

Manufacturer. The manufacture of hard gelatin capsules on a large scale has been made possible by automatic machines. Special noncorroding stainless steel molds,

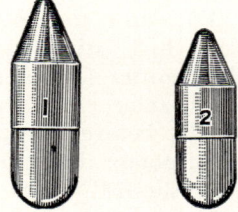

Fig. 167. Rectal suppository capsules.

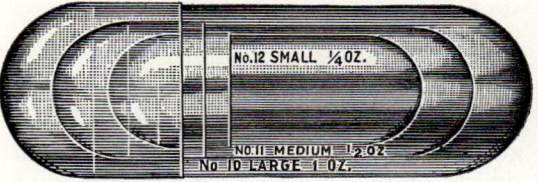

Fig. 168. Veterinary capsules.

traveling on a slow conveyor, are dipped in a gelatin mixture. As the conveyor continues, the gelatin film dries, forming the capsule which is cut to proper length. In like manner, the top part is made and then fitted on the lower part. Coloring is accomplished by adding a suitable certified dye to the gelatin bath. As the capsules leave the machine, they are inspected under a strong light to eliminate defective ones. Many factors are important in the process, such as exactness of size of molds (pins), composition and temperature of the gelatin bath, temperature and humidity of the room. Air-conditioned rooms are necessary. Sanitary conditions prevail. Hands do not touch them.

Storage. When storing empty capsules, extremes of humidity and high temperatures should be avoided. A dry atmosphere brings about a loss of moisture in the gelatin, producing a tendency to crack. Screw-top bottles are admirable for storing capsules as they are sanitary and moisture- and dust-proof. Visibility enables supplies of them to be checked easily for reorders.

Sanitary Conditions. Before filling capsules, the pharmacist should wash his hands to remove bacteria, dirt and perspiration. The latter can easily soil capsules. On humid days, it is found advantageous to wet the hands with alcohol and thoroughly dry with a towel just prior to handling the capsules. Rubber gloves or latex finger cots are used by some pharmacists.

DISPENSING CAPSULES

Dispensing capsules containing powders involves the following:

1. **Preparing the Powder.** The methods discussed on page 409 under the heading "Powders" are used.

2. **Choosing the Correct Size and Color of Capsules.** The manufacturer usually supplies a table on the side of the box which gives the correct size of capsules to use for quantities of different drugs. Inasmuch as all drugs cannot be incorporated in such tables, they must be used as general guides for correct sizes to enclose drugs of similar bulk. The usual method is to make trial weighings of filled capsules in order to ascertain the proper size. Tice and Moore have designed a slide rule for this purpose, whereas Cooper uses a marked cylinder. Both methods are based on the measurement of the volume of the powder. The correct size is that which is filled conveniently by the correct amount. Sometimes large sizes must be avoided if the patient has difficulty in swallowing them. This can be overcome by getting the physician's consent to dispense twice the number of capsules with half the dosage in each, with directions that the patient take 2 capsules per dose instead of 1. Colorless capsules are used unless otherwise specified by the physician. Pink capsules can be purchased by the pharmacist. Other colors such as red, green, yellow, blue and black are used by manufacturers for their specialties. Some are marketed with different colored tops and bottoms. If the dispenser will write the size number on the prescription as well as the color, this will assist in compounding refills.

3. **Filling Capsules.** At the prescription counter, filling capsules usually is done by the method of "punching." The required number of capsules is taken from stock. The powder is placed on a paper or pill tile and smoothed with a spatula so as to have a depth of one fourth to one third the length of the bottom of the capsules. The empty capsule bottom is held between the thumb and the forefinger and repeatedly pressed vertically into the powder until filled. The amount of compression used is important because, the greater the compression, the greater will be the amount packed into the capsule. The pharmacist should fill all of the capsules with the same compression so that the content of each capsule weighs the correct amount. If the amount should vary in each, there may be too little or too much powder to fill the last capsule. The cap is then placed on the capsule, after which it is inverted and tapped on the counter so that the powder fills the cap. In some cases, the cap may be filled partially before putting the capsule together. If potent drugs are involved, the pharmacist should weigh each filled capsule, using an empty capsule on the opposite pan for the tare. When filling

for deliquescent bodies, is of no assistance in overcoming liquefaction of eutectic mixtures.

Deliquescent Bodies. Not only will deliquescent bodies absorb moisture from the air, but also they will abstract a small amount of water from the capsule, causing it to crack. Husa and Becker found that 3 or 4 grains per capsule of magnesium carbonate, light or heavy magnesium oxide would keep most drugs in this class stable in capsules for at least 2 weeks. Their research indicated poor efficiency for lactose and starch. The use of talc gave fair results. Because magnesium oxide causes hydrolysis of esters in the presence of moisture, the mixing of it with such compounds should be avoided in deliquescent mixtures. If the inert absorbents cause too large a bulk, twice as many capsules may have to be used and the patient instructed to take twice as many per dose, as indicated on the prescription. Consent of the physician should be obtained before doing this. Capsules containing deliquescent substances should be dispensed in screw-on or snap-cap vials or bottles.

Powders That Do Not Pack Well. These usually can be put into capsules with the aid of a spatula which holds the powder in place while the capsule is moved toward the spatula horizontally to the prescription counter. Another method of solving the problem is to moisten the powder with alcohol. When powders such as cinchophen and amidopyrine become electrified and fluff around in the mortar, several drops of alcohol may be added and the mixing will be accomplished in one third the usual time. Mineral oil is recommended for glandular products exhibiting this property.

Liquids. Liquids should be dispensed in soft gelatin capsules which are easier to swallow; however, hard capsules can be used if necessary. The liquids must be limited to those such as oils which will not dissolve gelatin. Creosote dissolves gelatin and must be diluted with 2 or 3 times its volume of a vegetable oil. Liquids of low viscosity may be dropped into the capsules from a medicine dropper or pipet. Viscid liquids can be poured. Care should be taken not to get any of the liquid on the outside of the capsule. Should this occur the liquid should be wiped off carefully with a pledget of cotton. The cap preferably should be sealed on. This is done by moistening the lower half of the inside of the cap of the capsule with water, using a small camel's-hair brush or a stirring rod. As the cap is put on, a slight twisting motion should be applied. This facilitates a complete seal. Before dispensing liquid-filled capsules, they should be checked for leaks which can be observed by laying them on a blotter or filter paper. It will aid the filling process to stand the capsules in perforations in a powder-box top.

Enteric Coatings. Such coatings may be applied to capsules in much the same manner as pills and tablets. For details, the student is referred to the research of Husa and Magid in 1932 and to Chapter 24, "Masses, Pills, Troches and Tablets."

Weight Variation Test

The *U.S.P. XVI* provides a weight variation test for the contents of hard capsules. It is a 2-stage procedure whereby the sample may pass a simple first-stage test if the variation between capsules is small enough to neglect the rather negligible variation in the empty capsules. In cases where that test fails the analyst then applies the *U.S.P. XV* procedure which in itself is a sequential, 2-stage operation. Limits of variation have been reduced materially in the *U.S.P. XVI*. The test is as follows:

Weigh collectively 20 intact capsules, and calculate the average gross weight. Taking each capsule individually, balance it against weights representing 90 per cent and 110 per cent of the average, respectively: if each capsule weighs between 90 per cent and 110 per cent of the average gross weight, the sample meets the requirements.

If not all of the capsules fall within the aforementioned limits, weigh the 20 capsules individually and remove the contents of each capsule with the aid of a small brush or pledget of cotton. Combine and weigh the total contents and calculate the average weight. Weigh the emptied shells individually and calculate for each capsule the net weight of its contents by subtracting the weight of the shell from the respective gross weight. Determine the difference between the net weight and the average weight: the sample meets the requirements if (1) not more than two of the differences are greater than 10 per cent and (2) in no case is the difference greater than 25 per cent.

If more than 2 but less than 7 capsules deviate from the average between 10 per cent and 25 per cent, determine the net weights of an additional 40 capsules and determine the average content of the entire 60 capsules. Determine the 60 deviations from the new average: in not more than 6 of the entire 60 capsules does the difference exceed 10 per cent of the average, and in no case does the difference exceed 25 per cent.

Elastic Capsules

Apparently, the demand for empty elastic (soft) capsules has decreased to such an extent that it is no longer profitable for any American manufacturer to produce them. However, the author believes that the student should have some knowledge of them in case empty elastic capsules are needed and become available from domestic or foreign sources.

They are olive-shaped with a sealed elongated neck which prevents their collapse and the possibility of the walls sticking together. They are made by dipping molds into a warm bath of glycerogelatin composition. After drying, the molds are stripped, and the capsule necks are sealed. Elastic capsules are used primarily for the administration of liquids so prescribed. On rare occasions, some powder may be included in the liquid, e.g., salol and santal oil. As previously stated, the liquids must be limited to those which will not dissolve gelatin. Fixed and volatile oils commonly are dispensed in this manner. Stronger mercurial ointment is sold in soft capsules by some manufacturers. It is squeezed out by the patient at the time of application and represents a measured dose. Elastic capsules are easier to swallow than hard capsules; therefore, they are desirable for large volumes of liquids.

Filling Elastic Capsules. The necks are cut off and may be melted on a water bath and used for sealing. The capsules are filled by a dropper, pipet or buret, taking care not to get any of the liquid on the orifice. (If this occurred it might interfere with the seal.) A small air space should be left which is necessary if the capsule is to be compressible.

Sealing Elastic Capsules. This usually is done by one of two methods. A drop of warm glycerogelatin or solution of the melted capsule necks is applied to the opening with a previously warmed stirring rod and allowed to dry. If a small portion of the neck is permitted to remain on the capsule, the blade of a hot spatula may be pressed on it, causing the gelatin to flow into a seal. The latter method requires more practice. If the spatula is too hot or too cold, failure will result. The ideal temperature for the spatula blade is several degrees higher than the melting point of the capsule. Seals should be smooth and should be checked for leaks.

Packaging Elastic Capsules. Some provision should be made to prevent elastic capsules from sticking together, especially in a warm humid climate. This can be done by using boxes with partitions made

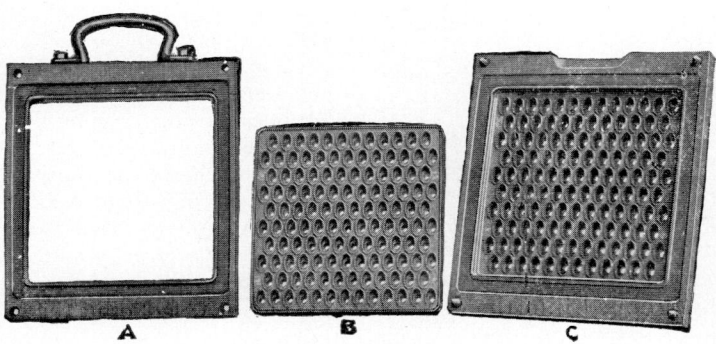

Fig. 171 Frame and molds for pearls.

for this purpose. Another method is to dust the capsules with an inert powder such as lycopodium, using a technic like that for dusting pills. (See p. 432, Chap. 24.)

Pearls and Globules

Pearls and globules are round or oval capsules made by enclosing liquids in a shell of glycerogelatin composition. Solids and even tablets may be included. They contain no air, thus are not so elastic as the soft capsules filled at the prescription counter. Their sizes range from 3 to 80 minims. The popularity of vitamin preparations has greatly increased the use of pearls and globules for the administration of these products. They are factory-made.

Manufacture. Two methods of manufacture are used. The older method utilizes 2 plates and a mechanical press. Each plate contains a specified number of depressions or molds the shape of the pearls or the globules to be made. A sheet of soft gelatin is fitted over the bottom plate, and the correct quantity of liquid poured on top (Fig. 172). A second sheet of gelatin is laid

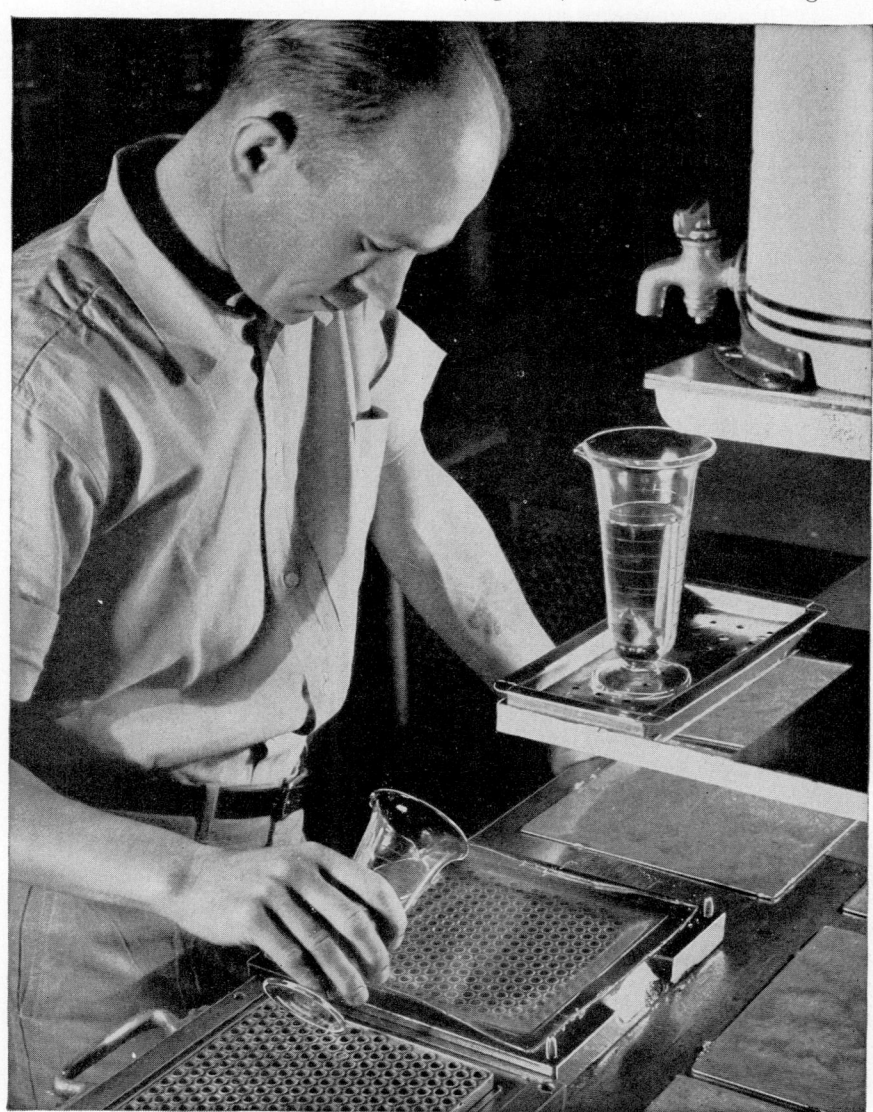

Fig. 172. Pouring liquid on the gelatin sheet.

carefully on top of the liquid, so as to exclude air. The top plate is then fitted on with the help of guides, and the combined set placed in the press. Powerful pressure is applied, forming the pearls. After separating the plates, the pearls are removed from the excess gelatin and washed with a suitable solvent such as acetone. Imperfect ones are discarded. A special device is available for enclosing tablets in globules.

The plate-method for making pearls and globules has been almost totally superseded in this country by a newer continuous process.

The newer method produces pearls by patented continuous automatic machines (Fig. 173). The liquid is injected between 2 ribbons of gelatin while passing between revolving dies. This method is faster and more economical than the former. Within recent years equipment has been invented to enclose dry powders in soft gelatin capsules.

Official Capsules

Capsules became official for the first time in *U.S.P. XII* and *N.F. VIII*. Those now official are:

U.S.P. XVI:
  Amobarbital Sodium
  Calciferol
  Chloral Hydrate
  Chloramphenicol
  Decavitamin
  Diphenhydramine Hydrochloride
  Diphenylhydantoin Sodium
  Ephedrine Sulfate
  Novobiocin Sodium
  Oleovitamin A
  Pentobarbital Sodium
  Phenoxymethyl Penicillin
  Procainamide Hydrochloride
  Secobarbital Sodium
  Sodium Radio-iodide
  Tetrachloroethylene
  Tetracycline Hydrochloride

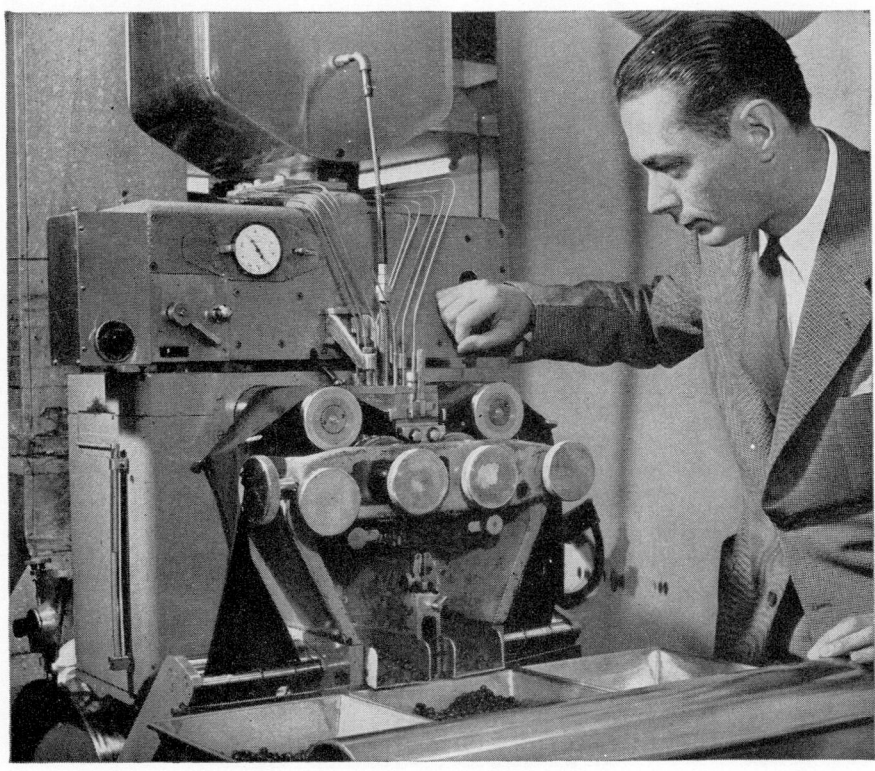

Fig. 173. Rotary die machine to make pearls.

Trimethadione
Water-miscible Vitamin A

National Formulary XI:
Acetylsalicylic Acid
Acetylsalicylic Acid, Acetophenetidin and Caffeine
Bishydroxycoumarin
Butabarbital Sodium
Carbarsone
Chlorotrianisene
Chlortetracycline Hydrochloride
Choline Bitartrate
Choline Dihydrogen Citrate
Digitalis
Ephedrine Hydrochloride
Ephedrine Sulfate and Phenobarbital
Ethchlorvynol
Glutamic Acid Hydrochloride
Halibut Liver Oil
Hexavitamin
Liver with Stomach
Menadione
Mephenesin
Methionine
Nicotinamide
Oleandomycin Phosphate
Oleovitamin A and D
Ox Bile Extract
Oxytetracycline Hydrochloride
Paramethadione
Pentathienate Bromide
Quinidine Sulfate
Quinine Sulfate
Racephedrine Hydrochloride
Theobromine Sodium Acetate
Triacetyloleandomycin
Triasyn B
Vinbarbital
Vitamin B_{12} with Intrinsic Factor Concentrate

WAFERS, CACHETS, KONSEALS

Wafers, cachets and konseals represent stages of improvement in the continual efforts of European apothecaries to mask the taste of powders in a shell that will break up quickly in the stomach. Although these dosage forms are little used in American pharmacy today, nevertheless we must recognize them.

The term "wafer" has been applied to all 3 forms. In a strict sense, the term refers to wafer paper which is made of rice flour and cut into small round or square sheets. The patient places the wafer in a tablespoon containing a little water. After the water is absorbed and the wafer becomes soft, the powder is poured in the center of the wafer and covered by folding in the corners or sides. The wafer is further moistened and swallowed with the aid of water.

Cachets were invented by Limousin with the idea of improving on the wafer. They are made in several different sizes which will hold from 0.5 to 1.0 Gm. of powder. A cachet consists of 2 circular rice-flour wafers each formed into a concave-convex shape. The halves are usually identical and formed with flanged edges which can be easily fitted together, as illustrated in Figure 174. The measured powder is poured in one half. The flanged edge of the top half is moistened slightly with water and pressed on the bottom half, thereby causing a seal. The amount of moisture used should be controlled carefully as too little will not permit a tight seal and too much will cause the edges to shrink on drying. For this purpose, moisture may be applied with a small camel's hair brush to the edge (or flange) of the upper half, or the upper half may be brought in contact with a damp cloth, such as bandage gauze, a moistened filter paper or blotter.

Cachet-filling machines have been invented for use at the prescription counter but rarely are used in America today. These consist of a set of hinged metal plates containing perforations in which the cachet parts will fit. A funnel is used for filling and a roller for moistening. The plate containing the empty half shells is brought against the plate containing the filled half shells, thereby effecting a seal. If the phar-

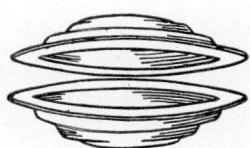

FIG. 174. Cachet.

macist lacks such a device, he may facilitate the procedure by using a perforated pill box to hold half the cachet while filling and sealing. Another aid can be 2 wide-mouth bottles; the mouth of one supports half the cachet while filling. The second bottle is inverted, and its mouth used to press on the other half of the cachet.

Cachets are administered by momentarily dipping them in a tablespoonful of water for softening, after which they are swallowed with more water.

Konseals are said to be an improved form of cachet. In American pharmacy, these terms have become synonymous. Modifications in the structure of cachets have been made. One with a dry seal has been invented, using a cap in the fashion of a capsule. Another type contains a partition for the separation of incompatible powders. Cachets and konseals sometimes are called starch capsules.

OIL-SUGARS

Oil-sugars (oleosacchara or Elaeosacchara) were designed in Germany to be used for flavoring powders or as correctives. They are not popular in American pharmacy. Their use in flavoring powders, particularly for children, has been overlooked by most physicians and pharmacists. Oil-sugars are not recognized in *U.S.P. XVI* or *N.F. XI*. *N.F. VII* gave a general formula for them as follows:

The Prescribed Volatile Oil.......... 2 cc.
Sucrose, in fine powder............... 100 Gm.

Triturate the sucrose with the volatile oil until uniformly mixed.

In prescribing oil-sugars, the oil must be named, e.g., Oleosaccharum Menthae Piperitae, Oleosaccharum Anisi, etc. As far as possible, it is advisable to prepare oil-sugars just before dispensing. This will minimize possible chemical changes in the oils which would detract from their flavor.

CANDY MEDICATION

Candy medication as advocated by Dr. Bernard Fantus deals largely with the incorporation of water-insoluble drugs in candylike tablets. A cocoa-sugar tablet base is always used and sometimes a solution of tolu balsam and saccharin or an alcoholic solution of saccharin. The *Pharmaceutical Recipe Book III* recognizes this dosage form under the name Sweet Tablets and gives formulas for the basic ingredients and 11 different kinds of them. These include the following drugs: Acetophenetidin, Albumin Tannate, Quinine Ethylcarbonate, Atropine Sulfate, Calcium Iodobehenate, Digitalis, Ipecac, Saccharated Ferrous Carbonate, Arsenic Trioxide and Saccharated Ferrous Carbonate, Methenamine and Terpin Hydrate. In handling them, care must be taken that children do not have access to any such tablets which are toxic. Fantus suggested that this problem could be solved by dispensing only a limited number at a time. The possibilities of this mode of administration may well be explored by pharmacists and physicians alike.

TRITURATIONS

Triturations (Latin, *triturationes*) represent powders that have been diluted with 9 parts of milk sugar. Every 10 Gm. of finished product represents 1 Gm. of active medicating agent. Each grain contains $\frac{1}{10}$ gr. of the drug. They were designed originally by the homeopaths for convenience in measuring small doses accurately. This is their primary function today. Triturations also offer some advantage by presenting an increase in the surface of the medicinal substance which hastens absorption. *U.S.P. XIV* gives the following directions for their preparation:

Unless otherwise directed, triturations are to be prepared according to the following formula:

Take of:
The Medicinal Substance............ 10 Gm.
Lactose, in fine powder.............. 90 Gm.
    To make .... 100 Gm.

Place the medicinal substance, previously reduced, if necessary, to a moderately fine powder, in a mortar. Add about an equal measure of lactose, and triturate the powders thoroughly together. Then add successive portions of the lactose from time to time, until the whole is added, and continue the trituration after each addition until the medicinal substance is intimately mixed with the lactose and reduced to a fine powder.

Low percentage triturations sometimes are compounded as stock preparations to assist in weighing very small amounts of potent drugs accurately. Thus, if 1 gr. of atropine sulfate were diluted with 99 gr. of lactose, the pharmacist would weigh 1 gr. of the finished product to get $\frac{1}{100}$ gr. of atropine sulfate. Stock bottles of such products must be labeled plainly indicating the concentration.

BIBLIOGRAPHY

Andrews, M. J.: Determination of the reasonable or permissible margin of error in dispensing, J. Am. Pharm. A. **22**:755, 838, 1933; ibid., **27**:374, 1938.

Auch, R. H.: Manufacture of powders, Amer. Perfumer **32**:79, 1936.

Bellafiore, I. J.: Stabilization of capsules of eutectic mixtures against liquefaction, J. Am. Pharm. A. (Pract. Ed.) **14**:580, 1953.

Cooper, M. L.: A capsule size selector, J. Am. Pharm. A. (Pract. Ed.) **15**:300, 1954.

Davis, N. S.: The administration of certain deliquescent and liquid drugs in capsules, J. Am. Med. A. **67**:1160, 1916.

Fantus, Bernard: General Technic of Medication, Chicago, American Medical Association, 1938.

Husa, W. J., and Becker, C. H.: The use of inert powders in capsules to prevent liquefaction due to formation of a eutectic mixture, J. Am. Pharm. A. **29**:78, 1940.

———: The use of inert powders to prevent liquefaction of the contents of capsules due to deliquescence, J. Am. Pharm. A. **29**:136, 1940.

Husa, W. J., and Macek, T. J.: The use of tribasic calcium phosphate and silica gel in capsules to prevent liquefaction, J. Am. Pharm. A. **31**:213, 1942.

Husa, W. J., and Magid, L.: Enteric coating of capsules, J. Am. Pharm. A. **21**:1030, 1932.

Lee, J. W.: Accuracy and speed factors in hand filling capsules, J. Am. Pharm. A. **24**:469, 1935.

Tice, L. F., and Moore, A. W.: A slide rule for selecting capsule size, J. Am. Pharm. A. (Pract. Ed.) **15**:296, 1954.

Urdang, G.: The invention of gelatin capsules, Pharm. Arch. **14**:58, 1943.

H. GEORGE DeKAY, PH.D.
Professor of Pharmacy, Purdue University

24

Masses, Pills, Troches and Tablets

MASSES
PILLS
    PILLS OF THE U.S.P.
    PILLS OF THE N.F.
    NONOFFICIAL PILLS
TROCHES

TABLETS
    COMPRESSED TABLETS
    MOLDED TABLETS
    PILL AND TABLET COATING
    OFFICIAL TABLETS

MASSES

Masses are pharmaceutical preparations composed of medicinal substances combined with other materials in such proportions that the products are plastic semisolids, capable of being shaped into pills with little or no further treatment. They are relatively permanent pill masses from which the pharmacist may make pills from time to time without the necessity of preparing the mass repeatedly.

The art of making masses is gradually disappearing because of the trends of modern medicine. There are no masses still official in our books of standards, yet the student of pharmacy should be familiar with the art and the skill needed in preparing good products. Even though the making of a mass in prescription work may be remote, it is well to be prepared to render the service and to produce a good product when called upon to do so by the medical needs of the moment. The manufacture of a mass is of little difficulty because the formula specifies the proper amount of liquid necessary to produce a plastic semisolid.

Ferrous Carbonate Mass, *N.F. X* (Vallet's Mass) has survived the changes in modern-day medicine.

There are 2 types of masses still in use. These types may be called the chemical preparation (Mass of Ferrous Carbonate) and the other the galenical preparation (Mass of Mercury).

The preparation of masses, in general, differs in no important respect from the initial steps in the preparation of pills and will be discussed later in this chapter, under the title of "Pills."

MERCURY MASS, N.F. IX
Massa Hydrargyri; Blue Mass, Blue Pill

Mercury Mass contains not less than 31 per cent and not more than 35 per cent of mercury.

Mercury .... 330 Gm.
Mercury oleate .... 10 Gm.
Glycyrrhiza, in very fine powder .... 100 Gm.
Althea, in very fine powder .... 150 Gm.
Glycerin .... 90 Gm.
Honey .... 320 Gm.

Triturate the mercury oleate in a mortar, gradually add the mercury, then a small amount of honey, and triturate the mixture until globules of mercury no longer are visible under a lens magnifying 10 diameters. Incorporate the remainder of the honey and the glycerin, gradually add the glycyrrhiza and the althea, and continue the trituration until the mass is homogeneous.

Usual dose, 0.2 Gm. (approximately 3 gr.).

The Mass of Mercury manufactured by

hand is a skillful and laborious procedure because the mercury has a tendency to coalesce or run together when the mass is made. The objective is to break the mercury into globules so small that they are not visible under the glass magnifying 10 diameters. This is said to be "extinguishing the mercury." If the trituration is stopped before the addition of the glycerin, the powdered althea and glycyrrhiza, the mercury will coalesce.

The product is a dark, slate-colored mass which, when recently made, can be shaped into pills readily, but which tends to become hard and rather dry on aging and exposure to air. It should be kept in a tightly closed container. Its condition will be improved if a small piece of bibulous paper, moistened from time to time, is placed within the container.

Occasionally, Mercury Mass is prescribed as one of several ingredients in a pill mass. When compounding such a prescription, the pharmacist should use as little pressure as possible in incorporating the Mercury Mass, since undue pressure may cause the globules of mercury to coalesce and thus reduce the effectiveness of the preparation.

An unofficial dry preparation containing a similar concentration of mercury is available on the market under the name of "Mercury Mass Powder." Its chief advantage lies in its greater stability.

FERROUS CARBONATE MASS, N.F. X

Massa Ferri Carbonatis; Vallet's Mass

Pills containing ferrous carbonate were listed in the *London Pharmacopœia* of 1809 under the title of *Pilulae Ferri Compositae*. In 1831, the French physician, Blaud, submitted to the French Royal Academy of Medicine the formula for his *pilules antichloratiques;* and, in 1837, his colleague, Vallet, submitted the formula that he had elaborated. The formula of the *London Pharmacopœia* called for sodium bicarbonate and ferrous sulfate, that of Blaud for potassium carbonate and ferrous sulfate. It was Vallet who recommended the use of monohydrated sodium carbonate as best suited for the double decomposition with ferrous sulfate resulting in the formation of ferrous carbonate.

Ferrous Carbonate Mass contains not less than 36 per cent and not more than 41 per cent of $FeCO_3$. For its preparation and further details, see the monograph in N.F. X.

Ferrous carbonate is made by chemical reaction during the manufacture of this preparation. The ferrous carbonate so prepared in the moist state oxidizes readily in the presence of even small amounts of air. This can be noted readily as the ferrous carbonate will be changed to a red-brown subcarbonate of iron, which is a mixture of ferrous carbonate and ferrous oxide. This oxidation is minimized during the manufacture by using boiling purified water and by introducing syrup into the wash water.

The ferrous carbonate is made by the following chemical reaction: $FeSO_4 + Na_2CO_3 \longrightarrow FeCO_3 + Na_2SO_4$

The precipitated ferrous carbonate is washed by decantation to remove the soluble sodium sulfate, using the syrup water. The syrup water is used for this purpose until the washings no longer have a salty taste. The presence of sugar in the water aids in preventing the oxidation of the green ferrous carbonate. The precipitate is now drained onto a muslin strainer to remove as much water as possible, then mixed quickly with the honey and the syrup which tends to stabilize the preparation chemically.

This preparation has been replaced almost entirely, in practice, by an unofficial dry "Ferrous Carbonate Mass" containing approximately the same concentration of ferrous carbonate. Its chief advantages over the official preparation are its greater stability and the greater ease with which it may be dispensed, as it usually is, in capsules.

PILLS

Pills are globular or ovoid dosage forms, intended for oral administration. They are prepared by incorporating medicinal agents with other material in such proportion that a cohesive, plastic mass is formed. Then this mass is divided into the requisite number of portions, and each portion is formed into the desired shape. Pills vary considerably in weight, the usual range being from

0.10 Gm. to 0.30 Gm. An exceptionally large pill, one of 0.60 Gm. or more, sometimes is referred to as a *bolus*. Very small pills, of 0.06 Gm. or less, are known as *parvules* or *granules*. The term "granule" also is used to designate small spheres of sugar which are saturated with liquid medication before being swallowed.

For the past several hundred years and, indeed, until rather recently, pills occupied a most important place in pharmacy. As an example, the prescription files of a Charlestown, Mass., pharmacy for the years 1872–75 reveal that over half of the prescriptions dispensed were for pills. Thus, at one time pill-making was considered to be the highest expression of the art of the apothecary. It is still a necessary accomplishment, because prescriptions for pills, while not common are encountered occasionally in retail practice.

The decline in the popularity of pills is due chiefly to the development of 2 comparatively new dosage forms. These are the compressed tablet and the hard gelatin capsule. The former can be produced on a manufacturing basis at only a fraction of the cost of pills; at the dispensing counter, the latter can be filled in much less time than would be needed to make pills from similar ingredients.

In addition to the time and the labor needed for the manufacture of pills, there are other disadvantages. They are not suitable when rapid action is desired, since a pill firm enough to retain its shape will disintegrate slowly in the alimentary tract. Some pills lose moisture and become so hard that they actually may pass unchanged through the tract and be eliminated in the feces. A further disadvantage lies in the possibility of chemical reaction between ingredients of the pill formula, since moisture is necessary, in most instances, for preparation of the mass.

Many of the advantages once possessed by pills no longer exist. Thus, smallness of bulk with consequent ease of administration, concealment of taste and relative permanence are objectives realized more economically and more efficiently by using other dosage forms, such as the capsule and the compressed tablet. However, certain recipes are suitable for neither tablets nor capsules; for these, pills may offer the only practicable means of dispensing.

Preparation of Pills

Mixing the Ingredients. Since pills often contain very potent substances, great care must be used in mixing the ingredients to ensure accurate and uniform dosage. The most reliable method is that of geometric dilution. The most potent substance, which is usually the smallest in bulk, is placed in the mortar first. To this is added an equal bulk of the substance which is next in potency, and the 2 portions are mixed thoroughly by trituration. This process is repeated, as many times as is necessary, adding the ingredients in the order of decreasing potency, the bulk of each added portion being approximately equal to that of the material in the mortar, at the time it is added.

Dry ingredients should be in as fine a form as is practicable. It may be necessary, in some cases, to reduce the particle size of a substance by trituration in a mortar previous to incorporation with the other ingredients. If an ingredient is a pilular extract or a substance of similar physical nature, a considerable error may be incurred in transferring it from the paper on which it has been weighed to the mortar. To reduce the error to negligibility, the following method may be used. Lightly grease a portion of a weighing paper with petrolatum and then tare the paper. Weigh the semisolid substance on the greased portion of the paper and transfer it to the head of the pestle with a lightly greased spatula.

Making the Pill Mass. To produce satisfactory pills, it is necessary that the ingredients be formed into a plastic mass, soft enough to permit manipulation into the desired shape, yet sufficiently firm to retain that shape. This ordinarily is accomplished by the addition of a substance called the *excipient*. The ideal excipient is one that imparts the requisite degree of plasticity by its adhesive character, by a slight solvent action on the pill ingredients, or by a combination of these qualities. It should be pharmacologically and chemically inert and should be capable of producing a mass which retains its plasticity for long periods of time. It should not retard disintegration of the pill in the alimentary tract. There is no excipient which can be used in all cases, but liquid glucose is suitable for nearly all pills prepared extemporaneously. Other excipients which have been found useful are honey, syrup, tragacanth mucilage, soap, glycerin, alcohol and water, or combinations of these. The selection of the proper excipient is an important part of the art of pill-making and one that ordinarily is learned only after considerable experience.

The utensils best suited for the efficient preparation of a pill mass are a relatively deep and narrow mortar, a pestle with a fairly long, wooden handle, and a steel spatula having a short, stout blade (Fig. 175). The previously mixed ingredients are placed in the mortar, and a portion of the chosen excipient is added. If the excipient is a liquid, it may be added by means of a graduate or a pipet; if it is a viscid substance, such as glucose or honey, it is customary to transfer it to the head of the pestle by means of a spatula. The correct amount of excipient to use in a given situation is learned only after long experience. The novice would do well to use it sparingly, since the usual practice of the beginner is to use too much.

Considerable pressure is required to make a good pill mass. The pharmacist may exert the necessary pressure with a minimum of effort by using the pestle as a lever, with the rim of the mortar as the fulcrum. If the pestle handle is of sufficient length, and if the force is applied with a twisting motion, even those of slight physical strength will not find it difficult.

During the forming of the pill mass, it will be found necessary, from time to time, to collect the material by scraping it from the inner surface of the mortar and from the head of the pestle. For this purpose, the stout spatula previously mentioned should be used, since an ordinary spatula would bend or break. When the mass is finally of the proper consistency, it will tend to collect of itself, by rolling away from the surface of the mortar under the pressure of the pestle.

Dividing the Mass. The finished mass is removed from the mortar, as completely as possible, is kneaded in the hands until no fissures are visible and then is shaped into a ball by rolling in the palms. The ball is placed on a *pill tile* and is rolled into a cylinder, the *pill pipe*, by means of a *pill roller*, which is simply a flat, thin board with rounded edges. Since the accuracy of division depends in large measure on the uniformity of the pill pipe, the pipe must be of the same diameter throughout its length, and its ends must be kept square.

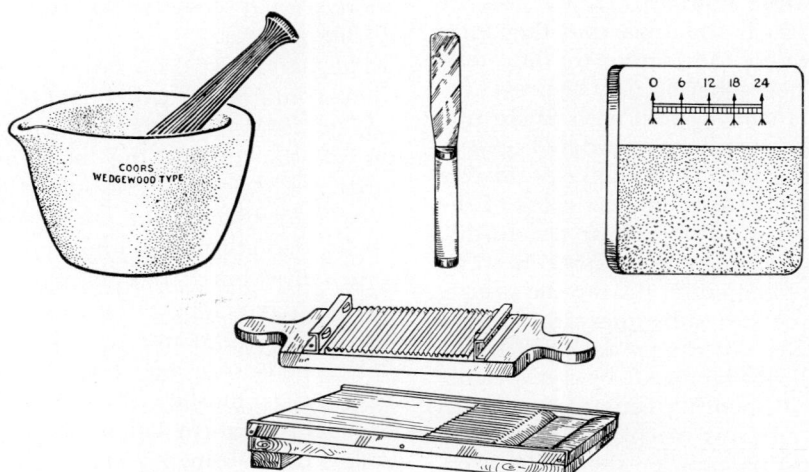

Fig. 175. Utensils used in making pills: mortar and pestle, pill spatula, pill tile and pill machine.

When the pill pipe has been rolled to the desired number of spaces on the scale of the tile, it is scored lightly to correspond with the divisions of the scale. To attempt to divide the pipe without first scoring it would result in distortion of the pipe and consequent inaccurate division. When inspection reveals that the pipe has been scored properly, it is divided by cutting with a sharp instrument, preferably a razor blade, held carefully at right angles to the pipe.

Shaping and Finishing the Pills. The segments of the pipe are rolled with the fingers into approximately globular shape, making certain that the surfaces roughened by cutting are made smooth. Then they are subjected to the action of the *pill finisher,* a wooden disk having a flange on each side, one flange being somewhat deeper than the other. The pills are gathered beneath the finisher, using that side of the finisher which permits complete support by the pills. Then, cupping the finisher in the hand, and using only the degree of pressure indicated by the condition of the mass, it is rotated rapidly in a figure-of-eight or eccentric movement until the pills are uniformly globular with smooth surfaces. Uneven division of the pill pipe will be revealed during this process by the tendency of the large portions to become spindle-shaped and by the failure of the small portions to become smooth and globular.

Using Dusting Powders. Unless pills are dispensed in such a manner that they form a single layer in the container, they tend to cohere. Their cohering may be prevented by dusting them lightly with such substances as lycopodium, powdered glycyrrhiza, starch or talc. The choice of dusting powder depends chiefly on the color of the pill, the objective being to have the dusting powder as inconspicuous as possible. The powder is applied either during the process of finishing or just subsequent to it. Any dusting powder not closely adherent to the pills should be removed before placing them in the dispensing container. If pills are to have any sort of coating applied to them, no dusting powder should be used.

The foregoing discussion is concerned with the making of pills on a small scale, as in compounding prescriptions. The manufacturer, in making pills on the grand scale, follows the procedures outlined above, but with different equipment. Instead of mortar and pestle, tile, roller and finisher, he uses machines which are almost wholly automatic.

INDUSTRIAL PRODUCTION OF PILLS

The industrial production of pills follows the general pattern of hand production except that larger equipment is used. The making of the pill mass is performed by using large massing machines which are similar to those used in bread-making. The mass is completely mixed to a dough consistency which is pliable yet is a semiplastic mass. This dough is a uniform mixture of all of the ingredients comprising the formula.

There are 2 machines used in industry for completing the dough mass described above into completed pills. These machines are dependent upon each other. The first is a ball-cutting machine in which the semiplastic dough mass is cut into balls of uniform size before being transported to the pill-making machine. This ball-cutter has 2 hoppers: the first is filled with a dusting powder to prevent the mass from sticking to the ball cutter; the second contains the pill mass. This mass is carried to the ball-cutter by means of a worm-gear feeding device, where it is cut into small balls and covered with the dusting powder.

The balls now drop down a chute onto a belt containing small hoppers. They are now carried by this belt to a hopper at the top of the pill-making machine. These dough balls now fall through the hopper onto a movable belt and are passed between 2 belts, one above the other moving in opposite directions. The balls are thereby rolled out and elongated into a cylinder or a pipe of uniform diameter. It is rolled many times as it advances between the belts. When the pipe is finished it will have passed through the entire length of the pathway designed for piping.

The pipe now drops between 2 revolving cutter blades, where it is divided into small cylinders of uniform size and weight. These pieces now drop onto a tray which transports them between 2 pill-rolling belts. They are thoroughly rolled and shaped by the motion of the moving belts and the agitator attachment.

The pills pass through this path and reach the separator rollers, where the finished pills are now automatically sorted. Those meeting the proper size will be retained, while the smaller ones will pass into a waste container. The waste pills are reworked and passed through the machine a second time. The pills which have been retained are now dried and prepared for coating. The capacity of this machine is 300,000 2-grain pills per day.

While this may seem to be very efficient, it is not nearly so efficient as the modern tablet machine. Comparatively speaking, then, pills are an expensive and inefficient form of medication, whether prepared by hand or by machine.

Pill Coating

Pills are coated with various substances by methods similar to those used for tablets, and for similar purposes. A general discussion of coating will be found under the heading "Tablets."

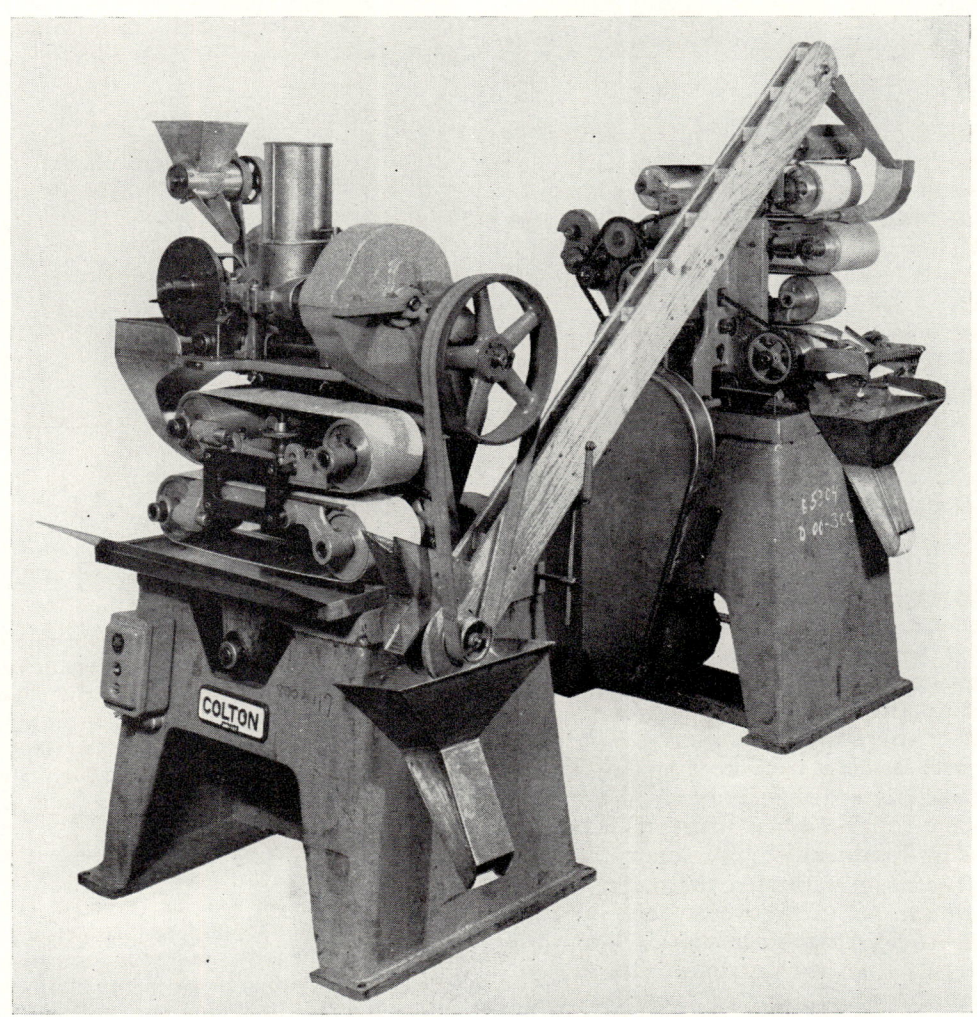

Fig. 176. Automatic pill machine. At the left side is a ball cutter and on the right is the pill machine. (Arthur Colton Co., Detroit)

PILLS OF THE U.S.P.

HEXYLRESORCINOL PILLS

These consist of hexylresorcinol covered with a rupture-resistant coating that is dispersible in the digestive tract. The coating used is gelatin, and it must be sufficiently tough and elastic to withstand a pressure of 10 Kg., gradually applied, without fissuring. Hexylresorcinol pills are used as an anthelmintic.

PILLS OF THE N.F.

Three formulas for pills are listed; only one requires special directions for its preparation.

FERROUS CARBONATE PILLS

Chalybeate Pills, Blaud's Pills, Ferruginous Pills

The history of these pills is discussed on page 429 under the heading "Ferrous Carbonate Mass." For the ingredients and the method of preparation, see *N.F. XI* (p. 144). Each pill contains not less than 60 mg. of $FeCO_3$.

The official formula may be modified to advantage by omitting the glycerin and the purified water, since the water of crystallization of the ferrous sulfate is more than sufficient to moisten the mass. The reaction is started, in the absence of water and glycerin, by submitting the mixture of ferrous sulfate, sucrose and potassium carbonate to heavy pressure with the pestle.

After the pill mass has been formed, it should be allowed to stand for at least half an hour before attempting to divide it into pills, in order to permit development of the desired plasticity and firmness.

Potent substances such as strychnine sulfate and arsenic trioxide frequently are prescribed as added ingredients of Ferrous Carbonate Pills. When such prescriptions are being compounded, the potent ingredients should be triturated thoroughly with one of the dry ingredients, such as the sucrose, before carrying out the reaction between the ferrous sulfate and the potassium carbonate. This procedure is followed to ensure uniform distribution of the potent material throughout the mass.

One of the disadvantages of Ferrous Carbonate Pills is their tendency to become so hard that disintegration in the alimentary tract may not occur. To overcome this disadvantage, pharmaceutical manufacturers have placed on the market a product known as Blaud Pills, Soft Mass, in which a small amount of petrolatum has been incorporated in the pill mass. Pills so made will remain soft indefinitely.

The other 2 pills official in *N.F. XI* are:
1. Aloin, Belladonna, Cascara and Podophyllum Pills, Hinkle's Pills.
2. Compound Mild Mercurous Chloride Pills, Compound Cathartic Pills.

Each of the foregoing is directed to be prepared by the general directions for making pills on page 444 of *N.F. XI*.

NONOFFICIAL PILLS

Of pills that formerly were official, only one, Pills of Phosphorus, U.S.P. X, needs to be mentioned.

PILLS OF PHOSPHORUS, U.S.P. X

Pilulæ Phosphori

Phosphorus	0.06 Gm.
Althea, in very fine powder	6.00 Gm.
Acacia, in very fine powder	3.00 Gm.
Chloroform, Glycerin, Water, Tolu, Ether	q.s.
To make	100 pills

Dissolve the phosphorus in a test tube in 5 ml. of chloroform, with the aid of a very gentle heat, replacing from time to time any of the chloroform that may be lost by evaporation. Mix the althea and the acacia in a mortar, next add the solution of phosphorus, then immediately afterward a sufficient quantity (about 4 ml.) of a mixture of 2 volumes of glycerin and 1 volume of water, and quickly form a mass. Divide it into 100 pills.

Dissolve 10 Gm. of tolu in 15 ml. of ether, shake the pills with a sufficient quantity of this solution until they are uniformly coated and put them on a plate to dry, occasionally rolling them about until the drying is completed. Preserve in a well-stoppered bottle. The usual dose is 1 pill.

TROCHES

Troches (derived from the Greek word *trochos,* anything round or circular, e.g., a wheel) are dosage forms intended to be placed in the mouth and allowed to dissolve or disintegrate slowly. They usually consist of medicinal substances incorporated with sugar and an adhesive such as tragacanth. Flavor and color also may be included. Most of the troches marketed under brand names have a base of hard candy; others are hard glycerogelatins. Troches usually are formed as flat disks, but other shapes are permissible. Most of the trade-marked varieties have a distinctive shape. The usual weight of a troche is about 1 Gm.

Once a fairly common prescription item, troches declined in popularity until a prescription for a troche became a rarity. However, the advent of new medicinal agents, especially the antibiotics, has restored their former popularity, and prescriptions for troches no longer are rare. Most of these prescriptions specify trade-marked specialties, but, occasionally, the prescribed troche must be prepared extemporaneously.

Extemporaneous Preparation of Troches

The troche mass is prepared in much the same fashion as a pill mass. The medicinal substances, an adhesive such as tragacanth, and powdered sugar are mixed properly and then moistened with an excipient, usually water or syrup. When the proper amount of excipient has been added, the mass should have the consistency of rather firm dough; and a small piece, flattened into a thin sheet, should not show marked fissures at the margins.

The troche mass must now be divided into the prescribed number of doses. There are several ways of making this division; but the most accurate and convenient method is by the use of a troche board, roller and cutter.

The troche board consists of a piece of smooth-finished, hard wood approximately 10 in. by 16 in. Thin strips of wood are attached to the longer sides in such manner that they may be adjusted at varying heights parallel with the surface of the board. The troche roller is simply a rolling-pin. When in use, it is supported wholly by the adjustable flanges of the troche board, and thus forms the troche mass into a sheet of uniform thickness. The troche cutter is a steel punch attached to a hollow, metal cone (Fig. 177). As successive troches are cut, they accumulate in the cone, which may be emptied from time to time by inverting it.

The most critical point in the accurate division of a troche mass lies in the forming of the mass into a sheet of exactly the correct thickness. The correct thickness may be ascertained by weighing the entire mass and dividing the weight by the number of troches to be made, thus obtaining the weight of one troche in the moist state. This amount of the troche mass is weighed, dropped into the troche cutter, and pressed down with the aid of some blunt instrument. The troche thus formed is removed carefully from the cutter and used as a guide in adjusting the flanges of the troche board.

With the flanges at the proper height, the mass is placed on the troche board and is formed into a sheet with the roller, using a dusting powder, such as starch or pow-

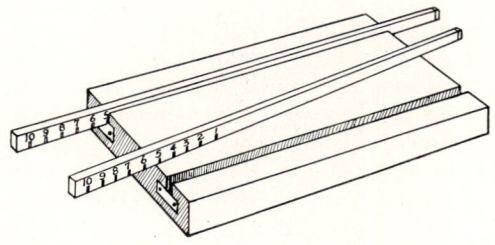 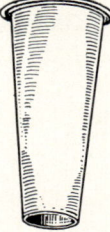 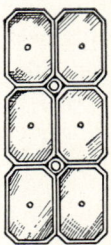

Fig. 177. Equipment for making troches. (*Left*) lozenge board, (*center*) single punch, (*right*) end view of multiple lozenge cutter.

dered sucrose, rather liberally to prevent the mass from sticking to the utensils. When the maximum number of troches possible have been cut, the net which remains is collected, remoistened if necessary, and the process of rolling and cutting repeated until the entire mass is divided.

Lacking the equipment described above, the troche mass may be divided into the requisite number of portions by rolling it into a cylinder and slicing it with a sharp blade, using the scale on the tile as a guide. Any distortion in the slices caused by pressure of the blade can be removed by manipulating the slices with the fingers. Troches so prepared will have neither the finish nor the uniformity of those prepared with proper equipment, but no doubt they are as useful therapeutically.

Troches must be dried thoroughly before packaging, since they will support the mold if any appreciable amount of moisture remains.

There is 1 troche now official:

Tyrothricin Troches, N.F. XI

These are flavored, compressed tablets containing either 1 mg. or 2 mg. of tyrothricin.

Of troches recently official, 2, Penicillin Troches and Troches of Eucalyptus Gum, N.F. V, are still in use.

Penicillin Troches, N.F. X

These appear on the market in 2 forms, both differing considerably from the type described above. The more common variety is in reality a compressed tablet; the other is a solid, plastic at body temperature, intended for mastication.

The penicillin troches ordinarily available contain either 1,000 or 5,000 units of penicillin.

Troches of Eucalyptus Gum, N.F. V

Trochisci Eucalypti Gummi; Troches of Red Gum

Eucalyptus gum, in fine powder...	6.0 Gm.
Tragacanth, in fine powder.......	6.0 Gm.
Acacia, in fine powder...........	12.0 Gm.
Sucrose, in fine powder..........	40.0 Gm.
Oil of orange...................	0.3 Gm.
Fluidextract of rose.............	3.0 Gm.
Water, a sufficient quantity,	
To make	100 troches

Triturate the powders together until well mixed, then incorporate the oil and the fluidextract and form a mass with water. Divide this into 100 troches and dry them in a current of warm air.

TABLETS

Tablets are dosage forms prepared by molding or compressing medicinal substances in dies. They vary widely in shape, but the most common form is discoid. They vary widely in weight, also, but those intended for administration by mouth usually weigh between 0.06 Gm. and 0.60 Gm.

A comparison of the many prescription surveys which have been made during the past year shows a very close relationship with that of previous years. A breakdown of the surveys shows that 74 per cent of the prescriptions are written for solid medication, of which 47.6 per cent is for tablet medication. There has been a gradual increase each year in the percentage of tablets being used.

A tablet may be defined as "a unit dosage form of medication containing one or more medicinal agents, with or without diluents, made by moulding the mixture in the form of a fine powder, or compressing it in the form of a granular powder into a suitable shape." They vary in shape and size, some of which are distinctive for a particular company, but as a rule they are discoid. They naturally vary in weight according to the amount of medication contained in each dose.

The tablets used for oral administration must be of a reasonable size and weight to ensure the patient's accepting them. Some tablets have been made for the purpose of chewing them and are larger in size and are heavier than those used for oral administration.

Two classes of tablets, in general, are recognized. Those prepared by forcing dry material into a die, under pressure which may reach several tons per square inch, are known as compressed tablets. Those which are made by forcing moistened material into a die, under manual pressure only, are known as molded tablets. Each of these general classes can be divided into subclasses, as will be seen later in the discussion.

Tablets, both molded and compressed, are comparative newcomers to pharmacy and medicine. The first patent for a compressed tablet device was granted in 1843; the molded tablet was originated somewhat later. Although, at first, both forms were slow to gain favor, the last 50 years have seen a great increase in their popularity.

Surveys are being made each year on the use of medication on prescription, and they have proved continually that tablet dosage forms are on the increase and that the tablet is a favored form of medication. There must be reasons for this increase in use.

A study of our official books of standards in Pharmacy reveals a rapid increase in the tablets that have become official. Prior to 1940 there were only 3 *U.S.P.* tablet dosage forms, while in 1955 there were 113. The new *United States Pharmacopoeia XVI* contains monographs for 141 tablets. The *National Formulary* of 1936 listed 36 monographs for tablet dosage forms, and in 1955 92 were listed. The *N.F. XI* shows monographs for 125 tablets.

The official recognition of so many tablet dosage forms shows clearly the trend in this type of solid medication. The advent of the 2 latest types of tablets, the triple-layer tablet and the tablet within a tablet or press-coated tablet will further the use of this type of medication.

There must be reasons for the increased use of this form of medication. One of the natural causes is the tremendous developments in the fields of antibiotics, antihistamines, tranquilizers, hypertensive drugs and hormones. When new products are approved, one form of use is that of the tablet. Many factors favor the use of tablet medication, and its popularity may be due to the advantages inherent in this form of medication. The most common advantages lie in the ease with which tablets can be transported. This is accomplished readily in small containers, and one can carry them on his person to be administered at any hour of the day as prescribed by the physician.

The general public have come to accept with favor this form of medication because of its convenience and because of the psychological advantage which tablets have over other types of medication. The cost of one dozen tablets over other types of medication is strongly in its favor from an economically minded populace. The knowledge that 1 tablet represents 1 dose and that the dosage form is stable adds to the psychological value.

Compressed tablets have many uses in the field of food and medicine. They offer accuracy of dose, combined with a homogenous preparation for use in the fields of medicine and veterinary practice. They are used also in confectionery with convenient wrappings to give a candied preparation which is pleasing and attractive to the eye.

We also find compressed tablets of a type used in foods: soup cubes, malted milk tablets, flavoring tablets, sugar tablets, dehydrated food tablets and a variety of drink tablets used to dissolve in cold water to produce a palatable preparation.

Compressed tablet manufacture is a process requiring long years of experience and a high degree of skill. There exists a belief that to make tablets all one needs is to purchase a tablet machine, feed the material into the hopper and thence to the die, and the machine will do the rest. This belief is erroneous, although there are a few chemical substances that can be fed directly to the hopper, and tablets can be compressed without any additional treatment. The best examples of this are the halides of sodium, potassium and ammonium, and a few others.

The discussion which follows is intended for the purpose of giving the reader an insight into the problems and the processes involved in the making of the tablet on a large batch or manufacturing scale. The details will be found in the pharmaceutical literature or in the *Textbook of Pharmaceutical Compounding and Dispensing* by Lyman and Sprowls.*

Certain steps are involved in the making of tablets such as:

1. Weighing the ingredients
2. Mixing the ingredients
3. Moistening and massing the ingredients
4. Granulating the mass
5. Drying the granules

---

* Lyman, R. A. and Sprowls, J. B.: Textbook of Pharmaceutical Compounding and Dispensing, Philadelphia, Lippincott, 1955.

6. Sizing the dried granules
7. Adding the lubricant and the running powder
8. Compressing the tablet
9. Sorting and analyzing the tablets
10. Bottling and storage of the finished tablets.

The 3 main essentials in successful tablet making are:

1. The material should be free-flowing or "flow like sand" which is the common expression used by tablet men.
2. It should have binding properties.
3. It should not adhere to the punches or the die.

Examining these 3 essentials, one can see readily that when granules "flow like sand" they do not entrap air, and they have the property of squeezing or interlocking together. The fact that it has binding properties causes the granules to adhere to each other when compressed, and these granules must be lubricated to prevent sticking to the punch or the die.

Weighing the Ingredients

The dry ingredients are weighed on various types of balances of a sensitivity equivalent to good practices so that a fairly high degree of accuracy is involved. When the tablet has been assigned by production planning, work sheets or formula sheets are prepared and sent to the departments involved. One of the work sheets is consigned to the chemical stores where the dry or liquid ingredients are weighed or measured by those in charge of this phase of production. All weighings and measurements are checked carefully by this department before the entire assignment is ready for the production department. The material is transported to the proper department and is now ready for the second step.

Mixing the Ingredients

All of the dry ingredients of the formula should be in powdered form, as uniformly fine as is possible. The chemical companies have aided the manufacturer in this by producing chemicals in the form of very fine powder so that a more uniform mixture is obtained more easily than in the earlier years of this industry. Particular care must be exercised in mixing because of the larger amounts ordinarily involved. The primary use of the mixer is to mix all of the ingredients so that a uniform tablet can be made. The process of mixing follows the method of geometric dilution.

To ensure rapid disintegration of the tablet in the alimentary tract, a substance known as a disintegrator usually is included among the dry ingredients of the tablet formula. The disintegrator most commonly used is cornstarch; its grains swell rapidly when moistened, thus breaking the tablet apart.

Granulating the Mixture

A tablet mixture can be granulated by 2 different processes known as: (1) the wet granulation method, and (2) the dry granulation method, precompression or slugging. It is extremely important at this step to determine several factors: namely, the size of the tablet to be made, the type of tablet to be made, the chemical composition of the tablet, the tablet machine to be used, and others. Granulation is carried out in our modern production laboratories by means of 1 of 3 different machines: (1) the oscillating granulator, (2) the Fitzpatrick comminutor, (3) the upright granulator, and (4) by hand. The amount of liquid granulating agent added will be different for each process. It has been assumed in our practice that 150 cc. of a liquid binder (gelatin, gelatin-acacia solution, starch paste, sucrose solution, glucose, etc.) will be sufficient for each 1,000 grams of powder. This is not a positive quantity but approximate. The liquid must be thoroughly worked into the mass before granulation. The equipment commonly used in this step is dependent upon the size of the batch. Small batches can be worked in a Hobart mixer, a Readco mixer, a Mass mixer or dough mixer. When the mass has become wet enough, then it is forced through a granulator. The granulators are usually stainless steel or Monel metal, which are not reactive to most of the substances used in tablet making.

The size of the finished tablet also indicates the type of granulating sieve to use.

For very small tablets such as 1/8" to 5/32", it would be advisable to use a 20- to 30-mesh sieve.

Up to 3/8" in diameter, a 16-mesh sieve would be sufficient.

For 3/8" to 7/16", it would be best to use a 12- to 20-mesh sieve.

For larger tablets, a larger sieve size would do.

Another factor affecting sieve size is the type of tablet machine being used for compression. We have found that the 12-mesh will work well on a rotary tablet press and not do so well on a single punch. Our experience has led us to predict that a larger mesh size can be used for a rotary tablet machine than for a single punch machine for the same size tablet. The finished granule should contain a minimum of fine powder, known as fines. The presence of a limited amount of fines is necessary for the proper working of the tablet machine.

Another method of granulation, and one which is of increasing importance, is that of precompression or *slugging*. In this method, the mixed ingredients, in finely powdered form, are compressed into rather large disks, or slugs. Then these slugs are broken and passed through a sieve of the proper size. This process is more economical than the wet method of granulation, since fewer operations are necessary, and no expensive drying apparatus is required. It has the further advantage of avoiding chemical reactions which, in the wet method, would require that separate granulations of the reacting substances be made.

The wet granules are dried in appropriate drying ovens under suitable conditions, after which they are again passed through a sieve to break up the large lumps and the agglomerated particles. The dry granules are now mixed with the proper lubricating agent. The principal objectives of a lubricant are: (1) to assist the ejection of the tablet from the die, (2) to prevent the tablet's sticking to the punches or the die and (3) to give an attractive finish to the tablet. Lubrication is an important function in tablet-making. A few of the lubricating agents commonly used are stearic acid and its salts, talc, and liquid petrolatum.

Compressing the Tablet

The machines used for making a tablet vary from the single punch hand machine to the double-rotary high-speed machines.

1. The simplest machine is the "Eureka" tablet machine (Fig. 178) which is available in either a table-top or stand model and can be operated either by hand or driven by a motor. It will make tablets ranging in size from 1/8" to 1/2" in diameter at a maximum speed of about 100 tablets per minute.

2. The single punch tablet machine is used for tablets ranging in size from 1/8" to 1" in diameter. The usual machine makes tablets 1/8" to 1/2" in diameter; a heavier and more powerful machine is used to make the larger tablets. The speed of this machine can be varied by means of a variable pulley to make from 65 to 125 tablets per minute.

3. These machines may have a multiple punch consisting of 3 upper punches and 3 lower punches and a die with 3 holes which make 3 tablets at every revolution of the machine; hence, the number of tablets per minute will increase correspondingly.

4. The rotary press generally has 16 punch and die sets, making approximately

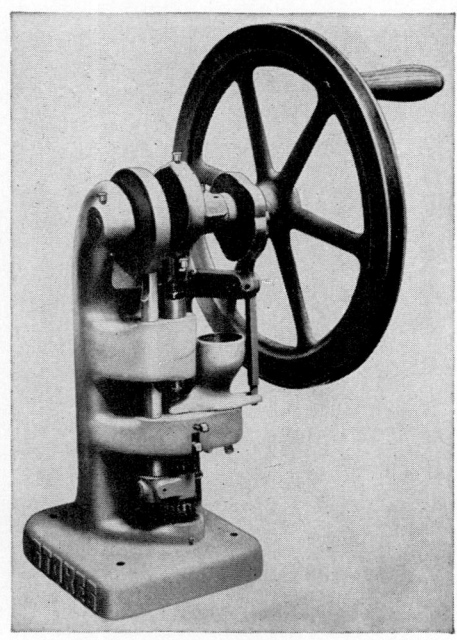

Fig. 178. Tablet-making machine, hand-powered.

440 Masses, Pills, Troches and Tablets

350 to 650 tablets per minute. The machine will make tablets up to $5/8''$ in diameter. It is an economical machine for the manufacturing of pharmaceutical tablets.

5. The double rotary uses 27, 33 or 37 sets of dies and punches. The 27-set machine will make from 750 to 1,400 tablets per minute, ranging in size up to $5/8''$ in diameter. It has 2 complete mechanisms for making the tablet, and each die set makes 2 tablets (double) per revolution of the machine.

6. The 2 most recent machines are known as the press-coater, or tablet within a tablet, machine, and the multiple-layer tablet machine.

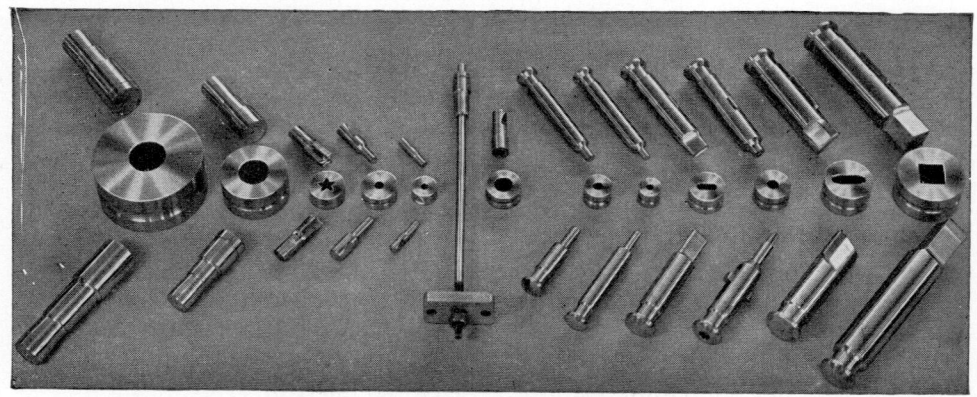

Fig. 179. Tablet die and punches.

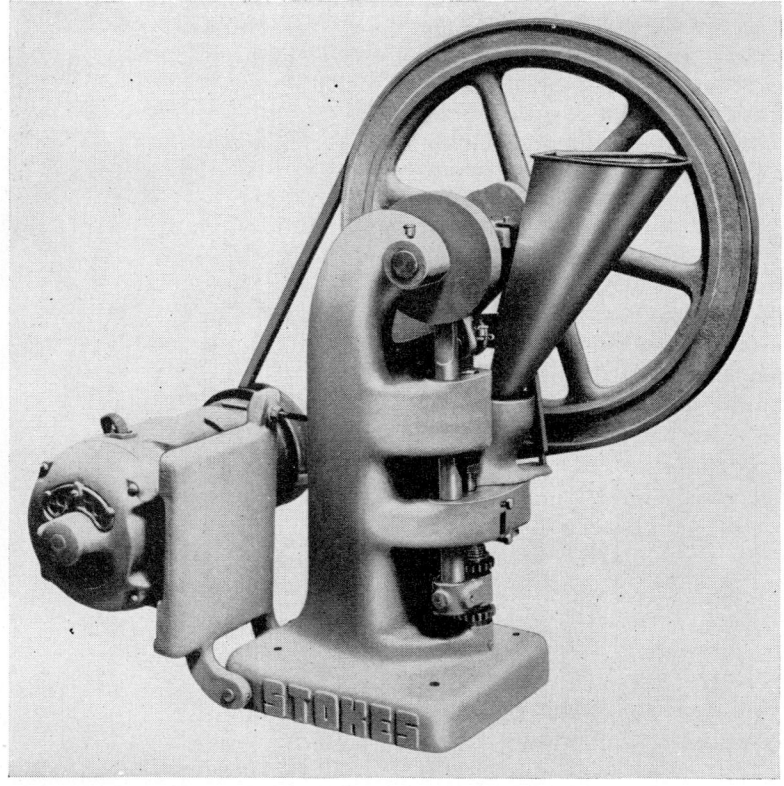

Fig. 180. Motor-driven single-punch tablet press. (Stokes, Philadelphia.)

All tablet compressors, of whatever power or capacity, are basically similar. The element common to them all is a die, or dies, each one fitted with an upper and a lower punch (Fig. 179). These operate in the following manner. With the upper punch out of and above the die and the lower punch at the lowest point of descent within the die, a charge of the granulated material flows into the die, completely filling the cavity. The upper punch then descends, compressing the material against the lower punch, which remains stationary. The upper punch then ascends, followed at an interval by the lower punch, which rises until it is flush with the upper surface of the die, thus ejecting the tablet. The lower punch then descends within the die, and the cycle of operations begins again.

One of the most serious difficulties encountered in tablet compression is the sticking of the material to the die and to the faces of the punches. This difficulty has

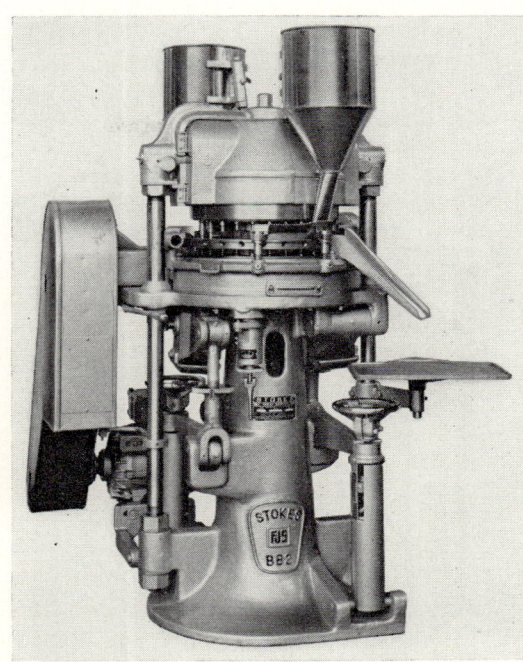

FIG. 182. Twenty-seven station rotary press. (Stokes, Philadelphia.)

been overcome to some extent by the use of specially hardened and highly polished dies and punches, but it still is necessary to add a lubricant to many tablet formulas. Liquid petrolatum and magnesium stearate are commonly used. Where these are not suitable as, for instance, in a tablet intended to be placed in solution, often a water-soluble lubricant will achieve the desired result.

COMPRESSED TABLET TRITURATES

Nearly all the compressed tablets used for medicinal purposes are discoid in shape with their opposing surfaces convex. Compressed tablet triturates differ from most compressed tablets in that their opposing surfaces are flat. In appearance, the compressed tablet triturate is almost exactly the counterpart of the molded tablet triturate, which will be discussed later in this chapter. However, there is a very important difference between them. Although a disintegrator may have been used in making the compressed tablet triturate, the disintegration time of the compressed tablet triturate is slow when compared with that

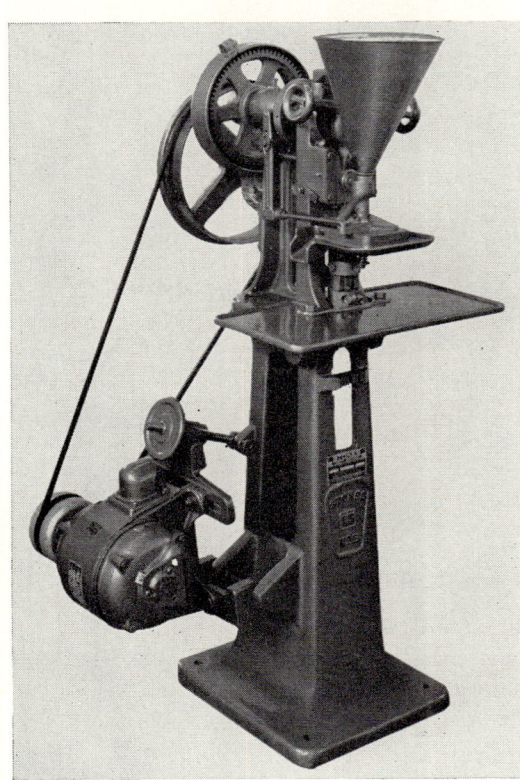

FIG. 181. Single punch press. (Stokes, Philadelphia.)

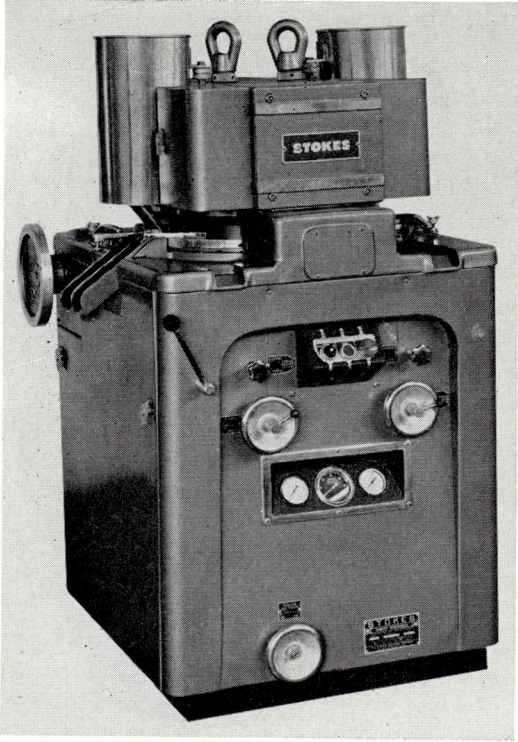

Fig. 183. Rotary machine, 41-station. (Stokes, Philadelphia.)

or less accurate fractions. The tablet ingredients are usually such that a clear solution in water may be obtained.

It is difficult to see why a competent pharmacist should purchase dispensing tablets. Since most of them contain lethal doses, it is dangerous to keep them on hand even though they may be of distinctive shape. If the pharmacist has an accurate and sensitive balance, as he should, there is little to be gained by using a dispensing tablet, particularly when it is considered that it is pure chance whether the amount of a potent substance needed for a prescription corresponds exactly to that in a dispensing tablet or one of its segments.

of the molded tablet triturate, which disintegrates almost instantaneously on contact with moisture. This distinction is one which must be kept in mind by the pharmacist, since some tablet triturates contain substances which must be available instantly upon administration, whereas others are dissolved or allowed to disintegrate in small quantities of water before administration. The sole advantages which may be claimed for the compressed form are that they are cheaper and less fragile.

Dispensing Tablets

These are either molded or compressed tablets, containing large amounts of potent substances not intended for administration but rather for a convenience at the prescription counter. To lessen the risk of their being dispensed by mistake for other tablets, they are always of an angular rather than a discoid shape. They usually are scored to facilitate their division into more

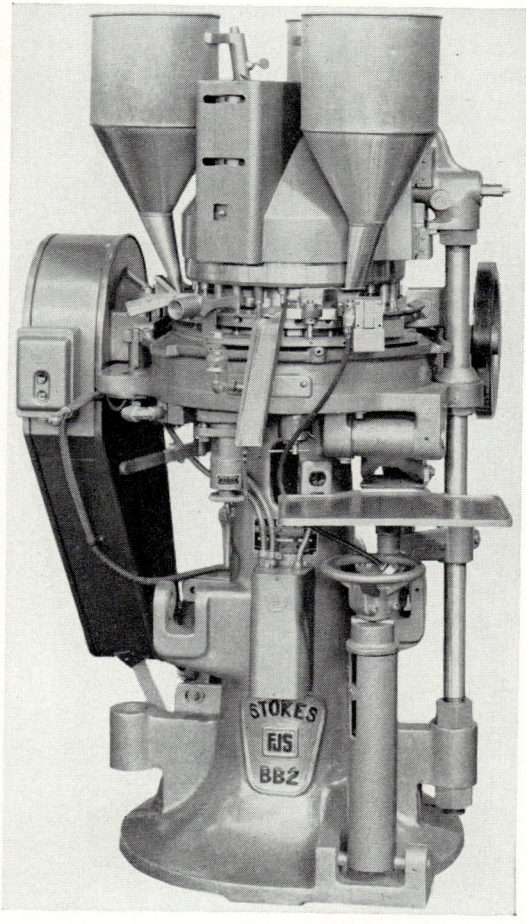

Fig. 184. Twenty-seven station, 3-layer rotary tabletting machine. (Stokes, Philadelphia.)

SUBLINGUAL OR BUCCAL TABLETS

These are compressed tablets which are placed in the sulci (alveolabial, alveolingual, buccal) of the mouth and there allowed to dissolve. They are used for the administration of substances—certain steroids, for example—which would be destroyed by enzymatic action if swallowed, and readily enter the circulation by absorption from the oral sulci. Most of these tablets have a base consisting of the high molecular weight polyethylene glycols. Because salivary stimulation might result in undue loss of the medicinal substance, the tablets are neither flavored nor sweetened. The time required for solution varies with the size and the degree of compression of the tablet, but if it is allowed to remain undisturbed in the sulcus, complete solution usually results within 30 minutes.

MOLDED TABLETS

Molded tablets are disks of medicinal substances prepared by forcing the moistened material, by manual pressure, into a die. They are known as *tablet triturates*

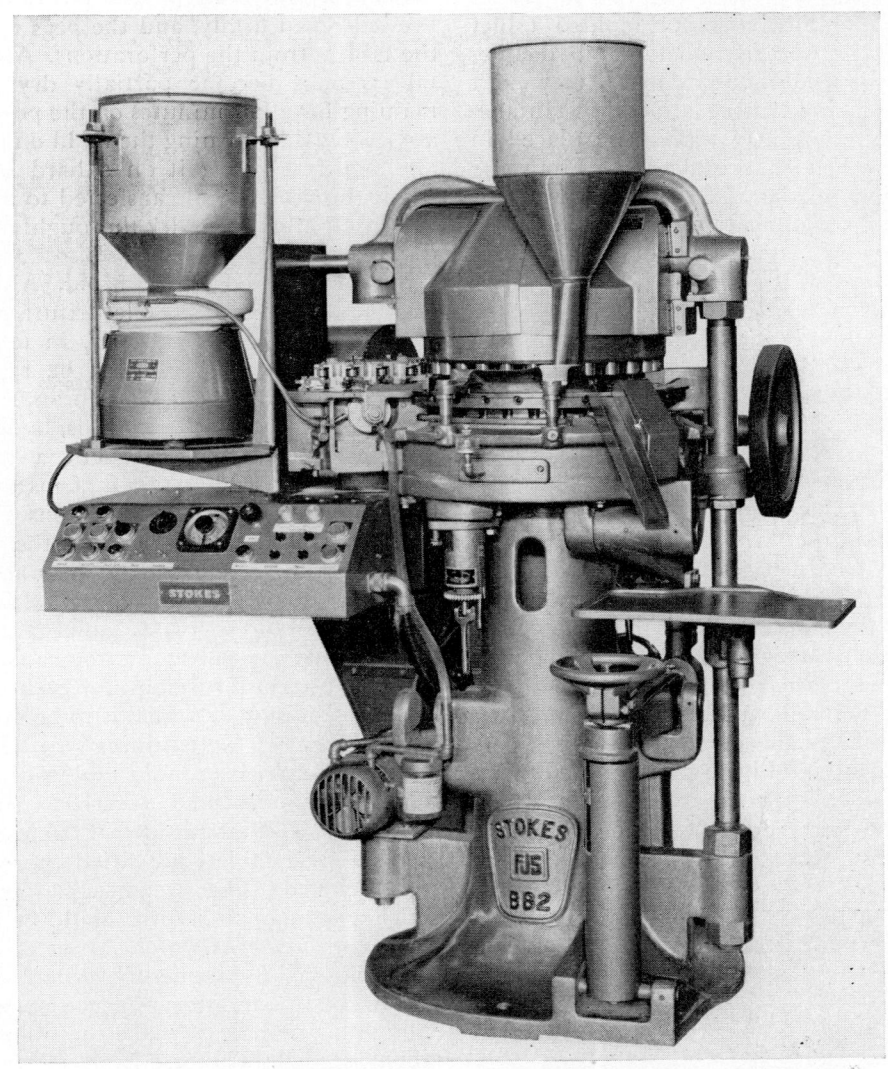

FIG. 185. Twenty-seven station, press-coating, rotary tabletting machine. (Stokes, Philadelphia.)

because originally they were devised as a means of administering triturations of potent substances.

Although it is possible to make molded tablets in many shapes and sizes, nearly all of those made by the manufacturer or the retail pharmacist are round disks weighing approximately 0.06 Gm. In addition to the medicinal substance, which only rarely accounts for the entire weight, molded tablets contain a diluent or base. With few exceptions, the base used is an especially finely powdered lactose or a mixture of lactose and sucrose.

The chief advantage of molded tablet triturates is their extremely rapid disintegration when moistened. Hence, they exert their medicinal effect almost instantaneously, and they may readily be placed in solution when that is desired. From the standpoint of the dispensing pharmacist, a further advantage lies in the fact that they may be made easily in the prescription laboratory. They have 2 disadvantages, neither of which, however, is serious: they are more fragile than compressed tablets, and their small size makes them unsuitable for substances which are not effective in small doses.

Preparation of Molded Tablet Triturates

The mold used in preparing these tablets is made of hard rubber or metal and consists of 2 parts (Fig. 186). The upper portion, or the *die,* is a thin plate in which have been drilled, in regular alignment, a number of perforations of uniform diameter, the number varying from 50 to 200. At each end of the plate, there is one perforation considerably larger than the others. On one side of the die, the edges are beveled. The lower portion, or the *base,* is a fairly thick plate in which pegs are set

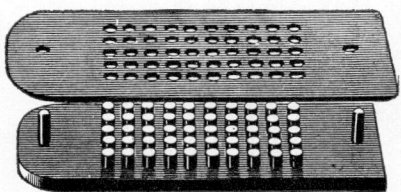

Fig. 186. Tablet triturate mold.

conforming in pattern to the perforations in the die. The pegs are of such size that they fit snugly into the perforations. For convenience in fitting the 2 parts of the apparatus together, both the base and the die have one square and one tapered end.

When the mold is used, the perforations in the die are filled with the moistened tablet material. Then the die is placed on the base with the beveled edge down and with the square and the tapered ends matching. The 2 large pegs of the base are inserted into the 2 large perforations of the die. When the die is in proper position, it is pressed down firmly, and the pegs displace the tablets from the perforations. After the tablets have become partially dry by remaining for a few minutes on the pegs, they are removed by turning the mold on its side and lightly tapping it on a hard surface. Then the tablets are transferred to a warm place and allowed to dry thoroughly before dispensing.

Standardization of the Mold. Although the manufacturer of a tablet triturate mold usually indicates its capacity, in terms of weight, this indication must be regarded by the pharmacist simply as an approximation. The capacity of a mold is, by weight, not an absolute quantity but a relative quantity. Thus, the volume of material in the completely filled perforations is constant, but the weight varies with the nature of the material. Since there is no accurate and convenient way of measuring the volume of substances such as tablet materials, it is necessary to determine the capacity of a mold, in terms of weight, for each combination of substances which is to be molded.

One way of determining capacity in terms of weight is to mold tablets of a substance commonly used as a base, such as lactose or a combination of lactose and sucrose. The tablets are dried thoroughly and weighed. The weight obtained, of which a permanent record should be made, is the capacity of the mold in terms of the base chosen. Subsequently, when tablets are to be made, the pharmacist weighs enough of the base to make the number of tablets needed. The base is placed on a tile and near it is put the quantity of medicinal substance required for the tablets. Then an amount of the base, equal in bulk to the medicinal substance, is removed. The tablets are made from the remaining base and the medicinal substance. Although, with sufficient practice, it is possible to achieve a fair degree of accuracy with this method, the estimation of relative bulks is always subject to a potential error of considerable magnitude. Furthermore, it would hardly be practicable to standardize the mold for the many bases that would be necessary to provide for all contingencies.

Another method, and one which does not have the disadvantages of the procedure just described, is as follows. Mix the medicinal substance with an amount of the base which is known to be insufficient. Moisten the mixture and place it in the required number of perforations of the die, making no attempt to fill the perforations evenly. Completely fill the perforations with a sufficient amount of the moistened base containing no medication. Punch out the tablets, mix thoroughly, moisten if necessary and fill into the die again. The tablets first made must be mixed very carefully to ensure uniform distribution of the medicinal substance in the finished tablets.

Choice of Base and Excipient. The base ordinarily used for molded tablets is an especially finely powdered lactose or lactose containing from 5 to 20 per cent of sucrose, the latter being added to make a firmer tablet. A small amount of acacia sometimes is added to the lactose; but its use is not recommended, for tablets containing it are likely to be exclusively hard, and white tablets are made dingy. Medicinal substances which would react chemically with sugars require special bases. Some of the special bases that have been used are precipitated calcium carbonate, precipitated calcium phosphate, kaolin and bentonite.

The liquid used to moisten the tablet mixture is known as the *excipient*. Mixtures of alcohol and water in varying proportions usually are employed—the alcohol to hasten drying of the tablets, the water to bind the tablet by its solvent action on the base. In most tablets, a mixture of equal parts of alcohol and water is satisfactory. However, if a tablet is to contain a substantial amount of a substance which is very soluble in water, some or all of the water must be omitted. Thus, if a tablet weighing 0.06 Gm. is to contain 0.03 Gm. of sodium nitrite, the excipient should contain not more than 20 per cent of water; if the tablet is to contain 0.06 Gm. of sodium nitrite, only alcohol should be used as the excipient. The probability of a chemical reaction sometimes precludes the use of water in the excipient as, for instance, in a tablet containing calomel and sodium bicarbonate. With these substances, if water is used, black oxide of mercury is formed. The reaction is avoided by using alcohol, which is not a solvent for either chemical. Conversely, in making tablets containing oxidizing agents, alcohol should not be used, for the oxidizing agents would be reduced by it.

Molding the Tablets. While this topic has been anticipated to some degree by the foregoing discussion, certain parts of the procedure remain to be described.

The medicinal ingredients, in very fine condition, should be mixed with the base by the method of geometric dilution, preferably in a glass mortar. Then the mixture is moistened with the chosen excipient. The proper amount of excipient to be added must be learned by experience; but, as a guide to the beginner, enough should be used to form a stiff paste, yet not so much that it can be forced out of the paste by pressure.

With the die lying flat on a tile or other clean, nonabsorbent surface and held firmly by the spread fingers, the paste is forced into the perforations with a spatula. Great care must be used to ensure complete filling, particularly of the marginal perforations. Both sides of the die should be inspected to make certain that the spaces are filled. If considerable pressure is exerted on the blade of the spatula while it is being moved in circular fashion on the die, the exposed surfaces of the tablets are made flat and smooth.

Then the tablets are ejected from the mold and are dried as described previously.

HYPODERMIC TABLETS

These are molded tablet triturates intended to be dissolved in water to make a solution to be injected parenterally. To ensure rapid and complete solution, they are made with a base of specially recrystallized lactose. The usual weight of hypodermic tablets is about 0.03 Gm. A larger size is unnecessary in view of the dosages usually employed parenterally, and the smaller size is desirable for distinguishing hypodermic tablets from ordinary tablet triturates.

Although hypodermic tablets are not intended to be sterile (sterility of the solution being achieved by the physician or the nurse at the time of administration), they are manufactured under very rigid precautions against contamination. The tablets are molded under hoods in air-conditioned rooms, by operators who wear gowns and masks. The air entering the room is filtered to protect the tablets from dust particles.

Hypodermic tablets are marketed in glass tubes of 20 tablets, 5 tubes to a "case," and in bottles of 100, 500 and 1,000. When it is necessary to dispense less than an original container, the pharmacist should take every precaution possible against contamination in transferring the tablets to the dispensing container.

Abbreviations Commonly Used for Tablets

The type of tablet intended is often expressed in prescriptions, price lists and other forms of pharmaceutical literature by means of an abbreviation. These abbreviations should be thoroughly familiar to the pharmacist. The following is a list of the more important ones and their meanings:

C.T., Compressed tablet.
C.T.T., Compressed tablet triturate.
T.T., On a prescription, this may be interpreted as meaning either the molded or the compressed tablet triturate. Seldom, if ever, does the physician specify which type is wanted, although in some instances it would be to the advantage of the patient for him to do so.
H.T., Hypodermic tablet.
D.T., Dispensing tablet.

PILL AND TABLET COATING

Many substances are used, or have been used, to coat pills and tablets. Sugar, either plain or colored with chocolate or certified dyes, is the most commonly used coating. Gelatin is used to some extent but is decreasing in popularity. Gold leaf and silver leaf were once the acme of elegance in pill coating but are now obsolete. Salol, shellac, casein, cellulose acetate phthalate, combinations of vegetable fiber and wax, and combinations of n-butyl stearate and wax also are used.

The coatings may be applied for a number of reasons. The usual objectives are improvement of appearance and concealment of taste; however, preservation of the pill or the tablet ingredients also may be an important consideration. Increasing numbers of pills and tablets now are being coated by substances which prevent or retard disintegration in the stomach but permit it in the intestinal tract. Pills or tablets treated in this manner are said to be *enteric-coated*.

Methods of Application of Coatings

The successful application of coatings to pills and tablets is an operation requiring great skill and long experience and, in most cases, the installation of expensive machin-

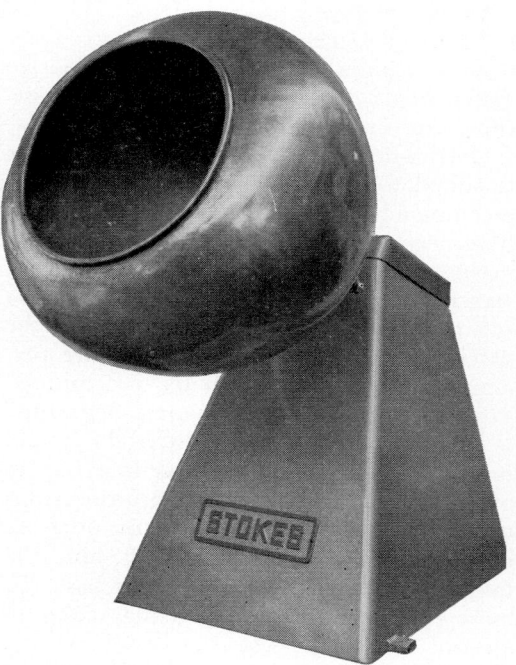

Fig. 187. Machine for coating tablets and pills. (Stokes, Philadelphia.)

ery. With the exception of certain enteric coatings, satisfactory coatings for pills and tablets cannot be applied by the retail pharmacist. He does not have the necessary means at his disposal. Therefore, the brief descriptions of methods of application which follow, are intended, with 2 exceptions, to furnish only general information to the student on commercial methods of coating. More detailed explanation of the processes involved may be obtained from many sources in the literature.

Sugar Coating. Only in this description, tablets will be mentioned, since the process by which pills are coated is essentially the same as that for tablets.

The apparatus used consists of a series of copper, motor-driven, coating pans. The pans, which resemble bean-pots in shape, are mounted at an angle of about 45° and are capable of being operated at varying speeds.

The tablets, freed from powder and broken pieces, are placed in one of the pans, which is then made to revolve. A small amount of heavy syrup containing about 5 per cent of gelatin is added and, when the tablets are partially dry, they are sprinkled with a dusting powder. This powder usually consists of a mixture of powdered sugar and starch but also may contain talc and acacia. A blast of warm air is now directed into the pan, which continues to revolve until the tablets are thoroughly dry. This process is known as subcoating. From 3 to 5 subcoats are usually necessary to give tablets the rounded form desired.

When the tablets have been properly subcoated, they are given from 5 to 10 coats with a very heavy syrup, each coat being dried thoroughly before the application of another. In order to obtain a very smooth surface, the tablets usually are transferred to a clean pan for the final, or finishing, coats.

The final step in the process is waxing and polishing. This process is carried out in a copper pan lined with canvas; or in a wooden tub or pan. The wax used is carnauba, or carnauba and beeswax, dissolved in acetone or petroleum benzin. The wax solution is added to the tablets in the polisher, and, when the solvent has evaporated completely, talc is added. It may be necessary to repeat this operation once or twice to develop a high luster.

Coatings of any desired color may be obtained by adding certified dyes to the syrup which is used for the finishing coats. For chocolate coating, powdered cocoa is added to the dusting powder used in the subcoats, and chocolate syrup is used for the finishing coats.

A comparatively recent development in tablet coating is the inclusion of one or more of the medicinal components of a tablet in the coatings. By this means, it is possible to effect physical separation of substances which would be incompatible if in contact with each other. The process also makes possible the construction of a single dosage form which exhibits a series of pharmacologic effects as successive layers are exposed in the digestive tract.

The more nearly tablets approach the spherical form, the more easily are they coated. It follows, then, that tablets with highly convex surfaces and thin edges are the most easily coated of the various tablet types. Tablet triturates, because of their flat surfaces and thick edges, cannot be coated satisfactorily.

ENTERIC COATING OF PILLS AND TABLETS

A pill or tablet is said to be enteric-coated when the coating will prevent disintegration in the stomach but will permit disintegration in the intestinal tract. A coating of such nature is desirable when the medicinal substances contained in the dosage form would be decomposed or otherwise rendered inactive by the gastric enzymes, when they would irritate the gastric mucosa or when their presence in concentrated form in the intestinal tract is necessary.

A number of substances have been used for enteric coating, among them salol, keratin, stearic acid, casein, shellac and combinations of these. The use of these substances is based on the theory that, being acid-insoluble, they will not dissolve in the stomach; but, being alkali-soluble, they will dissolve in the intestine. Since it is now known that stomach acidity varies widely both as to the individual and as to time, and since it is known that the duodenum frequently has an acid reaction, the use of these substances is no longer on a rational basis. Many investigations of the efficacy of enteric coatings have been made and reported in the pharmaceutical literature. The usual method employed has been to prepare pills or tablets of barium sulfate or bismuth subnitrate, and to follow their progress through the alimentary tract by means of the fluoroscope or by roentgenography. While the reports reveal a considerable difference of opinion, the weight of evidence seems to be against reliance on the substances mentioned above as enteric coatings.

New types of enteric coatings have been developed by pharmaceutical companies. While the substances and the methods employed are, for the most part, trade secrets, it is known that, in some instances, their use is based on the time required for the disintegration of the coating rather than on the acidity or the alkalinity of portions of the alimentary tract. In at least one instance, a mixture of finely powdered waxes and vegetable fiber is applied as a coating; and the tablets are then passed through a flame, which fuses the waxes and forms a continuous, smooth coat. When the tablet so coated is placed in contact with moisture, as in the stomach, the vegetable fiber swells and begins the disintegration of the coating. By varying the thickness of the wax coating, the time required for exposure of the material in the tablet can be controlled. Although not invariably successful in preventing disintegration of the tablet in the stomach, this type of enteric coating is of very high efficiency.

Salol. While most enteric-coated tablets and pills dispensed by the retail pharmacist are products of large-scale pharmaceutical manufacturing, it is not unusual for the pharmacist to receive a prescription, usually for capsules or pills, in the compounding of which an enteric coating must be applied extemporaneously. Of the substances previously mentioned as enteric coatings, salol, until recently, was the one used most commonly by the dispensing pharmacist because of the ease of application and the attractive appearance of the finished product. It may be applied by the following method, the directions given being for not more than 25 pills. (If a larger number is to be coated, the operation should be carried out in units of 25 or less.)

PROCEDURE. Prepare a series of 3 or more thin-walled flasks of about 150 ml. capacity. Place about 2 Gm. of salol in each flask. Heat the flasks in a water bath, in succession, just long enough to melt the salol. Cool the flask first heated to the point at which, although the salol remains liquid, there is scarcely any sensation of warmth. Drop the pills into the flask, immediately begin rotating the flask, and continue the rotation until the salol has crystallized, but not beyond that point. Repeat the process a sufficient number of times to obtain a satisfactory coating. To give the pills a smooth, finished appearance, heat one of the flasks until distinctly warm, pour out the excess salol, drop the pills into the flask while it is being rotated, and immediately cool the flask by rotating it under a stream of cold water.

In using salol as an enteric coating, care must be exercised to apply no more than is necessary to achieve the result desired, since salol is an active medicinal agent.

n-Butyl stearate, carnauba wax and stearic acid, which comprise a newly developed coating, to some extent replace the traditional salol coating. All of these resist the action of the gastric contents but, with the exception of the carnauba wax, are hydrolyzed readily in the intestine. It was found, experimentally, that none of the dosage forms so coated disintegrated in the stomach. The coating is nontoxic, pharmacologically inactive and comparatively easy to apply. Because it is best adapted for the coating of capsules, this dosage form will be used as the illustration in the discussion of procedure which follows.

PROCEDURE. To 45 parts, by weight, of n-butyl stearate, add 30 parts of carnauba wax and 25 parts of stearic acid. Fuse the mixture, bring the temperature to 75° C. and maintain this temperature during the coating process. Grasp one of the capsules at one end with tweezers and dip it for somewhat more than half its length into the coating mixture. Withdraw the capsule, touch its free end to the lip of the dish to remove the rundown and place it on a tile. Repeat this operation until one end of each of the capsules has been coated. Then complete the coating by grasping each capsule carefully at the coated end and dipping it in such fashion that the coats will overlap. The cycle should be repeated once to ensure that the coating will be adequate.

Although it is possible to coat tablets and pills by modifying the procedure outlined above, it is difficult to achieve results that are acceptable pharmaceutically.

OFFICIAL TABLETS

Two classes of tablets are now official: Poison Tablets (*Toxitabellae*) and Tablets. The former appellation is reserved solely for tablets of mercury bichloride, which first became official in *U.S.P. IX*. Two strengths were official in *N.F. X*. The one designated as "Mercury Bichloride Large Poison Tablets" contains from 420 mg. to 520 mg. of $HgCl_2$ and produces a solution of approximately 1:1,000 concentration when 1 tablet is dissolved in 475 ml. (1 pint) of water. The other, designated as "Mercury Bichloride Small Poison Tablets," contains from 110 mg. to 140 mg. of $HgCl_2$ and produces a solution of approximately 1:1,000 concentration when 1 tablet is dissolved in 120 ml. (4 fluidounces) of water.

The *N.F. XI* recognizes only 1 of these, Mercury Bichloride Large Poison Tablet, containing not less than 420 mg. and not more than 520 mg. of $HgCl_2$ with a sufficient quantity of a suitable excipient or diluent.

Tablets first appeared in *N.F. V* in the place of certain troches. In subsequent revisions of the *N.F.*, and in *U.S.P. XI* and subsequent revisions, many other tablets have been admitted, chiefly in order to establish standards to which manufacturers of the tablets must conform.

Conformity with 4 types of standards is required. The first type is concerned with the identity and the purity of the medicinal substances present. The second requires that the tablet disintegrate within a certain time, under the conditions of the official test for disintegration. In general, the disintegration times required by *U.S.P. XV* are much lower than those of *U.S.P. XIV*. The third type stipulates that the tablets must meet the requirements of the official "Weight Variation Test for Tablets." The fourth type establishes quantitative limits for the active constituent or constituents of the tablets. These vary with the identity of the substance, its physical and chemical stability and the amount of it present in the tablet. Generally speaking, the most exacting requirement is a quantitative deviation no greater than ±5 per cent from the labeled strength, and the most liberal is a permitted error of ±10 per cent.

Tablets of the following substances are now official. Included in this list are 3 substances, Desoxycorticosterone Acetate, Estradiol and Testosterone, the official tablet forms of which are entitled "Pellets." These are compressed tablets formed without the presence of any binder, diluent or excipient. They are not intended for oral administration but rather for implantation in the tissues from whence they are absorbed into the circulation.

LIST OF OFFICIAL TABLETS
United States Pharmacopoeia

Acetazolamide
Acetophenetidin
Acetylsalicylic Acid
Aluminum Hydroxide Gel, Dried
Aminophylline
Aminosalicylic Acid
Ammonium Chloride
Amobarbital
Amobarbital Sodium
Amodiaquine Hydrochloride
Amphetamine Sulfate, Dextro
Ascorbic Acid
Atropine Sulfate
Bethanechol Chloride
Bishydroxycoumarin
Bismuth Sodium Triglycollamate
Busulfan
Calcium Cyclamate, Compound
Calcium Gluconate
Calcium Pantothenate
Carbarsone
Chlorcyclizine Hydrochloride

Chloroquine Phosphate
Chlorothiazide
Chlorpheniramine Maleate
Chlorpromazine Hydrochloride
Codeine Phosphate
Colchicine
Compound Calcium Cyclamate
Cortisone Acetate
Cyclizine Hydrochloride
Decavitamin
Dehydrocholic Acid
Desoxycorticosterone Acetate
Dextro Amphetamine Sulfate
Dienestrol
Diethylcarbamazine Citrate
Diethylstilbestrol
Digitalis
Digitoxin
Digoxin
Dihydromorphinone Hydrochloride
Diiodohydroxyquin
Dimenhydrinate
Doxylamine Succinate
Dried Aluminum Hydroxide Gel.
Ergonovine Maleate
Ergotamine Tartrate
Erythromycin
Ethinyl Estradiol
Ethisterone
Ferrous Gluconate
Ferrous Sulfate
Folic Acid
Glyceryl Trinitrate
Glycobiarsol
Homatropine Methylbromide
Hydrocortisone
Hydroxychloroquine Sulfate
Iodochlorhydroxyquin
Iopanoic Acid
Iophenoxic Acid
Isoniazid
Isoproterenol Hydrochloride
Magnesium Trisilicate
Mecamylamine Hydrochloride
Meclizine Hydrochloride
Menadiol Sodium Diphosphate
Menadione
Meperidine Hydrochloride
Mephobarbital
Meprobamate
Mercaptopurine
Methadone Hydrochloride

Methenamine Mandelate
Methimazole
Methylrosaniline Chloride
Methyltestosterone
Methylthiouracil
Morphine Sulfate
Neomycin Sulfate
Neostigmine Bromide
Nicotinamide
Nicotinic Acid
Nitrofurantoin
Nystatin
Papaverine Hydrochloride
Penicillin G
Penicillin, Phenoxymethyl
Penicillin, Phenoxymethyl, Potassium
Phenindamine Tartrate
Phenobarbital
Phenoxymethyl Penicillin
Phenoxymethyl Penicillin, Potassium
Phthalylsulfathiazole
Phytonadione
Piperazine Citrate
Polymyxin B Sulfate
Potassium Chloride
Potassium Phenoxymethyl Penicillin
Potassium Permanganate
Prednisolone
Prednisone
Primaquine Phosphate
Primidone
Probenecid
Prochlorperazine Maleate
Progesterone
Promethazine Hydrochloride
Propantheline Bromide
Propylthiouracil
Pyridostigmine Bromide
Pyridoxine Hydrochloride
Pyrilamine Maleate
Pyrimethamine
Quinacrine Hydrochloride
Quinidine Sulfate
Reserpine
Riboflavin
Saccharin Sodium
Sodium Aminosalicylate
Sodium Bicarbonate
Sodium Carboxymethylcellulose
Sodium Chloride
Sodium Levothyroxine

Sodium Liothyronine
Sodium Salicylate
Sodium Sulfoxone
Sulfadiazine
Sulfamethoxypyridazine
Sulfapyridine
Sulfisoxazole
Thiamine Hydrochloride
Thyroid
Tolazoline Hydrochloride
Tolbutamide
Trihexyphenidyl Hydrochloride
Tripelennamine Hydrochloride
Trisulfapyrimidines
Urethan

LIST OF OFFICIAL TABLETS
National Formulary, XI

Acetaminophen
Acetarsone
Acetylsalicylic Acid, Acetophenetidin and Caffeine
Amisometradine
Amphetamine Phosphate
Dextro-Amphetamine Phosphate
Dibasic Amphetamine Phosphate
Dibasic Dextro-Amphetamine Phosphate
Amphetamine Sulfate
Apomorphine Hydrochloride
Arecoline Hydrobromide
Azacyclonol Hydrochloride
Barbital
Barbital Sodium
Benzestrol
Benztropine Methanesulfonate
Bismuth Subcarbonate
Bismuth Subnitrate
Three Bromides
Bromisovalum
Butabarbital Sodium
Citrated Caffeine
Calcium Aminosalicylate
Calcium Carbonate
Calcium Lactate
Carbinoxamine Maleate
Cascara Sagrada Extract
Chiniofon
Chlorothen Citrate
Choline Bitartrate
Choline Dihydrogen Citrate
Cocaine Hydrochloride
Codeine Sulfate
Cyclobarbital Calcium
Cycrimine Hydrochloride
Desoxycorticosterone Acetate (Pellets)
Dextromethorphan Hydrobromide
Diethylstilbestrol Dipropionate
Dihydrocodeinone Bitartrate
Dihydroxyaluminum Aminoacetate
Diphemanil Methylsulfate
Diphenadione
Ephedrine Hydrochloride
Ephedrine Sulfate
Estradiol (Pellets)
Estradiol
Ethinamate
Glutethimide
Halazone
Hexavitamin
Hexestrol
Hydralazine Hydrochloride
Hydroxyzine Hydrochloride
Iodoalphionic Acid
Lanatoside C
Levorphanol Tartrate
Magnesium Hydroxide
Tribasic Magnesium Phosphate
Mephenesin
Mercurophylline
Mild Mercurous Chloride
Mercury Bichloride Large Poison
Mersalyl and Theophylline
Methacholine Bromide
Methamphetamine Hydrochloride
Methantheline Bromide
Methapyrilene Hydrochloride
Metharbital
Methenamine
Methenamine and Sodium Biphosphate
Methionine
Methylergonovine Maleate
Methyprylon
Morphine and Atropine Sulfates
Neocinchophen
Nylidrin Hydrochloride
Ox Bile Extract
Para-aminobenzoic Acid
Penthienate Bromide
Pentobarbital Sodium
Pheniramine Maleate
Phenobarbital Sodium
Phenolphthalein

Phentolamine Hydrochloride
Phenyl Salicylate
Phthalylsulfacetamide
Piperazine Estrone Sulfate
Pipradol Hydrochloride
Potassium Iodide
Procaine Hydrochloride
Quinine Sulfate
Rauwolfia Serpentina
Rescinnamine
Rutin
Salicylamide
Santonin
Santonin and Mild Mercurous Chloride
Scopolamine Hydrobromide
Sodium Bicarbonate and Calcium Carbonate
Sodium Bicarbonate and Magnesium Oxide
Sodium Bromide
Sodium Chloride and Dextrose
Compound Sodium Cyclamate
Sodium Nitrite
Strychnine Sulfate
Succinylsulfathiazole
Sulfacetamide
Sulfacetamide, Sulfadiazine and Sulfamerazine
Sulfadiazine and Sulfamerazine
Sulfaguanidine
Sulfamerazine
Sulfamethizole
Sulfanilamide
Sulfathiazole
Testosterone (Pellets)
Tetracycline Hydrochloride
Thenyldiamine Hydrochloride
Theobromine Calcium Salicylate
Theobromine Sodium Acetate
Theophylline
Theophylline Sodium Acetate
Theophylline Sodium Glycinate
Thonzylamine Hydrochloride
Triasyn B
Tridihexethyl Chloride
Trimethadione
Tyrothricin (Troches)
Vitamin B_{12} with Intrinsic Factor Concentrate
Dried Yeast
Zoxazolamine

BIBLIOGRAPHY

Bauer, C. W., and Gerraughty, R. J.: Enteric coatings in dispensing pharmacy: I. The preliminary investigation, J. Am. Pharm. A. (Pract. Ed.) 14:504, 512, 1953.

Chatten, L. G.: Tablet disintegration, Can. Pharm. J. 85:494, 1952.

Clarkson, R.: Tablet Coating, New York, Drug & Cosmetic Ind., 1951.

Doerr, D. W., Serles, E. R., and Deardorff, D. L.: Tablet coatings: cellulosic high polymers, J. Am. Pharm. A. (Sc. Ed.) 43:433, 1954.

Evanson, R. V., and DeKay, H. G.: A study of the disintegration of tablets, Bull. Nat. Formulary Comm. 18:45, 1950.

Filleborn, V. M.: A new approach to tablet disintegration testing, Am. J. Pharm. 120:233, 1948.

Gans, E. H., and Chavkin, L.: The use of polyethylene glycol in tablet coating, J. Am. Pharm. A. (Sc. Ed.) 43:483, 1954.

Goldstein, S. W.: Accuracy and tolerances in pharmaceutical compounding: IX. Powders, J. Am. Pharm. A. (Pract. Ed.) 9:477, 509, 1948.

Grim, W. M., and Gordon, W. E., Jr.: Comparative study of the disintegration time determination of compressed tablets according to the U.S.P. XIV and a modified British Pharmacopoeia (1948) method, Am. J. Pharm. 124:410, 1952.

Gross, H. M., and Becker, C. H.: A comparative study of tablet disintegrating agents, J. Am. Pharm. A. (Sc. Ed.) 41:157, 1952.

Hammerness, F. C., and Waldon, C. H.: A method of evaluating enteric coatings using the white rat, J. Am. Pharm. A. (Sc. Ed.) 43:357, 1954.

Holstius, E. A., and DeKay, H. G.: A statistical study of some disintegrating and binding agents in certain compressed tablets, J. Am. Pharm. A. (Sc. Ed.) 41:505, 1952.

Hooper, R. L., and Walker, G. C.: Sublingual administration, Bull. Ontario Coll. Pharm. 4:13, 1955.

Lezberg, T. C., and Murphy, J. T.: A study of the U.S.P. requirements for disintegration of tablets, Bull. Am. Soc. Hosp. Pharm. 11:397, 1954.

Little, A., and Mitchell, K. A.: Tablet Making, Liverpool, Northern Pub. Co., 1949.

Miller, B., and Chavkin, L.: The use of polyethylene glycol as a binder in tablet compression, J. Am. Pharm. A. (Sc. Ed.) 43:486, 1954.

Silver, J. A., and Clarkson, R.: Manufacture of Compressed Tablets, Philadelphia, F. J. Stokes Machine Co., Publisher, 1944.

Stoklosa, M. J., and Ohmart, L. M.: Enteric coatings in dispensing pharmacy: II. A practical method of extemporaneous enteric coating, J. Am. Pharm. A. (Pract. Ed.) 14:507, 514, 1953.

H. GEORGE DeKAY, Ph.D.
Professor of Pharmacy, Purdue University

25

Effervescent Salts

THE OFFICIAL EFFERVESCENT SALT
METHODS OF MANUFACTURE
  PREPARING THE FORMULA
  PREPARING AND MIXING THE INGREDIENTS
  MOISTENING AND GRANULATING
  DRYING THE MOIST GRANULES
  PACKAGING AND STORING
COLORING EFFERVESCENT SALTS

Effervescent salts are mixtures of a medicinal agent with citric acid, tartaric acid, or both, and a bicarbonate, usually sodium bicarbonate. Mixtures of this kind usually are dissolved in water for purposes of administration and are taken during effervescence or immediately thereafter. This supplies a medicinal agent dissolved in carbonated water which is more acceptable than a noncarbonated saline draught.

The reaction between the acids and the bicarbonate may be indicated by the following equations:

$$3NaHCO_3 + H_3C_6H_5O_7 \rightarrow Na_3C_6H_5O_7 + 3CO_2 + 3H_2O$$

$$2NaHCO_3 + H_2C_4H_4O_6 \rightarrow Na_2C_4H_4O_6 + 2CO_2 + 2H_2O$$

Powdered mixtures of this kind react very rapidly when added to water, and in many cases part of the draught is lost due to the violence of the effervescence. Therefore, they are made into granular form in order to retard solution and violent effervescence. The size of the granules is a factor in this retardation as the large granules dissolve more slowly than do the small ones or fine powders. They are divided conveniently into small, medium and large granules according to the size of the sieves used in the granulating procedures. A retarded effervescence results in a more thorough carbonation of the finished solution. Reactions of this kind take place more slowly in cold water than in warm. The rapidity of solution of such mixtures depends on 2 factors: (1) the temperature of the water and (2) the size of the granular particles.

Effervescent salts have been known for many years. The French pharmacist, G. A. Quesneville (1810–1889) is said to have been the first to prepare such salts or at least to make them known in the scientific world as well as among laymen. In 1838, he published a recommendation for the administration of ferrous sulfate in the form of a granulated effervescent salt. Although these salts apparently attained their peak in medicine in the early part of the 20th century, they are still in demand, as indicated by the advertisements one sees and by the many products of this kind on the market. The basic constituents of this class of products are practically always the same, with variations in the amounts of each ingredient and of the medicinal agent used.

Many of the early formulas for this class of preparations contained sucrose in addition to the active ingredients. It was used to give the preparations a more pleasant flavor as well as to act as a binder for the moistened mass, thereby making it possible to obtain a better granulation. Because of the disadvantages of the use of sucrose, saccharin has replaced it in many of these formulas.

THE OFFICIAL EFFERVESCENT SALT

The *U.S.P. XIV* formula for Effervescent Sodium Phosphate was dropped from *U.S.P. XV* and appeared in *N.F. X* as the only official effervescent salt. Effervescent Potassium Citrate N.F. IX was deleted in the *N.F. X*. The formula for the official preparation is as follows:

EFFERVESCENT SODIUM PHOSPHATE, N.F. XI

Exsiccated Sodium Phosphate, dried and powdered	200 Gm.
Sodium Bicarbonate, in dry powder	477 Gm.
Tartaric Acid, in dry powder	252 Gm.
Citric Acid (uneffloresced crystals)	162 Gm.
To make about	1,000 Gm.

Powder the citric acid, mix it intimately with the exsiccated sodium phosphate and the tartaric acid, and thoroughly incorporate the sodium bicarbonate.

Place the mixed powders on a plate or in a suitable dish in an oven previously heated to between 93° C. and 104° C. Manipulate the mixture carefully with a spatula which is acid resistant, and, when it has become moist, rub it through a No. 6 tinned-iron sieve. Dry the granules at a temperature not exceeding 54° C.; transfer the salt to suitable containers, and seal them tightly.

Note: The proportion of tartaric acid and citric acid may be varied if desired, but their combined acidity must be equivalent to the acidity indicated in the official formula.

EFFERVESCENT POTASSIUM CITRATE, N.F. IX

Potassium Citrate	200 Gm.
Sodium Bicarbonate, in dry powder	477 Gm.
Tartaric Acid, in dry powder	252 Gm.
Citric Acid (uneffloresced)	162 Gm.
To make about	1,000 Gm.

Note: The proportions of tartaric acid and citric acid may be varied if desired, but their combined acidity must correspond to the acidity indicated in the official formula, and the percentage of potassium citrate must be maintained.

Dry the potassium citrate on a water bath until it ceases to lose weight, and powder the dried salt. Mix this intimately with the powdered citric and tartaric acids, and thoroughly incorporate the sodium bicarbonate. Place the mixed powders on a plate of glass or in a suitable dish in an oven, previously heated to between 93° C. and 104° C. Manipulate carefully with a spatula which is acid-resistant, until the mixture becomes moist; rub it through a No. 6 tinned-iron sieve and dry the granules at a temperature not exceeding 54° C. Transfer the salt immediately to suitable containers and seal tightly. Care must be taken to prevent the product from coming in contact with air containing moisture.

The procedure for these official salts is practically the same, but, if a pharmacist were attempting to make these in his own prescription room, he would not have the oven for maintaining the temperature at which the water of crystallization is released and would have to resort to the wet method of manufacture. He could use the water-bath method by means of a double boiler, as explained later (p. 457).

METHODS OF MANUFACTURE

The preparation of effervescent salts on either a small or a large scale follows more or less the same general procedure and can be divided into a number of steps: (1) preparing the formula, (2) preparing and mixing the ingredients, (3) moistening and granulating, (4) drying the moist granules and (5) packaging and storing.

The two general methods for making effervescent salts are commonly known as the *fusion method* and the *wet method*. In the case of the fusion method, the mixed powders are moistened by heating in an electrically controlled oven or over an actively boiling water bath. The wet method consists in dampening the mixed powders by means of some nonsolvent moistening agent. In both cases, the moistened mass is passed through a suitable sieve, and then the granules are dried carefully at a low temperature prior to packaging. The industrial process of making effervescent salts by the wet method follows this same procedure essentially, except that the powders are placed in a mixer such as a large Pony Mixer or a Mass Mixer before the addition of the moistening agent. A known quantity of alcohol mix is added while the mixers are in operation, and, when a thorough mixing has taken place, the mass is passed through the appropriate sieve.

The author has found, in his small laboratory, that if approximately 150 ml. of liquid per 1,000 Gm. of powder is used, a suitable mass can be made which gives a good uniform granule. The steps to be followed in either case are the same.

PREPARING THE FORMULA

The proportion of acids used in making the salt must be governed by the chemical reaction between them and the bicarbonate. The amounts necessary for neutralization can be calculated as follows:

I. $2NaHCO_3 + H_2C_4H_4O_6 \rightarrow Na_2C_4H_4O_6 + 2H_2O + 2CO_2$

According to this reaction, 2 molecular weights of sodium bicarbonate will be neutralized by 1 molecular weight of tartaric acid.

II. $3NaHCO_3 + H_3C_6H_5O_7 \cdot H_2O \rightarrow Na_3C_6H_5O_7 + 3H_2O + 3CO_2$

The citric acid is the uneffloresced crystals and contains 1 molecule of water. Three molecular weights of sodium bicarbonate will be neutralized by 1 molecular weight of citric acid.

It is a well-known fact that effervescent salts prepared with tartaric acid for total acidity will produce granules which are powdery and chalky, and the finished product will have a salty taste. It will be necessary to granulate this mixture with some nonsolvent liquid because tartaric acid contains no water of crystallization. On the other hand, when the total acidity is citric acid containing 1 molecule of water of crystallization, the mass is decidedly sticky and difficult to manipulate.

A combination of these two acids will make a better granulation mixture. The proportions of each are varied according to the preparation desired and the formula to be used. It has been found that a good working formula should contain citric acid 19 per cent, tartaric acid 28 per cent and sodium bicarbonate 53 per cent. The percentage of acids can be interchanged so as to retain approximately the acidity indicated above. A comparison with the N.F. preparation for effervescent salt shows a close proximity to these proportions with an interchange of acids according to the preparation.

The amount of medicinal agent should be determined according to the dose desired. The usual procedure for the physician is to prescribe a teaspoonful dose or a multiple of that amount. Four Gm. of the finished salt is considered to be a teaspoonful. If the dose of medicament is 0.25 Gm., then the finished product should contain 3.75 Gm. of the effervescent salt mixture to each teaspoonful. The total amount of preparation then can be calculated on the basis of the number of doses to be prescribed.

PREPARING AND MIXING THE INGREDIENTS

The sodium bicarbonate and the tartaric acid should be dried to constant weight at a temperature of 100° to 110° C. and the medicinal agent should be dried at a suitable temperature until constant weight has been reached to remove all of the moisture that might be present. Then they are powdered and passed through a No. 60 sieve.

The chemical reaction will be produced by any moisture which may be present, thus producing a greater loss in carbon dioxide during the preparation of the salt. According to a number of experiments, it has been shown that part of the sodium bicarbonate is lost by chemical reaction during the preparation of an effervescent salt, part of which is dissipated as carbon dioxide. This loss is compensated for in the formula.

The moisture content of the mixed powders must be controlled carefully to ensure a good product. The citric acid should be in the uneffloresced condition, thus giving access to its 1 molecule of water of crystallization which is released by heating and is used in producing the moistened mass for granulation purposes. The acid should be finely powdered prior to mixing with the bicarbonate mixture.

The sodium bicarbonate, the sweetener (if used) and the medicinal agent are mixed by placing the powdered chemicals into a suitable container. Then these are mixed intimately by stirring them with a wooden paddle or a mechanical mixer or by rolling them in a closed container such as a mixing jar or a ball or pebble mill (see Fig. 75, p. 82). The powders should be passed through a No. 30 to 60 noncorrosive sieve to ensure proper fineness and thorough mixing. The sieves should be made of a noncorrosive metal or alloy such as well-tinned iron, silverplate, stainless steel, Monel metal or other suitable material. The tartaric acid and the citric acid are powdered and mixed according to the above procedure, then passed through the same noncorrosive sieve as used above. The two powders are transferred to a suitable container and mixed thoroughly. They are passed quickly through the No. 30 to 60 sieve to ensure uniform mixing.

The temperature and the humidity of the room must be considered in the manufacture of effervescent salts. If the room has a high humidity, the powders will pick up the moisture, thereby causing a partial solution of the sodium bicarbonate and the acids, after which they will begin to react. If the reaction is started during the mixing process, there will be a distinct gumming or lumping of the material, making it difficult to get a uniform mixture and thereby creating a greater loss of the effervescing properties of the salt.

Moistening and Granulating

Moistening or massing of the ingredients may be produced in one of two ways. The first is by releasing the water of crystallization contained in the citric acid by means of heat. This may be done by an oven or an actively boiling water bath. A double boiler is good equipment for this purpose. The second method is to produce a mass by adding some nonsolvent moistening agent, such as alcohol, to the dry powdered mixture. If all of the powders are in the anhydrous condition, the moistening agent should contain a small amount of water to produce a satisfactory mass.

The fusion method is the one followed by most of the manufacturers of granular effervescent salts. The equipment is comprised of a large steam-heated hot plate with a slightly raised rim or a large electrically controlled oven (Fig. 188). When

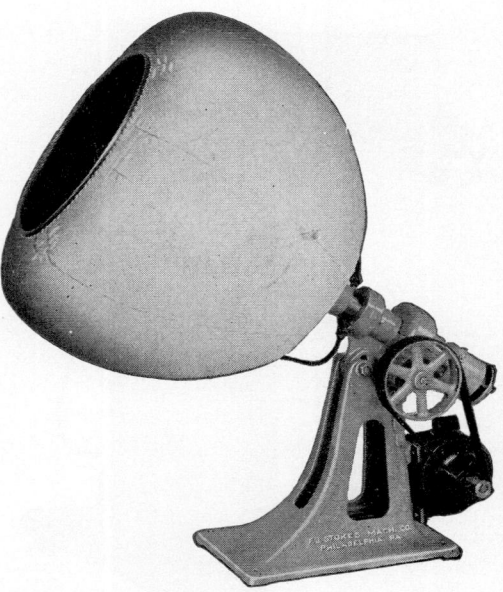

Fig. 188. Fusion pan. (Stokes, Philadelphia.)

the steam-heated hot plate is used, the powdered mixture is placed on the plate to a depth ranging from $\frac{1}{2}$ to $1\frac{1}{2}$ inches. The heat from the hot surface releases the water of crystallization from the citric acid, and this in turn dissolves part of the active ingredients, causing the chemical reaction to take place. The powders next to the hot plate become sticky due to this release of moisture. The carbon dioxide which is released by the chemical reaction causes the mass to become spongy, like raised bread dough. Then the mass is stirred by means of a trowel or other device until the entire mass reaches the proper consistency. This moistened mass is removed quickly and forced through a sieve. The size of the sieve varies according to the particle size desired. During this process of granulating, the mass is cooled by the removal of the heat, and the chemical reaction subsides.

The most important step of this entire procedure is that of moistening or massing of the ingredients prior to granulation. Frequently the experienced operator will take a handful of the moistened mass and squeeze it into a ball. If the ball sticks together and is of sufficient hardness, it has become sufficiently moist and immediately is removed to the granulators, where it is forced

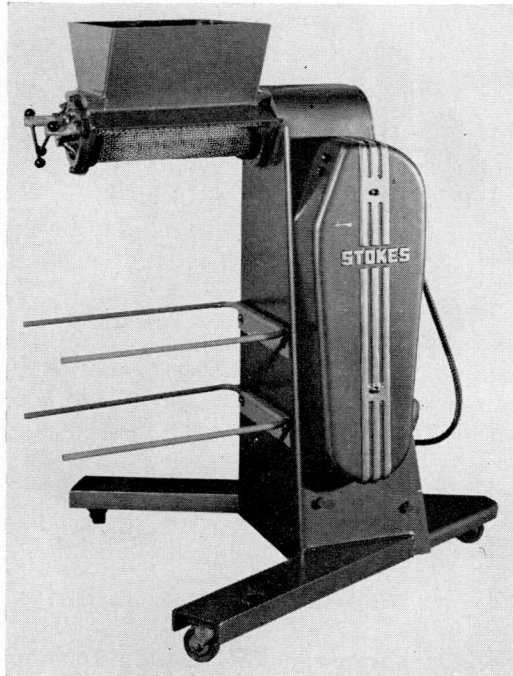

Fig. 189. Oscillating granulator. (Stokes, Philadelphia.)

through the sieve and then removed to the drying chamber.

The oscillating granulator (Fig. 189) and the upright granulators are very good pieces of equipment to use for making uniform granulations. The author has found that the granules made by hand-sieving require a mass which is more moist than the same mass which is to be used for machine granulation. The pressure applied by the granulators is sufficient to force the liquid from the moistened mass, which in turn causes it to become wetter as it is granulated. The mass which is too wet will clog the machine at times. The mass also should be forced through a sieve which is one size larger than the end-product desired. The dried granules can be resieved through the oscillator, using the desired sieve size. The Colton upright granulator cannot be used for the sieving of dried granules.

The oven-heating procedure is similar to the hot-plate method of heating. The mixed powders on suitable trays are placed in a preheated oven where the water is released from the citric acid as stated above. When the mass has reached a proper consistency, it is removed from the trays, kneaded into a dough and then passed through the granulator. Then, the granules are removed to the drying chamber (Fig. 190).

It is essential to stir the powders in the hot-plate method because the mass next to the steamed surface will be heated and react before the external surface has reached that temperature. This is overcome partially by having the mixture at a minimum depth on the heated surface. In the oven-heating process, the trays are usually at a lower temperature than the oven, and the powder on the upper surface will be preheated and react before the powder next to the trays releases its water of crystallization. This is overcome by having the trays preheated and by occasionally stirring the heated mass with a wooden spoon or other suitable device. When the mass has reached the proper consistency, it is removed and granulated as stated above.

The type of sieve used for granulation will depend on the particle size of the product desired. Large granules are obtained from a No. 3 or 4 sieve, medium granules from a No. 6 or 8 sieve and small granules from a No. 10 or 12 sieve.

The second method of massing is known as the wet method. This procedure is appropriate for the average pharmacist and is used by a number of manufacturers who produce small quantities of effervescent salts. The powders are mixed thoroughly, then the moistening agent is added in small portions. Alcohol usually is used as the nonsolvent liquid. The mass is mixed carefully and rubbed together after each addition of the liquid. This mixing is continued until the mass will retain its shape when molded into a ball. It then is forced through a sieve of the suitable size. The granules will have a more uniform shape if there is a fair amount of pressure applied when the mass is forced through the sieve.

A third method of massing has come to the fore recently: namely, that of using steam under a given pressure for the moistening of the granules. The dried mixed powders are weighed carefully into a large Pony Mixer container, after which this container is attached to the Pony mixing equipment where a steam tube reaches to within 2 inches of the bottom of the container.

Then the steam is transmitted to the mix until a known weight of condensed moisture has been transmitted to the powders. The Pony Mixer has been in operation all of this time, after which this moistened mass is passed immediately through the oscillating granulator and then dried. This procedure has been successful and does save considerable time in this step of moistening and granulating. The granules when dried are of excellent quality and effervesce freely when placed in water.

Drying the Moist Granules

The moistened granules are transferred to a suitable tray and are dried by one or two general methods. Most effervescent salts are dried by placing the trays into a drying chamber where a uniform and constant temperature is maintained, not to exceed 54° C. The granules are allowed to remain in this chamber until dry, when they are removed and quickly passed over a sieve to remove the fine powder before packaging.

The granules also may be dried in the open air if the drying-room temperature is between 30° and 50° C. and the humidity is low. The granules are placed on trays and put into a suitable rack or placed on papers spread on the table top. A good product can be obtained in this way by drying the granules obtained by the wet method.

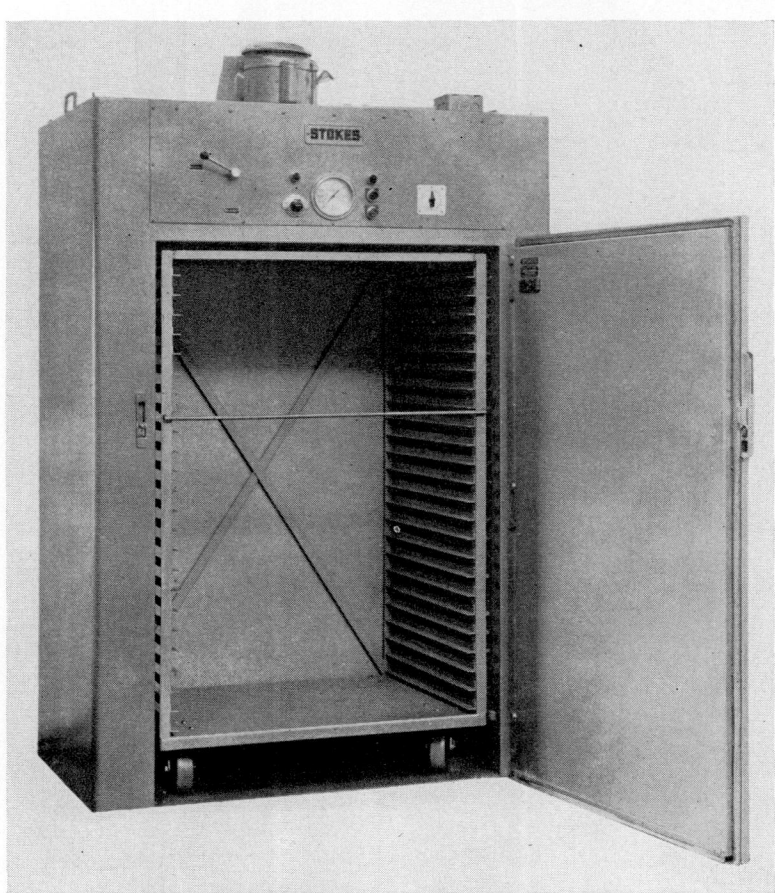

Fig. 190. Drying cabinet. (Stokes, Philadelphia.)

460 Effervescent Salts

These granules also can be dried by passing them on belts through a current of dry air and maintaining a uniform temperature until dried.

PACKAGING AND STORING

The dried sifted granules are removed from the drying trays and bottled in wide-mouth, clear or colored, dry-glass bottles. These bottles are sealed tightly to exclude air and moisture. They usually are stored in a cool place.

COLORING EFFERVESCENT SALTS

Some pharmacists may desire a product that is distinctive in appearance and more pleasing to the eye. This can be produced easily and conveniently by means of acceptable coloring agents. The coloring agents which can be used are those dyes permitted by the Federal Food, Drug and Cosmetic Act and by the individual state laws to be used for internal administration.

Also, the coloring agent should be one that will not be altered by any of the ingredients of the effervescing mixture. It also will be necessary to determine the quantity of color needed to produce the desired shade or tint. The color should be added to the powders and mixed intimately before the addition of the moistening agent; it should be a color that is soluble in the

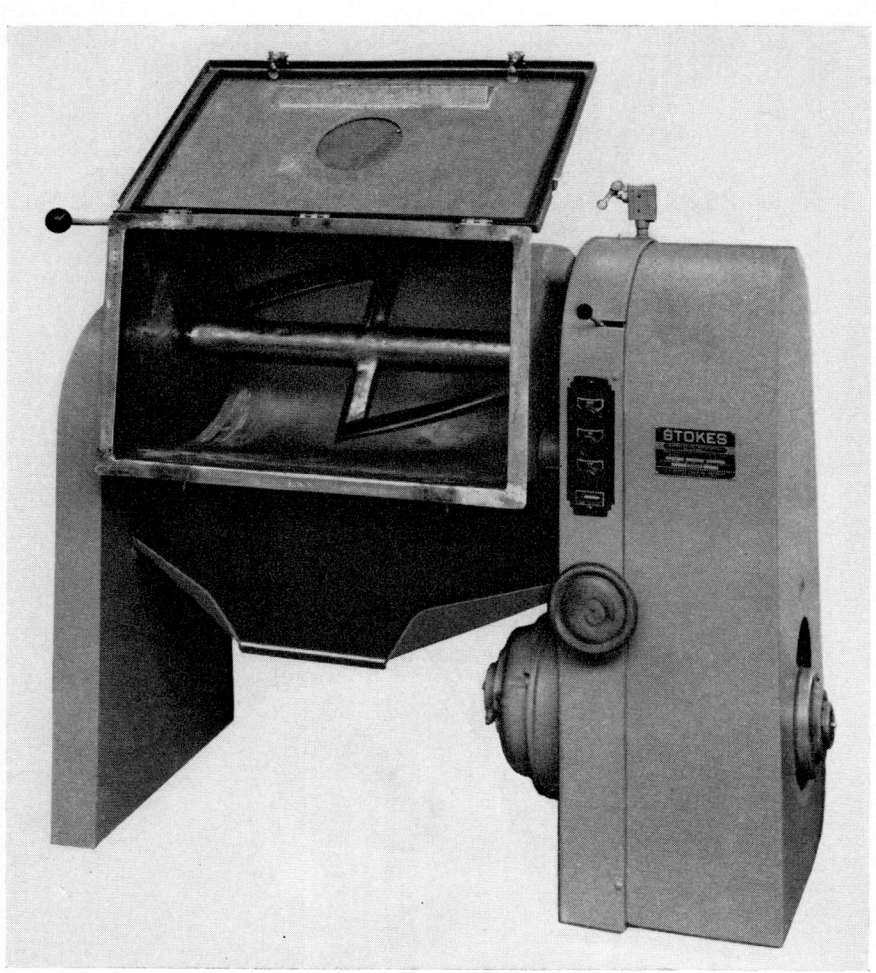

Fig. 191. Mixer for granulated drugs. (Stokes, Philadelphia.)

liquid used. This causes the color to be mixed uniformly so that when the moistening agent is added the color is in intimate contact with all of the powder and will give a uniformly colored granule when pressed through the sieve. The granules are dried and packaged according to the usual procedures.

BIBLIOGRAPHY

Cook, E. F.: Granular effervescent salts, Am. J. Pharm. **75**:464, 1903.

Lunan, G.: Granular effervescent preparations, Pharm. J. **77**:665, 675, 1906.

White, R. C.: The manufacture of effervescent salts, J. Am. Pharm. A. **10**:609, 1921.

DONALD M. SKAUEN, Ph.D.
*Professor of Pharmacy, School of Pharmacy,
University of Connecticut*

26

Radioactive Pharmaceuticals

FUNDAMENTAL CONCEPTS
METHODS OF PRODUCTION OF RADIOACTIVE
    ISOTOPES
      THE CYCLOTRON
      THE NUCLEAR REACTOR
METHODS OF DETECTION
UNITS OF MEASUREMENT

TYPE OF RADIATION
RADIOACTIVE HAZARDS AND PROTECTION
    THEREFROM
OFFICIAL AND NON-OFFICIAL RADIOISOTOPES
    USED IN PHARMACY AND MEDICINE
PROCUREMENT OF RADIOACTIVE ISOTOPES
DISTRIBUTORS

Radioactive isotopes no longer are considered to be scientific curiosities by the medical and the pharmaceutical professions. Sufficient knowledge has been gained through an intensive research program to indicate that radioactive isotopes have therapeutic value, are excellent diagnostic agents and are worth-while research tools.

When radioactive materials first were used for medical purposes, their solutions were prepared and administered to patients without regard to bacterial or mold contamination. With increased understanding of isotope therapy came the realization that these materials were actually pharmaceuticals and as such should be prepared under the control of the Food and Drug Administration. Now, commercial products for isotope therapy must conform to the same regulations of the Food and Drug Administration assigned to any drug, in addition to meeting Atomic Energy Commission requirements.

Several manufacturers are producing sterile, pyrogen-free, assayed radioactive parenteral drugs and preparations suitable for oral use.

FUNDAMENTAL CONCEPTS

In order to understand fully the applications of radioactive materials in pharmacy, it is important to review briefly certain aspects of atomic structure.

The building blocks for all matter, as we know it, are atoms. Atoms consist of a number of parts arranged in an orderly fashion. The nucleus, within which is concentrated most of the mass of the atom, is made up of protons, carrying a unit positive charge, and neutrons, having the same mass as protons but carrying no charge. The number of protons is equal to the atomic number of the element; for example, helium with atomic number 2 has 2 protons. There are enough neutrons present in the nucleus to make up the proper mass number of the element when added to the number of protons. In the case of helium, with a mass number of 4, it requires 2 neutrons to make up this difference. Rotating in orbits about the nucleus are particles known as electrons which bear a unit negative charge. The electron is considerably smaller in size than the proton and the neutron, being about $1/1850$ of their weight.

The number of electrons in the orbits surrounding the nucleus of the atom is equal to the number of protons within the nucleus. This means that the total positive charge of an atom is equaled by the total negative charges in the orbital electrons.

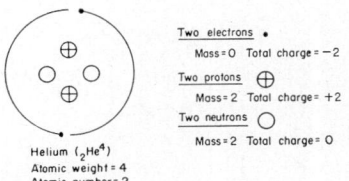

FIG. 192. Diagrammatic conception of the important components of a typical atom.

Figure 192 illustrates diagrammatically the important components of a typical atom.

All naturally occurring elements, excepting the common isotope of hydrogen, contain at least 1 neutron for each proton. Hydrogen has only 1 proton in its nucleus and 1 electron in its orbit, and is devoid of neutrons. Those elements containing more than 16 protons have a greater number of neutrons than protons, yet maintain their stability. For example, the mercury atom has 80 protons and 118 neutrons in the nucleus. While each element has a fixed number of protons in the nucleus and a fixed number of electrons in the outer shell, it is possible to vary the number of neutrons in the nucleus. Alteration of the neutron content of the nucleus changes the mass of the atom but has no effect on the electric charge or the atomic number. The change in mass affects the physical properties of the atom to a considerable extent without altering the chemical characteristics. Those substances which have the same number of protons but have varying numbers of neutrons are called *isotopes*. If we take the element hydrogen, for example, and add a neutron to its nucleus, the resulting element is still hydrogen chemically, but its mass has been doubled. The physical behavior of the new hydrogen isotope called deuterium is different from its parent. If a second neutron is added to the first, another isotope of hydrogen known as tritium would be produced which differs physically from either of the other hydrogens as it is unstable and therefore radioactive but reacts chemically as hydrogen. The isotopes of hydrogen described above are shown in Figure 193.

Isotopes are classified as stable or unstable. Those which are unstable are radioactive because their nuclei undergo a rearrangement while changing to a stable state, and energy is given off in one of the forms of ionizing radiation. The rearrangement of the unstable hydrogen isotope, tritium, to form the stable helium atom is shown in Figure 193. One of the neutrons of the nucleus of tritium is converted to a proton during the rearrangement, and an electron is acquired. The resulting atom is the stable helium isotope. Energy is released during this transformation in the form of a beta particle.

All of the atoms of an unstable or radioisotope do not completely rearrange or disintegrate at the same instant. The time required for one half of a given number of atoms to disintegrate to a more stable form is called the *half-life* of the isotope. Since the half-life is different for each isotope, this serves as a convenient method of distinguishing between the various isotopes.

The importance of radioactive isotopes in pharmacy and medicine is associated directly with the nuclear instability and its accompanying ionizing radiation. When administered, radioisotopes are utilized by the body mechanisms or eliminated by the body without differentiation from stable

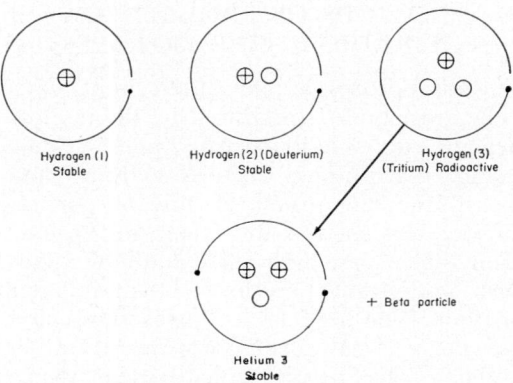

FIG. 193. The isotopes of hydrogen.

isotopes. However, the fact that they yield radiations which can be detected by suitable instruments means that these isotopes can be followed through the complicated body processes until they are utilized in the body or eliminated. An entirely new approach to diagnosis has thus been made possible through the development of radioactive pharmaceuticals. As an example, studies based on rate of transfer are illustrated by the determination of circulation time. An isotope can be injected into one area of the body and its arrival at another place observed by a detecting device.

In a similar manner, since radioactive isotopes give off radiations which are destructive, it is possible to administer an isotope which will be absorbed selectively by a certain tissue and ultimately destroy it. Various isotopes have been employed in this way for therapeutic purposes. One of the iodine isotopes, I^{131}, is assimilated after administration by thyroid tissue to a major extent. In certain cases, after a thorough diagnostic preparation, a dose of iodine[131] is administered to the patient in sufficient concentration to destroy part of the thyroid tissue. In such cases, this method replaces surgical procedures.

In other areas of basic and applied research, the ionizing rays of the isotopes have aided in solving many problems which might well have remained unsolved without this useful tool. An illustration of such uses is the study of the disintegration time of enteric coatings using radioactive sodium[24] as the tracing material.

METHODS OF PRODUCTION OF RADIOACTIVE ISOTOPES

Radioisotopes are produced in 2 ways. The great bulk is produced by the nuclear reactor or "chain-reacting pile." Some radioactive isotopes, such as sodium[22] and beryllium[7], are produced only by particle accelerators such as the cyclotron. Production difficulties, high costs and low yields are undesirable features of the latter method. The particles or "projectiles" used for nuclear transformations are several in number. They may be alpha particles, which are actually the nuclei of helium atoms since they possess 2 protons and 2 neutrons; they may be protons, which are nuclei of the hydrogen atom; they may be deuterons, which are the nuclei of heavy hydrogen with 1 proton and 1 neutron; they may be neutrons; or they may be a number of other particles.

THE CYCLOTRON

To enable a particle to penetrate the electric-force barrier protecting the nucleus, the particle must be accelerated to a very high velocity. This is accomplished in the cyclotron by injecting the particle to be accelerated into the center of an evacuated chamber, which, in turn, is located between the poles of an electromagnet. The particles move at a low velocity initially and are deflected by the strong magnetic field into a circular path. After moving through the first half-circle, the particle receives a push before starting the next half-circle. This impetus or push is produced by a large potential difference between the two sides of the evacuated chamber. In the second half-circle, the particle moves at a greater speed and through a larger half-circle. Another push is received at the next half-circle, and the particle moves at greater speed and through an even larger half-circle. The process continues until the particle is moving so rapidly that it has

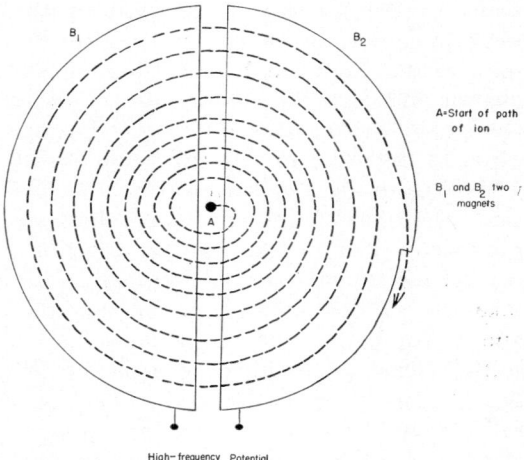

FIG. 194. Path of an ion or particle in a cyclotron.

acquired an energy of a few million electron volts. Then the ions are deflected to the outside of the chamber by means of a mirrorlike arrangement and focused onto the target. The beam of high-energy particles collides directly with the material fixed to the target and produces nuclear transformations. The identity of the resulting element will depend on the target and the type of particle accelerated. The path of an ion or particle in a cyclotron is represented schematically in Figure 194.

THE NUCLEAR REACTOR

With the development of the nuclear reactor, an abundance of neutrons became available for use in the production of radioactive isotopes.

Very simply stated, the nuclear reactor is composed of a latticelike arrangement of graphite or other moderating material within which is placed uranium. Uranium atoms under the influence of neutrons disintegrate and liberate additional high-velocity neutrons. Since it does not have an electric charge, the neutron can pass the electric-force barrier of the nucleus without the necessity of high velocity. Low-velocity neutrons are capable of producing a greater number of reactions than high-velocity neutrons; therefore, those resulting from uranium fission are slowed down by materials known as moderators. When the neutrons are captured by an atom, the nucleus becomes unstable, and a radioactive isotope is formed with simultaneous emission of energy in the form of ionizing radiation. Because of the abundance of neutrons produced in the pile, it is possible to obtain high activity yields in a short period of time, with considerably less expense, than by the cyclotron.

METHODS OF DETECTION

Any device or instrument which will be affected by ionizing radiations so that the resulting reaction can be recorded may be used for the detection of radioactivity. The Geiger-Müller counter and its refinements have been utilized most widely. In recent years, the scintillation counters, which make use of the light produced in various crystals and liquids when acted upon by ionizing radiations, have become quite important for measurements of radioactive materials for diagnostic and therapeutic purposes. The scintillation counters are much more sensitive than any of the other devices now used for radioactive measurements. For this reason, they offer a distinct advantage in diagnositic work because a much smaller dose can be given to the patient with less radiation damage.

The electrometer is another instrument used for assay work which is finding increased application in counting of low level betas such as carbon[14] and tritium.

Photographic films also are used for detecting radioactive particles particularly in the area of autoradiographic technics.

UNITS OF MEASUREMENT

The amount of radioactivity possessed by an unstable isotope is expressed in terms of curies (c), millicuries (mc) or microcuries (μc). A *curie* of an isotope is defined as that quantity in which 3.7×10^{10} atoms disintegrate per second. This means that if an isotope has a long half-life, 1 curie of it will have to contain more atoms than if it has a short half-life, in order to keep up the supply of disintegration. A millicurie is 10^{-3} curies (3.7×10^7 disintegrations per second). A microcurie is 10^{-6} curies (3.7×10^4 disintegrations per second).

The *roentgen* is another unit which is used in work with radioactivity and is defined as the quantity of x-rays or gamma rays that will produce, as a consequence of ionization, 1 electrostatic unit of electricity of either sign. The roentgen-equivalent-physical (r-e-p) is the amount of radiation resulting in the dissipation of 83.8 ergs per gram of tissue.

The rad is that quantity of radiation which results in the dissipation of 100 ergs per gram of tissue.

TYPE OF RADIATION

The 3 important types of radiation for medical and pharmaceutical purposes are the alpha and the beta particles and the gamma rays. All 3 of these types possess in common the property of causing the atoms of the material through which they pass to ionize.

Alpha particles consist of 2 neutrons and 2 protons and can be considered as the nucleus of the helium atom stripped of orbital electrons. Because it is a large particle, it produces a great number of ionizations along its path and thus has a low penetrating power. Most alpha particles are unable to pierce the outer layers of skin and can be stopped by a thin layer of paper.

Beta particles may be either electrons with unit negative charge or positrons with unit positive charge. Like alpha particles, betas cause ions to be produced along their path. However, they do not cause the same extent of ionization and, therefore, are capable of traveling greater distances than alphas of comparable energy. High-energy betas are able to penetrate as much as 2 cm. of animal tissue.

Gamma rays are electromagnetic vibrations comparable with light but of much shorter wavelength. Similar to x-rays, they penetrate deeply into matter and cause fewer ionizations along their path than do either the alpha or the gamma particles.

RADIOACTIVE HAZARDS AND PROTECTION THEREFROM

Any quantity of radioactivity used for medical and pharmaceutical research can be handled safely provided that a reasonable degree of caution is exercised and that the individuals are equipped and trained properly.

Living cells may be damaged by all radiations. The extent of damage inflicted is dependent on the type and the amount of radiation and the length of exposure. Exposure to ionizing radiation is divided into 2 classes—external and internal. External exposures are limited to those in which the radiation source remains outside the body. Damage such as severe burns, cellular changes and genetic effects can occur. Many of these changes are of the latent variety and may not manifest themselves for a number of years. A limited area of the body may be involved, such as a hand or a foot, or the entire body may suffer exposure. The danger from external exposure is slight when working with isotopes for medical diagnostic purposes and for pharmaceutical research if proper precautions are observed. Some of these precautions are: to ensure adequate shielding, to limit the time spent in the vicinity of an energetic source, the use of remote controlled handling devices and the usual good habits of cleanliness. On the other hand, many of the radioisotopes used for therapeutic purposes are of considerably greater hazard and are capable of causing tissue damage because of their energetic character and the larger amounts employed. The isotope of cobalt, Co^{60}, for example, is used in kilocurie amounts in much the same way as an x-ray apparatus for destroying tumorous tissue. In these large amounts, and with such high energies, it is necessary to prepare extensive shielding to prevent overexposure to technical personnel.

The internal hazards associated with the use of radioactive materials are of considerable importance. Deposition in the body may result from ingestion, inhalation or absorption through the intact or injured body surface. After ingestion, the hazard may be due to a direct irradiation of the gastro-intestinal tract. Many of the isotopes concentrate in the organs of the body with inevitable irradiation of that organ (iodine isotopes localize in thyroid tissue, strontium deposits in bone). Inhalation of active gas, vapor, spray or dust is considered to be particularly dangerous because of the retention of such contamination in the lungs. In the laboratory, therefore, extreme personal cleanliness must be maintained to avoid internal exposure. Materials must not be spilled or scattered, and work areas must be kept neat and uncluttered. Skill in radiation protection is as important to the worker in the field of radioactivity as skill in bacterial protection is important to the bacteriologist.

RADIOISOTOPES IN PHARMACY AND MEDICINE

Radioactive Iodine[131]

Radioactive iodine (I^{131}) is produced in the nuclear reactor by the transformation of tellurium. It has a half-life of 8 days and emits both beta and gamma radiations. It is used for preparing the iodine solutions discussed below.

Sodium Radio-iodide Solution
U.S.P. XVI
(Radioactive Iodine Solution)
(Sodium Radioiodine [I^{131}] Solution
U.S.P. XV)

The radioactive iodine^{131} procured from the Atomic Energy Commission generally is in the form of a solution of both radioactive iodide and radioactive iodate. This solution is neither sterile nor pyrogen-free and does not meet other U.S.P. standards for purity, quality, etc. Before it can be employed for therapeutic or diagnostic purposes, it must be converted to a sterile, pyrogen-free solution standardized to contain no more than 5 per cent iodate I^{131} since the iodate I^{131} does not contribute to the medicinal action. The solution usually is dispensed in hard-glass single- or multiple-dose vials with sodium bisulfite added as a stabilizing agent. A bacteriostatic agent may be added to the multidose vials.

The label of each container must show the number of millicuries or microcuries represented at the time indicated in the labeling. This makes it possible to calculate the activity at any future time by using available tables or by using the half-life formula.

The commercial samples for diagnostic use are supplied generally in 10-ml. vials containing 250 μc, while the vials for therapeutic use are considerably stronger, ranging up to 100 millicuries in 30-ml. vials.

Since I^{131} is a source of the highly penetrating gamma rays, the glass vials containing it usually are placed in hermetically sealed tins which are enclosed in thick-walled lead containers for transportation and handling purposes.

Sodium Radio-iodide Capsules U.S.P. XVI
(Radioactive Iodine Capsules)

Aqueous oral solutions of radioactive sodium iodide easily may be spilled by the patient, causing difficulties in removing the radioactive contamination on the spilled area. This danger was overcome by placing the minute amount of radioactive salt in a capsule after dilution with a suitable inert powder. This method of formulation, while overcoming one problem, presented another hazard. During the process of diluting the radioactive iodide with inert powder, an appreciable quantity of dust was produced which was potentially dangerous. To overcome this objectionable feature, capsules are now made by adsorbing the small amount of radioactivity on the interior walls of the capsule, leaving essentially an empty capsule shell. The capsule is sealed, and a hazard-free preparation is obtained. The patient need not fear spilling the contents, and the manufacturer is not concerned with contamination by radioactive dust.

Uses. In microcurie amounts, sodium iodide I^{131} is used both orally and parenterally for special diagnostic studies in patients suspected of exhibiting thyroid disease. It also has been used to seek out metastatic growths which result from thyroidal carcinoma. Therapeutically, sodium iodide I^{131} is administered in millicurie doses for the treatment of thyrotoxicosis. Also, it is used in attempts to treat thyroid carcinoma.

In pharmaceutical research, sodium iodide I^{131} has been used to determine the rate of release of iodide ion from a variety of ointment bases. In this study, various ointments were prepared containing identical quantities of sodium iodide I^{131}, and the ointments were applied to the skin of rats. After a suitable exposure period, the animals were sacrificed, the thyroids removed, and the quantity of radioiodide in the thyroid was used to estimate rate of absorption. In another study using sodium iodide I^{131}, the effect of astringents on normal permeability of frog skins was observed.

Radiodiiodo (I^{131}) Fluorescin

Another compound of radioactive iodine (I^{131}) which is important medicinally is diiodo (I^{131}) fluorescein. This dye, labeled with I^{131}, is prepared as a sterile, pyrogen-free solution so that it can be administered intravenously. The material localizes in tumor tissue to a greater extent than in normal tissue and thus affords a technic of detecting tumors of the brain. The labeled compound is injected intravenously, and the site and the extent of localization determined with a scintillation or Geiger counter, since the emitted rays are energetic enough to pass through the skull and the tissues of the head.

Radio-iodinated Serum Albumin U.S.P. XVI
(Radio-iodinated [I^{131}] Serum Albumin [Human])

Radioactive iodinated (I^{131}) serum albumin is prepared by the incorporation of not more than 1 atom of iodine per 60,000 molecular weight of albumin. In order to minimize protein decomposition, the iodine is introduced by mild iodination at low temperatures in a dilute reaction mixture. The iodinated albumin solution, which is neutral and approximately isotonic, is sterilized, standardized and placed in multiple-dose containers. To provide bacteriostatic activity, 0.09 per cent benzyl alcohol is added to the sterile product. It is also recommended that the vials of iodinated albumin solution be kept in a cool location, but they must not be frozen. Accurate assay information is also included in the labeling.

Uses. Radioactive iodinated (I^{131}) serum albumin has been established as one of the most valuable diagnostic agents. It is the agent most frequently used for brain-tumor studies. It is used for the determination of blood volumes and plasma volumes. Experimental studies on blood circulation indicate that the iodinated albumin solution may be very useful, possessing the advantages of low cost and desirable half-life.

Radioactive Gold^{198}

Gold^{198} is prepared from gold foil by irradiation in the nuclear reactor for a period of about 7 days. In the reactor, neutrons are captured by the nucleus of the gold^{197}, and gold^{198} is produced. The resultant gold^{198} has a half-life of about 2.7 days, and emits both beta particles and gamma rays.

Uses. Radioactive gold (Au^{198}) metal in the form of small pieces of sterile wire called "seeds" is used in the treatment of cancer. For convenience, the gold seeds are inserted in nylon thread, and the thread containing gold metal is implanted directly at the site to be irradiated.

Radiogold Solution U.S.P. XVI
(Sterile Radioactive Gold Colloid)
(Sterile Radiogold [I^{198}] Colloid)

The radioactive gold^{198} metal obtained from the reactor is dissolved in aqua regia with the formation of gold chloride, $AuCl_3$. This gold chloride solution is then neutralized and reduced with ascorbic acid in the presence of a highly select pyrogen-free gelatin. A cherry-red colloidal solution results with particle sizes ranging between 0.002μ and 0.2μ. The colloidal solution may be diluted with saline solution, pectin and other colloids and is stable to reasonable degrees of heat. It should not be treated with steam under pressure. Certain metallic salts such as aluminum and iron create an unstable condition with gold colloid solutions.

After the colloidal solution has been prepared, it is assayed for radioactivity, then pipetted with remote-handling devices into hard-glass vials which are sealed and then sterilized by heat. Shipment is made in lead-shielded cases of suitable thickness to minimize exposure to transportation workers.

Therapeutic effects of gold colloid (Au^{198}) are due largely to the beta particles rather than the gamma rays which are given off. However the gamma component is very penetrating in animal tissue and increases the danger in handling and administering the solution. Gold^{198} colloid is given in much larger doses than are most of the short-lived isotopes, thus further increasing the hazard. For these reasons, elaborate precautions are exercised in the preparation, the dilution, the administration and the storage of radioactive gold^{198} to ensure that overexposure does not occur.

Uses. Radioactive gold (Au^{198}) colloid is employed to destroy tumorous growth by direct infiltration technics.

Radioactive Sodium^{24}

Radioactive sodium^{24} is prepared in the uranium reactor by the irradiation of stable sodium^{23} in the form of sodium carbonate (Na_2CO_3). The half-life of radioactive sodium^{24} thus produced is 14.8 hours. This half-life is advantageous in some experiments, since decay may proceed to a point where hazard is insignificant before any damage to tissue can occur. On the other hand, its half-life is a disadvantage in scheduling experiments.

The strong beta-particle and gamma-ray

emission by sodium^{24} make it useful as a diagnostic aid and a valuable research tool. Its radiations are not readily shielded out by tissues as is the case with low-energy radiations from some of the other isotopes.

Adequate precautions must be taken to protect against excessive exposure to laboratory and clinical workers.

Radioactive Sodium (Na^{24}) Chloride Solution

Radioactive sodium (Na^{24}) chloride solution is a pyrogen-free solution of the radioactive salt in purified water, sterilized by autoclaving.

Use. The principal use for radioactive sodium (Na^{24}) chloride solution in medicine has been as a diagnostic aid. Among other uses, it has been utilized to determine blood-circulation time. The radiosodium solution is injected in one extremity, such as the arm, and a counter is placed over another extremity, such as the leg. As soon as the counting chamber detects the radioactivity, the time is noted. Then calculations and comparisons with normal circulation times are made. A method of differentiation between heart disease and other diseases with similar manifestations has been worked out, using Na^{24} and utilizing a technic known as "radiocardiography." With this method, when Na^{24} is injected into a vein of the arm it finds its way to the heart. If a counting device, connected to an automatic recorder, is located suitably over the heart, it will pick up the radiations forced into the heart and will record a rapid peak or pulse on the chart. If the heart muscle is damaged, the recording will show a more gradual, less extensive peak.

Radioactive sodium chloride (Na^{24}) was one of the first radioactive isotopes to be used in solving a pharmaceutical problem. The isotope contained in enteric-coated capsules was administered to human subjects. The time elapsing before the appearance of activity in the urine was taken as an indication of the effectiveness of the enteric coating.

In another study, radioactive sodium chloride (Na^{24}) was made into pills which were coated and administered to rats. The time and the place of disintegration were established by noting the appearance of radioactivity in the circulation and by direct observation of the intestinal tract.

Radioactive Sodium (Na^{22})

Radioactive sodium (Na^{22}) is prepared in the cyclotron, since no nuclear reactions are available for its production by the pile. During its decay, sodium^{22} emits 2 sets of gamma rays which are moderately energetic. The longer half-life of sodium^{22}, 3 years, is much more convenient than that of sodium^{24}. This permits studies of a more extended nature.

Radiosodium (Na^{22}) Chloride Solution

Sodium chloride Na^{22} solution is prepared by purifying the sodium chloride Na^{22} received from the cyclotron, dissolving in appropriate quantities of water. After radioactive assay, the solution is filtered and sealed in sterile vials and sterilized by autoclaving. The usual precautions for handling moderately active gamma emitters are observed with sodium chloride Na^{22}.

Use. Sodium chloride Na^{22} solution is used therapeutically for diagnostic and research purposes in blood-circulation studies, retention studies and radiocardiography.

Radioactive Phosphorus (P^{32})

Phosphorus^{32} is a pure beta emitter of high enough energy to classify it as one of the most powerful of the beta emitters employed in medicine. The half-life of 14.3 days is convenient for many diagnostic, therapeutic and research purposes.

Sodium Radiophosphate Injection U.S.P. XVI
(Radioactive Phosphorous Solution)
(Sodium Radiophosphate [P^{32}] Solution [U.S.P. XV])

A sterile buffered isotonic solution of radioactive sodium phosphate (P^{32}) is prepared from the material obtained by irradiation of elemental sulfur in the nuclear reactor. This solution at a pH of 6.5 is placed in borosilicate vials fitted with rubber closures for the purpose of withdrawing accurate doses in a hypodermic syringe. It has been demonstrated that glass is capable of adsorbing measurable amounts of radioactive sodium phosphate. Since such a very small quantity of phosphate is in the solutions for therapeutic and diagnostic use, a slight amount or ordinary carrier sodium phosphate is added. This helps to minimize the loss of radioactive phosphate by adsorption on the glass. As an additional precaution the U.S.P. recommends the use of a sodium hydroxide solution (1 in 1,000) to rinse all containers used to handle Sodium Radiophosphate Injection followed by rinsing with purified water until the rinsings are neutral to litmus.

The vials usually are protected by lead-shielded hermetically sealed cans. This permits laboratory workers to handle the solutions safely without unduly exposing themselves.

Uses. Radiophosphorus as sodium phosphate is reported in the literature to be the agent of choice in the treatment of the blood disease polycythemia vera. It is also useful in the treatment of chronic leukemia.

In a pharmaceutical research problem, labeled phosphorus as phosphate was injected intraperitoneally into rats, which were sacrificed when their teeth became radioactive. The effect of certain mouthwashes, beverages, juices, tap water and distilled water on the phosphorus depletion of the teeth was determined.

Radioactive Chromic (P^{32}) Phosphate

Several methods have been advanced for preparing a suitable suspension of this insoluble salt. In one of the methods, the phosphorus as obtained from Oak Ridge* is added to a phosphoric acid solution; then chromic nitrate solution is added slowly. The chromic phosphate resulting from this reaction is dried in a furnace at about 500° C., cooled to about room temperature and ground in a ball mill for about 1 day. The particle size is thus reduced to 1 micron or less.

During this entire process, great care must be exercised to prevent workers from becoming contaminated with even minute quantities of dust.

The finely divided chromic phosphate

* Oak Ridge, Tenn., is the location of one of the nuclear reactors operated by the Atomic Energy Commission to furnish isotopes for industrial and medical purposes.

then is dispersed as an aqueous colloidal suspension, which may be diluted with saline and gelatin. The autoclaved colloidal particles settle out on standing and should be resuspended prior to removal of the calculated dose.

Use. Radioactive chromic (P^{32}) phosphate suspension has been advocated for the treatment of prostate tumors, for the destruction of tumor masses generally and in the management of myelogenous leukemia. The advantages of chromium phosphate P^{32} over gold colloid therapy are that its beta ray is simpler and safer to handle, and its half-life is more satisfactory.

Radiocobalt^{60}

Cobalt metal and Co_2O_3 are activated by placing them in the nuclear reactor for approximately 28 days. Radioactive cobalt^{60} resulting from this reaction has a half-life of 5.3 years and 2 energetic gamma-ray patterns.

Uses. Radioactive cobalt^{60} metal, because of the high-energy gamma radiation and its moderately long half-life, is being used as a replacement for radium. The cobalt isotope is considerably less expensive and less difficult to produce than radium.

The gamma rays of cobalt^{60} are being investigated very intensively as a potential means of sterilization of drug and food products. Both the food processing industry and the pharmaceutical industry have been searching for a method to destroy micro-organisms without the use of heat, for many of their products are thermolabile. Workers in this field report notable progress to date.

The stability of vitamin B_{12} in a multivitamin mixture has been determined by using cobalt^{60} as the labeling agent. The vitamin B_{12} labeled with cobalt^{60} was prepared by microbial synthesis for use in this study.

Radiocyanocobalamin Solution U.S.P. XVI
(Rdiocyanocobalamin [Co^{60}] Solution)

Radiocyanocobalamin Solution is a solution which contains cobalt^{60} labeled cyanocobalamin in which a portion of the molecules contain radioactive cobalt (Co^{60}) in the molecular structure. The solution as usually marketed contains a bacteriostatic agent and is administered in 0.5 microcurie doses.

This preparation is employed as a diagnostic agent for pernicious anemia.

RADIOCARBON[14]

Radioactive carbon[14] is a pure beta emitter with rays so "soft" that they may be shielded out by a thickness of paper. This low energy diminishes hazards in handling the isotope, since the usual glass vial or bottle will adequately prevent radiation from reaching the exterior.

The calculated half-life for carbon[14] is about 5,600 years, which allows adequate time for any of the biologic or the pharmaceutical research problems.

Uses. In medical therapy and diagnosis, radioactive carbon[14] has been used less than other isotopes, but, in pharmaceutical and related research areas, numerous studies have been conducted.

Attention has been directed to the use of carbon[14] in the synthesis by plants of carbon[14] labeled products such as alkaloids and glycosides. In one study, the glycosides of digitalis were labeled with carbon[14]. In another, the labeled alkaloids of colchicum were prepared and in yet another the active labeled narcotic principles of opium were isolated. A recent publication lists the successful labeling of ergot alkaloids.

A number of compounds of importance in pharmaceutical as well as medical research have been developed which have been C^{14}-labeled. Among these are the silicone fluids, ethylenediaminetetraacetic acids, Pentothal, thiourea and others. Obvious applications in research in many areas readily can be seen for each.

SODIUM RADIOCHROMATE INJECTION
U.S.P. XVI
(STERILE RADIOACTIVE CHROMIUM SOLUTION)
(STERILE SODIUM RADIOCHROMATE (Cr^{51}) SOLUTION)

Sodium Radiochromate Injection is a clear, slightly yellow, solution containing a bacteriostatic agent. The chromium[51] used to prepare the sodium chromate in this preparation is produced by neutron bombardment of chromium[50] and has a half-life of 27.5 days.

Sodium Radiochromate Injection is used to estimate blood volume as a diagnostic aid.

PROCUREMENT OF RADIOACTIVE ISOTOPES

Federal regulations set forth the application procedure for obtaining radioisotopes and limit the procurement, the possession and the use of radioisotopes to those persons validly authorized by the Atomic Energy Commission.

All persons desiring to obtain radioisotopes must first file an "Application for Radioisotope Procurement," Form AEC-313, with Isotopes Division, U.S. Atomic Energy Commission, Oak Ridge, Tenn. A separate form AEC-313 must be completed for each radioisotope and special irradiation service desired. The technical staff of the Isotopes Division reviews the applica-

TABLE 35. SOME ADDITIONAL RADIOACTIVE MATERIALS USED IN PHARMACY AND MEDICINE

NAME	ISOTOPE	USE
Calcium chloride	Calcium[45]	Metabolic studies
Streptomycin	Carbon[14]	Study of drug action
Diodrast	Iodine[131]	Urinary clearance studies
l-Thyroxine, sodium	Iodine[131]	Thyroid function
Rose Bengal	Iodine[131]	Liver function
Tritium oxide	Hydrogen[3]	Total body water
Sodium sulfate	Sulfur[35]	Extracellular space studies
Penthothal	Sulfur[35]	Studies on the metabolic fate of Penthothal
Sucaryl	Sulfur[35]	Biological studies
Iron globulin complex	Iron[59] and Iron[55]	Iron turnover studies
Ferrous sulfate	Iron[59] and Iron[55]	Iron turnover studies
Ferrous citrate	Iron[59] and Iron[55]	Iron turnover studies
Yttrium phosphate	Yttrium[90]	Pleural and peritoneal effusions

tion and the proposed use to decide whether the applicant is equipped to use the requested isotope in a manner which will not endanger health and safety. The experience and the training of the applicant, the facilities, the safety procedures and the equipment as stated in the application are evaluated.

An "Authorization for Radioisotope Procurement," Form AEC-374, is issued to the applicant, and this allows him to purchase, possess and use the radioisotope for which he has applied. Then Form AEC-374 is sent to the supplier or the distributor along with the purchase order for the isotopes named on the form.

DISTRIBUTORS

The supply sources for radioactive isotopes and compounds containing them for medical and pharmaceutical purposes are limited.

The Atomic Energy Commission facilities such as those at Oak Ridge, Tenn., furnish many of the chemically processed isotopes to qualified users. It must be emphasized that these isotopes are not developed pharmaceutically and so they require additional processing.

The AEC now requires that medical users procure materials from a secondary supplier or demonstrate the ability and the facilities to prepare an acceptable pharmaceutical product.

The largest supplier for most of the radioactive pharmaceuticals for medical use is the Abbott Laboratories, Radioactive Isotope Division, Oak Ridge, Tenn. As a manufacturer of these materials, the Abbott facilities have made it possible for even small clinics and hospitals to participate in the medical isotope field without the necessity of establishing elaborate, expensive, processing facilities.

BIBLIOGRAPHY

Glasstone, S.: Sourcebook on Atomic Energy, New York, Van Nostrand, 1950.
Jarvis, A. E., Christian, J. E., Edwards, L. D., and Jenkins, G. L.: A comparative study of the effect of various solutions on the phosphorus depletion of the rat tooth using radioactive phosphorus, J. Am. Pharm. A. (Sci. Ed.) **38**:206, 1949.
Kamen, M. D.: Radioactive Tracers in Biology, New York, Academic Press, 1947.
Lux, R. E., and Christian, J. E.: A study of the effect of certain astringents on the permeability of frog skin using radioactive tracer techniques, J. Am. Pharm. A. (Sci. Ed.) **40**:160, 1951.
Morton, M. E.: Colloidal chromic radiophosphate in high yields for radiotherapy, Nucleonics **10**:92, 1952.
Parke, Davis and Co.: Modern Pharmacy, November, 1948.
Peterson, C. F., Lee, C. O., and Christian, J. E.: A study of an *in vivo* method of testing coatings using radioactive tracer techniques, J. Am. Pharm. A. (Sci. Ed.) **39**:607, 1950.
Quimby, E. H.: Radioactive isotopes as aids in medical diagnosis, New England J. Med. **252**:1, 1955.
Rosenblaum, C., and Woodbury, D. T.: The determination of the stability of vitamin B_{12} in a multivitamin mixture by a radioactive indicator method, J. Am. Pharm. A. (Sci. Ed.) **41**:368, 1952.
Sacks, J.: The Atom at Work, New York, Ronald, 1951.
Skauen, D. M., Cyr, G. N., Christian, J. E., and Lee, C. O.: A study of the absorption of radioactive sodium iodide from a variety of ointment bases, J. Am. Pharm. A. (Sci. Ed.) **38**:618, 1949.
Tabern, D. L., Taylor, J. D., and Gleason, G. I.: Radioisotopes in pharmaceutical and medical studies, Nucleonics **7**:3, 40, 1950; **8**:60, 1951.
Tabern, D. L., and Storey, R. W.: Use of iodine[131] capsules in thyroid-uptake studies, Nucleonics **13**:58, 1955.
Tutin, J.: Atomic Energy Year Book, New York, Prentice-Hall, 1949.
United States Atomic Energy Commission: Radioisotopes—Uses, Hazards, Controls, Oak Ridge, Tenn., 1954.
United States Atomic Energy Commission: Isotopes, A Five-Year Summary of U.S. Distribution, 1951.
United States Atomic Energy Commission: Isotopics, 1954.
United States Department of Commerce, National Bureau of Standards: **Safe** Handling of Radioactive Isotopes, Handbook No. 42, 1949.

Index

Abbreviations, apothecaries'
  weight, Roman origin, 4
  English systems, 3-6
  gram and grain, 3
  metric system, 2-3
  in prescriptions, molded tablets, 446
Absorbable Dusting Powder, 414
Absorbable Gelatin Sponge, 131
Absorption, vs. adsorption, 124
  bases for ointments, 333
  of gases by solid as method of separation, 58
Acacia as emulsifying agent, 291
Acacia Mucilage, 250
Acacia Syrup, 188
A. C. D. Solution, 216
Acetic Larkspur Tincture, 387
Acetone as solvent, in extraction, 156
  for pharmaceutical use, 100
Acetyl Sulfisoxazole Oral Suspension, 266
Acetylene as source of heat, 26
Achromycin Ophthalmic Powder, Sterilized, 220
Acids as base of ointments, 320, 324
Acon Drops, 209
Aconite Tincture, 386-387
Activated charcoal, 125
Adsorbate, 124
Adsorbent, 124
Adsorption, vs. absorption, 124
  chromatographic, separation of components of solutions, 74-75
  of colloidal dispersions, 124-127
  definition, 124
  dependence of surface films on, 127
  in emulsions, films, 134
  formation and stability, emulsifiers, mixed, 135
    solid, 135-136
    theories, oriented wedge, 135
  of gases by solid as method of separation, 58
  of ions on colloidal particles, 125-126
  of liquids, industrial applications, 125
  mechanism, theories, 124
  positive and negative, 124
  selectivity and specificity, 125
Aeration, separation of gas from liquid by, 58
Aerosols, 122-124
  definition, 122
  dispensers, 123

Aerosols (Continued)
  dust explosions, 124
  flocculation devices, 124
  pioneer work of Lister, 123
  preparation methods, 123
  smogs,
  smokes, 123-124
  treatment of respiratory conditions, 123
Agar, 251
Agitator, mechanical, separation of particle sizes of drugs by, 90-91
Alcohol(s), absolute, as solvent for pharmaceutical use, 99
  addition to syrups, 183
  aliphatic, as base of ointments, 320, 322-323
  as base of ointments, 320, 322-323
  cyclic, as base of ointments, 320, 323-324
  dehydrated, as solvent for pharmaceutical use, 99
  denatured, as source of heat, 25
  distillation from wine, 150
  in elixirs, 369-370
  isopropyl, as solvent for pharmaceutical use, 99
  long-chain, as emulsifying agents, 138
  monoatomic, esters of, 320, 324-325
  polyhydric, esters of, 320-321, 325-328
    natural triglycerides, 326
    oils, hydrogenated, 327
      vegetable, 326-327
    Polysorbate 80, 327-328
    synthetic compounds, 325-326
  as solvent, in extraction, 156
    for pharmaceutical use, 99
  specific gravity, legal requirements, 17
  sulfated fatty, in emulsions, 296
  in thermometers, 27
Alcohol-ethers (cellosolves) as base of ointments, 320, 324
Alcoholometer, 18
Alkaline Aromatic Solution, 199
Alkaline Sulfur Ointment, 340
Aloin, Belladonna, Cascara and Podophyllum Pills, 434
Alum, 256
Aluminum Acetate Solution, 209
Aluminum Hydroxide Gel, 113, 125, 271-272
Aluminum oxide, 125

Aluminum Paste, 343
Aluminum Phosphate Gel, 272
Aluminum Subacetate Solution, 209-210
Amaranth Solution, 198
American Chemical Society, standards and tests of purity of drugs, 54-55
American Standard Teaspoon, 5
American Standards Association, 5
Aminoacetic Acid Elixir, 374
Aminophylline, administration by various routes, blood levels, 349
Aminophylline Injection, 229
Aminopyrine, in-vitro release from cocoa butter suppositories, 352
Ammoniacal Silver Nitrate, Howe, 214
Ammoniacal Silver Nitrate Solution, 214
Ammonium Acetate Solution, 222
Amobarbital Elixir, 372
Ampul(s), cleaning before filling, 231
  filling, 230-233
  glass, types, standards for, 230-231
  invention by S. Limousin, 225
  Iodine, 225
  sealing, 233-234
  sizes and styles, 230
Analysis, chromatographic, separation of components of solutions, 74-75
Antacids, recent investigations, 272-273
Antazoline Phosphate Ophthalmic Solution, 217
Antepar Syrup Multifuge, 186-187
Antibiotics, ointments, 339
Anticoagulant Acid Citrate Dextrose Solution, 216
Anticoagulant Sodium Citrate Solution, 216-217
Antifreeze, freezing point, 53
Antihistaminics, elixirs, 374
Antistine Ophthalmic Solution, 217
Aquasol A, 209
Archimedes' principle, 6, 16, 17
Argentamine, 108
Argonin, 108
Aristotle, description of leaching, 150
Arnaldus of Villanova, first reference in European pharmacy to spirit made from wine, 367
Arnica Tincture, 382-383
Aromatic Ammonia Spirit, 368-369
Aromatic Cascara Sagrada, 391

Index

Aromatic Elixir, 370, 371
Aromatic Eriodictyon Syrup, 189-190
Aromatic Rhubarb Tincture, 385-386
Aromatic Yerba Santa Syrup, 189-190
Arsenic trisulfide, colloid particle stabilized by HS− ions, 118
Arsenious Acid Solution, 214
Asafedita Tincture, 387
Ascorbic Acid Injection, 229
Aspidium Oleoresin, 405-406
Association of Official Agricultural Chemists, standards and tests of purity of drugs, 54-55
Atomic Energy Commission, 471-472
Aureomycin Ophthalmic Powder, Sterilized, 220
Aurothioglucose Injection, 229
Autoclave, 235, 236
  in extraction, 157
  for sterilization, 32
Autoclaving, injections, 235-236
  solutions, ophthalmic, 197
Avertin Fluid, 208
Avertin with Amylene Hydrate, 208
Azure A Carbacrylic Resin, 404
Azuresin, 404

Balance(s), 6-9
  analytical, 8, 9
  counter, 9
  hand, 6-7
  Mohr-Westphal, 16-18
  with parallel beams, 6-8
  prescription, torsion, 7-9
    Troemner, 7, 8
  solution, 9
  weights for, 9-11
  Westphal, 16
Balsam, Friar's, 380
  Traumatic, 380
Barbiturates, in elixirs, 372-373
Barton, description of preparation of emulsions (1747), 276-277
Basham's Mixture, 113, 222
Basic Ferric Sulfate Solution, 211
Baths for distribution of heat, 29-32
  constant-temperature, 30-31
  glycerin, 30
  oil, 30
  salt-water, 31
  sand, 29-30
  steam, 31-32
  water, 30
Baumé, Antoine, development of modern hydrometer, 16
  discovery and development of cocoa butter as suppository base, 348

Baumé hydrometer, 18
Bechhold, ultrafiltration of colloidal dispersions, 117
Beckman, origin of Latin word *sapo*, 304
Beef Extract, 398
Belladonna, Extract, 398
  Leaf Fluidextract, 171, 392
  Leaf Tincture, 380
  Root Fluidextract, 392
  Tincture, 380
Benoxinate Hydrochloride Ophthalmic Solution, 217-218
Bentonite, 125
  as emulsifying agent, 298
  Magma, 270-271
Benzalkonium Chloride Solution, 199-200
Benzene, as solvent for pharmaceutical use, 100-101
Benzethonium Chloride Solution, 200
Benzin, purified, as solvent for pharmaceutical use, 100
Benzoate, addition to syrups, 183
Benzoic acid, addition to syrups, 183
Benzoin, discovery of preservative action on lard, 326
  Tincture, 383
Benzyl Benzoate Lotion, 311
Berkefeld filter, 117
Bismuth, Cream, 271
  Glycerite, 256
  Magma, 271
  Milk of, 271
Bitter Almond Water, 181
Bitter Apple Extract, 399
Bitter Orange Peel Tincture, 388
Bitters, elixirs, 373
Bitumen, Sulfonated, 257
Black Draught, 247
Blaud's Pills, 434
Blender, laboratory twin-shell, 409
Blowing, separation of particle sizes of drugs by, 91
Blue Mass, 428-429
Blue Pill, 428-429
Bogardus mill, 83
Boiling point, 39-41
  curves, completely immiscible liquids, 61-63
    partially immiscible liquids, 62, 63
  definition, 39
  determination, 40-41
  and pressure, 39-40
  of solution, 103
  Torricellian tube, 39, 40
  vaporization at and below, 35-36
  variations due to elevations other than sea level, 40
Borax, 256

Boric Acid Solution, 200-201
Boroglycerin Glycerite, 255
Bottle, emulsification by, 285
  graduated percolation, 158
  wide-mouth, use in extraction, 157
Boullays, use of displacement in extraction of drugs, 150
Boulton's Solution, 212
Boutron and Robiquet, account of extraction with ether, 150
Boyle, law of, 56
Brandy, 369
Braun, O., discovery of hydrophilic properties of wool fat, 323
Breddin diacolator, 161
Breddin, H., description of diacolation, 151
Bredic arc method of preparation of colloidal dispersions, 114
British Thermal Unit (B.T.U.), definition, 26
Bromethol, 208
Bromides, in elixirs, 372
  Syrup, 188-189
Brown, Robert, brownian movement of particles, 116
Brownian movement, colloidal dispersions, 116
Bruehl receiver, 46
Bruising, comminution of drugs by, 80
Brunschwygk (Brunschwig, Brunschwyk), Hieronymus, books on distillation, 178
Buchner, J. A., quoted, definition of "liquor," 195
  suggestion for name oleoresin, 405
Buchu Fluidextract, 393
Buffer solutions, 105-106
  preparation, directions in *U.S.P. XVI*, 106
Burets, 13
Burow's Solution, 209
Burton, Henry, cataphoresis apparatus of, 119
Busse, L. W., and T. Higuchi, sterilization of procaine, 236
Butabarbital Sodium Elixir, 372
Butane as source of heat, 26
n-Butyl stearate, as enteric coating for pills and tablets, 448-449

Cacao Syrup, 184-185
Cachets, 425-426
Calamine Lotion, 311
Calciferol Solution, 201
Calcination, 33

Index   475

Calcium, Gluconate Injection, 228, 229
  Hydroxide Solution, 201
    toleration of soaps, 295
Calorie, definition, 26
Cameron, D. H., and H. N. Holmes, preparation of chromatic emulsions, 144
Camphor, Liniment, 309
  and Soap Liniment, 309
  Spirit, 369
  Water, 180, 181
Camphorated Oil, 309
Camphorated Opium Tincture, 382
Camphorated Tincture of Soap, 308
Candy medication, 426
Cantharides, 257
  Cerate, 341
  Tincture, 387
Capillary attraction in extraction of dried drugs, 153
Capryl Alcohol, 131
Capsicum, Oleoresin, 157, 406
  Tincture, 383
Capsules, 416-425
  advantages, 417
  dispensing, 418-420
    choosing correct size and color, 418
    cleaning filled capsules, 419
    filling, 418-420
    packaging, 420
  elastic, 422-423
  hard, 417-418
  official, N.F., 425
    U.S.P., 424-425
  Radioactive Iodine, 467
  Sodium Radio-iodide, 467
  special problems, 420-421
  weight variation test, 421-422
Caramelization of sucrose, 183
Carbohydrates, as emulsifying agents, 138
Carbol-Fuchsin Solution, 201-202
Carbolic Acid Glycerite, 255
Carbolized Iodine Solution, 212
Carbon, disulfide, as solvent for pharmaceutical use, 101
  tetrachloride, as solvent for pharmaceutical use, 100
Carbon[14], 471
Carbonization, 33
Carbowax as ointment base, 334
Carey-Lea, production of concentrated sols of silver, 113
Carfusin, 202
Carnauba wax as enteric coating for pills and tablets, 448-449
Caryl and Ericks, classification of wetting agents, 128, 129
Cascara Sagrada, Extract, 398
  Fluidextract, 392

Castellani's Paint, 201-202
Cataphoresis, apparatus of Burton, 119
  separation of colloids by, 75
Ceepryn Chloride Aqueous Solution, 202
Celsius, Anders, Centigrade scale, 27
  De Medicina, plasters listed in, 343
Centigrade scale, 27-28
  conversion to Fahrenheit, 28
Centrifugation, separation of liquid from solid, 72-73
Centrifuges, 50, 51, 72, 73
Cerates, 340-341
  Cantharides, 341
  unofficial, 341
Cetylpyridinium Chloride Solution, 202
Chalk Mixture, 260, 268
Chalybeate Pills, 434
Charcoal, activated, 125
  adsorptive power, 125
  source of heat, 24
Charles, law of, 56
Chemical reactions as sources of heat, 23
Chemicals, grades for various specifications, 55
Cherry Juice, 193
Cherry Syrup, 185
Chevreul, M. E., studies of chemical constitution of fats, 304
Chloramphenicol, 197
  for Ophthalmic Solution, 220
  Palmitate Oral Suspension, 266
Chloroazodin Solution, 222
Chloroform, Liniment, 308-309
  as solvent, in extraction, 157
  for pharmaceutical use, 100
  Water, 175, 180
Chloromycetin Ophthalmic, 220
Chlorpheniramine Maleate Syrup, 185
Chlorpromazine Hydrochloride Syrup, 185
Chlortetracycline Hydrochloride for Injection, 229
Chlor-Trimetron Maleate Syrup, 185
Cholesterol, as emulsifier, 283, 284
  in Hydrophilic Petrolatum, 324
  in wool fat, discovery of, 316
Chondrus Extract, 398-399
Chondrus Mucilage, 251
Chopping, comminution of drugs by, 80
Chromic phosphate, radioactive, 470
Chromatograph, pharmaceutical uses, 126
Chromatography, in research problems, 126

Chromatography (Continued)
  separation of components of solutions, 74-75
Chrysarobin Ointment, 338
Cinnamon Water, 180
Citric Acid Syrup, 185
Clarification, 78
Clopane Hydrochloride Solution, 202-203
Clorox, 215
Clowes, inversion of phases of an emulsion, 137
Coagulation, definition, 119
Coal, gas, as source of heat, 25
  as source of heat, 24
Coal Tar Ointment, 339
Coal Tar Solution, 202
Coatings, enteric, of capsules, 421
Cobalt[60], 470
Cocoa butter, cooling curves, 355-356
  melting characteristics of meta stable crystalline forms, 352-354
  photomicrographs, 354
  solubility in certain drugs, 355, 356
  substitutes, 356-359
    commercial base ingredients, 356-358
  triglyceride composition, 352
Cod Liver Oil Emulsion with Malt, 290
  with Pectin, 290-291
Coke as source of heat, 24
Colation, separation of liquid from solid by, 69
Colchicum Seed, Fluidextract, 393
  Tincture, 387
Collargol, 108
Collodion(s), 256-257
  flexible, 256
  salicylic, 257
  Styptic, 257
Colloid(s), 108-131
  adsorption, 124-127
  aerosols. See Aerosols
  agents, surface-active, 127-130
    in commercial processing of foods, 130
    dispersions of oil-soluble vitamins A and D, 130
    in ointment bases, 129-130
    in sewage treatment, 130
    as wetting agents, 127-129
      in antiseptics, 129
      classification, 128, 129
      qualifications, 128
  applications in pharmacy, 146
  artificial, 112
  dispersions, preparation, 112-114
    methods, condensation, 113-114

476 Index

Colloid(s), dispersions, preparation, methods (*Continued*)
    Bredig arc method, 114
    changed conditions of solution, 113
    double decomposition reactions, 113-114
    hydrolysis, 113
    oxidation, 113
    reduction, 113
  dispersion, 114
  properties, 114-119
    deviations from solution laws, 117-118
    differences, optical, 114-116
      brownian movement, 116
      electron microscopy, 115-116
      turbidity, 114
      Tyndall effect, 114-115
      ultramicroscopy, 115
    size, 116-117
      dialysis, 116-117
      electrodialysis, 117
      ultracentrifuge, 117
      ultrafiltration, 117
    electric, 118-119
  sol, 112
  systems, 112
  terminology, 112
foams, 130-131
gels, 121-122
history, 108-109
hydrophilic, 263-265
iso-electric point, 120
lyophilic, 120
natural, 112
phase, 109
  disperse or continuous, 111-112
  interface, 112
precipitation, 119-120
protection, 120-121
separation, methods, 75
stability, pH as factor, 120
state, 109-112
  surface, absolute and specific, 110
Sterile Radioactive Gold, 468
Sterile Radiogold (Au^{198}), 468
surface films, dependence on adsorption, 127
system(s), boundaries and overlapping, 110
  corpuscular, 112
  difform, 112
    fibrillar, 112
    laminated, 112
  disperse, classification, 110, 111
  heterogeneous, 109
Colloidal Aluminum Hydroxide, 271-272

Colloidal Silver Iodide, 121
Colocynth Extract, 399
Colophony, 404
Colors, in powders, compounding, 414
Combustion as source of heat, 23-24
Comminution, 79-85
  definition, 79
  extraction, 79-80
  mechanical aids, Mead disintegrator, 83
  mills. *See* Mills
  methods, 80-82
    bruising, 80
    chopping, 80
    contusion, 80
    cutting, 80
    grating, 80
    grinding, 81-82
    levigation, 81
    pulverization by intervention, 80-81
    rasping, 80
    slicing, 80
    trituration, 81
  objects, 79
  rate of solution, 79
  reduction to powder, 80
Compazine Syrup, 187
Compound, Aconite and Iodine Dental Liniment, 310
  Amaranth Solution, 198
  Benzaldehyde Elixir, 370, 372
  Benzoin Tincture, 380
  Calcium Cyclamate Solution, 201
  Cardamon Spirit, 368
  Cardamon Tincture, 383
  Cathartic Pills, 434
  Colocynth Extract, 399
  Cresol Solution, 210
  Digestive Elixir, 373
  Dimethyl Phthalate Solution, 222
  Effervescent Powders, 414-415
  Gentian Tincture, 384-385
  Icthyol Glycerite, 256
  Infusion of Senna, 247
  Iodine Solution, 203-204
  Iodochlorhydroxyquin Powder, 414
  Lavender Tincture, 387-388
  Mild Mercurous Chloride Pills, 434
  Myrcia Spirit, 369
  Orange Spirit, 368
  Pepsin Elixir, 373-374
  Sarsaparilla Syrup, 191
  Senna Powder, 415
  Sodium Borate Solution, 214-215
  Sodium Cyclamate Solution, 207
  Syrup of Hypophosphites, 183
  White Pine Syrup, 192

Compound (*Continued*)
  with Codeine, 192
  Zinc Sulfate Powder, 416
Condensation, preparation of colloidal dispersions by, 113-114
  separation of gases by, 57
Congealing point, 53
Containers, disposable, for parenteral preparations, 231, 232
Contusion, comminution of drugs by, 80
Cortisone Acetate Ophthalmic Suspension, 266
Cosmolin and Paraffin Ointment, of A. W. Miller, 316
Cottrell precipitator, 124
Council on Pharmacy and Chemistry (A.M.A.), use of metric system in publications, 1
Cream(s), 252-254
  Bismuth, 271
  cold, 330-331
  definition, 252-253
  general considerations, 253
  history, 253
  properties and uses, 253-254
  shaving, 254
  Sun, 253
  vanishing, 253, 329-330
Creaming, emulsions, 298-299
Crede, description of Collargol, 108
Crushing, preparation of colloidal dispersions by, 114
Cryoxcide Gas as sterilizing agent, 237
Crystal Violet, 204
Crystallization, fractional, components of mixture of solids, 77
  separation of mixtures of solids, 77-78
  water of, as cause of liquefaction of powders, 413
Curie, definition, 465
Cutting, comminution of drugs by, 80
Cyclaine Hydrochloride Solution, 203
Cyclogyl, 218
Cyclopentamine Hydrochloride Solution, 202-203
Cyclopentolate Hydrochloride Ophthalmic Solution, 218

Dandelion Root Fluidextract, 393
Decantation, separation of liquid from solid by, 68-69
  washing of precipitates by, 88
Decoction(s), 247-248
  extraction by, 165
Deflagration, 33
Deflocculating agents, 263
Deliquescence, 51
Density of substance, 21

Dentiliniments, 310
Deschamps, discovery of preservative action of benzoin on lard, 326
Desiccation, 48-51
  centrifuges, 50, 51
  purposes, facilitation of comminution, 49-50
    preservation, 48-49
    reduction of bulk and weight, 49
    separation of liquid from solid, 73-74
Desiccators, 50, 51, 74
Dew point, 41
Dextran, 117
Dextromethorphan Hydrobromide Syrup, 189
Dextrose, 183
  and Sodium Chloride Injection, 228
Diabetes mellitus, syrups for diet, 192
Diacolation, description by Breddin, 151
Diacolator, Breddin, 161
Diagnex Blue, 404
Dialysis, application to colloids, 116-117
  separation of colloids by, 75
Diaphragms, rubber, cleaning, 231-232
Dicodid Bitartrate, 189
Diehl, contribution to development of percolation, 150
Diethylcarbamazine Citrate Syrup, 185
Digestants, elixirs, 373-374
Digestion, extraction by, 166
Digitalis Infusion, 247
Digitalis Tincture, 383-384
Digitoxin Injection, 229
Dihydrocodeinone Bitartrate Syrup, 189
Dihydroxyaluminum Aminoacetate Magma, 272
Diluted Ammonia Solution, 198
Diluted Lead Subacetate Solution, 222
Diluted Sodium Hypochlorite Solution, 215-216
Dimenhydrinate Syrup, 185-186
Dimethisoquin Hydrochloride Lotion, 312
Dimethyl ketone, as solvent for pharmaceutical use, 100
Dioscorides, use of suppositories advocated by, 348
Diphenhydramine Hydrochloride Elixir, 374
Dish, evaporating, 59
Disintegrator, Mead, 83
Dispersion, colloidal, 92, 109
  definition, 92

Displacement, circulatory, effect on solubility, 93
Distillation, 42-47
  apparatus, 42-44
  destructive, 46-47
  fractional, 45-46
    of immiscible mixtures of liquids, 59-63
    fractionating columns, 63-64
    scrubbers, 63-64
  molecular, of liquids, 65-66
  by reduced pressure, liquids, 65
  reflux, 44-45
  separation of liquids by, 59-66
    falling-film still, 66
    fractional method, 59-63
    fractionating columns, 63-64
    molecular process, 65-66
    reduced pressure, 65
    scrubbers, 63-64
    steam, 64-65
  steam, 43, 44
    liquids, immiscibles, 64-65
  vacuum, 46
  water, 177
    aromatic, 178-179
Distilled Water, 176
Distilled Witch-hazel Extract, 181
Distribution ratio or constant, 154
Dobell's Solution, 214-215
Dorsacaine Hydrochloride Ophthalmic Solution, 218
Dramamine Liquid, 185-186
Dried Aluminum Hydroxide Gel, 272
Drisdol, 201
Drop, as unit of liquid measure, 6
Dry Liver Extract, 399-400
Dublanc, improvement of soft gelatin capsules, 416
Duffield, S. P., description of vacuum maceration and expression for preparation of fluidextracts, 150
Duhammel, Augustine, published first American paper on percolation, 150
Du Nouy tensiometer, 132, 133
Durand, Elias, first American pharmacist to employ percolation for extraction of drugs, 150
Dust explosions, 124

Effervescent Potassium Citrate, 455
Effervescent salts. *See* Salts, effervescent
Effervescent Sodium Phosphate, 455
Efflorescence, 51
Egg oil hand lotion, 297
Egg yolk, as emulsifying agent, 291
  Glycerite, 256
Electricity, as source of heat, 26

Electrodialysis, colloidal dispersions, 117
Electro-endosmosis, separation of colloids by, 75
Electrolysis, separation of components of solutions, 75
Electrolytes, effect on stability of emulsions, 143-144
  precipitation, separation of colloids by, 75
  washing out, preparation of colloidal dispersions by, 114
Electron microscopy, colloidal dispersions, 115-116
Elixir(s), 369-375
  Aminoacetic Acid, 374
  Amobarbital, 372
  Aromatic, 370, 371
  barbiturates in, 372-373
  bromides in, 372
  Butabarbital Sodium Elixir, 372
  classification, medicated, 372-374
    nonmedicated, 370-372
  Compound Benzaldehyde, 370, 372
  Compound Digestive, 373
  Compound Pepsin, 373-374
  definition, 369-370
  Diphenhydramine Hydrochloride, 374
  Ferrous Sulfate, 374
    and Thiamine Hydrochloride, 374-375
  Glycerinated Gentian, 373
  Glycyrrhiza, 370, 372
  history, 370
  Iron, Quinine and Strychnine, 373
    Phosphates, 373
  Iso-Alcoholic, 371-372
  Lactated Pepsin, 373
  medicated, 372-374
    antihistaminics, 374
    digestants, 373-374
    expectorants, 374
    sedatives and hypnotics, 372 373
    stomachics (bitters), 373
  Methypyrlon, 373
  nonmedicated, 370-372
  Pentobarbital, 372
  Red Aromatic, 370, 371
  Secobarbital, 372
  Sodium Bromide, 372
  Terpin Hydrate, 374
    and Codeine, 374
  Thiamine Hydrochloride, 374
  Three Bromides, 372
  Tripelennamine Citrate, 374
  unofficial, 374
  Vitamin B Complex, 374, 375
Elutriation, separation of particle sizes of drugs by, 89

Emulsification, dual, 278
  purpose, 277-279
Emulsion(s), 131-145, 276-301
  administration, external application, 279
    intravenous injection, 278-279
    oral, 278
  agents, 138-140
    classification, 138
    Hydrophile-Lipophile Balance (HLB), 139
  applications in pharmacy, 146
  bases for ointments, 333-334
  chromatic, 144
  Cod Liver Oil, with Malt, 290
    with Pectin, 290-291
  composition, 279-285
    emulsifying agents, 280-285
      antagonistic, 284-285
      classification, 282, 283
      lecithin and cholesterol, 283, 284
      mixed, 282-284
      natural, 282
      properties, 280-281
        hydrophil-lipophil balance, 280-281
      stabilizers or auxiliary, 282, 283
      synthetic, 282
      true or primary, 282
    phase, aqueous, 279
      oil, 279-280
  cracking or de-emulsification, 142-143
    chemical, 143
    physical, 143
  creaming, 142
  definition, 131, 276
  deterioration and preservation, 298-300
    coalescence and breaking, 299-300
    flocculation and creaming, 298-299
    micro-organisms, 300
    physical and chemical changes, 300
  formation and stability, 132-138
    adsorbed films, 134
    electric charges, 137-138
    globule size, 138
    inversion, 137
    "quasi-emulsions," 135-136
    tension, interfacial, 132-133
      measurement, 132, 133
      surface, 132
    theories, 132
      Fischer hydration, 134
    viscosity, 133-134
    volume effect, 136-137
  history, 276-277
  internal use, 277-279
  of liniments, 309

Emulsion(s) (Continued)
  Liquid Petrolatum, 300
    Phenolphthalein in, 300-301
  Mineral Oil, 300
  official, 300-301
  phases, 131
  preparation, 141-142, 285-299
    agitation, by hand, 141
      mechanical, 141
    colloid mills, 142
    devices and machines, 285-287
      bottle, 285
      colloid mill, 286-287
      homogenizers, 286
      mixers, high-speed impeller-type, 285-286
      mortar and pestle, 285
    emulsifying agents, anionic, 293-296
      alcohols, sulfated fatty, 296
      compounds, sulfated, 296
      oils, sulfated, 296
      soaps, 293-295
    auxiliary, for internal use, 293
    cationic, 296
    for externally used products, 293-297
    finely divided solids, 297-298
    for internally used products, 291-293
    natural, 297
    nonionic, 296-297
    sequestering, 295-296
  homogenizers, 142
  large-scale, 141-142
  methods, addition of external to internal phase containing emulsifying agent, 287-288
    addition of internal to external phase containing emulsifying agent, 288-289
    bottle, 277
    dry gum (continental), 277, 287-288
    early, 277
    variations, 290-291
    wet gum (English, American), 277, 288-289
  mixing and stirring equipment, 142
  preservatives in, Rdzok method of testing efficiency of, 279
  stability, effect of electrolytes on, 143-144
  stabilizers, 139
  sterile, parenteral preparations, 224
  Sterile Phytonadione, 301
  transparent, 144

Emulsion(s) (Continued)
  types, 132, 140
Energy, heat as form of, 22
  kinetic, of molecules, 56
Engelmann, pioneer work in colloids, 109
English systems of weights and measures, 3-6
  apothecaries, 4-5
    fluid measure, 4
    weight, 5
  drop, 6
  equivalents of metric system, 5
  historical background, 3-4
  household, 5-6
  imperial, 4
  lack of uniformity and integration, 4
  length, 4
  troy, 3-4
  volume, 4-6
  weight, 3-5
dl-Ephedrine Hydrochloride Solution, 206
Epinephrine, Bitartrate Ophthalmic Solution, 218
  Sulfate Jelly, 251, 273-274
  Sulfate Solution, 203
  Sulfate Syrup, 189
Epinephrine, addition to local anesthetic drugs, 228
  Inhalation, 313
  Solution, 197, 221
  Solution 1:1,000, 221
Ergot Fluidextract, 151, 156, 392-393
Ericks and Caryl, classification of wetting agents, 128, 129
Erlenmeyer flask, use in extraction, 157
Erydictyon Fluidextract, 393
Erythromycin Oral Suspension, 266
Esters, of alcohols, monoatomic, 320, 324-325
  polyhydric, 320-321, 325-328
    natural triglycerides, 326
    oils, hydrogenated, 327
      vegetable, 326-327
    Polysorbate, 80, 327-328
    synthetic compounds, 325-326
  as base of ointments, 320-321, 324-328
Ether, pioneer use in extraction, 150
  as solvent, 100
  in extraction, 156
Ethereal Tinctures, 388
Ethyl Nitrite Spirit, 369
Ethyl oxide, as solvent for pharmaceutical use, 100
Ethylenediamine Solution, 203

Ethylene-glycol-water mixtures, freezing points, 53
Eucalyptus Gum, Troches of, 436
Eucerin, introduction as base for ointments, 316, 323
Evacolation, description by Kessler, 151
Evaporation, 37-38
concentration of solutions by, 37
definition, 37
dish, 59
hastening, 37
hoods for removal of undesirable vapors, fumes and odors, 37-38
pans, 31-32
separation, of gas from liquid by, 58
of liquids by, 59
spontaneous, 37
under reduced pressure, of immiscible mixtures of liquids, 59
Expectorants, elixirs, 374
Exsiccation, 50-51, 74
Extract(s), 395-401
Beef, 398
Belladonna, 398
Bitter Apple, 399
Cascara Sagrada, 398
Chondrus, 398-399
Colocynth, 399
Compound Colocynth, 399
Distilled Witch-hazel, 181
Dry Liver, 399-400
Glycyrrhiza, 399
Goulard's, 222
history, 395-396
Hyoscyamus. *See* Belladonna Extract
Irish Moss, 398-399
Licorice Root, 399
Liquid Liver, 221
Liver, 399-400
Malt, 400
N.F., 398-401
nonofficial, 401
Nux Vomica, 400
Opium, 401
Ox Bile, 400-401
pilular, in powders, compounding, 413
Powdered Cascara Sagrada, 398
Powdered Nux Vomica, 400
Powdered Opium, 401
Powdered Ox Bile Extract, 400-401
Powdered Rhubarb, 401
preparation, 396-397
Pure Glycyrrhiza, 397-398
Pure Licorice Root, 397-398
Rhamnus Purshiana, 398
Rhubarb, 401

Extract(s) *(Continued)*
Rice Bran, 401
Rice Polishings, 401
Stramonium. *See* Belladonna Extract
Tikitiki, 401
U.S.P., 397-398
Extraction, 149-171
apparatus, 157-163
autoclave, 157
bottle, 157, 158
flask, Erlenmeyer, 157
improvised, 162-163
infusion pot, 157
kettle with jacket, 158
Lloyd, 163
percolators. *See* Percolators
Soxhlet, 162-163, 171
tank, maceration, 158
in comminution, 79-80
conversion of solid to liquid phase, 77
definition, 149
dried drugs, capillary attraction, 153
force of gravity, 153
osmosis, 152
theory of, 152-154
history of process, 149-151
methods, 163-171
decoction, 165
digestion, 166
infusion, 165-166
maceration, 163-165
theory of, 153, 154
percolation. *See* Percolation
pressure, development by Husa, 151
purposes, 151
recovery of menstrua, 171
solvents as agents, 155-157
acetone, 156-157
alcohol, 156
chloroform, 157
ether, 156
glycerin, 156
hexane, solvent, 156
hydroalcoholic menstrua, 156
immiscible, 171
water, 155-156
substances from liquors, theory of, 154-155
theory, 151-155
Extractive, definition, 149

Fahrenheit, Gabriel Daniel, temperature scale, 27
Fahrenheit scale, 27, 28
conversion to Centigrade, 28
Faraday, Michael, sensitivity of colloidal dispersions to impurities, 119
Farina, J. Maria, introduction of eau de cologne, 368

Fathergill, John, investigations of emulsions, 277
Fermentation, clarification of solution by, 78
Ferric Ammonium Citrate, 121
Ferric Chloride Solution, 210-211
Ferric Chloride Tincture, 384
Ferric Citrochloride Tincture, 384
Ferric Subsulfate Solution, 211
Ferrous Carbonate Mass, 429
Ferrous Carbonate Pills, 434
Ferrous Iodide Syrup, 190
Ferrous Sulfate Elixir, 374
Ferrous Sulfate Syrup, 190
Ferrous Sulfate and Thiamine Hydrochloride Elixir, 374-375
Ferruginous Pills, 434
Figuier, studies in adsorptive power of carbon, 124
Filter(s), Berkefeld, 117
retentive, pyrogen and bacterial, 178
Filtration, continuous, 71-72
hot, 72
injections, 227
pressure, 72
separation of liquid from solid by, 69-72
sterilization by, 238-240
suction, 72
Firm Zinc Glycerogelatin, 254
Fischer hydration theory of formation of emulsions, 134
Fitzpatrick mills, 84
Flask(s), distilling, 59
Erlenmeyer, use in extraction, 157
filter, 72
suction, 72
volumetric, 11, 13
Flavors, in powders, compounding, 414
Flaxseed, 250, 251
Flocculation, of aerosols, devices, 124
definition, 119
emulsions, 298-299
Fluid, Sabouraud Medium, 240
Thioglycollate Medium, 240
Fluidextract(s), 388-394
Aromatic Cascara Sagrada, 391
Belladonna Leaf, 392
Belladonna Root, 392
Buchu, 393
Cascara Sagrada, 392
Colchicum Seed, 393
Dandelion Root, 393
Ergot, 392-393
Eriodictyon, 393
Gentian, 393
Ginger, 394
Glycyrrhiza, 392
Goldenseal, 394
Grindelia, 394

Fluidextract(s) (*Continued*)
  history, 389
  Hydrastis, 394
  Ipecac, 392
  Licorice Root, 392
  N.F., 392-393
  nonofficial, 393-394
  Nux Vomica, 393
  preparation, 389-391
  Rhubarb, 393
  Sarsaparilla, 393
  of Seneca Snakeroot, 394
  Senega, 394
  Senna, 393
  Squill, 394
  Taraxacum, 393
  U.S.P., 391-392
  Wild Cherry, 394
  Yerba Santa, 393
Fluidglycerates, 394-395
Fluorescein Sodium Ophthalmic Solution, 218
Foams, 130-131
Forbes, introduction of bottle method of preparing emulsions, 277
Formaldehyde Solution, 211-212
Formalin, 211
Formol, 211
Fowler's Solution, 214
Freezing, conversion of liquid to solid by, 66-67
Freezing point, 53
  determination, 53
  ethylene-glycol-water mixtures, 53
  of solution, 103
French, investigations of emulsions, 277
Fresh Drug Tinctures, 388
Freundlich, terminology for gels, 121
Friar's Balsam, 380
Friction, as source of heat, 22-23
Fuels as sources of heat, gas, 25-26
  liquid, 24-25
  solid, 24
  values, 26
Fuller's Pharmacopoeia, emulsions in, 276
Funnel, separatory, 58
Furazolidone and Nifuroxime Powder, 415
Furnace, muffle, 34
Fusion, 34
  latent heat of, 57

Galen, first description of soap suppository, 348
Galenos, Claudius, formula for an ointment, 315-316
Gallon, imperial, defined, 4
  wine, 4

Gantrisin Ophthalmic Solution, 219
Garbling, separation of particle sizes of drugs by, 89
Gas(es), Cryoxcide, as sterilizing agent, 237
  fuel, as source of heat, 25-26
  in liquids, solutions, 98-99
  pressure by, on sides of container, 56
  separation, 57-58
    from liquid, 58
    methods, absorption by solid, 58
      adsorption by solid, 58
      condensation, 57
      solution, 57-58
  as state of matter, 56
  thermometers, 29
Gasoline as source of heat, 25
Geiger, P. I., definition of "liquor," 195
Gel(s), 121-122, 269-273
  Aluminum Hydroxide, 271-272
    Dried, 272
  Aluminum Phosphate, 272
  classification, 121-122, 269
  definition, 121, 269
  elastic and inelastic, 121-122
  heat-reversible and heat-irreversible, 121
  inorganic, 270-272
  official, 270-272
  organic, 273-274
  silica, 332
  structure, 122, 270
  thixotropic, 271
Gelatin, as emulsifying agent, 291-293
  glycerinated, as base for suppositories, 359-360
Gelatin Solution, Special Intravenous, 117
Gentian Fluidextract, 393
Gentian Violet, 204
Gerding, P. W., and G. J. Sperandio, studies of suspending agents, 145
Gershenfeld, Louis, classification of wetting agents, 128
Ginger, Fluidextract, 394
  Oleoresin, 157, 406
Glassware, sterilization, 237, 238
Glauber, 195
Globules, manufacturing methods, 423-424
Glycerin, 256
  addition to syrups, 183
  anhydrous, 256
  baths for distribution of heat, 30
  in elixirs, 370
  as solvent, 99-100, 156

Glycerin (*Continued*)
  and starch as ointment base, first use, by Schacht, 316
Glycerinated Gentian Elixir, 373
Glycerite(s), 255-256
  Bismuth, 256
  Boroglycerin, 255
  Carbolic Acid, 255
  Compound Icthyol, 256
  Egg Yolk, 256
  of Hydrogen Peroxide, 256
  Iodine and Zinc Iodide, 255
  Magnesium Sulfate, 256
  Pepsin, 256
  Phenol, 255
  Starch, 255
  Tannic Acid, 255
  Tragacanth, 255
Glycerogelatin(s), 254-255
  Firm Zinc, 254
Glycerol, as solvent for pharmaceutical use, 99-100
Glycols, polyethylene, as substitute bases for cocoa butter in suppositories, 358
Glycyrrhiza, Elixir, 370, 372
  Extract, 399
  Fluidextract, 168, 392
  Syrup, 186
"Gold Number" as measure of protective power of colloidal dispersions, 121
Gold[198], 468
Goldenseal Fluidextract, 394
Goulard's Extract, 222
Graduates, conical, 11-12
  cylindrical, 12
  legal requirements, 12-13
  pharmaceutical, 12
Graham, Thomas, application of dialysis to colloids, 116
  as father of colloidal chemistry, 108
  syneresis, 122
Grahame, Israel, G., pioneer work in pharmacy, 150
Gram, definition, 2-3
  as unit of weight in metric system, 2
Granulation, 89
Grating, comminution of drugs by, 80
Gravity, force of, in extraction of dried drugs, 153
  specific. See Specific gravity
Green Soap, 306-307
Grew, emulsions for medicinal use first prepared by, 276
Grindelia Fluidextract, 394
Grinding, comminution of drugs by, 81-82
  preparation of colloidal dispersions by, 114
Guaiac, 256

Index 481

Guillemond, superiority of displacement over maceration, 150
Gum, karaya, 251
 sterculia, 251

Hagen, studies in adsorptive power of carbon, 124
Hager, Herman, stearic acid in preparation of ointments, 316
Hammamelis Water, 175, 179-181
Hard Soap, 307
Hartman, cholesterol and oxycholesterol in wool fat, 323
Hatschek, effect of electrolytes on emulsions, 145
 inversion of phases of an emulsion, 137
Heat, 22-47
 applications in pharmacy, 22, 32-33
  chemical changes involved, inorganic materials, 33
   organic materials, 33-34
  physical changes involved, evaporation, 37-38
   fusion, 34
   vapor pressure, 38-39
   vaporization. See Vaporization
 boiling point, 39-41
 distillation. See Distillation
 exsiccation, 50-51
 as form of energy, 22
 humidity. See Humidity
 measurement, 26-29
  qualitative, 26
  quantitative, 26-29
   pyrometers, 29
   thermometers. See Thermometers
 melting point, 41
 regulation and distribution, 29-32
  methods, 29-32
   autoclave, 32
   baths, constant-temperature, 30-31
    glycerin, 30
    oil, 30
    salt-water, 31
    sand, 29-30
    steam, 31-32
    water, 30
   coil, steam, 32
   evaporating pan, 32
   necessity for, 29
 sources, chemical reactions, 30
  combustion, 23-24
  electricity, 26
  fuels, gas, 25-26
   liquid, 24-25
   solid, 24
   values, 26

Heat, sources (Continued)
  physical, friction, 22-23
  theories, 22
Heating, liquids, effect on solubility, 93
Helmholtz, Hermann, double-layer concept for arrangement of electric charges of colloids, 118
Henry, law of, 60
Herbs, extraction of active constituents, 149
Hetrazan Syrup, 185
Hexachlorophene Liquid Soap, 307-308
Hexane, solvent, use in extraction, 156
Hexylcaine Hydrochloride Solution, 203
Hexylresorcinol Pills, 434
Higuchi, T., and L. W. Busse, sterilization of procaine, 236
Hinkle's Pills, 434
Hippocrates, indications for suppositories and enemas, 348
 record of use of acacia, 250
History of the National Formulary, 370
Hofmeister or lyotropic series of ions, 122
Holmes, H. N., and D. H. Cameron, preparation of chromatic emulsions, 144
Homogenizers, 142, 286
Household measures, 5-6
Humidity, 41-43
 absolute, 41
 dew point, 41
 hygrometers, 41-42
 psychrometers, 41-42
 relative, 41
Hunter, Charles, popularization of hypodermic syringe, 225
Husa, W. J., development of pressure method of extraction, 151
 study of emulsifying agents, 139
Huyck, C. L., and M. Woo, formulas for nonnutritive "syrups," 192
Hyclorite, 215
Hycodan, 189
Hydrastis Fluidextract, 394
Hydriodic Acid Syrup, 190-191
Hydrocarbons, as base of ointments, 320, 322
Hydrogen, Dioxide Solution, 212
 Peroxide Solution, 212
Hydrolysis, of salts of weak bases or weak acids, preparation of colloidal dispersions by, 113
 of sucrose, 182-183
Hydrometer, Baumé, 18

Hydrometer (Continued)
 determination of specific gravity of liquids, 17-18
 historical developments, 16
 Twaddle, 18
Hydrophilic Ointment, 338-339
Hydrophilic Petrolatum, 324
Hydrosols, oil, 280
Hygrometers, 41-42
Hygroscopic drugs, as cause of liquefaction of drugs, 413
Hyoscyamus, Extract. See Belladonna Extract
 Tincture. See Belladonna Tincture
Hypnotics, elixirs, 372-373

Ichthammol Ointment, 339-340
Ignition, 33
Imferon, 121
Incineration, 33-34
Infusion(s), 245-247
 Compound, of Senna, 247
 concentrated, 247
 Digitalis, 247
 extraction by, 165-166
 history, 245
 nonofficial, 247
 preparation, 245-247
 of Senna with Magnesium Sulfate, 247
Inhalant, Prophylhexedrine, 313-314
Inhalation, Epinephrine, 313
 Isoproterenol Hydrochloride, 313
Injection(s), Aminophylline, 229
 Ascorbic Acid, 229
 Aurothioglucose, 229
 Calcium Gluconate, 228, 229
 Chlortetracycline Hydrochloride for, 229
 Dextrose and Sodium Chloride, 228
 Digitoxin, 229
 Lidocaine Hydrochloride, 229
 Mercurophylline, 229
 Methylglucamine Diatrizoate, 229
 nonaqueous, sterilization, 238
 official, miscellaneous products, N.F., 243
  U.S.P., 243
  N.F., 243
  U.S.P., 241-242
 parenteral preparations, 224
 Picrotoxin, 229
 preparation, 227-241
  added substances, 228, 229
  filling of ampuls and vials, 230-233
   mechanical devices, 223-225
  filtration of solution, 227
  labeling, 241

Injection(s), preparation (*Cont.*)
    oils as vehicles, 230
    preservative agents, 228
    sealing ampuls, 233-234
    solvents, 227
    stabilizing agents, 228-230
    sterilization, 230, 234-238, 240
    stock solutions, 227
    testing of sterility, 240-241
    water-soluble materials, 228
  previous classification as sterile solutions for parenteral administration, 197
  Quinidine Gluconate, 229
  Repository Corticotropin, 229
  Reserpine, 229
  Ringer's, 227, 228
    Lactated, 228
  Sodium Acetrizoate, 228, 229
  Sodium Chloride, 227, 228
  Sodium Psylliate, 229
  Sodium Radiochromate, 471
  Sodium Radiophosphate, 469-470
Insulins, labeling, color code, 241
International Prototype Kilogram, 3
International Prototype Meter, 2
Iodine, Ampuls, 225
  Iodoform and Croton Oil, 257
  Ointment, 340
  Solution, 203
  Tincture, 380-381
    and Zinc Iodide Glycerite, 255
Iodine[131], 466-468
Ion(s), effect, common, separation of components of solutions, 74
  exchange, purification by, 75
  Hofmeister or lyotropic series, 122
Ipecac, Fluidextract, 169, 392
  and Opium Powder, 415
  Syrup, 186
Ipomea Resin, 403
Iron, and Ammonium Acetate Solution, 113, 222
  Perchloride Solution, 210-211
  Quinine and Strychnine, Elixir, 373
    Phosphate, 256
    Phosphates Elixir, 373
  Tincture, 384
Irish Moss Extract, 398-399
Iso-Alcoholic Elixir, 371-372
Isocholesterol, discovery in wool fat, 316, 323
Iso-electric point, colloids, 120
Isoflurophate Ophthalmic Solution, 218-219
Isoproterenol Hydrochloride Inhalation, 313
Isotopes, fundamental concepts, 463-464

Isotopes (*Continued*)
  radioactive, methods of manufacture, 464-465
    cyclotron, 464-465
    nuclear reactor, 465

Jalap Resin, 403-404
Jar, canning, use in extraction, 157
Jelly(ies), 269-270, 273-274
  definition, 121
  Ephedrine Sulfate, 251, 273-274
  and gelatinous precipitates, 270
  official, and recent investigations, 273-274
  Pramoxine Hydrochloride, 274
Jesuit's Drops, 380
Juice(s), 193
  Cherry, 193
  Raspberry, 193
  U.S.P. XVI, 193

Kaolin, Cataplasm, 345
  mixture with Pectin, 260, 268-269
Kelvin scale, 28
Kerosene (coal oil) as source of heat, 25
Kessler, description of mulcolation and evacolation, 151
Kettle with jacket, use in extraction, 158
Kilogram, International Prototype, 3
King, A., effect of electrolytes on emulsions, 145
  stabilization of o/w emulsions, 139
Konseals, 425-426

Labarraque's Solution, 215
Lactated Pepsin Elixir, 373
Lactated Ringer's Injection, 228
Lactometer, 18
Lanette Wax, 140
Langmuir theory, 127
Lanolin, origin of term and rediscovery of therapeutic value, 316, 323
Larkspur Tincture, 387
Laudanum, Deodorized Opium Tincture, 381-382
Law(s), of Boyle, 56
  of Charles, 56
  of Henry, 60
  of Nernst, 154
  of Raoult, 101-102
  solutions, deviations from, 117-118
  of Stokes, 145
Lead Subacetate Solution, 222
Lead Water, 222
Lecithin as emulsifying agent, 283, 284

Lémery, Nicolas, *Pharmacopée Universelle*, 150
Lemon Peel Tincture, 381
Lemon Syrup, 185
Lemon Tincture, 381
Le Mort, introduction of paregoric, 382
Length, ancient measures, 4
  English measures, 4
  metric system, 2
  redefinition by English-speaking nations, 5
Levigation, comminution of drugs by, 81
Licorice, 399
  Root, Extract, 399
    Fluidextract, 392
  Syrup, 186
Lidocaine Hydrochloride Injection, 229
Liebreich, Oscar, rediscovery of therapeutic value of wool fat, renamed "lanolin," 316, 323
Liesegang rings, 122
Lifschuetz, discovery of isocholesterol and oxycholesterol in wool fat, 316, 323
Lime Water, 201
Limousin, S., invention of ampul, 225
Liniment(s), 308-310
  Camphor, 309
  and Soap, 309
  Chloroform, 308-309
  classification, 308-309
  Compound Aconite and Iodine Dental, 310
  definition, 308
  emulsions and suspensions, 309
  history, 308
  Medicinal Soft Soap, 309
  Soft Soap, 309
  solutions, alcoholic, 308-309
  oily, 309
Lipomul, 229
Liquid(s), boiling point, 57
  in capsules, dispensing, 421
  at equilibrium with its vapor, 57
  in liquids, solutions, 98
  Liver Extract, 221
  mixtures, binary, types, 60
    miscible, completely, vapor tension, and pressure, changes at constant temperature, 60-61
    types of behavior, 60-61
Opodeldoc, 308
Parazine, 186-187
Petrolatum Emulsion, 300
  in powders, compounding, 413
  separation, 58-68
    colloidal suspensions, 75

Liquid(s), separation (Continued)
 of gas from, 58
 mixtures, immiscible, 58-59
  soluble, 59-68
   conversion to gaseous phase, 59-66
    distillation, 59-66
    evaporation, 59
   conversion to immiscible liquid, 67-68
    by extraction, 67-68
    by salting-out, 68
   conversion to solid, 66-67
    by chemical reaction, 67
    by lowering temperature, 66-67
  solid from liquid, 68-75
   components of solutions, 74-75
   mixtures, insoluble, 68-73
    centrifugation, 72-73
    colation, 69
    decantation, 68-69
    filtration, 69-72
    siphoning, 69
   soluble, 73-74
    conversion to vapor, 73-74
 settling of particles, facilitation of, 78
 soluble, distribution or partition coefficient, 67
 specific gravity, determination methods, 17-19
  hydrometer, 17-18
  Mohr-Westphal balance, 17, 18
  pycnometer or specific gravity bottle, 18-19
  Sprengel tube, 19
 as state of matter, 56-57
 sterility test, 177, 178
 vapor pressure of, 57
 vapor tension of, 56-57
Liquor(s), definitions, 195-196
 origin of pharmaceutical use, 195
 See also Solutions
Liquores, early classification, U.S.P. (1860), 195
Lister, Joseph, sterilization of air in operating room with antiseptic materials, 123
Liter, definition, 2
Liver, Extract, 399-400
 Solution, 197, 221
Lloyd, extractor, 163
 reagent of, 126
Lloyd, John Uri, contribution to development of percolation, 150
 discovery of adsorptive power of a hydrous aluminum

Lloyd, John Uri (Continued)
 silicate for alkaloids, 126
 Elixirs, formulas, 370
Lobella Tincture, 388
Lotion(s), 310-312
 bases, 254
 Benzyl Benzoate, 311
 Calamine, 311
  Phenolated, 311-312
 Dimethisoquin Hydrochloride, 312
 hand, egg oil, 297
 medicated, 254
 Monobenzone, 312
 Vleminckx', 212-213
 White, 312
Lowitz, studies in adsorptive power of carbon, 124
Luer, improvement of hypodermic syringe, 225
Lugol's Solution, 203-204
Lullus, Raimundus, 150
Lyophilization, 47-48

Macerate liquid or solution, definition, 149
Maceration, apparatus, 163, 164
 definition, 163
 extraction by, 163-165
 of infusions, 246
 as period in percolation, 168
 process, 163-165
 tank, 158
 theory of, 153, 154
 vacuum, description of process by S. P. Duffield, 150
Magma(s), 269-272
 Bentonite, 270-271
 Bismuth, 271
 Dihydroxyaluminum Aminoacetate, 272
 Magnesia, 271
 official, 270-272
Magnesia, Magma, 271
 Milk of, 271
Magnesium, Citrate Solution, 213-214
 Sulfate Glycerite, 256
Malt Extract, 400
 as emulsifying agent, 293
Manometer for vacuum distillation, 46
Marc, definition, 149
Martial, first use of word sapo, 304
Mass(es), 428-429
 Blue, 428-429
 in capsules, 420
 Ferrous Carbonate, 429
 Mercury, 428-429
 Vallet's, 429
Mastic, 404
Matter, phase, definition, 55

Matter (Continued)
 states, 55-57
  gaseous, 56
  liquid, 56-57
  solid, 57
 systems, 55-56
Mead disintegrator, 83
Medicinal Soft Soap, 306-307
 Liniment, 309
Medicine droppers, 13-14
Melting point, 41
Menstruum(a), definition, 149
 hydroalcoholic, as solvent in extraction, 156
 recovery after percolation, 161
Mephyton, 229
Merbromin Solution, 204
Mercurochrome, 204
Mercurophylline Injection, 229
Mercury, Mass, 428-429
 Oleate, 313
 in thermometers, 27
Merthiolate Solution, 208
Mesue, Jr., origin of cold cream, 316
Metaphen, 205
Meter, International Prototype, 2
 as primary unit of length, 2
Methenamine as source of heat, 24
Methyl Violet, 204
Methylcellulose, 251-252
Methylglucamine Diatrizoate Injection, 229
Methylrosaniline Chloride Solution, 204
Methyprylon Elixir, 373
Metric system, 1-3
Metrology, 1-14
 definition, 1
 English systems. See English systems of weights and measures
 metric system, 1-3
Micelle, 130, 260
Microgram, definition and abbreviations, 3
Micro-organisms, deterioration of emulsifying agents by, 300
Mild Naphazoline Hydrochloride Solution, 204-205
Mild Silver Protein, 113, 121
Milk, of Bismuth, 271
 of Magnesia, 271
Mill(s), ball, 82
 Bogardus, 83
 Burrstone, 82
 chaser, 82
 colloid, 114, 142
  for emulsification, 286-287
 in comminution of drugs, 82-85
 Fitzpatrick, 84
 hand, 84-85
 high-speed, separation of particle sizes of drugs by, 89

Mill(s) *(Continued)*
  ointment, 336
  roller, 82
  Wiley, 83
Miller, A. W., "Cosmolin and Paraffin Ointment" (petrolatum), 316
Milliliter, 2
Millipore filters, 238, 240
Mineral Oil Emulsion, 300
Mixers, high-speed impeller-type, for emulsification, 285-286
Mixture(s), 259-262
  Basham's, 222
  Chalk, 260, 268
  eutectic, in capsules, 420-421
    as cause of liquefaction of powders, 413
  explosive, as problem in compounding powders, 413-414
  Kaolin, with Pectin, 260, 268-269
  official, 260, 261
  solubilizing agents, 260-262
Modified Dakin's Solution, 215-216
Mohr, Carl Friedrich, development of balance, 16
  Lehrbuch der Pharmazeutischen Technik, early method of preparing emulsions, 277
Mohr-Westphal balance, 16-18
Mold, suppository, 364
Molecules, characteristics, 56
  kinetic energy, 56
Monobenzone Lotion, 312
Monsel's Solution, 211
Mortar and pestle, emulsification by, 285
  in manufacture of pills, 431
  in preparation of ointments, 335-336
Mothes, inventor of soft gelatin capsules, 416
Mucilage(s), 249-252
  Acacia, 250
  Chondrus, 251
  definition, 249
  general considerations, 250
  history, 250
  properties and uses, 252
  Tragacanth, 250, 251
Muffle furnace, 34
Mulcolation, description by Kessler, 151
Münzel, K., emulsifying agents for preparations for internal administration, 139
Murdock, patenting of 2-piece hard gelatin capsule, 416
Mustard Plaster, 345
Myrrh Tincture, 385

Naphazoline Hydrochloride Solution, 204-205
National Bureau of Standards, recognition of household measures, 5-6
  specifications, balances, 9
  graduates for measuring liquids, 12-13
National Formulary (N.F.), method of expressing solubility, 95
Neisser, introduction of Protargol, 109
Neo-Synephrine Hydrochloride Solution, 206
Nernst, law of, 154
New York and Brooklyn Formulary, 370
Newton, Isaac, proposed temperature scale, 27
N.F. Antiseptic Solution, 199
N.F. Dentifrice, 416
N.F. Tooth Powder, 416
Nitrofurantoin Oral Suspension, 266
Nitrofurazone Solution, 205
Nitromersol, Solution, 205
  Tincture, 385
Nomenclature in pharmacy and colloid science, 259
Novobiocin Calcium Oral Suspension, 266
Nux Vomica, Extract, 400
  Fluidextract, 393
  Tincture, 385
Nystatin for Oral Suspension, 266

Ohmart, L. M., and M. J. Stoklosa, base for medicated lotions, 254
  use of Tween 20 as solubilizing agent, 261
Oil(s), baths for distribution of heat, 30
  Camphorated, 309
  essential, in powders, compounding, 413
  hydrogenated, as ointment bases, 327
  hydrosols, 280
  as source of heat, 24-25
  sulfated, in emulsions, 296
  sulfonated and sulfated, as emulsifying agents, 138
  theobroma. *See* Cocoa butter
  vegetable, as ointment bases, 326-327
  as vehicles for parenteral preparations, 230
Oil-sugars, 426
Ointment(s), 315-340
  Alkaline Sulfur, 340
  antibiotic, 339
  application, 317

Ointment(s) *(Continued)*
  bases, 317-334
    absorption, 333
    acids, 320, 324
    alcohol-ethers (cellosolves), 320, 324
    alcohols, 320, 322-324
      aliphatic, 320, 322-323
      cyclic, 320, 323-324
    chemicophysical properties, 320
    emulsion, 333-334
    esters, 320-321, 324-328
      of alcohols, monoatomic, 320, 324-325
        polyhydric, 320-321, 325-328
        hydrogenated oils, 327
        natural triglycerides, 326
        polysorbate 80, 327-328
        synthetic compounds, 325-326
        vegetable oils, 326-327
    hydrocarbons, 320-322
    soaps, 321, 328-330
      creams, cold, 330-331
        vanishing, 329-330
      silicon derivatives, 331-333
      water-soluble, 334
  Chrysarobin, 338
  classification, 317-334
    bases. *See* Ointments, bases
  Coal Tar, 339
  Cosmolin and Paraffin of A. W. Miller, 316
  definition, 315, 316
  demulcents, 317
  diadermic, 318
  emollients, 317
  endodermic, 318
  epidermic, 318
  history, 315-317
  Hydrophilic, 338-339
  Ichthammol, 339-340
  Iodine, 340
  N.F., 338
  packaging, storage and labeling, 336-338
  Penicillin, 339
  preparation, 335-336
    mill, 336
    mortar and pestle, 335-336
    slab and muller, 335
  Stainless Iodine, 340
  Stronger Mercurial, 339
  Sun Tan, 253
  Tannic Acid, 339
  U.S.P., 337
  of Wool Alcohols, 324
Oldberg, contribution to development of percolation, 150
  percolator, 159
Oleate(s), 312-313

Index   485

Oleate(s) (*Continued*)
  Mercury, 313
Oleoresin(s), 404-406
  Aspidium, 405-406
  Capsicum, 406
  Ginger, 406
  history, 405
  N.F. galenical, 405
Ophthalmic Chlortetracycline Hydrochloride, 197, 220
Ophthalmic Oxytetracycline Hydrochloride, 197, 220
Opium, Extract, 401
  Tincture, 381-382
Oral Oxytetracycline for Suspension, 266-267
Orange Flower Water, 175, 179
Orange Syrup, 186
Osmosis, 102-103
  in extraction of dried drugs, 152
Ostwald, Wolfgang, boundaries of colloid systems, 110
  classification of disperse systems of colloids, 110, 111
  pioneer work in colloids, 108
Ox Bile Extract, 400-401
Oxidation, preparation of colloidal dispersions by, 113
Oxycholesterol, discovery in wool fat, 316, 323

Pala as Indian unit of weight, 3
Paracelsus, 150
Paramethadione Solution, 205
Para-nitrosulfathiazole Suspension, 267
Parazine Liquid, 186-187
Paregoric, 382
Parenteral preparations (parenterals), 224-243
  advantages and uses, 225-226
  definition, 224
  forms, 224
  general considerations, 226-227
  historical, 224-225
  injections. *See* Injections
  official, N.F., 243
    U.S.P., 241-243
  pyrogens in, 225
  undesirable reactions, 225
Parrish, contribution to development of percolation, 150
Parsons and Wilson, inversion of phases of an emulsion, 137
Particle sizes of drugs, change, accompanied by change in color, 111
  magnification, highest obtainable under ordinary microscope, 110
  powders, 91
  separation, 89-91
    blowing or air sifting, 91
    by elutriation, 89

Particle sizes of drugs, separation (*Continued*)
  by garbling, 89
  by mills, high-speed, 89
  by sifting, 89-91
Partition coefficient, 154
Paste(s), 341-343
  Aluminum, 343
  N.F., 343
  unofficial, 343
  U.S.P., 343
Pearls, manufacturing methods, 422-424
Pectin, 251
Penetrol, 329
Penicillin, Ointment, 339
  Troches, 436
Pentobarbital Elixir, 372
Peppermint, Spirit, 368
  Water, 180
Pepsin Glycerite, 256
Peptization, preparation of colloidal dispersions by, 114
Percolate, definition, 149
Percolation, definition, 166
  early descriptions of process, 151
  extraction by, 166-171
  fractional, 169-170
  historical developments, 149-151
  of infusions, 246
  pressure, 170-171
  stages, 166-169
    dampening the drug, 167-168
    packing percolator, 167, 168
    period of maceration, 168
    preparation of drug, 166-167
    regulation, 168-169
  theory of, 152-153
Percolator(s), bottom, flat or rounded, 162
  Breddin diacolator, 161
  closed, 159, 161, 162
  in extraction, 158-163
  fractional, 160-161
  glass, 159-160
  metal, 159, 160
  Oldberg, 159
  open, 159-162
  outlets, 159-160
  pressure, development by Count Réal, 150
  regulation of flow, 159
  Soxhlet, 162-163, 171
  Squibb well-tube, 161
Peschier, first application of name galenical, 405
Petrol as source of heat, 25
Petrolatum, Hydrophilic, 324
  origin of, 316
Petroleum benzin, as solvent for pharmaceutical use, 100
  as source of heat, 25
Petroloxins, 310, 329
Pfaudler evaporating pan, 32

pH, determination, colorimetric, 104-105
  potentiometric, 104, 105
  as factor in stability of colloids, 120
  measurement, pharmaceutical applications, 103-104
  meter with glass electrode, 104, 105
Pharmacopée Universelle of Nicolas Lémery, 150
Pharmagels A and B as emulsifying agents, 292
Phenergan Hydrochloride Syrup, 187
Phenergan Syrup Fortis, 187
Phenindamine Tartrate Syrup, 186
Pheniramine Maleate Ophthalmic Solution, 219
Phenol Glycerite, 255
Phenolated Calamine Lotion, 311-312
Phenolated Iodine Solution, 212
Phenolated Water, 181
Phenolphthalein in Liquid Petrolatum Emulsion, 300-301
Phenoxymethyl Penicillin for Oral Suspension, 267
Phenylephrine Hydrochloride Solution, 205-206
Phosphorus Pills, 434
Phosphorus^{32}, 469
Pickering, preparation of emulsions of petroleum oil in water, 135-136
Picrotoxin Injection, 229
Pills, 429-434
  Aloin, Belladonna, Cascara and Podophyllum, 434
  Blaud's, 434
  Chalybeate, 434
  coating, 433, 446-449
    application methods, 446-447
    enteric, 447-449
    sugar, 447
  Compound Cathartic, 434
  Compound Mild Mercurous Chloride, 434
  Ferrous Carbonate, 434
  Ferruginous, 434
  Hexylresorcinol, 434
  Hinkle's, 434
  industrial production, 432-433
  N.F., 434
  nonofficial, 434
  of Phosphorus, 434
  preparation, 430-432
    dividing the mass, 431-432
    dusting, 432
    making the mass, 430-431
    mixing ingredients, 430
    shaping and finishing, 432
  U.S.P., 434

Pine Tar, 256
Piperazine Citrate, 186
Pipets, 13
Pipizan Citrate Syrup, 186-187
Plantago seed, 251
Plaster(s), 343-345
  Mustard, 345
  N.F., 345
  preparation, 344-345
  U.S.P., 345
Plate, theoretical, definition, 64
Pliny the Elder, *Historia Naturalis,* first authentic record of soap, 303-304
Pliny, report on gums, 250
Pluronics, 229
Podophyllum Resin, 402-403
Polyethylene glycol, suppositories, formulas, 361
Polyethylene Glycol 400, 139
  as solvent for pharmaceutical use, 100
Polyethylene Glycol 4,000, 139
Polyoxyethylene sorbitan monolaurate, 261
Polyoxyl 40 Stearate as ointment base, 328
Polysorbate 80, 261
  as ointment base, 327-328
Pot, infusion, use in extraction, 157
Potassium Arsenite Solution, 214
Potassium Iodide Solution, 206
Pound, new international, 5
  tower, as English unit of weight, 3
  troy, 4
Powder(s), 408-416
  Absorbable Dusting, 414
  Achromycin Ophthalmic, Sterilized, 220
  administration, 409
  advantages, 408-409
  Chloromycetin Ophthalmic, 220
  Compound Effervescent, 414-415
  Compound Iodochlorhydroxyquin, 414
  Compound Senna, 415
  Compound Zinc Sulfate, 416
  compounding, special problems, colors, 414
    essential oils, 413
    explosive mixtures, 413-414
    flavors, 414
    liquefaction, 413
    liquids, 413
    pilular extracts, 413
    small quantities of ingredients, 412-413
  definition, 408
  dispensing, 410-412
    in bulk, 410
    divided powders, 410-412
      packaging, 411-412

Powder(s) (*Continued*)
  dry, sterilization, 238
  Furazolidone and Nifuroxime, 415
  Ipecac and Opium, 415
  liquefaction, causes, 413
  mixing, methods, 409-410
  N.F., 414-416
  N.F. Tooth, 416
  ophthalmic, 197
  Seidlitz, 414-415
  sizes, 91
  specific gravity, 20
  Starch-Derivative Dusting, 414
  U.S.P., 414
Powdered Cascara Sagrada Extract, 398
Powdered Nux Vomica Extract, 400
Powdered Opium Extract, 401
Powdered Rhubarb Extract, 401
Pramoxine Hydrochloride, Jelly, 274
  Solution, 206
Pravez, C. G., invention of hypodermic syringe, 225
Precipitates, collection of, 87
  types, 87
  washing, 87-89
    decantation, 88
    lotion or displacement, 87-88
    siphoning, 88-89
Precipitation, 85-89
  definition, 85
  iso-electric point, 86-87
  methods, cooling, 85
    crystallization, 86
    heating, 85
  purification by, 85
  of suspended particles of liquid, clarification by, 78
  types of precipitates, 87
Precipitator, Cottrell, 124
Prefixes, metric system, Latin and Greek, 1-2
Prescription(s), balance, torsion, 7-9
  Troemner, 7, 8
Preservation, of infusions, 247
Preservatives, in injections, 228
  for syrups, 183-184
Press, suppository, 364
Pressure, atmospheric, effect on boiling point according to elevation above sea level, 40
  osmotic, 102-103
Privine Hydrochloride Nasal Solution, 204-205
Procaine hydrochloride, in-vitro release from cocoa butter suppositories, 352
Prochlorperazine Ethanedisulfonate Syrup, 187

Proctor, contribution to development of percolation, 150
Promethazine Hydrochloride Syrup, 187
Propane as source of heat, 26
Prophenpyridamine Maleate Ophthalmic Solution, 219
Propylene glycol as solvent, for injections, 227
  for pharmaceutical use, 100
Propylhexedrine Inhalant, 313-314
Protargol, 109
Protegin, 323-324
Proteins, as emulsifying agents, 138
Pseudosublimation, conversion of solid to vapor phase, 76
Psychrometer, sling, 42
  wet and dry bulb, 41-42
Psyllium seed, 251
Pulverization by intervention, in comminution of drugs, 80-81
Pump, vacuum, molecular distillation of liquids by, 65
Pure Glycyrrhiza Extract, 397-398
Pure Licorice Root Extract, 397-398
Purification, 54-77
  biologic methods, 78
  definition, 54
  by manufacturer, 54
  matter, states, 55-57
  methods, 55
  by pharmacist, 54
Purification, separation, of liquids. *See* Liquids, separation
  separation, solids. *See* Solids, separation
  standards and tests, 54-55
  sterilization. *See* Sterilization
Purified Water, 175-177
Pycnometer, 18-19
Pyoktanin, 204
Pyrogens, 177
  in parenteral preparations, 225
  test, 177, 178
Pyrometers, optical, 29
  thermocouple, 29

Quesneville, G. A., effervescent salts first prepared by, 454
Quincy's Pharmacopoeia (1718), emulsions in, 276
Quinidine Gluconate Injection, 229

Racephedrine Hydrochloride Solution, 206
Radioactive Iodine, Capsules, 467
  Solution, 467
Radioactive pharmaceuticals, 462-472
  detection methods, 465
  fundamental concepts, 462-464

Radioactive pharmaceuticals (*Continued*)
  hazards and protection, 466
  measurement units, 465
  methods of production of isotopes, 464-465
    cyclotron, 464-465
    nuclear reactor, 465
  radioisotopes. *See* Radioisotopes
  types of radiation, 465-466
Radioactive Phosphorus Solution, 469-470
Radioactive Sodium (Na^{24}) Chloride Solution, 469
Radiocarbon^{14}, 471
Radiocobalt^{60}, 470
Radiocyanobalamin Solution, 470-471
Radiodiiodo (I^{131}) Fluorescin, 467-468
Radiogold Solution, 468
Radio-iodinated (I^{131}) Serum Albumin, 468
Radioisotopes, distributors, 472
  in pharmacy and medicine, 466-471
    carbon^{14}, 471
    chromium^{50} and chromium^{51}, 471
    cobalt^{60}, 470
    gold^{198}, 468
    iodine^{131}, 466-468
    phosphorus^{32}, 469-470
    sodium^{22} and sodium^{24}, 469
  procurement, 471-472
Radiosodium (Na^{22}) Chloride, 469
Raoult, law of, 101-102
Raspberry, Juice, 193
  Syrup, 187
Rasping, comminution of drugs by, 80
Rdzok method of testing efficiency of preservatives in emulsions, 279
Réal, Count, development of pressure percolator, 150
Reaumur, René A. F., temperature scale, 27-28
Reaumur scale, 27-28
Red Aromatic Elixir, 370, 371
Red Gum, Troches of, 436
Red Mercuric Oxide, 111
Refrigeration, 47-50, 52-53
  congealing point, 53
  desiccation. *See* Desiccation
  freezing point, 53
  lyophilization, 47-48
Refrigerators, 52
Remington, *The Practice of Pharmacy*, English method of preparing emulsions, 277
Repercolation, introduction by Squibb, 150
Repository Corticotropin Injection, 229

Reserpine Injection, 229
Resin(s), 402-404
  Azure A Carbacrylic, 404
  galenical, 403
  history, 402
  Ipomea, 403
  Jalap, 403-404
  natural, 404
  Podophyllum, 402-403
  synthetic, 404
Resina, 404
Retort, tubulated, 59
Rezifilm, 257
Rhamnus Purshiana Extract, 398
Rhubarb, Extract, 401
  Fluidextract, 169, 393
Rice Bran Extract, 401
Rice Polishings Extract, 401
Ringer's Injection, 227, 228
Ringer's Solution, 217
  No. 1, 217
Robiquet and Boutron, account of extraction with ether, 150
Roentgen as unit of measurement of radioactivity, 465
Romilar Hydrobromide Syrup, 189
Rose Water, 175, 180
Rosin, 404
Rota-Film, molecular still, 66

Salicylic Acid and Fluidextract of Cannabis in Compound Salicylic Collodion, 257
Salts, effervescent, 454-461
  coloring, 460-461
  definition, 454
  manufacturing methods, 455-460
    drying moist granules, 459-460
    formula preparation, 456
    fusion, 455
    ingredients, preparing and mixing, 456-457
    moistening and granulating, 457-459
    packaging and storing, 460
    wet, 455
  official, 455
  hydroxyalkylamine, as emulsifying agents, 138
  quaternary, as emulsifying agents, 138
Sand baths for distribution of heat, 29-30
Saponated Cresol Solution, 210, 293
Sarsaparilla Fluidextract, 393
"Saturated" Boric Acid Solution, 200-201
Saturated Potassium Iodide Solution, 206

Schacht, glycerin and starch as ointment base, 316
Scheele, studies in adsorptive power of carbon, 124
Schönbein, discovery of guncotton, 256
Schulze, cholesterol and oxycholesterol in wool fat, 323
Schulze-Hardy rule, 119
Scott's Solution, 204
Scrubbers, separation of immiscible mixtures of liquids by, 63-64
Secorbarbital Elixir, 372
Sedatives, elixirs, 372-373
Seidlitz Powders, 414-415
Selas microfilter, 238, 239
Selenium Sulfide Detergent Suspension, 267
Seneca Snakeroot, Fluidextract of, 394
Senega Fluidextract, 394
Senna, Fluidextract, 393
  Syrup, 191
Sifter, hand, 90
Sifting, separation of particle sizes of drugs by, 89-91
  methods, hand sifter, 90
  mechanical agitator, 90-91
Silica gel, 125, 332
Silicate, colloidal magnesium aluminum silicate, 332
Silication of glass, 230
Silicon derivatives as ointment bases, 331-333
Silicones, 332-333
Silver Nitrate Ophthalmic Solution, 219
Simple Syrup, 184
Siphoning, separation of liquid from solid by, 69
  washing of precipitates by, 88-89
Sirup, 184
Slab and muller, in preparation of ointments, 335
Slicing, comminution of drugs by, 80
Smogs, 124
Smokes, as aerosols, 123-124
  in chemical warfare, 124
  control ordinances, 124
  in mines, 124
Soap(s), 303-308
  amino, in emulsions, 294-295
  calcium tolerance, 295
  Camphorated Tincture of, 308
  definition, 303
  as emulsifying agents, 138, 293-295
  Green, 306-307
    Tincture of, 309
  Hard, 307
  Hexachlorophene Liquid, 307-308

488 Index

Soap(s) (*Continued*)
  history, 303-304
  manufacture, 304-305
  Medicinal Soft, 306-307
  official, 306-308
  as ointment bases, 321, 328-330
  organic, in emulsions, 294-295
  properties, 305-306
  sequestering agents in emulsions, 295-296
  uses, 306
Sodium, Acetrizoate Injection, 228, 229
  Bromide Elixir, 372
  Carboxymethylcellulose, 252
  Chloride, Injection, 227, 228
    Solution, 217
  Hypochloride Solution, 215
  Phosphate Solution, 207
  Psylliate Injection, 229
  Radiochromate Injection, 471
  Radio-iodide, Capsules, 467
    Solution, 467
  Radioiodine (I^{131}) Solution, 467
  Radiophosphate, Injection, 469-470
    Solution, 469-470
Sodium^{22}, 469
Sodium^{24}, 468-469
Soft Soap Liniment, 309
Sol, definition, 112
Solid(s), absorption of gases as method of separation, 58
  adsorption of gases as method of separation, 58
  conversion to soluble liquid, 66-67
  as emulsifying agents, 138
  insoluble in water, and heavier than water, specific gravity, 20
    and lighter than water, specific gravity, 20
  melting point, 41
  separation, 75-78
    conversion, to liquid phase, 76-77
      to vapor phase, 76
    crystallization, 77-78
    from liquids. *See* Liquids, separation, solid from liquid
  soluble, conversion to insoluble, 74
    in water, and heavier than water, specific gravity, 20
      and lighter than water, specific gravity, 20
  specific gravity, determination methods, apparent loss of weight, 19-20
    displacement, 19
  as state of matter, 57

Solubility, determination, 96
  effect of various substances on, 94-95
  expression, 95-96
  factors affecting, 93-94
    circulatory displacement, 93
    heating liquids, 93
    increase in temperature, 94
    rate of solution, 93
    supersaturation, 93
  molar, 95
  product, 96
Solubilization, 260
Solute, definition, 92
Soluthricin Concentrate, 208-209
Solution(s), 92-106, 195-222
  A. C. D., 216
  Alkaline Aromatic, 199
  Aluminum, Acetate, 209
    Subacetate, 209-210
  Amaranth, 198
    Compound, 198
  Ammonia, Diluted, 198
    Strong, 198-199
  Ammoniacal Silver Nitrate, 214
  Ammonium Acetate, 222
  Ammonium Hydroxide, Stronger, 198-199
  Anticoagulant Acid Citrate Dextrose, 216
  anticoagulant and physiologic, 216-217
  Anticoagulant Sodium Citrate, 216-217
  Arsenious Acid, 214
  balance, 9
  Basic Ferric Sulfate, 211
  Benzalkonium Chloride, 199-200
  Benzethonium Chloride, 200
  Boric Acid, 200-201
    "Saturated," 200-201
  Boulton's, 212
  buffer, 105-106
    directions for preparation, in U.S.P. XVI, 106
  Burow's, 209
  Calciferol, 201
  Calcium Hydroxide, 201
  Carbol-Fuchsin, 201-202
  Carbolized Iodine, 212
  Ceepryn Chloride Aqueous, 202
  Cetylpyridinium Chloride, 202
  Chloroazodin, 222
  classification, 196-198
  Clopane Hydrochloride, 202-203
  Coal Tar, 202
  colloidal, 92
  Compound Calcium Cyclamate, 201
  Compound Cresol, 210
  Compound Dimethyl Phthalate, 222
  Compound Sodium Borate, 214-215

Solution(s) (*Continued*)
  Compound Sodium Cyclamate, 207
  Cyclaine Hydrochloride, 203
  Cyclopentamine Hydrochloride, 202-203
  Dakin's, Modified, 215-216
  definition, 92, 195-196
  Diluted Lead Subacetate, 222
  Dobell's, 214-215
  of Drisdol, 201
  dl-Ephedrine Hydrochloride, 206
  Ephedrine Sulfate, 203
  Epinephrine, 197, 221
  Epinephrine 1:1,000, 221
  Ethylenediamine, 203
  Ferric Chloride, 210-211
  Ferric Subsulfate, 211
  Formaldehyde, 211-212
  Fowler's, 214
  Gantrisin Ophthalmic, 219
  gases in liquids, 98-99
  general considerations, 195-198
  Hexylcaine Hydrochloride, 203
  Hydrogen Dioxide, 212
  Hydrogen Peroxide, 212
  Iodine, 203
    Compound, 203-204
    Strong, 203-204
  Iron, and Ammonium Acetate, 222
    Perchloride, 210-211
  Labarraque's, 215
  laws, deviations from, 117-118
  Lead Subacetate, 222
  liquids in liquids, 98
  Liver, 197, 221
  Lugol's, 203-204
  Magnesium Citrate, 213-214
  Merbromin, 204
    Surgical, 204
  Merthiolate, 208
  Methylrosaniline Chloride, 204
  Monsel's, 211
  Naphazoline Hydrochloride, 204-205
    Mild, 204-205
  Neo-Synephrine Hydrochloride, 206
  N.F. Antiseptic, 199
  Nitrofurazone, 205
  Nitromersol, 205
  ophthalmic, 217-220
    Antazoline Phosphate, 217
    Antistine, 217
    autoclaving, 197
    Benoxinate Hydrochloride, 217-218
    Chloramphenicol for, 220
    Cyclopentolate Hydrochloride, 218
    Dorsacaine Hydrochloride, 218

Solution(s), ophthalmic (*Cont.*)
   Epinephrine Bitartrate, 218
   Fluorescein Sodium, 218
   Isoflurophate, 218-219
   Pheniramine Maleate, 219
   prepared from sterile ophthalmic powders, 220-221
   preservatives in, 197
   Prophenpyridamine Maleate, 219
   Silver Nitrate, 219
   sterile, 197
   Sulfacetamide Sodium, 219
   Sulfisoxazole Diethanolamine, 219-220
   Tetracycline Hydrochloride for, 220-221
   Trimeton Maleate, 219
Paramethadione, 205
percentage, 96-98
  liquids in liquids, 97-98
  solids in liquids, 97
  volume in volume, 96
  weight, in volume, 96
    in weight, 96
pH determination, 104-105
  colorimetric, 104-105
  pharmaceutical applications, 103-104
  potentiometric, 104, 105
Phenolated Iodine, 212
Phenylephrine Hydrochloride, 205-206
Potassium Arsenite, 214
Potassium Iodide, 206
  Saturated, 206
Pramoxine Hydrochloride, 206
preparation, 196-198
  by chemical reaction, 196-197, 209-216
  by extraction, 196, 221
  simple solution, 196, 198-209
  with sterilization, 196, 197, 216-221
Privine Hydrochloride Nasal, 204-205
properties, 101-105
  boiling point, 103
  diffusion in solution, 102
  freezing point, 103
  osmosis and osmotic pressure, 102-103
Racephedrine Hydrochloride, 206
Radioactive Iodine, 467
Radioactive Phosphorus, 469-470
Radioactive Sodium (Na^{24}) Chloride, 469
Radiocyanocobalamin, 470-471
Radiogold, 468
Radiosodium (Na^{22}) Chloride, 469
Ringer's, 217

Solution(s), Ringer's (*Cont.*)
   No. 1, 217
  Saponated Cresol, 210, 293
  saturated, 92
  Scott's, 204
  separation of gases by, 57-58
  Sodium Chloride, 217
  Sodium Hypochlorite, 215
    Diluted, 215-216
  Sodium Phosphate, 207
  Sodium Radio-iodide, 467
  Sodium Radioiodine (I^{131}), 467
  Sodium Radiophosphate (P^{32}), 469-470
  Sorbitol, 207
  sterile, for parenteral administration. *See* Injections
  Sterile Radioactive Chromium, 471
  Sterile Sodium Radiochromate (Cr^{51}), 471
  sterilization, Berkefeld filter, 117
  Sucaryl Calcium Sweetening, 201
  Sucaryl Sodium Sweetening, 207
  Sulamyd Sodium, 219
  Sulfacetamide Sodium, 219
  Sulfurated Lime, 212-213
  Talbot's, Diluted, 255
  Tetrahydrozoline Hydrochloride, 207
  Thimerosal, 208
  Tribromoethanol, 208
  Trimethadione, 208
  Tronothane Hydrochloride Topical, 206
  Tyrothricin, 208-209
  Tyzine, 207
  unofficial, 222
  unsaturated, 92
  uses, 196
  Valangin's, 214
  Water-Miscible Vitamin A, 209
Solvent(s), definition, 92
  immiscible, extraction by, 171
  modern, 101
  for pharmaceutical use, 99-101
Sorbitol, 193
  Solution, 207
Sorbo, 193
Soxhlet extraction apparatus, 45, 162-163, 171
Span 80, 138
Spans compounds as ointment base, 328
Specific gravity, 15-20
  apparent vs. true, 15-16
  as a constant of a pure substance, 16
  definition, 15
  determination, 16-17
    liquids, hydrometer method, 17-18
      Mohr-Westphal balance, 17, 18

Specific gravity, determination, liquids (*Continued*)
    pycnometer or specific gravity bottle, 18-19
    Sprengel tube, 19
   powders, 20
   solids, method, apparent loss of weight, 19-20
    displacement, 19
  liquids, 17-19
  powders, 20
  solids, 19-20
  true vs. apparent, 15-16
Sperandio, G. J., and P. W. Gerding, studies of suspending agents, 145
Spirit(s), 367-369
  Aromatic Ammonia, 368-369
  Camphor, 369
  Compound Cardamom, 368
  Compound Myrcia, 369
  Compound Orange, 368
  definition, 367
  Ethyl Nitrite, 369
  history, 367-368
  Mindererus, 222
  official, 368-369
  Peppermint, 368
Spray(s), 313-314
  Tyrothricin, 314
  Tyzine, 207
Sprengel tube, 19
Squibb, E. R., carbolic acid as preservative in parenteral solutions, 225
  introduction of repercolation, 150
  well-tube percolator, 161
Squill, Fluidextract, 394
  Vinegar, 376
Stainless Iodine Ointment, 340
Standards and tests for purity of drugs, general, 54-55
  specific, 55
Starch Glycerite, 255
Starch-Derivative Dusting Powder, 414
Steam, baths for distribution of heat, 31-32
  coil, 32
  distillation by, liquids, immiscible, 64-65
  superheated, 31
Stearic acid, as enteric coating for pills and tablets, 448-449
  in preparation of ointments, 316
Stere as metric unit of dry volume, 2
Sterile Phytonadione Emulsion, 301
Sterile Procaine Penicillin G, with Aluminum Stearate Suspension, 229-230
  Suspension, 229

Sterile Radioactive Chromium Solution, 471
Sterile Radioactive Gold Colloid, 468
Sterile Radiogold (Au^{198}) Colloid, 468
Sterile Sodium Radiochromate (Cr^{51}) Solution, 471
Sterile Water for Injection, 178
Sterility, injections, testing, 240-241
  test for liquids, 177, 178
Sterilization, agents, heat, moist, 235
  apparatus, autoclave, 235-236
  definition, 177, 234
  emulsions, 230
  by filtration, 238-240
  fractional, 238
  injections, 234-238, 240
  intermittent, 238
  purification by, 78
  self-sterilizing drugs, 236-237
  suspensions, 230
Sterilizer(s), "cold," with Cryoxcide Gas, 237
  hot air, 237
  simple, household use, 38-39
Still(s), falling-film, molecular distillation of liquids by, 66
  molecular, 65-66
  pot, molecular distillation of liquids by, 65
  registration with Treasure Department, 47
  types, 44
Stokes, Law of, 145
Stoklosa, M. L., and L. M. Ohmart, base for medicated lotions, 254
  use of Tween 20 as solubilizing agent, 261
Stomachics, elixirs, 373
Stramonium, Extract. See Belladonna Extract
  Tincture. See Belladonna Tincture
Strong Ammonia Solution, 198-199
Strong Iodine Solution, 203-204
Strong Iodine Tincture. See Iodine Tincture
Strong Silver Protein, 121
Stronger Ammonia Water, 198-199
Stronger Ammonium Hydroxide Solution, 198-199
Stronger Mercurial Ointment, 339
Styptic Collodion, 257
Sublimation, conversion of solid to vapor phase, 76
  of volatile solids, 47
  by lyophilization, 47-48
Substances, surface-active and surface-inactive, 127

Sucaryl Calcium Sweetening Solution, 201
Sucaryl Sodium Sweetening Solution, 207
Sucrose, 182
  caramelization, 183
  hydrolysis, 182-183
  inversion, 182-183
Sugar, as coating for pills and tablets, 447
Sulamyd Sodium Solution, 219
Sulfacetamide Sodium Ophthalmic Solution, 219
Sulfacetamide Sodium Solution, 219
Sulfacetamide, Sulfadiazine and Sulfamerazine Suspension, 267
Sulfamethiazole Suspension, 267
Sulfisoxazole Diethanolamine Ophthalmic Solution, 219-220
Sulfonated Bitumen, 257
Sulfurated Lime Solution, 212-213
Sun Cream, 253
Sun Tan Ointment, 253
Supersaturation, effect on solubility, 93
Suppositories, 347-365
  absorption by system, stages, 350
  bases, 351-363
    cocoa butter, 351-356, 359
      substitutes, 356-359
    comparative evaluation, 362-363
    emulsifying, 357, 360-361
    glycerinated gelatin, 359-360
    water-soluble, 358, 361-362
  definition, 347
  history, 348
  manufacture, 348, 363-365
    processes, cold, 364
      fusion, 364-365
      hot, 363
    size and shape, 363-364
  rectal administration, factors affecting drug action, 348-351
Surfactants, 263, 280, 281
Surgical Merbromin Solution, 204
Surgical Spray Dressing, 257
Suspension(s), 144-146, 262-269
  applications in pharmacy, 146
  definition, 92, 109, 262
  deflocculating agents, 263
  dispersion stabilizers and other constituents, 263-265
  formulation, 265
  hydrophilic colloids, 263-265
  of liniments, 309
  official, 266-269
    miscellaneous products, N.F., 243
    U.S.P., 243
  Ophthalmic, Cortisone Acetate, 266
  Oral, Acetyl Sulfisoxazole, 266

Suspension(s), Oral (*Continued*)
  Chloramphenicol Palmitate, 266
  Erythromycin, 266
  Nitrofurantoin, 266
  Novobiocin Calcium, 266
  Nystatin for, 266
  Oxytetracycline for, 266-267
  Phenoxymethyl Penicillin for, 267
  Tetracycline, 267-268
  Trisulfapyrimidines, 268
Para-nitrosulfathiazole, 267
preparation, 265-266
properties, 262-263
rate of settling, factors, 109
Selenium Sulfide Detergent, 267
stability, 145
sterile, official, N.F., 243
  U.S.P., 242-243
  parenteral preparations, 224
  Procaine Penicillin G, 229
    with Aluminum Stearate, 229-230
Sulfacetamide, Sulfadiazine and Sulfamerazine, 267
Sulfamethiazole, 267
surfactants, 263
ultrasonic waves, application to, 146
Sweet Orange Peel Tincture, 382
Sydenham, Thomas, formulation of liquid preparations of opium, 381
Syneresis, 122
Syringe(s), disposable, types and sizes, 232
  hypodermic, invention and improvement, 225
Syrup(s), 182-193
  Acacia, 188
  Antepar, Multifuge, 186-187
  Aromatic Eriodictyon, 189-190
  Aromatic Yerba Santa, 189-190
  Bromides, 188-189
  Cacao, 184-185
  Cherry, 185
  Chlorpheniramine Maleate, 185
  Chlorpromazine Hydrochloride, 185
  Chlor-Trimetron Maleate, 185
  Citric Acid, 185
  Compazine, 187
  Compound Sarsaparilla, 191
  Compound White Pine, 192
    with Codeine, 192
  Dextromethorphan Hydrobromide, 189
  diabetic, 192
  Diethylcarbamazine Citrate, 185
  Dihydrocodeinone Bitartrate, 189
  Dimenhydrinate, 185-186
  Ephedrine Sulfate, 189

Syrup *(Continued)*
  Ferrous Iodide, 190
  Ferrous Sulfate, 190
  flavoring, 182
  general, 192-193
  Glycyrrhiza, 186
  Hetrazan, 185
  Hydriodic Acid, 190-191
  of Hypophosphites, 183
    Compound, 183
  Ipecac, 186
  keeping quality, control, 183
  Lemon, 185
  Licorice, 186
  medicated, 182
  N. F. XI, 188
  Orange, 186
  Phenergan, Fortis, 187
    Hydrochloride, 187
  Phenindamine Tartrate, 186
  Piperazine Citrate, 186
  Pipizan Citrate, 186-187
  preservatives, 183-184
  Prochlorperazine Ethanedisulfonate, 187
  Promethazine Hydrochloride, 187
  Raspberry, 187
  Romilar Hydrobromide, 189
  Senna, 191
  Simple, 184
  storage, 184
  Thephorin Tartrate, 186
  Thorazine Hydrochloride, 185
  of Tolu, 191-192
  Tolu Balsam, 191-192
  U.S.P. XVI, 184-188
  Wild Cherry, 187-188

Tablets, 436-452
  buccal or sublingual, 443
  classification, 436-437
  coating, 446-449
    application methods, 446-447
    enteric, 447-449
    sugar, 447
  compressed triturates, 441-442
  definition, 436
  dispensing, 442
  dosage forms, 437
  molded, 443-446
    abbreviations in prescriptions, 446
    hypodermic, 445-446
    preparation, 444-445
      choice of base and excipient, 445
      standardization of mold, 444-445
  official, 449-452
    N.F., 451-452
    U.S.P., 449-451
  preparation, compression, 439-443

Tablets, preparation *(Continued)*
  granulating the mixture, 438-439
  mixing ingredients, 438
  steps, 437-438
  weighing ingredients, 438
  triturates. *See* Tablets, molded
Tael as Chinese unit of weight, 3
Talbot's Solution, diluted, 255
Talent as Babylonian unit of weight, 3
Tank, maceration, 158
Tannic Acid, Glycerite, 255
  Ointment, 339
Taraxacum Fluidextract, 393
Ta-Verm, 186-187
Taylor, A. B., development of use of cocoa butter as suppository base, 348
Temperature, increase, effect on solubility, 94
  standard, for determination of specific gravity of alcohol, 17
Tensiometer, Du Nouy, 132, 133
Terpin Hydrate and Codeine Elixir, 374
Terpin Hydrate Elixir, 374
Terramycin Hydrochloride Ophthalmic, 220
Test, drop-dilution, for emulsions, 140
  dye or indicator, for emulsions, 140
  electric conductance, for emulsions, 140
  indicator or dye, for emulsions, 140
  pyrogen, 177, 178
  sterility, for liquids, 177, 178
  weight variation, capsules, 421-422
Tetracycline Hydrochloride, 197
  for Ophthalmic Solution, 220-221
Tetracycline Oral Suspension, 267-268
Tetrahydrozoline Hydrochloride Solution, 207
Theobroma oil. *See* Cocoa butter
Theophrastus, description of tragacanth, 250
Theory, kinetic-molecular, 56
  Langumir, 127
Thephorin Tartrate Syrup, 186
Thermometer(s), clinical, 28-29
  gas, 29
  liquid, 26-29
  resistance, 29
  scales, 27-28
    Centigrade, 27-28
    conversion, Fahrenheit and Centigrade, 28
    Fahrenheit, 27, 28
    Kelvin (absolute), 28

Thermometer(s) scales *(Continued)*
  Newton, 27
  Réaumur, 27-28
Thiamine Hydrochloride Elixir, 374
Thimerosal, Solution, 208
  Tincture, 386
Thixotropy, 122, 271
Thompson, Benjamin, first use of term percolation, 150
Thompson, W. M., description of extraction method, 151
Thorazine Hydrochloride Syrup, 185
Three Bromides Elixir, 372
Tikitiki Extract, 401
Tincture(s), 377-388
  Acetic Larkspur, 387
  Aconite, 386-387
  Arnica, 382-383
  Aromatic Rhubarb, 385-386
  Asafetida, 387
  Belladonna, 380
  Belladonna Leaf, 380
  Benzoin, 383
  Bitter Orange Peel, 388
  Camphorated Opium, 382
  Cantharides, 387
  Capsicum, 383
  Colchicum Seed, 387
  Compound Benzoin, 380
  Compound Cardamon, 383
  Compound Gentian, 384-385
  Compound Lavender, 387-388
  Digitalis, 383-384
  Ethereal, 388
  Ferric Chloride, 384
  Ferric Citrochloride, 384
  Fresh Drug, 388
  of Green Soap, 309
  history, 377
  Hyoscyamus. *See* Belladonna Tincture
  Iodine, 380-381
  Iron, 384
  Larkspur, 387
  Laudanum, Deodorized Opium, 381-382
  Lemon, 381
  Lemon Peel, 381
  Lobelia, 388
  Myrrh, 385
  N.F., 382-386
  Nitromersol, 385
  nonofficial, 386-388
  Nux Vomica, 385
  Opium, 381-382
  preparation, 377-379
  Stramonium. *See* Belladonna Tincture
  Strong Iodine. *See* Iodine Tincture
  Sweet Orange Peel, 382
  Thimerosal, 386

Tincture(s) (*Continued*)
  Tolu, 386
  Tolu Balsam, 386
  U.S.P., 380-382
  Vanilla, 386
Tolu Balsam, Syrup, 191-192
  Tincture, 386
Tolu Tincture, 386
Torrefaction, 34
Torricelli, Evangelista, demonstration of variations in atmospheric pressure, 40
Torricellian tube, 39, 40
Torsion prescription balance, 7-9
Tower pound as English unit of weight, 3
Tragacanth, Glycerite, 255
  Mucilage, 250, 251
Traumatic Balsam, 380
Tribromoethanol Solution, 208
Triglycerides, natural, as ointment bases, 326
  as substitute bases for cocoa butter in suppositories, 357
Trimethadione Solution, 208
Trimeton Maleate Ophthalmic Solution, 219
Tripelennamine Citrate Elixir, 374
Trisulfapyrimidines Oral Suspension, 268
Trituration(s), 426-427
  comminution of drugs by, 81
Troches, 435-436
  of Eucalyptus Gum, 436
  Penicillin, 436
  of Red Gum, 436
  Tyrothricin, 436
Troemner prescription balance, 7, 8
Tronothane Hydrochloride Topical Solution, 206
Tube, Sprengel, 19
  Torricellian, 39, 40
Turbidity, colloidal dispersions, 114
Turlington's Drops, 380
Twaddle hydrometer, 18
Tweens, 229
  as ointment bases, 328
Tween 20, 261
Tween 60, 261
Tween 80, 138, 140, 202, 261
Tween 81, 138
Tyndall effect, colloidal dispersions, 114-115
Tyndall, John, development of Tyndall effect, 115
Tyndallization, 238
Tyrothricin, Solution, 208-209
  Spray, 314
  Troches, 436
Tyzine, Pediatric Nasal Drops, 207

Tyzine (*Continued*)
  Solution or Spray, 207

Ultracentrifuge, estimation of sizes and masses of colloidal particles, 117
Ultrafiltration, colloidal dispersions, 117
Ultramicroscope, invention by Richard Zsigmondy, 108
Ultramicroscopy, colloidal dispersions, 115
United States Bureau of Standards, copies of International Prototype Kilogram, 3
  use of metric system for weights and measures, 1
United States Pharmacopoeia (*U.S.P.*), method of expressing solubility, 95
United States Revenue Department, standards, specific gravity of alcohol, 17
United States Wine Measure, 4
Unna, Paul G., introduction of Eucerin as base for ointments, 316, 323
U.S.P., definition of kinds of percentage solutions, 96, 97

Vacuum distillation, 46
Valangin's Solution, 214
Vallet's Mass, 429
Van der Waal, forces of, 132
Van Helmont, 195
Vanilla Tincture (extract, essence), 386
Vapor, equilibrium of liquid with, 57
  pressure, 38-39
  of liquid, 57
  tension, of liquid, 56-57
Vaporization, 34-37
  boiling point, 39-41
  determination, 40-41
  effect of pressure on, 39-40
  distillation. See Distillation
  evaporation, 37-38
  humidity, 41-43
  latent heat of, 56
  pressure of vapor, 38-39
  rate, at boiling point, 36
    below boiling point, 35-36
    effect of stirring, 36
  separation, of components of solution, 74
  of liquid from solid, 73-74
  sublimation, 47
Vasogen, 329
Veegum, 298, 332
Vermago, 186-187
Vials, cleaning before filling, 231
  filling, 230-233

Vials (*Continued*)
  glass, types, standards for, 230-231
Vibesate, 257
de Villanova, Arnaldus, introduction of distillation into Europe, 178
Vinegar(s), 376
  Squill, 376
Viscosity of emulsions, 133-134
Vi-Syneral, 130
Vitamin, A, water-miscible solution, 209
  Water Soluble, 209
  B Complex Elixir, 374, 375
  D, crystalline, 201
Vleminckx' Lotion, 212-213
Volume, 11-14
  burets, 13
  capacity, receiving vs. delivery, 11
  flasks, 11, 13
  graduates, conical, 11 12
    cylindrical, 12
    legal requirements, 12-13
    pharmaceutical, 12
  medicine droppers, 13-14
  metric system, 2
  pipets, 13
  specific, 20-21
  technic of measuring liquids, 12-14

Wafers, 425-426
Washing, conversion of solid to liquid phase, 76-77
Water(s), 175-181
  aromatic, 178-181
    application, 178
    definition, 175
    distilled, 180-181
    history, 178
    official, *N.F. XI*, 180
      U.S.P. XVI, 180
    preparation, 178-180
      distillation, 178-179
    storage and preservation, 181
    uses, 180
  baths for distribution of heat, 30
  Bitter Almond, 181
  Camphor, 180, 181
  Chloroform, 175, 180
  Cinnamon, 180
  of crystallization, as cause of liquefaction of powders, 413
  deionization methods, 176
  demineralization, 176
  distillation, 177
  Distilled, 176
    in injections, 227
  Hammamelis, 175, 179-181
  for Injection, 177-178, 227

Water(s), for Injection (*Continued*)
  Sterile, 178
  ion-exchange resins, 176-177
  Lead, 222
  Lime, 201
  Orange Flower, 175, 179
  Peppermint, 180
  Phenolated, 181
  Purified, 175-177
  purity, degrees, 175
  Rose, 175, 179, 180
    Stronger, 179, 180
  salt, baths for distribution of heat, 31
  as solvent, in extraction, 155-156
    for pharmaceutical use, 99
  standards, 175-178
  Sterile, for Injection, 178
  sterilization, 177
  Stronger Ammonia, 198-199
  U.S.P., 175
  Wintergreen, 181
  Witch-hazel, 181
Water-Miscible Vitamin A, 209
  solution, 130, 209
Weighing, technic, 10-11
Weight(s), 6-11

Weight(s) (*Continued*)
  apothecaries', 5
  apparent, vs. absolute, 6
    vs. true, 15-16
  apparent loss of, as method for determination of specific gravity of solids, 19-20
  Archimedes' principle, 6
  avoirdupois, 3-5
  Babylonian, 3
  balances. *See* Balances
  for balances, 9-11
  definition, 6
  imperial, 4
  metric system, 2-3
  physical factors affecting measurement, 6
  prehistoric, 3
  technic of weighing, 10-11
  troy, 3-4
  true vs. apparent, 15-16
Von Weimarn, pioneer work in colloids, 108
Weiser, H. B., colloid particle of arsenic trisulfide stabilized by HS− ions, 118
Westphal balance, 16
Whisky, 369
White Lotion, 312

Wild Cherry, Fluidextract, 394
  Syrup, 187-188
Wiler, Hans, dry gum method of preparing emulsions, 277
Wiley mill, 83
Wilson and Parsons, inversion of phases of an emulsion, 137
Wine gallon, 4
Wintergreen Water, 181
Witch Hazel, 181
  Water, 181
Woo, M., and C. L. Huyck, formulas for nonnutritive "syrups," 192
Wood, Alexander, popularization of hypodermic syringe, 225
Wood as source of heat, 24
Wool Alcohols, Ointment of, 324
Wool fat, disadvantages, 323
  See also Lanolin

Yerba Santa Fluidextract, 393

Zinc Gelatin, 254-255
Zsigmondy, Richard, inventor of ultramicroscope, 108
  protection of colloidal dispersions, 121

ROBERT J. PHELAN
45 Hamilton Street
Holyoke, Massachusetts

ROBERT J. PHELAN
45 Hamilton Street
Holyoke, Massachusetts